Micronutrients and Health

Micronutrients and Health

Molecular Biological Mechanisms

Editors

Kalanithi Nesaretnam
Malaysian Palm Oil Board
Malaysia

Lester Packer
University of Southern California
Los Angeles, California

AOCS PRESS

Champaign, Illinois

AOCS Mission Statement

To be a forum for the exchange of ideas, information, and experience among those with a professional interest in the science and technology of fats, oils, and related substances in ways that promote personal excellence and provide high standards of quality.

The paper used in this book is acid-free and falls within the guidelines established to ensure permanence and durability.

Library of Congress Cataloging-in-Publication Data

Micronutrients and health : molecular biological mechanisms / editors, Kalanithi Nesaretnam and Lester Packer.

p. cm.

Includes bibliographical references and index.

ISBN 1-893997-19-7 (alk. paper)

1. Trace elements in nutrition. 2. Trace elements—Pathophysiology. I. Nesaretnam, Kalanithi. II. Packer, Lester.

QP534.M515 2001
612.3'92—dc21 2001022752

Printed in the United States of America with vegetable oil-based inks.

05 04 03 02 01 5 4 3 2 1

Preface

A workshop on Micronutrients and Health: Molecular Biological Mechanisms brought together a small but select number of experts with a special interest in micronturients, molecular mechanisms, and the effects of oxidants and antioxidants on health. Research in these areas is experiencing unprecedented interest throughout the world in the fields of nutrition, biochemistry, molecular biology, medicine, agri-utlture, public health, and biotechnology, with important implications for human health and life style.

The meeting was held from July 27 to July 30, 2000. It brought together more than 200 researchers to discuss the latest developments in molecular aspects of nutrition and the role of free radicals. The workshop was held on the island paradise of Langkawi, off the west coast of peninsular Malaysia. Among the contributors were leading authorities in the field of antioxidant nutrition from the region, as well as from other parts of the world.

The workshop was organized by the Society of Free Radical Research ASIA/ASEAN in collaboration with COSTAM (Confederation of Scientific Technological Associations of Malaysia) and UNESCO-MCBN (Global Network of Molecular and Cell Biology).

The major objectives of the international workshop were

- The Scientific Program, whose main themes were
  - I. Free Radical Scavenging and Antioxidant Activities
  - II. Cell Regulation—Cell Growth and Differentiation
  - III. Signal Transduction and Gene Expression
  - IV. Health Effects: Aging and Degeneration Diseases
  - V. Vitamin E Action of Tocotrienols and Tocopherols
- Strengthening the disciplines relevant to bridging knowledge and understanding between nutrution, health, and disease by focusing the program on molecular mechanisms of micronutrients
- Strengthening collaboration links already established within the scholarly community as well as establishing new links
- Promoting the activities of the Society of Free Radical Research International (SFRRI) Asia-ASEAN.

The sponsors for the Workshop on the Island of Langkawi, Malaysia, were
UNESCO-MCBN
International Union of Biochemistry and Molecular Biology (IUBMB)
Oxygen Club of California (OCC)
Ministry of Science, Technology and Environment, Malaysia
Malaysian Palm Oil Promotion Council
Hovid Pharmacy Sdn Bhd

The Organizing Committee was composed of Prof. Lester Packer, USA; Tan Sri Datuk Dr. Augustine S. H. Ong, Malaysia; Dr. Kalanithi Mesaretnam, Malaysia; Prof. Angelo Azzi, Switzerland; and Prof. Helmut Sies, Germany.

The International Advisory Committee was composed of Datuk Dr. Yusof Basiron (Kuala Lumpur), Prof. Gloria Bernas (Manila), Prof. Fedi Freisleben (Jakarta), Prof. Goh Swee Hock (Singapore), Prof. Barry Halliwell (Singapore), Tan Sri Dató Dr. Mohd Yusof Hashim (Kuala Lumpur), Prof. Midori Hiramatsu (Yamagata), Prof. Qi Shui Lin (Shanghai), Prof. Catherine Pasquier (Paris), Prof. Catherine Rice Evans (London), Prof. Alex Sevanian (Los Angeles), Dr. Kalyana Sundram (Kuala Lumpur), Prof. Fulvio Ursini (Padua), Prof. Prapon Wilairat (Bangkok), Prof. Wenjuan Xin (Beijing), and Prof. Junji Yodoi (Kyoto).

The Local Organizing Committee was composed of Tan Sri Datuk Dr. Augustine S.H. Ong (Advisor), Dató Dr. M. Mohinder Singh, JP (Chairman), Dr. Ting Kueh Soon (Vice Chairman), Dr. Ooi Cheng Keat (Secretary), Prof. R. Perumal (Treasurer), and the following members: Dr. Kalanithi Nesaretnam, Prof. Mohd Ismail Noor, Prof. Khor Hun Teik, Dr. Kalyana Sundram, Dr. Koh Chu Sing, and Ms. S. Kanga Rani.

For those who were unable to be present with us at the workshop to enjoy the warm friendship and participate in the scientific discussions, it was decided to edit and publish the proceedings of the meeting. We the editors are grateful to Dr. Chong Yoon Hin, Dr. Perumal Ramasamy, and Dr. Chandrasekharan for assisting with the editing of the manuscript.

Kalanithi Nesaretnam
Malaysian Palm Oil Board

Lester Packer
University of Southern California

Contents

Micronutrients and Health

Chapter 1

Oxidative Damage, Antioxidants, and Human Sperm

Choon Nam Ong,[a] Sin Eng Chia,[a] Han Ming Shen,[a] Tay Sun Kuie,[b] and Qi Xuan Chen[c]

[a]Department of Community Medicine, Faculty of Medicine, National University of Singapore, Singapore
[b]Department of Obstetrics and Gynaecology, Singapore General Hospital, Singapore
[c]Department of Clinical Nutrition, School of Public Health, Zhongsan University, Guangzhou, China

Introduction

We have begun to realize that diet and lifestyle can affect many degenerative diseases, such as cardiovascular disease and cancer. However, little attention has been given to date to the effects these factors may have on the human reproductive system.

Under physiologic conditions, endogenous oxidants are produced at a high rate, resulting in oxidative damage to proteins, lipids, and DNA (1). Accumulating epidemiologic evidence also suggests that oxidative damage to tissues is further increased by an unhealthy lifestyle and exposure to certain toxic substances, and is decreased by the appropriate intake of antioxidants and a balanced diet. Recent biochemical findings have also suggested that the rates of cellular oxidative damage can be modulated by exogenous factors, such as the diet (2).

This paper attempts to provide an up-to-date assessment on how cellular oxidative stress affects human seminal quality and the role of antioxidants in preventing oxidative insults to the human male reproductive system.

Spermatozoa and Oxidative Damage

Semen analysis, both qualitative and quantitative, is regarded as a valid approach to the assessment of male reproductive function. It is predictive of male infertility and indicative of reproductive health status in general, and testicular function in particular. Furthermore, there are other good reasons to suggest that human semen parameters can serve as valuable indicators of the status of reproductive health because spermatozoa are produced in large numbers and carry important genetic material to the next generation.

Several recent epidemiologic studies have suggested that there has been a population-wide decline in the quality of human sperm during the past few decades (3,4); the mechanism, however, remains unclear. On the other hand, there is also evidence suggesting that oxidative sperm DNA damage is closely associated with impaired sperm function and male infertility. Interest has grown in recent years regarding the role of oxygen toxicity and free radical reactions in association with fertility potential. Biochemically, the generation of reactive oxygen species (ROS) such as superoxide radicals ($O_2^{-\bullet}$), hydrogen peroxide (H_2O_2), and hydroxyl radicals ($^{\bullet}OH$) are known to result in cellular oxidative damage, with lipid peroxidation leading to a loss of membrane integrity and causing increased cell permeability to electrolytes. This free radical–mediated process may also cause enzyme inactivation, structural damage to DNA, and cell death. If hydroxyl radicals ($^{\bullet}OH$), the most damaging ROS, are generated close to DNA, they can attack the purine and pyrimidine bases and cause DNA base changes. Mammalian spermatozoa are known to be highly sensitive to injuries caused by high oxygen concentration (5). The production of abnormal levels of ROS is now believed to be involved in many aspects of human male infertility, in which spermatozoa are rendered dysfunctional by lipid peroxidation, altered membrane function, as well as impaired metabolism. Mazzilli *et al.* (6) found a significantly high level of superoxide anion in infertile patients (87%) compared with fertile normospermic men (55%). Using the lucigenine method to study the generation of ROS, we showed that there are close associations among sperm motility, morphology, and the ROS in seminal plasma (Fig. 1.1*A* and *B*).

8-Hydroxydeoxyguanosine (8OHdG) has been regarded as a precise and sensitive biomarker of oxidative DNA damage. Our earlier data (7) showed that the mean concentration of 8OHdG in infertile men was significantly higher than that in healthy subjects (10.03 vs. 4.79 8OHdG/10^5dG, $P < 0.01$). Follow-up investigations showed that there was a significant positive correlation between sperm 8OHdG and sperm head defects, whereas sperm 8OHdG showed an inverse correlation with sperm density, total sperm number, and normal sperm morphology (8). These findings provide direct evidence suggesting that oxidative damage to sperm DNA is important in the etiology of male infertility.

The spontaneous formation of ROS has been associated with decreased sperm-egg interaction and reduced fertility *in vivo* (9). Oxidative damage to germline DNA may also lead to heritable mutations and increased incidences of birth defects, genetic diseases, and cancer in offspring. Although most DNA damage would be repaired, remaining damaged residues may be converted to mutations during the DNA replication that accompanies spermatogenesis, oogenesis, and embryogenesis.

Spermatogenesis may occur when men are exposed to environmental insults that lead to oxidant reproduction. Any damaged residues remaining in the sperm DNA will be delivered to the oocyte upon fertilization, which may increase the possibility of mutations when the zygotes divides. Hence, the male reproductive system is believed to be susceptible to oxidative stress.

Lifestyle and Oxidative Stress

Tobacco smoking exerts a severe oxidative stress; as a result of the high level of nitrogen oxides as well as many carcinogens in the smoke, smoking depletes bodily antioxidant levels. Cigarette smoking is regarded as a major cause of cancer and is a well-known contributing factor to male infertility. It has been shown that a low intake of antioxidants, such as ascorbate, is associated with oxidative damage to

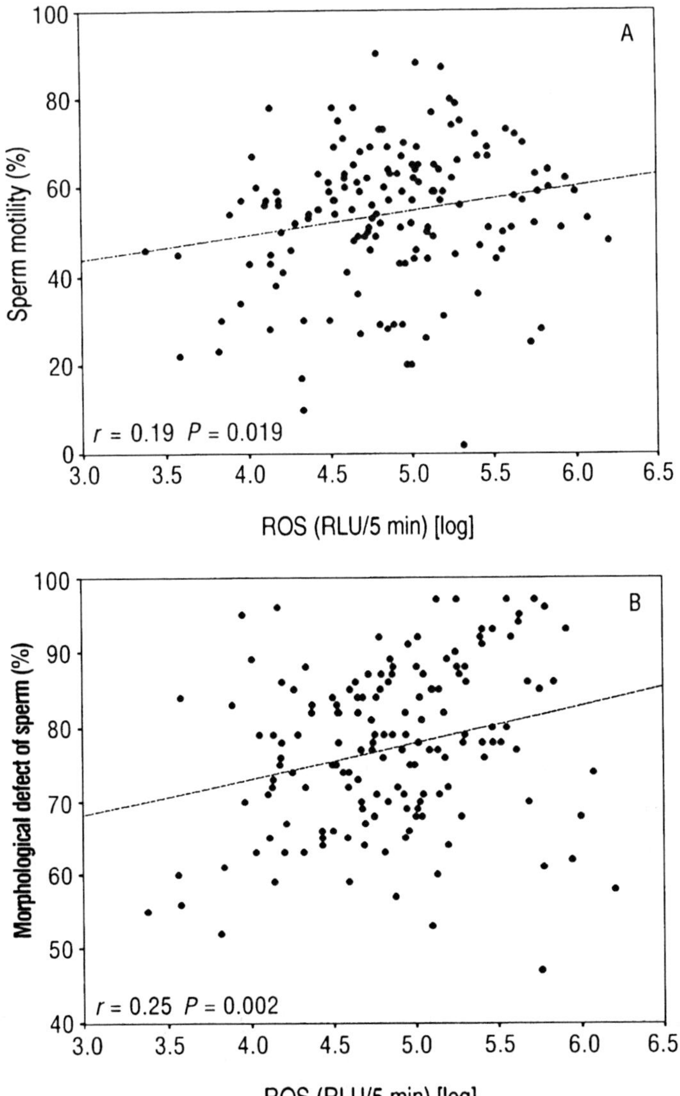

Fig. 1.1. Relationships between (*A*) reactive oxygen species (ROS) formation and sperm motility and (*B*) ROS formation and morphological defect of sperm.

sperm, and the mean 8OHdG levels in sperm DNA of smokers were higher than those of nonsmokers. Our recent epidemiologic study showed that the concentration of 8OHdG in the seminal fluid of smokers could be 1.5-fold higher than that of the nonsmokers (10). Furthermore, the level of 8OHdG was closely correlated with seminal continine concentrations. Smokers also have poorer seminal quality, with a higher percentage of sperm head defects and lower sperm density, compared with nonsmokers (8).

Antioxidant Nutrients and Oxidative Damage

Mammalian antioxidant defense mechanisms are located mainly intracellularly (e.g., superoxide dismutases, catalase, and glutathione peroxidases) and extracellularly (e.g., transferrin, ceruloplasmin, haptoglobin, and albumin). Despite the diversity and ubiquitous presence of antioxidants, some free radicals are still able to escape and cause damage. Thus, DNA undergoes constant oxidative damage, making it reasonable to believe that dietary antioxidants may diminish oxidative damage *in vivo*. The water-soluble antioxidant, ascorbic acid (AA), plays a critical role in protecting spermatozoa against oxidative damage. Laboratory findings have shown that a high concentration of AA is present in the seminal plasma, compared with blood plasma (60.25 ± 37.1 vs. 5.45 ± 3.1 mg/L, unpublished data). This reflects an important physiologic role for this antioxidant.

Ames and his colleagues (11) also showed that depletion of seminal plasma AA in male volunteers consuming controlled diets significantly increased the level of oxidative DNA damage, especially 8OHdG. Ascorbic acid serves as a powerful antioxidant in blood plasma, and it is believed that it would act in a similar manner in the seminal plasma. Administration of ascorbic acid has been shown to improve the sperm quality of heavy smokers (12). It is estimated that a smoker must consume two to three times as much AA compared with a nonsmoker to maintain a comparable blood plasma level (12). It is unclear, however, whether smoking depletes the seminal plasma AA pool directly, or indirectly as a consequence of blood plasma AA depletion. Nevertheless, the combined effects of a low intake of fruits and vegetables and smoking may suppress the reproductive tissue AA pool to such an extent that the level of oxidative stress in male germ cell DNA is increased.

It is clear that the cytotoxicity of ROS is held in check by the delicate balance between the rates at which ROS are generated and removed. Any shift in this equilibrium would lead to cellular damage.

Vitamin E (α-tocopherol), a major lipid-soluble antioxidant in human blood plasma, along with the water soluble AA, plays a vital role in limiting oxidative damage to cellular membranes and serum lipoproteins. It has been found that vitamin E *in vivo* can improve the fertilization rates of patients suffering from nuclear chromatin decongestion loss due to overoxidation of their chromatin by free radicals (13). Whether α-tocopherol has a definitive role in preventing oxidative damage to sperm or is depressed in the reproductive tissues without deleterious effect on sperm genome integrity requires further study. The spermatozoa cell membrane is known to contain an unusually high proportion of unsaturated fatty acids that are highly susceptible to peroxidation. Because the cell membrane is essential for sperm-egg fusion and in maintaining sperm cell viability and motility, it is possible that α-tocopherol could play the role of protecting the lipid membrane of the sperm cell. Further work is underway in our laboratory to establish the role of this vitamin, if any, in the protection of sperm against oxidative damage.

Coenzyme Q10 (CoQ10), a component of the mitochondrial respiratory chain, also plays a key role in energy metabolism and has potent antioxidant properties for cellular membrane integrity. This coenzyme is closely associated with Vitamin E, and its biomedical importance has attracted much attention in recent years. Earlier observations conducted on plasma low density lipoprotein (LDL) led to the conclusion that ubiquinol is a more efficient antioxidant than α-tocopherol and the carotenoids (14). It was recently confirmed that ubiquinol is ~2.5 and 1.9 times more reactive than α-tocopherol toward phenoxyl and peroxyl radicals, respectively (15). CoQ10 is present at remarkably high levels in the rat testis (16) and may play a role in seminal function, due to its antioxidant properties. In fact, it is known that a large amount of mitochondria is present in spermatozoa, although the functions of this coenzyme have not been fully elucidated. It is also important to mention that the mitochondrial genome is particularly susceptible to mutations because of the high level of ROS generation in this organelle, coupled with a relatively low DNA repair capability. The role of CoQ10 in protecting spermatozoa cannot be overlooked.

We conducted a study using a recently developed method (17) to study the concentrations of total CoQ10, ubiquinol, and the oxidized form of ubiquinol, ubiquinone of blood and seminal plasma of 115 men who attended a fertility screening clinic. The data demonstrated for the first time that there was a 10-fold increase in the level of ubiquinol compared with ubiquinone in blood plasma, but only a twofold increase in the seminal fluid (Table 1.1). The biological significance of this observation remains to be elucidated, although the ratio of ubiquinol to ubiquinone has been regarded at times as an index of antioxidant status or oxidative burden (18). The results further suggest that although there were no differences for the above

TABLE 1.1 Concentrations of Blood Plasma Cytochrome Coenzyme Q10 and Seminal Fluid Q10 in Normal Healthy Subjects

Plasma	(nmol/L)
Total Q10	0.88 ± 0.35
Ubiquinol	0.82 ± 0.33
Ubiquinone	0.06 ± 0.05
Seminal fluid	
Total Q10	0.12 ± 0.07
Ubiquinol	0.08 ± 0.04
Ubiquinone	0.03 (0.020, 0.046)[a]

[a] 25th and 75th percentiles.

three parameters measured in blood plasma, their levels were generally significantly higher in the seminal fluid of 96 fertile men, compared with the 19 infertile subjects (Fig. 1.2*A* and *B*).

Essential Trace Elements and Oxidative Stress

There is increasing epidemiologic evidence suggesting that some essential trace elements are critical for testicular development and spermatogenesis. Selenium (Se) is essential for normal spermatozoa development in both experimental animals and livestock, and probably in humans, although it is known to be toxic at high concentrations. Se is normally incorporated into the sperm mitochondria capsule and may thus play a major function in spermatozoan activity. In experimental animals, low Se levels affect fertility in males. Selenium is a known antioxidant, and we showed earlier that its metabolism in spermatogenesis is closely linked to another micronutrient, namely, zinc, in the male reproductive system (19). Furthermore, the levels of Se and Zn in the seminal fluid correlated closely with the sperm density (Table 1.2). A recent study of Scott *et al.* (20) further showed that Se supplementation in subfertile men with low selenium status can improve sperm motility and the chance of successful conception. The Se-containing enzyme phospholipid hydroperoxide glutathione peroxidase (PHGPx) is present in most mammalian tissues. It utilizes thiols such as glutathione to scavenge phospholipid hydroperoxides. The testis exhibits the highest PHGPx activity, and substantial amounts are present in sperm heads and tail midpiece mitochondria (21). These findings suggest a role of the selenium-containing enzyme in the maturation of spermatozoa through its free radical scavenging capability.

In livestock, the effects of Se supplementation, often in combination with other antioxidants, have been evaluated; however, no valid conclusion can be drawn. The only human investigation on supplementation of Se and vitamin E showed that there were significant increases in sperm motility, the percentage of live sperm, and normal spermatozoa in oligo-astheno-tetraozoospermic men (22). In general, it is believed that an adequate nutritional supply of selenium will secure optimal reproductive function, whereas additional supplementation may have a negative effect.

The ability of zinc to retard oxidative processes has been recognized for many years. In general, the mechanism of antioxidation can be divided into acute and chronic effects (23). Chronic zinc deprivation generally results in increased sensitivity to oxidative stress. Protection of cellular activity arises also by the induction of metallothionine, an effective antioxidant. The acute effects involve protection of sulfhydryls or through antagonism of transition metals such as cadmium.

In the male reproductive system, zinc is known to be an essential trace element for testicular development and spermatogenesis, although the exact mechanisms and its metabolism are not known. Deficiency of zinc leads to increased oxidative damage to testicular cells, gonadal dysfunction, decreased testicular weight, and shrinkage of seminiferous tubules (24). A recent study demonstrated that zinc is a potent scavenger of superoxide ions produced by defective spermatozoa (25).

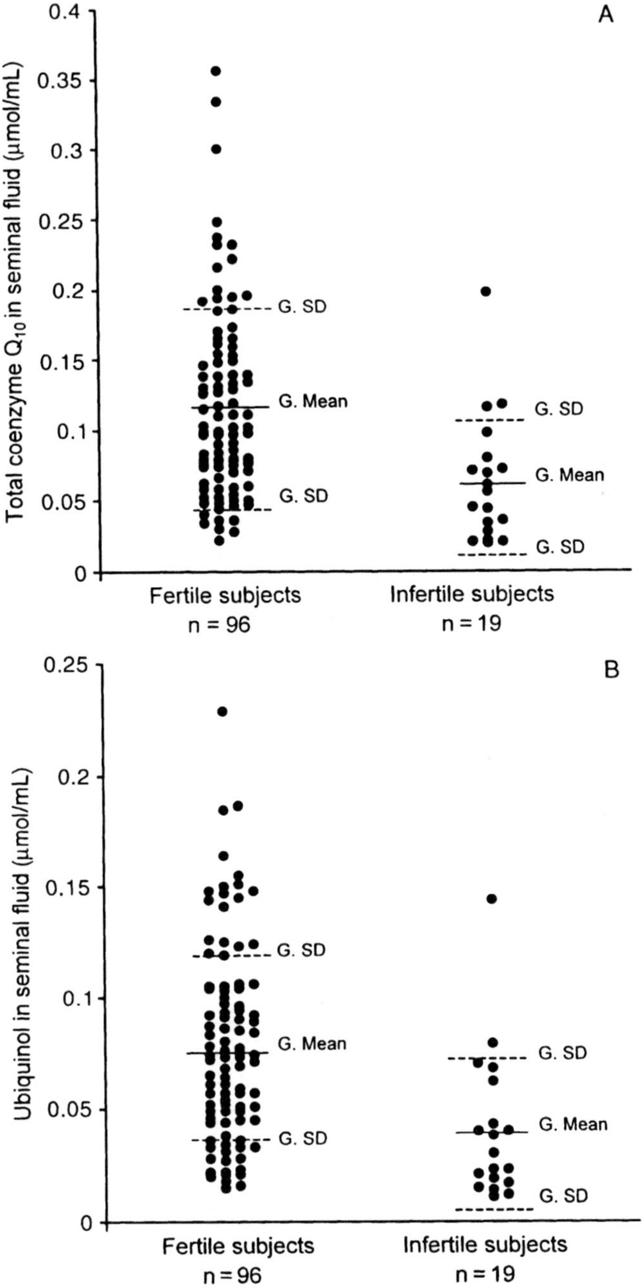

Fig. 1.2. Concentrations of (*A*) total coenzyme Q_{10} and (*B*) ubiquinol in the seminal plasma of 96 normal fertile men and 19 infertile men.

TABLE 1.2 Relationships Among Cadmium, Lead, Selenium, and Zinc in Seminal Plasma (SP), and Sperm Density in Normospermic and Oligozoospermic Men

	Linear correlation coefficient (sample size)			
Subject status	CdSP	PbSP	SeSP	ZnSP
Normospermic	0.27 (38)	–0.05 (41)	0.35[a] (34)	0.41[b] (54)
Oligozoospermic	–0.01 (36)	0.26 (42)	0.05 (43)	0.05 (58)

[a] $p < 0.05$.
[b] $p < 0.01$.

There was a significant relationship between seminal zinc concentration and the number of sperm in the seminal fluid (Fig. 1.3), suggesting that zinc may have a unique and specific function in protecting sperm or is involved in sperm production. Chia *et al.* (26) further showed that zinc in the seminal fluid of fertile men was ~36 times higher than that in the whole blood (274 vs. 7.6 mg/L). Although there was no significant difference of zinc in the blood for the fertile and infertile men (7.6 ± 1.0 vs 7.1 ± 1.0 mg/L), the zinc concentration of the seminal fluid in infertile men was significantly lower (183.6 ± 1.6 mg/L). These findings suggest that zinc has a crucial role in sperm production or viability and concur with some of the recent investigations showing that zinc therapy results in significant improvement in sperm quality, with an increase in density and improved conception and pregnancy outcome (27,28).

In short, although zinc does not have a direct role in the redox function in cellular activity, its remarkably high concentration in seminal fluid and close association with selenium suggest a potential role of this micronutrient in spermatogenesis.

Implications and Biological Significance

The above findings suggest that there are ample opportunities for disease prevention through a healthy diet and change of lifestyle. If the damage to sperm DNA from smoking is mainly oxidative, then diets low in antioxidant would exacerbate the risk of damage to sperm DNA, whereas diets rich in antioxidants would induce less risk. Cigarette smoke contains substantial quantities of mutagens that may reach the testes *via* the bloodstream to promote genetic lesions. It also contains high levels of nitrogen-related oxygen species that deplete serum antioxidants. The depletion of the blood antioxidant pool may lead to a depletion of antioxidants in other tissues and body fluids with which it is in equilibrium, including seminal plasma, testicular, and epididymal antioxidants, thus increasing the risk of oxidative damage during spermatogenesis and subsequent sperm storage.

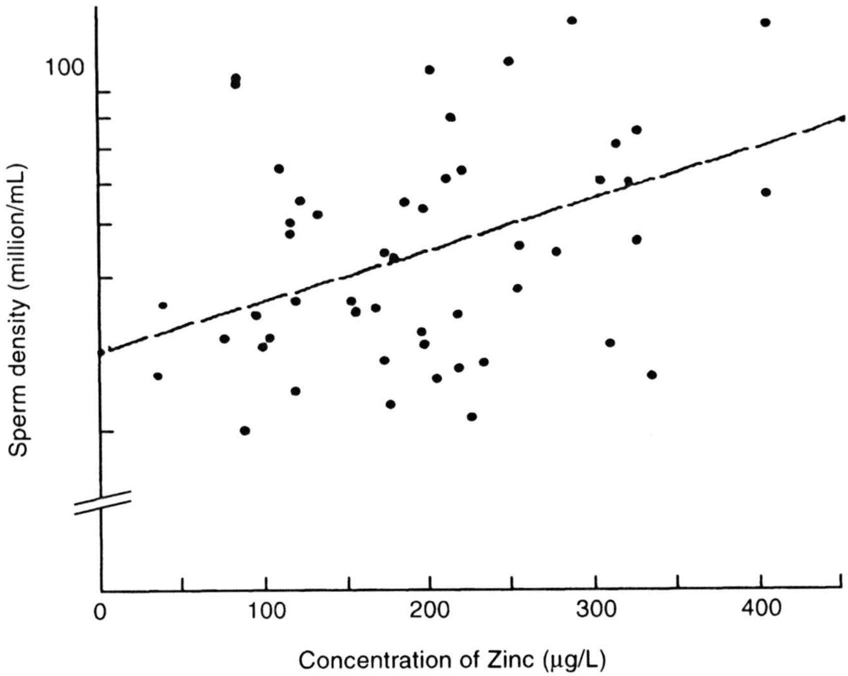

Fig. 1.3. Relationship between seminal plasma zinc concentration and sperm density (n = 114).

Spermatogenesis in mammals requires a considerable appropriation of resources that could otherwise be used to maintain somatic tissue viability. It requires large nutrient resources to support the high rate of germline cell division with high replicate accuracy. Thus, oxidative damage and/or limited resources of certain nutrients essential for accurate DNA replication may affect the protection of sperm DNA.

Oxidative damage to DNA has a deleterious effect on successful DNA replication and reproductive success; antioxidants allow organisms to limit oxidative damage in a number of ways, including the following: (i) prevention of free radical formation, e.g., chelation of damaging oxidative metals; (ii) destruction of oxidants enzymatically, e.g., superoxide dismutase (SOD), catalase, and glutathione reductase; and (iii) enzymatic removal of oxidant-damaged biomolecules, e.g., DNA glycosates.

In addition, this antioxidant defense process is reinforced by endogenous small molecule antioxidants that exist in the aqueous and lipid phases of cellular and extracellular fluids. These small molecules include glutathione, urate, and ubiquinol. These antioxidants are a vital component of the overall antioxidant defense, which acts by scavenging oxidants or by chelating oxidative transitional metals. Hence, there is a constant nutritional requirement to maintain an adequate antioxidant defense again oxidant injury to tissues.

Acknowledgments

We would like to acknowledge the following people for their valuable contributions to this work: D.X. Xu , B. Pang, B.L. Lee, H.Y. Ong, and J. Dai. The study was sponsored in part by the China Medical Board (New York) and National Medical Research Council (No. 0173).

References

1. Ames, A.N. (1998) Micronutrients Prevent Cancer and Delay Aging. *Toxicol. Lett. 103*, 5–18.
2. Halliwell, B., (2000) The Antioxidant Paradox. *The Lancet 355*, 1179–1180.
3. Carlsen, E., Giwercman, A., Keiding, N., and Skakkebaek, N.E. (1992) Evidence for Decreasing Quality of Semen During the Past 50 Years. *Br. Med.. J. 305*, 609–613.
4. Auger, J., Kunstmann, J.M., Czyglik, F., and Jouannet, P. (1995) Decline in Semen Quality Among Fertile Men in Paris During the Past 20 Years. *N. Engl. J. Med. 332*, 281–285.
5. Cummins, J.M., Jequier, A.M., and Kan, R. (1994) Molecular Biology of Human Male Infertility: Linked with Aging, Mitochondria Genetics, and Oxidative Stress? *Mol. Reprod. Dev. 37*, 345–362.
6. Mazzilli, F., Rossi, T., Marchesini, M., Roconi, C., and Dondero, F. (1994) Superoxide Anion in Human Semen Related to Seminal Parameters and Clinical Aspects. *Fertil. Steril. 62*, 862–868.
7. Shen, H.M., Chia, S.E., Ni, Z.Y., New, A.L., Lee, B.L., and Ong, C.N. (1997) Detection of Oxidative DNA Damage in Human Sperm and the Association with Cigarette Smoking. *Reprod. Toxicol. 11*, 675–680.
8. Shen, H.M., Chia, S.E., and Ong, C.N. (1999) Evaluation of Oxidative DNA Damage in Human Sperm and Its Association with Male Infertility. *J. Androl. 20*, 718–723.
9. Aitken, R.J., and Clarkson, J.S. (1987) Cellular Basis of Defective Sperm Function and Its Association with Genesis of Reactive Oxygen Species by Human Spermatozoa. *J. Reprod. Fertil. 81*, 459–469.
10. Ni, Z.Y., Liu, Y., Shen, H.M., Chia, S.E., and Ong, C.N. (1997) Does the Increase of 8-Hydroxyguanosine Lead to Poor Sperm Quality? *Mutat. Res. 381*, 77–82.
11. Fraga, C.G., Motchnik, P.A., Shigenaga, M.K., Helbock, H.J., Jacob, R.A., and Ames, B.N. (1990) Ascorbic Acid Protects Against Endogenous Oxidative DNA Damage in Human Sperm. *Proc. Natl. Acad. Sci. USA 88*, 11003–11006.
12. Fraga, C.G., Motchnik, P.A., Wyrobbek, A.J., Rempel, D.M., and Ames, B.N. (1996) Smoking and Low Antioxidant Levels Increase Oxidative Damage to Sperm DNA. *Mutat. Res. 351*, 199–203.
13. Vezina, D., Mauffette, F., Roberts, K.D., and Bleau, G. (1996) Selenium-Vitamin E Supplementation in Infertile Men: Effects on Semen Parameters and Micronutrient Levels and Distribution. *Biol. Trace Elem. Res. 53*, 65–83.
14. Stocker, R., Bowry, V.W., and Frei, A. (1990) Ubiquinol-10 Protects Human Low Density Lipoprotein More Efficiently Against Lipid Peroxidation than Does Alpha-Tocopherol. *Proc. Natl. Acad. Sci. USA 88*, 1646–1650.
15. Shi, H., Noguchi, N., and Niki, E. (1999) Comparative Study on Dynamics of Antioxidative Action of Alpha-Tocopheryl Hydroquinone, Ubiquinol, and Alpha Tocopherol Against Lipid Peroxidation. *Free Radic. Biol. Med. 27*, 334–346.

16. Kalen, A., Appelkvist, E.L., and Dallner, G. (1990) The Effect of Inducers of the Endoplasmic Reticulum, Peroxisomes and Mitochondria on the Amounts and Synthesis of Ubiquinone. *Chem.-Biol. Interact. 73*, 221–234.
17. Wang, Q., Lee, B.L., and Ong, C.N. (1999) Automated High-Performance Liquid Chromatographic Method with Precolumn Reduction for the Determination of Ubiquinol and Ubiquinone. *J. Chromatogr. B 726*, 297–302.
18. Lass, A., and Sohal, R.S. (2000) Effect of Coenzyme Q10 and α-Tocopherol Content of Mitochondria on the Production of Superoxide Anion Radicals. *FASEB J. 14*, 87–94.
19. Xu, B., Chia, S.E., and Ong, C.N. (1994) Concentrations of Cadmium, Lead, Selenium and Zinc in Human Blood and Seminal Plasma. *Biol. Trace Elem. Res. 40*, 49–57.
20. Scott, R., MacPherson, A., Yates, R.W., Hussain, B., and Dixon, J. (1998) The Effect of Oral Selenium Supplementation on Human Sperm Motility. *Br. J. Urol. 82*, 76–80.
21. Ursini, F., Heim, S., Maiorino, M., Roveri, A., Wissing, J., and Flohe, L. (1999) Dual Function of the Selenoprotein PHGPx During Sperm Maturation. *Science 285*, 1393–1396.
22. Suleiman, S.A., Ali, M.E., Zaki, Z.M., El-Malik, E.M., and Nasr, M.A. (1996) Lipid Peroxidation and Human Sperm Motility: Protective Role of Vitamin E. *J. Androl. 17*, 530–537.
23. Powell, S.R. (2000) The Antioxidant Properties of Zinc. *J. Nutr. 130*, 1447–1454.
24. Bedwal, R.S., and Bahuguna, A. (1994) Zinc, Copper and Selenium in Reproduction. *Experentia 50*, 626–640.
25. Gavella, M., and Lipovac, V. (1998) *In vitro* Effect of Zinc on Oxidative Changes in Human Semen. *Andrologia 30*, 317–323.
26. Chia, S.E., Ong, C.N., Chua, L.H., Ho, L.M., and Tay, S.K. (2000) Comparison of Zinc Concentration in Blood and Seminal Plasma and the Various Sperm Parameters Between Fertile and Infertile Men. *J. Androl. 21*, 53–57.
27. Kynaston, H.G., Lewis-Jones, D.I., Lynch, R.V., and Desmond, A.D. (1998) Changes in Seminal Quality Following Oral Zinc Therapy. *Andrologia 20*, 21–23.
28. Omu, A.E., Dashi, H., and Al-Othman, S. (1998) Treatment of Astenozoospermia with Zinc Sulphate: Andrologial, Immunological and Obstetric Outcome. *Eur. J. Obstet. Gynecol. Reprod. Biol. 79*, 179–184.

Chapter 2

The Ferric Reducing (Antioxidant) Power (FRAP) Assay, and Antioxidants in the Chinese Diet and Population

Y.T. Szeto, W.Y. Chung, and I.F.F. Benzie

Department of Nursing & Health Sciences, The Hong Kong Polytechnic University, Kowloon, Hong Kong SAR, China

Introduction

The ferric reducing antioxidant power (FRAP) assay (1) is a sensitive biomonitoring tool, which provides rapid and highly reproducible results of the "total antioxidant power" of biological fluids. The FRAP assay is suitable for use with plasma, and with aqueous and ethanolic extracts of whole foods, herbs, beverages and drugs, as well as solutions of purified antioxidants (1–4). In its modified form, known as FRASC, two indices of antioxidant status, the total antioxidant power (as the FRAP value) and the ascorbic acid concentration, are obtained within a few minutes (5,6).

The FRAP Assay

In the FRAP assay, a ferric-tripyridyltriazine (Fe^{III}-TPTZ) complex is reduced to its ferrous form, which absorbs light of 593 nm. The change from the colorless Fe^{III} form to the intensely blue-colored Fe^{II} form is caused by the combined action of the electron-donating antioxidants in the test sample. The change in absorbance at 593 nm is directly proportional, therefore, to the "total" reducing (antioxidant) power of these antioxidants. In the modified form, FRASC, ascorbic acid in the sample is selectively and specifically destroyed by ascorbate oxidase. The change in absorbance in these treated samples, therefore, is caused by the remaining antioxidants. In other words, the ascorbic acid concentration is calculated by determining the difference between the "total" and the total minus the ascorbic acid contribution [corrected for stoichiometry; the stoichiometric factor of ascorbic acid in the FRAP assay is 2.0 (7)].

The World Cancer Research Fund recommends five or more servings of fruits and vegetables daily to minimize the risk of chronic degenerative disease (8). However, most of us do not achieve this in our normal daily diet. To help design diets that might permit enhanced antioxidant status at more realistic quantities of intake, it is useful to know the "total antioxidant power" of different dietary agents. We used the FRAP and FRASC assays to measure the antioxidant power and ascorbic acid content of various fruits and vegetables, including some Chinese varieties not found in standard food tables, Chinese herbs, teas, fruit juices, and wines. Aqueous extracts of fresh, uncooked fruits and vegetables, infusions of tea and herbs, and "whole" juices were measured to assess their potential for improving *in vivo* antioxidant status. In addition, variability in antioxidant power and ascorbic acid content within the same type of fruit or vegetable purchased on different occasions was investigated.

Our preliminary results showed that the total antioxidant power (as the FRAP value) of plant-based dietary agents covers a wide range (Tables 2.1 and 2.2), and items purchased at different times can have widely differing results. Green tea is clearly very rich in antioxidant power (9). We estimate that a single cup of green tea in the strength usually made for drinking (~1.5%) would supply as much antioxidant power as 150 mg of pure vitamin C. Our preliminary data indicate that a 100-g serving of

TABLE 2.1 Total Antioxidant Power, as the Ferric Reducing Antioxidant Power (FRAP) Value, of Aqueous Extracts of Selected Fruits and Vegetables[a]

Fruit/Vegetable	(μmol/100 g fresh weight)
Strawberry	1594 (278)
Mandarin orange	540 (76)
Red apple	420 (42)
Pineapple	348 (142)
Chinese kale	1042 (282)
Onion	432 (126)
Garlic	268 (100)
Potato	144 (32)
Lettuce	88 (26)

[a]Values are the mean (SD) of at least triplicate readings.

TABLE 2.2 "Total Antioxidant Power" Content, as the Ferric Reducing Antioxidant Power (FRAP) Value, of Beverages in the Form and Volume Usually Ingested

Beverage	Amount (mL)	Antioxidant power (μmol/L)
Black tea (1% wt/vol)	200	500–900
"Semifermented" tea (1% wt/vol)	200	1000–1300
Green tea (1% wt/vol)	200	2000
Red wine		
Merlot	150	2900
Shiraz	150	2200
Cabernet sauvignon	150	3700
White wine		
Reisling	150	380
Sauvignon blanc	150	360
Chardonnay	150	520
Fresh orange juice	200	600

strawberries contains the same antioxidant power as almost 140 mg of vitamin C, and the same as that found in 1 kg of Chinese pears. One hundred grams of a commonly consumed Chinese leafy green vegetable (usually referred to in English as Chinese kale) was found to have as much antioxidant power as 90 mg of pure vitamin C, and as much as in 1.3 kg of iceberg lettuce.

The apparent richness in antioxidant power of traditional Chinese foods may help explain the relatively low rates of coronary heart disease (CHD) seen in the local Chinese population (10). It is interesting that a recently published paper (11) reported lower plasma FRAP values in a sample of adults in the United Kingdom, where CHD rates are much higher than those in Hong Kong (12). We did not detect lower plasma FRAP values in a small study of Caucasians living in Hong Kong, but their diet is likely to contain significant amounts of Chinese fruits and vegetables, and this may result in a different antioxidant profile from Caucasians consuming a more standard Western-style diet. We reported previously (3) that the ascorbic acid concentrations of Hong Kong Chinese do not show the male-female differences previously reported in literature, and that plasma ascorbic acid status is good, with mean levels of ~50 μmol/L for plasma ascorbic acid of subjects in the fasted state (3). We also reported that vitamin E levels in Hong Kong Chinese are lower than expected, considering the low CHD rate in this population, and that Caucasians living in Hong Kong appear to have higher lipid standardized vitamin E levels than Hong Kong Chinese (3). It is possible that the high antioxidant content of Chinese foods, or the regular ingestion of perhaps more bioavailable polyphenolic antioxidants in these foods, leads to an enhanced antioxidant status in our local population, with a greater contribution from, for example, flavonoid antioxidants (13–15). This warrants further study.

To determine bioavailability of antioxidants in food, some of which are likely to be currently unknown or incompletely characterized, a sensitive biomonitoring tool to determine postingestion changes in the total antioxidant status of body fluids is useful. By using this approach, and the FRAP or FRASC assay, the postingestion response can be monitored in terms of antioxidants, even though the individual antioxidant constituents may be unknown. We have employed this approach in investigating the bioavailability of single doses of vitamin C (ascorbic acid) and of green tea (16,17). Our results indicated that plasma ascorbic acid concentration peaked ~90 min after ingestion, and that the response was related to dose, but not to baseline (fasting) plasma ascorbic acid concentration. Furthermore, the responses to 1-, 2-, and 3-g doses were not significantly greater than that induced by a dose of 500 mg. Our results also showed that the plasma antioxidant power (as the FRAP value) increased significantly within 1 h of drinking green tea (Fig. 2.1). Our data are supported by two recent studies (11,18) that also used the FRAP assay to assess response to ingestion of tea. To date, however, there are no published studies that have determined the response to whole foods. Furthermore, storage and cooking effects on the antioxidant power of foods have not been investigated systematically.

In conclusion, oxidative damage is opposed *in vivo* by various, diverse antioxidant defense mechanisms, and enhanced antioxidant status may help delay or prevent

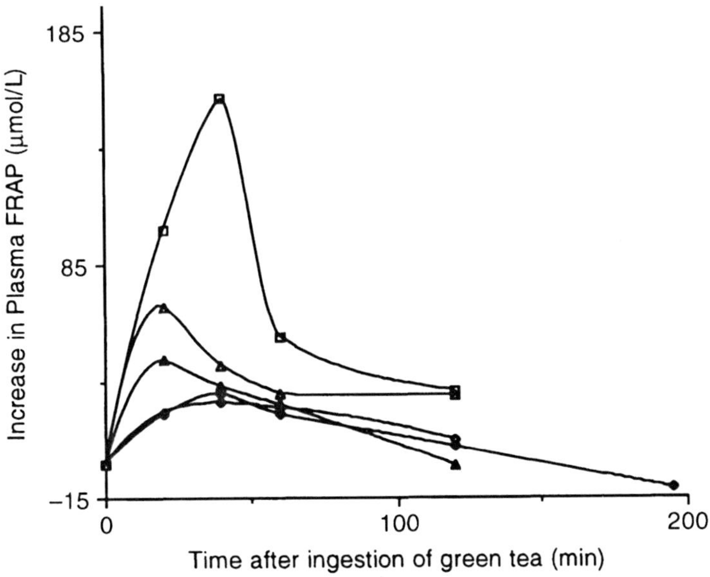

Fig. 2.1. Changes in plasma antioxidant power after ingestion of green tea by five individuals. Abbreviation: FRAP, ferric reducing antioxidant power.

pathologic changes to key biological sites, lowering the risk of cancer and heart disease (15,19–21). Assessing and optimizing antioxidant status, therefore, may be important in health maintenance, and determining absorption and systemic availability of dietary antioxidants is useful for planning nutritional strategies for optimizing antioxidant status. Strategic dietary planning to enhance antioxidant status requires an assessment of the antioxidant content of dietary constituents, knowledge of the effects of storage, processing, and preparation, as well as an evaluation of postingestion effects on antioxidant status. The FRASC assay will facilitate studies to aid in dietary planning and appraisal of dietary modification.

Acknowledgement

This work was supported financially by The Hong Kong Polytechnic University.

References

1. Benzie, I.F.F., and Strain, J.J. (1996) The Reducing Ability of Plasma as a Measure of "Antioxidant Power"—the FRAP Assay. *Anal. Biochem. 239*, 70–76.
2. Benzie, I.F.F., and Chung, W.Y. (1999) Total Antioxidant Power of Plasma: Male-Female Differences and Effect of Anticoagulant Used. *Ann. Clin. Biochem. 36*, 104–106.
3. Benzie, I.F.F., Janus, E.D., and Strain, J.J. (1998) Plasma Ascorbate and Vitamin E Levels in Hong Kong Chinese. *Eur. J. Clin. Nutr. 52*, 447–451.
4. Benzie, I.F.F., and Tomlinson, B. (1998) Antioxidant Power of Angiotensin-Converting Enzyme Inhibitors *in vitro*. *Br. J. Clin. Pharmacol. 45*, 168–169.

5. Benzie, I.F.F., and Strain, J.J. (1997) Simultaneous Automated Measurement of Total Antioxidant (Reducing) Capacity and Ascorbic Acid Concentration. *Redox Rep. 3*, 233–238.
6. Benzie, I.F.F., and Strain, J.J. (1999) Ferric Reducing (Antioxidant) Power as a Measure of Antioxidant Capacity: The FRAP Assay, in *Oxidants and Antioxidants, Methods in Enzymology*, (Packer, L., ed.) vol. 299, pp. 15–27, Academic Press, Orlando.
7. Benzie, I.F.F., Chung, W.Y., and Strain, J.J. (1999) Antioxidant (Reducing) Efficiency of Ascorbate in Plasma Is Not Affected by Concentration. *J. Nutr. Biochem. 10*, 146–150.
8. World Cancer Research Fund/American Institute for Cancer Research (1997) *Food, Nutrition and the Prevention of Cancer: A Global Perspective*. American Institute for Cancer Research, Washington.
9. Benzie, I.F.F., and Szeto, Y.T. (1999) Total Antioxidant Capacity of Teas by the Ferric Reducing/Antioxidant Power (FRAP) Assay. *J. Agric. Food. Chem. 47*, 633–637.
10. Hong Kong Department of Health Annual Report 1999.
11. Langley-Evans, S.C. (2000) Consumption of Black Tea Elicits an Increase in Plasma Antioxidant Potential in Humans. *Int. J. Food. Sci. Nutr. 51*, 309–315.
12. World Health Organization (1998) *World Health Statistics Annual*. WHO, Geneva.
13. Halliwell, B. (1996) Oxidative Stress, Nutrition and Health. Experimental Strategies for Optimization of Nutritional Antioxidant Intake in Humans. *Free Radic. Res. 25*, 57–74.
14. Duthie, G.G., Duthie, S.J., and Kyle, K.A.M. (2000) Plant Polyphenols and Heart Disease: Implications as Nutritional Antioxidants. *Nutr. Res. Rev. 13*, 95–106.
15. Strain, J.J., and Benzie, I.F.F. (1999) Diet and Antioxidant Defence. In: *The Encyclopedia of Human Nutrition*, (Sadler, M., Cabellero, B., and Strain, J.J., eds.) pp. 95–105, Academic Press, London.
16. Benzie, I.F.F., and Strain, J.J. (1997). Acute Post-Ingestion Changes in Plasma Ascorbic Acid Concentration: Relationship to Dose and to Existing Body Stores. *Nutr. Res. 17*, 187–190.
17. Benzie, I.F.F., Szeto, Y.T., Tomlinson, B., and Strain, J.J. (1999) Consumption of Green Tea Causes Rapid Increase in Plasma Antioxidant Power in Humans. *Nutr. Cancer 34*, 83–87.
18. Leenan, R., Roodenburg, A.J.C., Tijburg, L.B.M., and Wiseman, S.A. (2000) A Single Dose of Tea with or Without Milk Increases Plasma Antioxidant Activity in Humans. *Eur. J. Clin. Nutr. 54*, 87–92.
19. Collins, A.R. (1999) Oxidative DNA Damage, Antioxidants and Cancer. *Bioessays 21*, 238–246.
20. Ames, B.N., Gold, L.S., and Willet, W.C. (1995) The Causes and Prevention of Cancer. *Proc. Natl. Acad. Sci. USA 92*, 5258–5265.
21. Benzie, I.F.F. (1996) Lipid Peroxidation: A Review of Causes, Consequences, Measurement and Dietary Influences. *Int. J. Food Sci. Nutr. 47*, 233–262.

Chapter 3

Oxidant Damage in Haptoglobin Knockout Mouse

Yew-Koon Lim,[a] Andrew Jenner,[b] Azhar bin Ali,[a] Yanping Wang,[c] Heinz Baumman,[c] Barry Halliwell,[d] and Sai-Kiang Lim[a]

[a]National University Medical Institutes, The National University of Singapore, Singapore 117597, Singapore
[b]Guy's, King's and St. Thomas School of Biomedical Science, London Bridge Campus, London SE1 RT, UK
[c]Department of Molecular and Cellular Biology, Roswell Park Cancer Institute, Buffalo, NY 14263
[d]Department of Biochemistry, Faculty of Medicine, The National University of Singapore, Singapore 119260, Singapore

Introduction

Haptoglobin (Hp) is the major plasma protein that binds free hemoglobin (Hb) with high avidity (1). The strong avidity with which Hp binds Hb ($K_d \sim 1 \times 10^{-15}$ mol/L) and the high conservation of the Hp gene across species suggest that there must be important functions associated with Hp-Hb complex formation (1,2). Two major functions of Hb-Hp complex formation are thought to include hepatic clearance and degradation of free Hb (1–5) and retardation of passage of free Hb through the glomeruli into the renal tubular cells, resulting in renal damage (6). It has been observed that during severe intravascular hemolysis or transfusion of Hb solution, a common clinical complication is acute renal failure with a concomitant depletion of Hp (6,7), suggesting that Hp may have important functions in reducing Hb toxicity.

Using Hp-deficient (Hp–/–) mice that were generated by gene targeting, we showed that plasma Hb clearance in Hp–/– mice is as efficient as that of their normal Hp+/+ littermates (8). However, Hp–/– mice were more susceptible to hemolysis (8). Induction of severe hemolysis by phenylhydrazine caused death in 55% (n = 27) of Hp–/– mice and 18% of Hp+/+ (n = 17) mice. Like their Hp+/+ littermates, Hp–/– mice had a significant accumulation of Hb precipitates in the renal tubules as well as hydropic degeneration of the tubules. However, Hp–/– mice tended to suffer greater oxidative damage as indicated by their higher plasma malonaldehyde (MDA) and 4-hydroxy-2(*E*)-nonenal (HNE) levels, and greater general tissue damage as indicated by their serum α-glycoprotein (AGP) levels. This greater renal damage in Hp–/– mice also resulted in poorer renal regeneration as indicated by lower mitotic indices in the kidneys of surviving Hp–/– mice relative to their Hp+/+ littermates. Together, these results suggest that hemolysis causes oxidative tissue damage in the kidneys, and Hp can ameliorate some of this damage (8).

The cause of renal damage and the mechanism of the protective role of Hp in preventing renal damage in mice during hemolysis are not understood. Because Hb and its catabolic products, hemin and iron, are known to catalyze many potentially tissue-damaging oxidative reactions (8,9) and Hp has been shown to ameliorate oxidative damage mediated by Hb, particularly Hb-initiated lipid peroxidation (10–14), renal damage in Hp–/– mice during hemolysis and the protective role of Hp may be related to renal oxidative stress.

Materials and Methods

Analysis of Renal Tissues. Hemolysis was induced in mice by phenylhydrazine at 2 mg/10 g body weight as previously described (8). At various times after induction, mice were anesthetized with 0.1 mL/10 g body weight of a cocktail (1 part Hypnorm, 1 part Midazolom, and 2 parts distilled water) and perfused with 20 mL saline and 1 mmol/L EDTA through the heart. Kidneys were removed, washed in cold saline, and homogenized in ice cold 20 mmol/L Tris-HCl, pH 7.4, 1 mmol/L phenylmethylsulfonyl fluoride (10% wt/vol). The homogenate was centrifuged at 10,000 × *g*, 4°C, for 10 min and the supernatant was further centrifuged at 20,000 × *g*, 4°C, for 10 min. Protein concentration was assayed by Bio-Rad Protein Assay Kit II (# 500-0002, Bio-Rad, Hercules, CA). Hemoglobin in the extract was quantitated by a colorimetric assay (#S-527A, Sigma Chemical, St. Louis, MO). For Western-blot analysis, 10 mg of protein was separated on 10% SDS-PAGE, blotted onto nitrocellulose, and probed with antibodies against mouse Hb (# 55447, ICN, Costa Mesa, CA). The blot was then incubated sequentially with a biotinylated secondary antibody and a streptavidin-horseradish peroxidase conjugate before it was developed with a chemiluminescence substrate (# 34080, Pierce, Rockford, MD).

DNA Oxidation Analysis. DNA oxidation analysis was carried out essentially as described in Ref. 15. Brief details are as follows: Calf thymus DNA, 6-azathymine, 2,6-diaminopurine, 8-bromoadenine, 5-hydroxyuracil (isobarbituric acid), 4,6-diamino-5-formamidopyrimidine (FAPy-adenine), 2,5,6-triamino-4-hydroxypyrimidine, 5-(hydroxymethyl)uracil and guanase were purchased from Sigma Chemical (Poole, Dorset, UK). 8-Hydroxyguanine (8OHG) and ethanethiol were purchased from Aldrich (Gillingham, UK). 8-Hydroxyadenine and 2,6-diamino-4-hydroxy-5-formamidopyrimidine (FAPy-guanine) were synthesized (courtesy of Dr. H. Kaur, Kings College, London), respectively, by treatment of 8-bromoadenine with concentrated formic acid (95%) at 150°C for 45 min with purification by crystallization from water, and treatment of 2,5,6-triamino-4-hydroxypyrimidine with concentrated formic acid with purification by crystallization from water. Thymine glycol was synthesized by reaction of thymine with OsO_4 for 1 h at 60°C, and excess OsO_4 was removed by freeze drying. Purity of standards (>99%) was assessed by mass spectrometry (MS). Stable isotope–labeled [M + 4] 8-hydroxyguanine (*8-hydroxyguanine-1,3-15N2-(2-amino-15N)-2-13C*), 2-hydroxyadenine, 5-hydroxycytosine, 5-hydroxyhydantoin, and 5-hydroxy-5-methylhydantoin were kind gifts from Dr. M. Dizdaroglu (National Institute of Standards and Technology, Gaithersberg, MD). Silylation grade acetonitrile and bis(trimethylsilyl)trifluoracetamide (BSTFA) (containing 1% trimethylchlorosilane, TMCS) were obtained from Pierce Chemical (Rockford, IL) and ethanethiol was purchased from Fluka (Buchs, Switzerland). Distilled water passed through a purification system (Elga, High Wycombe, Bucks, UK) was used to make up all solutions.

DNA concentration was determined by ultraviolet (UV) absorbance; DNA was hydrolysed and derivatized for gas chromatography (GC)-MS analysis as previously described (15–17). *Caution: Ethanethiol has a very unpleasant odor.* Extracted DNA (100 μg) containing the internal standards, stable isotopically labeled 8OHG [M + 4] (0.2 nmol), 6-azathymine, and 2,6-diaminopurine (0.5 nmol), was lyophilized. Samples were hydrolyzed by the addition of 0.5 mL of 60% formic acid and heating at 140°C for 45 min in an evacuated, sealed hydrolysis tube, and then cooled and lyophilized. Samples were derivatized in poly(tetrafluoroethylene)-capped glass vials after purging with nitrogen by the addition of 75 μL of a BSTFA (+1% TMCS)/acetonitrile/ethanethiol (16:3:1 vol/vol) mixture at 23°C for 2 h and analyzed by GC-MS as described previously (15).

RNA and Protein Analysis. Kidney RNA extraction, and reverse transcription-polymerase chain reaction (RT-PCR) were carried out as previously described (8). Briefly, 2 mg RNA was reverse-transcribed to cDNAs. The cDNAs were diluted 1 and 10X, and amplified by PCR in the presence of ^{32}P-dCTP using gene-specific primers. Primers for triose phosphate isomerase (TPI), a housekeeping gene, were included as an internal control in the PCR reaction. The RT-PCR products were separated on a 5% polyacrylamide gel, quantitated by phosphorimaging, and exposed to autoradiography. All signals were normalized to that of TPI. The primers used were as follows: (i) erythropoietin (Epo) 5′-TCA TCT GCG ACA GTC GAG TTC-3′ and 5′-CGT GTA CAG CTT CAG TTT CCC-3′; (ii) TPI 5′-CCC TGG CAT GAT CAA AGA CTT-3′ and 5′-GAT GGG CAG TGC TCA TTG TTT-3′; and (iii) heme oxygenase-1 (HO-1) 5′GAA GAG GAG ATA GAG CGC AAC-3′ and 5′AGA GAA AGG AAA CAC AGG GAG-3′.

Renal Clearance of ^{3}H-Inulin. For every 20 g body weight, 3·7MBq of ^{3}H-Inulin (# NET 314L, NEN, Boston, MA) with 2 mg of unlabeled inulin (# I-3754, Sigma Chemical, St. Louis, MO) dissolved in 0.15 mL saline was injected into the left ventricle of anesthetized mice; 5 min after the injection was completed, the tip of the mouse tail was cut, a small aliquot of blood was collected in a heparinized capillary tube, and 10 mL of plasma was counted. This time point was designated 0 min. Thereafter, blood was collected at 15-min intervals for 1 h, and the amount of radioactivity was calculated as a percentage of that at time 0. For phenylhydrazine-treated mice, renal function was measured 48 h after induction of hemolysis with phenylhydrazine.

Results

Increased Renal Injury in Hp–/– Mice. The induction kinetics of erythropoietin and heme oxygenase-1 (HO-1) gene expression were also used to assess kidney-specific injury. It was shown previously that after ureteric obstruction, global ischemia, or focal needlestick injury, the number of erythropoietin-expressing interstitial cells in the kidney decreases (18). Within 48 h of phenylhydrazine treatment,

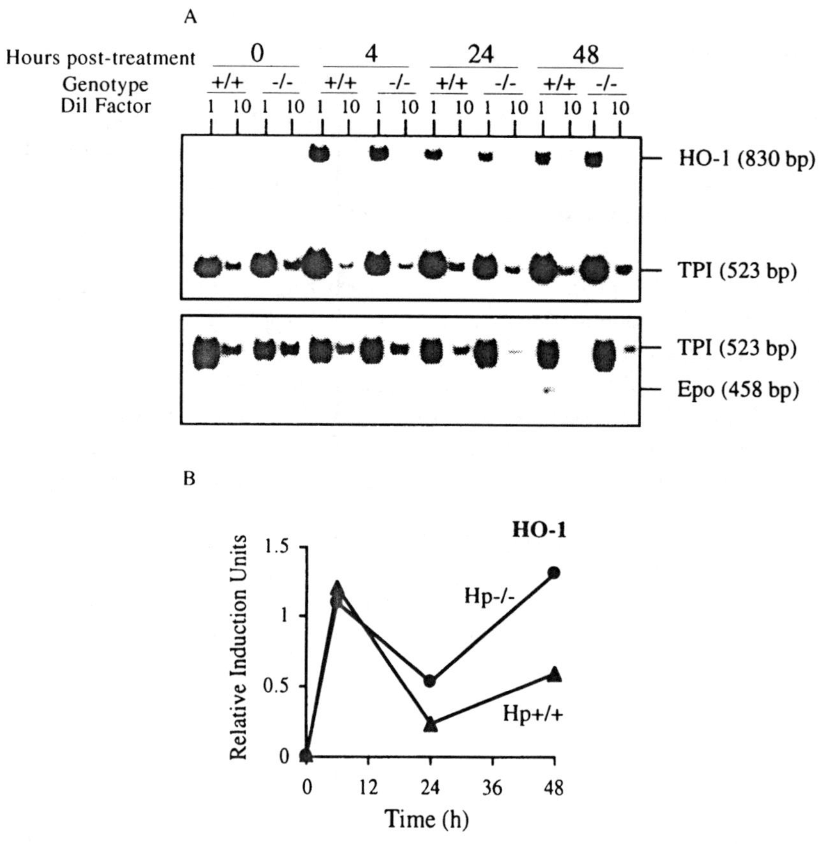

Fig. 3.1. Renal tissue injury during phenylhydrazine-induced hemolysis. (a) Renal induction kinetics of heme oxygenase-1(HO-1) and erythropoietin (Epo) gene expression. Total RNA was isolated from kidneys of mice at 0, 4, 24, and 48 h after treatment with phenylhydrazine (2 mg/10 g body weight) and analyzed by reverse transcription-polymerase chain reaction (RT-PCR) as described in Materials and Methods with triose phosphate isomerase (TPI) mRNA as an internal control. (b) Relative induction of HO-1. RT-PCR products were quantitated by phosphorimaging, and the signals were normalized to that of TPI.

erythropoietin mRNA was detectable in the kidneys of Hp+/+ mice but not Hp–/– mice, consistent with greater renal injury and/or delayed repair in Hp–/– mice during hemolysis (Fig. 3.1A).

Because HO-1 is an oxidative stress–responsive gene in many organs (19,20), its induction kinetics in the renal tissues were used to assess oxidative stress. Induction of renal HO-1 gene expression in both Hp–/– and Hp+/+ mice during phenylhydrazine-initiated hemolysis was biphasic, with the first phase peaking at ~4 h, followed by a second phase peaking at 48 h or thereafter (Fig.3.1b). In both Hp+/+ and Hp–/– mice, the first phase of HO-1 mRNA induction was similar in magnitude and kinetics but the second phase was greater in Hp–/– mice, suggesting that Hp–/– mice suffered greater oxidative stress.

Decreased Renal Function. Renal function was assessed by an inulin clearance assay. ^{3}H-inulin clearance from the plasma was measured by injecting a small aliquot of ^{3}H-inulin into the left ventricle of anesthetized mice 48 h after induction of hemolysis and measuring the rate of loss of radioactivity from the plasma. Both untreated Hp+/+ and Hp–/– mice demonstrated 60–70% clearance over 1 h (Fig. 3.2A). Induction of hemolysis by phenylhydrazine generally resulted in poor ^{3}H-inulin clearance in both wild-type and mutant mice, indicating a decline in renal function (Fig. 3.2B). From 0 to 30 min, Hp–/– mice exhibited poorer ^{3}H-inulin clearance than Hp+/+ mice ($P = 0.05$; Fig. 3.2b). At 60 min, Hp–/– mice continued to exhibit

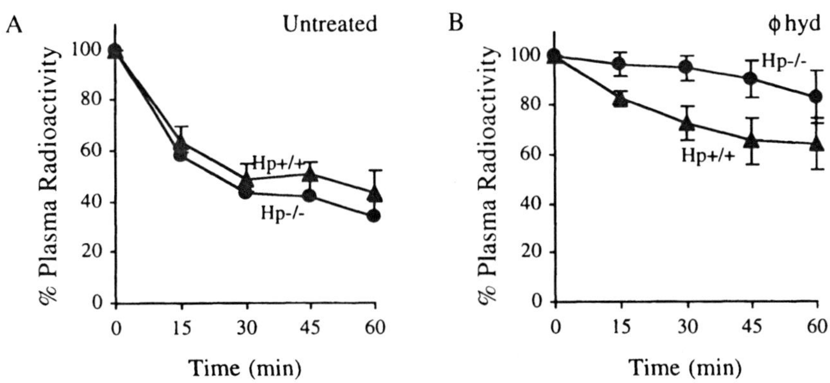

Fig. 3.2. Renal function during phenylhydrazine-induced hemolysis. As described in Materials and Methods, ^{3}H-inulin was injected into the heart of anesthetized mice. After 5 min, the mice were bled from the tail and plasma radioactivity was determined. This time point was designated 0 min. Thereafter, blood was collected at 15-min intervals over 1 h, and the amount of radioactivity was calculated as a percentage of that at time 0. (a) Untreated mice (Hp+/+ mice, *n* = 7; Hp–/– mice, *n* = 8); (b) mice treated with phenylhydrazine 48 h before assessment of inulin clearance (Hp+/+ mice, *n* = 5; Hp–/– mice, *n* = 6). Values represent the mean ± SEM.

a numerically poorer but statistically insignificant renal clearance than Hp+/+ mice [residual ^{3}H-inulin of 83 ± 21% (n = 5) vs. 64 ± 26% (n = 6); P = 0.177].

Increased Oxidative Damage in the Kidneys. Hemoglobin and its catabolic products, hemin and iron, are known to catalyze many potentially tissue-damaging oxidative reactions (9), and Hp has been shown to ameliorate oxidative damage mediated by Hb, particularly Hb-initiated lipid peroxidation (10–14).

Renal genomic DNA in Hp–/– mice and Hp+/+ mice was analyzed for multiple oxidized DNA bases using GC-MS. Levels of hypoxanthine and xanthine (which are not oxidation products but products of DNA base deamination) were also measured.

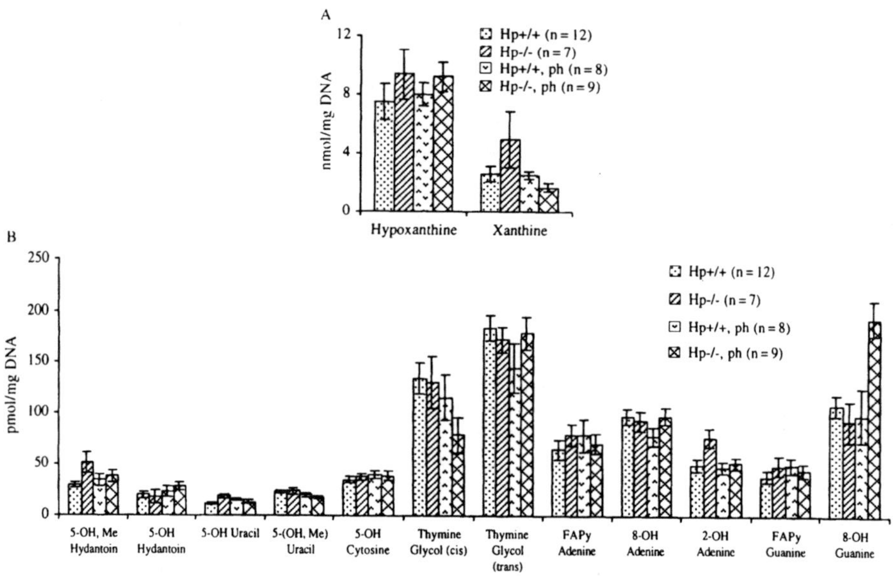

Fig. 3.3. Oxidative damage in renal tissues. At 0 and 48 h after induction of hemolysis, Hp+/+ and Hp–/– mice were anesthetized and perfused with saline. Kidneys were removed and used to prepare homogenates for lipid peroxidation assay or genomic DNA for analysis of modified DNA bases. (a) and (b) Levels of individual DNA base oxidation products analyzed. Genomic DNA from kidneys of Hp+/+ and Hp–/– mice with or without phenylhydrazine treatment was assayed for individual DNA base oxidation products as described in Materials and Methods. Data were plotted as the mean ± SEM. Sample size (n) for each group of mice is indicated on the figure. The results were presented as follows: (a) hypoxanthine and xanthine; (b) individual DNA base oxidation products analyzed were 5-OH Me hydantoin, 5-OH hydantoin, 5-OH uracil, 5-(OH, Me) uracil, 5-OH cytosine, 2-OH adenine, 8-OH adenine, 4,6-diamino-5- formamidopyrimidine (FAPy-adenine), thymine glycol (*cis* and *trans*), 2,6-diamino-4-hydroxy-5-formamidopyrimidine (FAPy-guanine), and 8-OH guanine. Data were plotted as the mean ± SEM. Sample size (n) for each group of mice is indicated on the figure.

A

	Hp+/+	Hp-/-	Hp+/+, ph	Hp-/-, ph
nmol Hb/mg protein	1.73 ± 0.27 ($n = 4$)	1.47 ± 0.29 ($n = 5$)	4.27 ± 1.17 ($n = 6$)	4.41 ± 1.22 ($n = 7$)

B

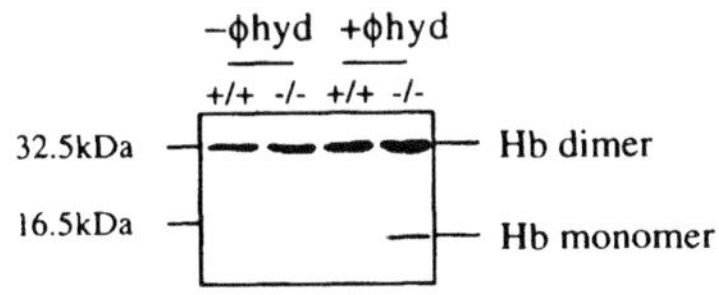

Fig. 3.4. Precipitation of hemoglobin (Hb) in renal tissue; 48 h after phenylhydrazine (ϕhyd) induction, mice were anesthetized, perfused with saline, and kidney extracts were prepared as described in Materials and Methods. (a) Kidney extracts were assayed for Hb levels biochemically as described in Materials and Methods. Values represent the mean ± SD. Sample size (n) for each group of mice is indicated on the figure; (b) Western-blot analysis. Kidney extracts (10 μg) from untreated Hp+/+, Hp–/– mice, and phenylhydrazine-treated mice were analyzed by Western blotting using antibodies against mouse Hb. A representative blot is shown.

Four groups of mice were used in this study: (i) untreated Hp+/+ mice; (ii) untreated Hp–/– mice; (iii) phenylhydrazine-treated Hp+/+ mice, and (iv) phenylhydrazine-treated Hp–/– mice.

The basal levels of DNA base oxidation or deamination products in Hp–/–mice and Hp+/+ mice were not significantly different, suggesting that the lack of Hp in mice did not result in increased levels of oxidative DNA damage in the kidneys of Hp–/– mice (Fig. 3.3). However, during phenylhydrazine-induced hemolysis, there was a significant increase in 8OHG in Hp–/– mice but not in Hp+/+ mice (99 ± 11.6 pmol/mg DNA in Hp+/+ mice vs. 195 ± 18.9 pmol/mg in Hp–/– mice, $P < 0.001$; Fig. 3.3). Basal levels of 8OHG in the renal DNA of untreated Hp+/+ and Hp–/– mice were similar (109 ± 10.8 pmol/mg in Hp+/+ mice vs. 93 ± 11.5 pmol/mg in Hp–/– mice; Fig. 3.3). The other DNA base oxidation or deamination products examined did not change (Fig. 3.3).

Hemoglobin Precipitation in Renal Tissues. It is generally thought that Hb contributes to renal injury during severe hemolysis by precipitating in the renal tissues and that Hp decreases this Hb-induced renal damage by preventing glomerular filtration of Hb through the formation of the large Hb-Hp complex (6). Therefore, we determined the level of Hb in saline-perfused kidneys of Hp–/– and +/+ mice during hemolysis. The amounts of Hb in the renal tissues of untreated Hp+/+ and Hp–/– mice were not significantly different (1.73 vs 1.47 nmol/mg protein, $P = 0.22$; Fig. 3.4A). During hemolysis, Hb precipitation in the kidneys increased dramatically, but it was not significantly different between Hp+/+ and Hp–/– mice (4.27 vs. 4.41 nmol/mg protein,

$P = 0.84$; Fig. 3.4A). These results were further verified by Western-blot analysis (Fig. 3.4B). Therefore, contrary to previous suggestions, Hp may not be important in preventing precipitation or deposition of Hb in renal tissues during severe hemolysis, at least in mice.

Discussion

This study shows that Hp decreases oxidative damage in renal tissues during hemolysis as evidenced by the induction kinetics of HO-1, an oxidative stress–responsive gene in the kidneys. Induction of HO-1 occurs in two phases; the first phase during the first 24 h may be due to the release of Hb from the lysis of erythrocytes. The kinetics and magnitude of the first phase in both genotypes of mice are similar, indicating a similar degree of hemolysis as indicated previously (8). The second phase at 48 h could be due to the release of cellular heme-containing proteins from damaged tissues and would be more indicative of tissue damage. Hp–/– mice have a greater second phase induction of HO-1, consistent with greater tissue damage. The more extensive renal damage in Hp–/– mice is further demonstrated by the failure of Hp–/– mice to induce erythropoietin expression as rapidly as Hp+/+ mice in response to the anemia induced by phenylhydrazine treatment. The more extensive renal tissue damage in Hp–/– mice during phenylhydrazine-induced hemolysis also resulted in a greater loss of renal function in Hp–/– mice.

Hemoglobin and its catabolic products, hemin and iron, are known to catalyze many potentially tissue-damaging oxidative reactions (9), and Hp has been shown to ameliorate oxidative damage mediated by Hb, particularly Hb-initiated lipid peroxidation (10–14). We postulate that the greater renal damage in Hp–/– mice is due to increased oxidative stress. To test this hypothesis, multiple products of oxidative damage to each of the four DNA bases were determined. They include 5-OH Me hydantoin, 5-OH hydantoin, 5-OH uracil, 5-(OH, Me) uracil, 5-OH cytosine, 2-OH adenine, 8-OH adenine, FAPy adenine, thymine glycol (*cis* and *trans*), FAPy guanine, and 8-OH guanine. Of these, only the 8OHG level in the renal DNA of Hp–/– mice was significantly elevated. We suggest that oxidative DNA damage in Hp–/– kidneys during phenylhydrazine-induced hemolysis is unlikely to have been initiated by hydroxyl radical ($^{\bullet}OH$), hypochlorous acid (HOCl) or peroxynitrite ($ONOO^-$). The extremely reactive hydroxyl radical ($^{\bullet}OH$) will react with all four DNA bases to produce a multiplicity of elevated oxidation products, including 8OHG (15–17,21), yet only increases in 8OHGwere seen. Peroxynitrite generates mainly base deamination and nitration products (e.g., xanthine from guanine, hypoxanthine from adenine) (22,23), whereas hypochlorous acid generally causes pyrimidine oxidation and chlorination (24). No increases in base deamination products were observed in this study, although the basal levels of deamination products in renal tissue appeared high. Nevertheless, this technique has led to the observation of increases in base deamination products in some other experimental situations (25). In addition, 8OHG, which is highly elevated in the renal DNA of Hp–/– mice, is usually a minor product in DNA oxidation by peroxynitrite and hypochlorous acid. Singlet oxygen, which is more selective for guanine oxidation or certain peroxyl radicals, could possibly be the species responsible for the increased DNA oxidation in Hp–/– mice (17). The identification of the radical species

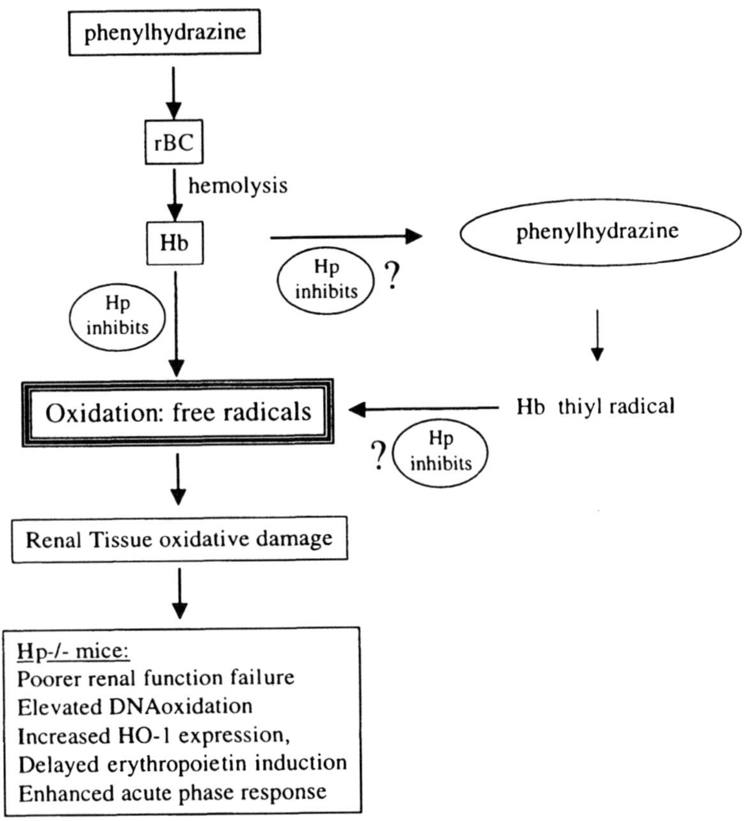

Fig. 3.5. Postulated events leading to increased oxidative tissue damage in haptoglobin (Hp)–/– mice. Induction of severe hemolysis by phenylhydrazine leads to massive release of hemoglobin (Hb). Hemoglobin and its breakdown products then initiate free radical formation, resulting in tissue oxidative damage. Haptoglobin decreases oxidative damage by binding Hb and inhibiting its oxidative potential. Lack of Hp in Hp–/– mice exacerbates oxidative stress, leading to increased DNA base oxidation, increased lipid peroxidation, and greater induction of heme oxygenase-1 (HO-1). Greater oxidative stress in Hp–/– mice causes greater tissue damage, leading to a delay in erythropoietin induction in response to the anemia induced by phenylhydrazine and a greater acute phase response as measured by the induction of acute phase response genes in the liver. Phenylhydrazine itself can also oxidize Hb to form the Hb thiyl radical. It is not known whether Hp inhibits oxidation of Hb by phenylhydrazine or whether Hp binds and reduces the reactivity of the Hb thiyl radical. Abbreviation: RBC, red blood cells.

will be important in elucidating the molecular mechanism by which Hp protects renal tissues from oxidative damage during hemolysis.

These data suggest that Hp is an important antioxidant that reduces renal oxidative damage especially during phenylhydrazine-induced hemolysis (Fig. 3.5). Treatment with phenylhydrazine causes severe hemolysis, which releases a large amount of Hb. Free plasma Hb and its catabolic products, hemin and iron, are potent catalysts of free radical damage (9). Phenylhydrazine itself is also a potent oxidizing agent and has been shown to cause the formation of the Hb thiyl radical (26). Therefore, the antioxidative effects of Hp can be mediated through Hp interactions with free plasma Hb released during hemolysis and/or reducing oxidation by phenylhydrazine. The high specific binding affinity of Hp for Hb and the previously documented inhibitory effects of Hp on Hb-initiated oxidation strongly suggest that some of the antioxidative effects of Hp must be mediated through Hp-Hb interactions (10–14). Hp could also reduce the oxidative effects of phenylhydrazine by preventing phenylhydrazine-mediated Hb oxidation or reducing the reactivity of the Hb thiyl radical. However, it remains to be determined whether Hb binding by Hp prevents phenylhydrazine oxidation of Hb or whether Hp binds the Hb thiyl radical, 8OHG.

Acknowledgments

This manuscript is an excerpt from a paper by Lim, Y.-K., Jenner, A., bin Ali, A., Wang,Y., Hsu, S.I.-H., Chong, S.M., Baumman, H., Halliwell, B., and Lim, S.-K. Haptoglobin Reduces Renal Oxidative DNA and Tissue Damage During Phenylhydrazine-Induced Hemolysis, *Kidney Int.*, *58(3)*:1033–44.

References

1. Bowman, B.H., and Kurosky, A. (1982) Haptoglobin: The Evolutionary Product of Duplication, Unequal Crossing Over, and Point Mutation. *Adv. Hum. Genet. 12*: 189–261.
2. McCormick, D.J., and Atassi, M.Z. (1990) Hemoglobin Binding with Haptoglobin: Delineation of the Haptoglobin Binding Site on the Alpha-Chain of Human Hemoglobin. *J. Protein Chem. 9*: 735–742.
3. Okuda, M., Tokunaga, R., and Taketani, S. (1992) Expression of Haptoglobin Receptors in Human Hepatoma Cells. *Biochim. Biophys. Acta 1136*: 143–149.
4. Oshiro, S., and Nakajima, H. (1988) Intrahepatocellular Site of the Catabolism of Heme and Globin Moiety of Hemoglobin-Haptoglobin After Intravenous Administration to Rats. *J. Biol. Chem. 263*: 16032–16038.
5. Oshiro, S., Yajima, Y., Kawamura, K., Kubota, M., Yokofujita, J., Nishibe, Y., Takahama, M., and Nakajima, H. (1992) Catabolism of Hemoglobin-Haptoglobin Complex in Microsome Subfractions. *Chem. Pharm. Bull. 40*: 1847–1851.
6. Glassock, R.J. (1995) Hematuria and Pigmenturia, in *Textbook of Nephrology*, 2nd edn., (Massry, S.G., and Glasock, R.J., eds.) vol. 1, pp, 557–566, Williams and Wilkins, Baltimore.

7. Tam, S.C., and Wong, J.T. (1988) Impairment of Renal Function by Stroma-Free Hemoglobin in Rats. *J. Lab. Clin. Med. 111*: 189–193.
8. Lim, S.K., Kim, H., Ali, A., Lim, Y.K., Wang, Y., Chong, S.M., Costantini, F., and Baumman, H. (1998) Increased Susceptibility in Hp Knockout Mice During Acute Hemolysis. *Blood 92*: 1870–1877.
9. Everse, J., and Hsia, N. (1997) The Toxicities of Native and Modified Hemoglobins. *Free Radic. Biol. Med. 22*: 1075–1099.
10. Miller, Y.I., Altamentova, S.M., and Shaklai N. (1997) Oxidation of Low-Density Lipoprotein by Hemoglobin Stems from a Heme-Initiated Globin Radical: Antioxidant Role of Haptoglobin. *Biochemistry 36*: 12189–12198.
11. Vercellotti, G.M., Balla, G., Balla, J., Nath, K., Eaton, J.W., and Jacob, H.S. (1994) Heme and the Vasculature: An Oxidative Hazard That Induces Antioxidant Defenses in the Endothelium. *Artif. Cells Blood Substit. Immobil. Biotechnol. 22*: 207–213.
12. Halliwell, B., and Gutteridge, J.M. (1990) The Antioxidants of Human Extracellular Fluids. *Arch. Biochem. Biophys. 280*: 1–8.
13. Gutteridge, J.M., and Smith, A. (1988) Antioxidant Protection by Haemopexin of Haem-Stimulated Lipid Peroxidation. *Biochem. J. 256*: 861–865.
14. Gutteridge, J.M. (1987) The Antioxidant Activity of Haptoglobin Towards Haemoglobin-Stimulated Lipid Peroxidation. *Biochim. Biophys. Acta 917*: 219–223.
15. Jenner, A., England, T.G., Aruoma, O.I., and Halliwell, B. (1998) Measurement of Oxidative DNA Damage by Gas Chromatography-Mass Spectrometry: Ethanethiol Prevents Artifactual Generation of Oxidized DNA Bases. *Biochem. J. 331*: 365–369.
16. Dizdaroglu, M., Aruoma, O.I., and Halliwell, B. (1990) Modification of Bases in DNA by Copper Ion-1,10-phenanthroline Complexes. *Biochemistry 29*: 8447–8451.
17. Halliwell, B. (1998) Can Oxidative DNA Damage Be Used as a Biomarker of Cancer Risk in Humans? Problems, Resolutions and Preliminary Results from Nutritional Supplementation Studies. *Free Radic. Res. 29*: 469–486.
18. Maxwell, P.H., Ferguson, D.J., Nicholls, L.G., Johnson, M.H., and Ratcliffe, P.J. (1997) The Interstitial Response to Renal Injury: Fibroblast-Like Cells Show Phenotypic Changes and Have Reduced Potential for Erythropoietin Gene Expression. *Kidney Int. 52*: 715–724.
19. Tyrrell, R.M. (1996) UV Activation of Mammalian Stress Proteins. EXS 77: 255–271.
20. Tyrrell, R.M. (1997) Approaches to Define Pathways of Redox Regulation of a Eukaryotic Gene: The Heme Oxygenase 1 Example. *Methods 11*: 313–318.
21. Mori, T., Tano, K., Takimoto, K., and Utsumi, H. (1998) Formation of 8-Hydroxyguanine and 2,6-Diamino-4-hydroxy-5-formamidopyrimidine in DNA by Riboflavin Mediated Photosensitization. *Biochem. Biophys. Res. Commun. 242*: 98–101.
22. Douki, T., and Cadet, J. (1996) Peroxynitrite Mediated Oxidation of Purine Bases of Nucleosides and Isolated DNA. *Free Radic. Res. 24*: 369–380.
23. Spencer, J.P., Wong, J., Jenner, A., Aruoma, O.I., Cross, C.E., and Halliwell, B. (1996) Base Modification and Strand Breakage in Isolated Calf Thymus DNA and in DNA from Human Skin Epidermal Keratinocytes Exposed to Peroxynitrite or 3-Morpholinosydnonimine. *Chem. Res. Toxicol. 9*: 1152–1158.

24. Whiteman, M., Jenner, A., and Halliwell, B. (1997) Hypochlorous Acid-Induced Base Modifications in Isolated Calf Thymus DNA. *Chem. Res. Toxicol. 10*: 1240–1246.
25. Spencer, J.P., Whiteman, M., Jenner, A., and Halliwell, B. (2000) Nitrite-Induced Deamination and Hypochlorite-Induced Oxidation of DNA in Intact Human Respiratory Tract Epithelial Cells. *Free Radic. Biol. Med. 28*: 1039–1050.
26. Jiang, J.J., Liu, K.J., Jordan, S.J., Swartz, H.M., and Mason, R.P. (1996) Detection of Free Radical Metabolite Formation Using *in vivo* EPR Spectroscopy: Evidence of Rat Hemoglobin Thiyl Radical Formation Following Administration of Phenylhydrazine. *Arch. Biochem. Biophys. 330*: 266–270.

Chapter 4

Study on Antioxidative Capacity of Flavonoids from Dried Balsam Flowers

Zhao-Feng Peng, Ngoh-Khang Goh, Tet-Fatt Chia, Ma Hnin Hnin Aung, and Lian Sai Chia

Nanyang Technological University, Singapore 637616, Republic of Singapore

Introduction

Over the years, flavonoids have become an important subject of research because they have been found to be powerful antioxidants; they are present in our daily diet and are considered an active principle in some medicinal plants. Much evidence exists in chemistry, biochemistry, and pharmacy to support the view that flavonoids play a vital role in scavenging reactive oxygen species (1–3). Chemically, flavonoids possess the following three remarkable characteristics as antioxidants (4): (i) the presence of hydrogen-donating substituents, hydroxyl groups attached to aromatic ring structures of flavonoids, making it much easier for the flavonoids to be involved in redox reaction to scavenge free radicals by virtue of their appropriate reduction potential; (ii) flavonoids are liable to form stable delocalization systems to delocalize the resulting radical because they contain aromatic and heterocyclic rings as well as multiple unsaturated bonds; and (iii) flavonoids possess certain structural groups capable of forming metal complexes, i.e., the transition metal–chelating potential.

In traditional Chinese medical practice, raw plant materials often serve as herbal medicines in dried form; thus they require a longer time to prepare compared with stewing. The effective antioxidative components that remain in the material under these conditions most likely are thermostable compounds. Obviously, flavonoids belong in this category because the enzymes are inactive under these conditions. This means that the antioxidative function of these plants, especially the dried species, likely comes from flavonoids. Another reason for their extensive study is the diversity and abundance of flavonoids in plants, which could lead to certain potential applications in the fields of biology and pharmacy. Fortunately, Singapore, which is located in the tropics and richly endowed by nature, contains many diverse species of plants. This cheap and plentiful source of plants is used extensively in studies on antioxidants from plants.

Balsam (scientific name: *Impatiens balsamina*, see Fig. 4.1) belongs to the Balsaminaceae family. It is a succulent annual herb with white, pink, purple, or variegated flowers. It is a native to Southeast Asia and exists as a common garden plant in Singapore, China and other places. The Chinese people use its seed to treat difficult labor, to relieve pain after labor, to increase the menstrual flow, to expel phlegm from the respiratory passages, and as an antidote to fish poisoning. The flowers are also

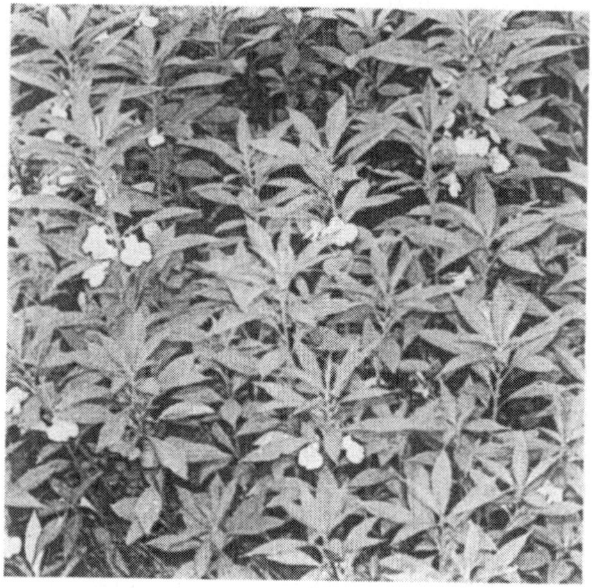

Fig. 4.1. A photograph of the balsam plant.

used to treat snake bite and lumbago. Its leaves are used to heal wounds in Malaysia, Indonesia, and the Philippines (5).

Experimental Procedures

Reagents and Instrumentation. The chemicals used were as follows: phosphate-buffered saline, pH 7.4 (PBS; Sigma Chemical), 0.4 g/L myoglobin (M-0630; Sigma); 0.1 g/L 2,2′-azinobis(3-ethylbenz-thiazolin-6-sulfonic acid) diammonium salt (ABTS; Sigma, Fluka); 10 and 4 mmol/L H_2O_2 (Fisher, Fluka); 0.1 unit/mL horseradish peroxidase (HRP; Sigma); 2.0 mmol/L etoposide (VP-16, $C_{29}H_{32}O_{13}$; Sigma). The spin-trapping agent was 100 mmol/L *N*-*t*-butyl-α-phenylnitrone (PBN; Sigma). The azo initiator (AI) was 100 mmol/L 2,2′-azobis (2-methyl propionamidine) dihydrochloride (Aldrich). The reference materials included 1, 10, and 50 mmol/L 6-hydroxy-2,5,7,8-tetramethylchroman-2-carboxylic acid (Trolox; Tokyo Kasei). The preparative high-performance liquid chromatography (HPLC) system for isolation was a Beckman System Gold equipped with a programmable solvent module-126NMP and a System Gold 168 dual-channel UV-visible (VIS) detector. The preparative column was a VP250/40 Nucleoprep 100-10 (Macherey-Nagel); length, 250 mm; i.d., 40 mm. The UV-VIS spectrophotometer was a HP-8452A Diode Array Spectrophotometer (Hewlett-Packard, U.S.A.), and the electron spin resonance (ESR) spectrometer was a JES-TE100 (JEOL, Japan).

Procedures. The experiments in this study can be classified into three categories, i.e., acquisition of pure flavonoids, identification of the compounds, and antioxidative activity assay. This paper focuses on the analysis of antioxidative activity. The acquisition of pure flavonoids from dried balsam flowers involved the following: (i) collection of plant samples; (ii) extraction; (iii) isolation with preparative HPLC; and (iv) final purification. The identification of isolated compounds was done by using various measurements, HPLC online-UV/VIS spectrometry, mass spectrometry and nuclear magnetic resonance spectrometry. In addition, a hydrolysis technique was used. The structural elucidation of each isolated flavonoid was conducted by comprehensively analyzing the data from the measurements and finally assembling a complete structure of the flavonoid on the basis of analytical chemistry, structural matter, and occurrence patterns of the flavonoids in plants (6–8).

For evaluation of the antioxidative activity of the isolated flavonoids, three assay methods were applied as follows:

Measurement of antioxidative capability (TEAC) of antioxidants. One of the commonly used methods for determining the radical-scavenging ability of antioxidants (such as flavonoids) as electron- or hydrogen-donating agents is to measure their ability to scavenge the ABTS radical, $ABTS^{\bullet +}$ (9,10). The basis of the method is the generation of a long-lived specific $ABTS^{\bullet +}$ radical cation chromophore and the determination of the relative abilities of antioxidants to quench (or to suppress the production of) the radical in relation to the abilities of standard materials. Here, Trolox, the water-soluble vitamin E analog, was used as a standard. Thus, Trolox equivalent antioxidant capability (TEAC), which is defined as the concentration of Trolox with the same antioxidant activity as a 1 mmol/L of the substance under investigation, is the unit representing antioxidative activity. The method, which is reported to be appropriate for both aqueous and lipophilic systems, can be carried out as a decolorization measurement in which the antioxidant is added to the performed radical solution produced on one-electron oxidation of ABTS by reduction of the ferryl myoglobin radical (10).

$$HX\text{-}Fe^{3+}\text{ (peroxidase)} + H_2O_2 \longrightarrow X^{\bullet}[Fe^{4+}{=}\,0] + H_2O$$

$$ABTS + X^{\bullet}[Fe^{4+}{=}0] \longrightarrow ABTS^{\bullet +} + HX\text{-}Fe^{3+}$$

$ABTS^{\bullet +}$ is a relatively stable green product of the above reaction. The TEAC value of a sample is calculated on the basis of the concentration change of $ABTS^{\bullet +}$ caused by the antioxidants (see Fig. 4.2). Experimentally, TEAC values of flavonoids are measured by using the following UV-ABTS assay: Transfer 2 mL of ABTS to a measuring tube. Add 200 μL myoglobin and dilute the solution with PBS to a volume of 6 mL. Add 80 μL of 10 mmol/L H_2O_2 and shake vigorously 10 times. Warm the resultant solution at 50°C in a water bath for 15 min to develop color. After removal, allow it to stand for an additional 20 min at room temperature. Finally, thoroughly mix the resulting solution with a sample; strictly control the final volume of the solution (e.g., 7 mL) and start a timer simultaneously. At exactly 2 min after shaking,

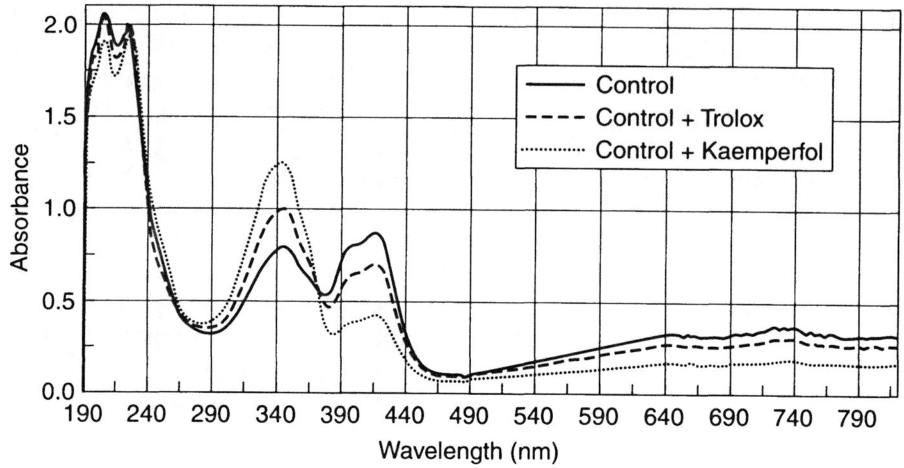

Fig. 4.2. Ultraviolet (UV)-visible spectral change of 2,2′-azino-bis(3ethylbenz-thiazoline-6-sulfonic acid) (ABTS)/$ABTS^{\bullet+}$ in the presence of antioxidants.

measure the absorbance of the solution at 414 nm or 730 nm. Finally, calculate TEAC values of the analyte in terms of a working curve calibrated by a series of standards.

For large-scale measurements (e.g. >20 portions), proportional amounts of PBS, ABTS, myoglobin, and H_2O_2 are added in a flask. Develop color under the same conditions as above. Take 7 mL of resultant solution as one portion, mix thoroughly with a given sample, and start a timer simultaneously. At exactly 2 min, measure the absorbance of the solution at 414 nm or 730 nm. The calculation of TEAC is as described above.

Estimation of antioxidative activities of antioxidants by ESR spectrometry. Using the ESR technique, antioxidative activity can be evaluated by monitoring its behavior in affecting the generation of certain free radicals. There are two free radical generation systems used in our ESR assay, i.e., the PBN-AI system and the etoposide (Et)-HRP-H_2O_2 system (11,12). For the former method, a water-soluble azo compound 2,2′-azobis(2-methylpropion-amidine) dihydrochloride is taken as an initiator to produce the initial free radical.

$$\underset{\text{(AI)}}{\text{R-N=N-R}} \longrightarrow N_2 + 2R^{\bullet}$$

In the presence of the spin-trapping reagent PBN, a nitroxide spin adduct is formed:

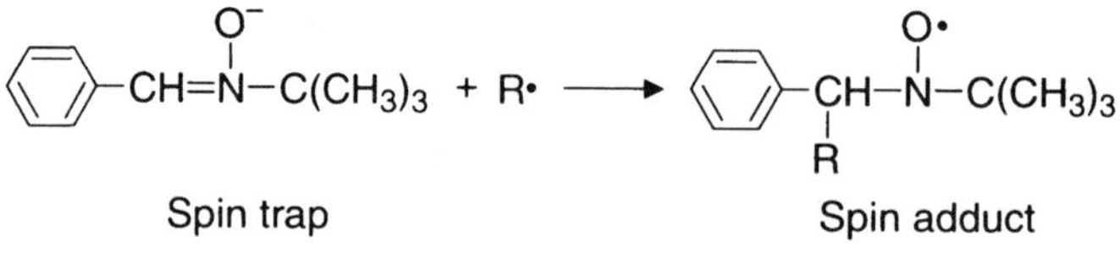

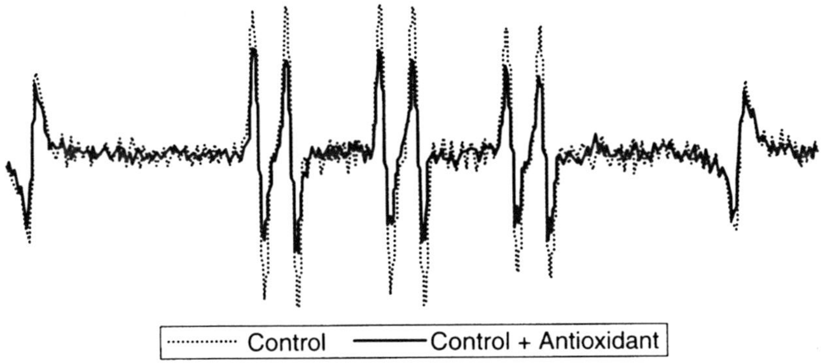

Fig. 4.3. Electron spin resonance (ESR) spectra of the *N-t*-butyl-α-phenylnitrone (PBN) radical.

The spin-trapping agent can trap free radicals rapidly to form more persistent radicals (spin adducts) detectable by ESR. Because the strength of an ESR signal is directly proportional to the number of radicals produced, spin trapping can be used as a quantitative tool for counting radical events in the system of interest as well as an effective way in which to study antioxidants. Here, evaluation of antioxidative capability is undertaken by monitoring the generation of the PBN spin adduct in the presence of the antioxidant (see Fig. 4.3).

Because spin trapping is a kinetic method, a successful assay depends critically on adduct formation and the rate of spin trapping, which must be much faster than the rate of other reactions of the radical. Moreover, the ideal spin trap would yield spin adducts that are perfectly stable and nonreactive to other reagents in the environment.

Evaluation of antioxidants with the method of one-electron oxidation of the Et-HRP-H_2O_2 system. By one-electron oxidation, horseradish peroxidase can make etoposide form an etoposide phenoxyl radical in the presence of hydrogen peroxide.

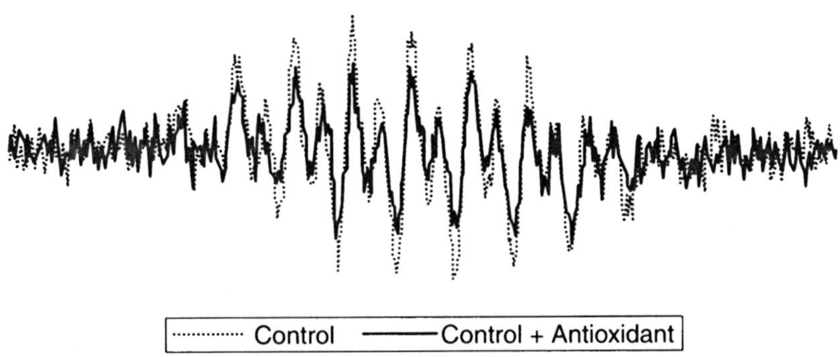

Fig. 4.4. Electron spin resonance (ESR) spectra of the etoposide phenoxyl radical.

TABLE 4.1 Parameters for Electron Spin Resonance (ESR) Measurements[a,b]

	PBN-AI system	Etoposide-H_2O_2-HRP
Magnetic field		
Center field	328.480 mT	328.654 mT
Sweep width	5.0 × 1	1.1 × 1
Sweep time	30 s	30 s
Amplitude parameters		
Modulation frequency	100 kHz	100 kHz
Modulation width	1.0 × 0.1 mT	0.5 × 0.1 mT
Amplification	5.0 × 100	10.0 × 100
Modulation	1st	1st
Phase	0	0
Time constant	0.03 s	0.03 s
Microwave status		
Frequency	9.208 GHz	9.207 GHz
Power	10 mW	10 mW
Phase	501	510
Digital marker	560	560

[a]Abbreviations: PBN-AI, *N-t*-butyl-α-phenylnitrone–azo initiator; HRP, horseradish peroxidase.
[b]The temperature was 25°C (room temperature).

This phenol intermediate possesses characteristic ESR absorption. Therefore, it is used for the study of antioxidative activity by detecting the formation of the etoposide phenoxyl radical in the presence of an antioxidant (see Fig. 4.4).

Experimentally, the ESR assays were conducted as follows:

1. Evaluation of antioxidant activities in aqueous PBN-AI system: Mix 20 μL PBS, 40 μL PBN and 20 μL of the sample or standard in a micro cell. Add 40 μL of AI [2,2′-azobis (2-methylpropion-amidine) dihydrochloride] and trigger a timer at once. Transfer the resultant solution to a flat cell for ESR measurement under the conditions listed in Table 4.1. Each minute, record the peak height readings, which reflect generation of the PBN radical. Plot the graph of time vs. amplitude.
2. Evaluation of antioxidant activities in the Et-HRP-H_2O_2 system. Mix 96 μL PBS, 40 μL etoposide, 20 μL H_2O_2 and 4 μL of the sample in a micro cell. Add 40 μL of HRP and start a timer immediately. Transfer the resultant solution to a flat cell for ESR assay under the conditions listed in Table 4.1. Record the peak height readings every 2 min and plot the graph of time vs. amplitude.

Results and Discussion

Flavonoids from Balsam Flowers. In dried balsam flowers, the types of flavonoids were relatively simple. Only kaempferol compounds were obtained. Flavonoids belonging to other classes were too small in quantity to be detected and extracted. The flavonoids isolated from dried balsam flowers are summarized in Table 4.2.

TABLE 4.2 Polyphenols from Balsam Flowers

Abbreviation	Structure (%)	Relative Amount	Source
B-KA	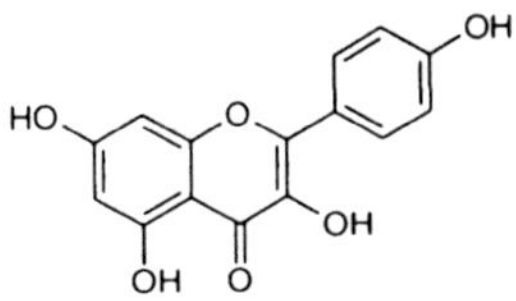 Kaempferol (Aglycone)	1.16	Fraction 5
B-KCG	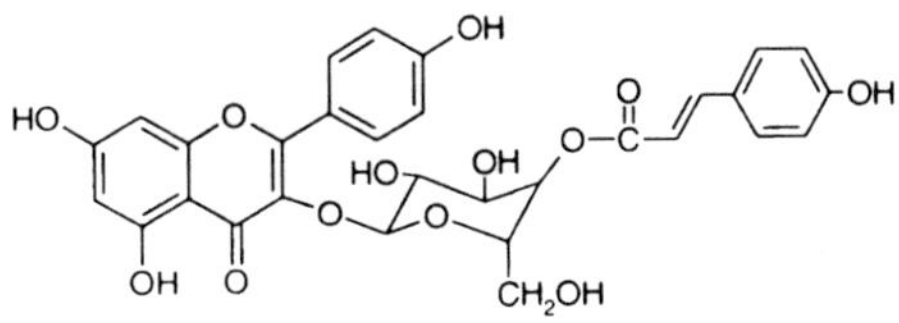 Kaempferol-3-*p*-coumaroyl glucoside	0.27	Fraction 4
B-KG	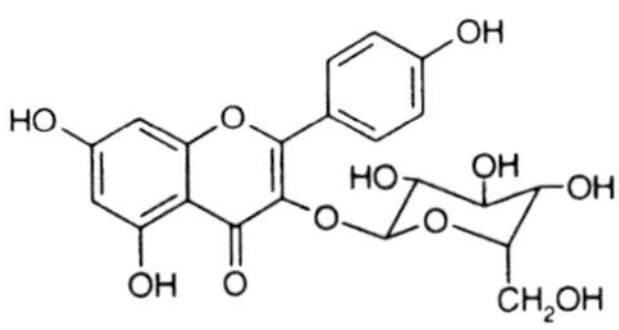 Kaempferol-3-glucoside	1.13	Fraction 3
B-KGR	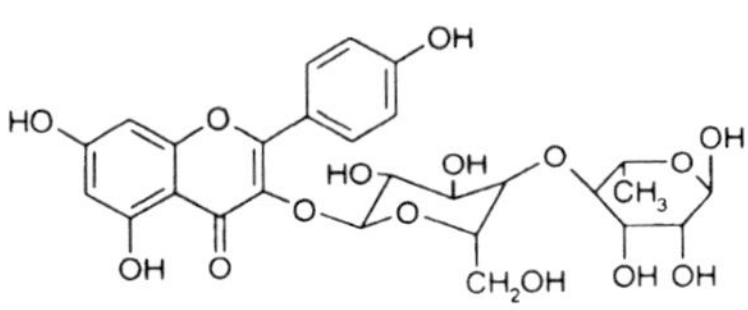 Kaempferol-3-glucosyl rhamnoside	0.56	Fraction 3
B-BA	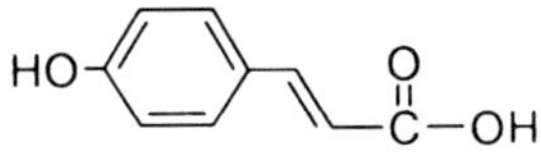 Benzoic acid	—	Fraction 2

Antioxidative Properties of the Isolated Flavonoids. The antioxidative properties of flavonoids extracted from balsam flowers were measured quantitatively and qualitatively by different estimation methods because, even for a flavonoid, different antioxidative behavior can be observed in the scavenging of various types of free radicals. For example, kaempferol glucoside, which possesses more powerful antioxidative capability against $ABTS^{\bullet+}$ radicals than Trolox (antioxidant reference material), showed lower antioxidative activity than Trolox in the PBN-AI system.

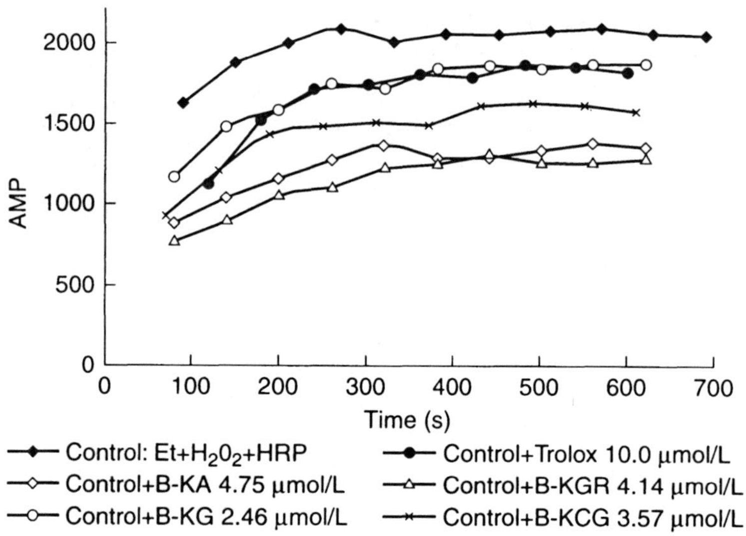

Fig. 4.5. Antioxidative capabilities of flavonoids from balsam flowers in the etoposide-H_2O_2-horseradish peroxidase (HRP) system. Abbreviations: B-KA, kaempferol; B-KGR, kaempferol-3-glucosyl rhamnoside; B-KG, kaempferol-3-glucoside; B-KCG, kaempferol-3-*p*-coumaroyl glucoside.

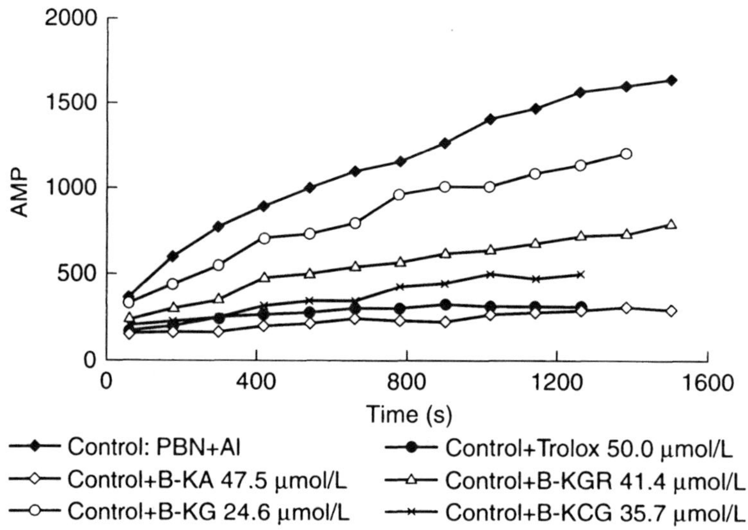

Fig. 4.6. Antioxidative capabilities of flavonoids from balsam flowers in the *N*-*t*-butyl-α-phenylnitrone (PBN)-azo initiator (AI) system. Abbreviations: B-KA, kaempferol; B-KGR, kaempferol-3-glucosyl rhamnoside; B-KG, kaempferol-3-glucoside; B-KCG, kaempferol-3-*p*-coumaroyl glucoside.

Thus, two semiquantitative assessments by ESR, which measured the antioxidative capability of flavonoids in PBN-AI and Et-H_2O_2-HRP systems, respectively, were carried out for general estimation. In addition, a quantitative assay approach, which measures scavenging capabilities of the flavonoids against the $ABTS^{\bullet+}$ radical, was used to determine the TEAC values of the flavonoids and to try to reveal a relationship between structures of the flavonoids and the antioxidative capabilities of these flavonoids. The results of the two semiquantitative assessments using ESR techniques, i.e., measuring antioxidative activities of the isolated flavonoids in the PBN-AI and Et-H_2O_2-HRP systems, are demonstrated in Figures 4.5 and 4.6, respectively.

All four flavonoids, kaempferol (B-KA), kaempferol-3-glucoside (B-KG), kaempferol-3-glucosyl rhamnoside (B-KGR), and kaempferol-3-*p*-coumaroyl glucoside (B-KCG), showed stronger antioxidative activity than Trolox. As shown in Figure 4.5, their concentrations (<5 mmol/L) were lower than Trolox (10 mmol/L), but their inhibition of Et radicals was stronger than that of Trolox. In the PBN-AI system, similar antioxidative behavior was also observed (see Fig. 4.6). But these flavonoids demonstrated almost identical antioxidative activities as Trolox, except for B-KCG, which demonstrated slightly weaker antioxidative activity than the other three compared with its behavior in the Et-H_2O_2-HPR system. Comparing the two series of

TABLE 4.3 Trolox Equivalent Antioxidant Capacity (TEAC) Values of Flavonoids from Balsam Flowers

Abbreviation	Name	Structure	TEAC value
B-KA	Kaempferol (Aglycone)	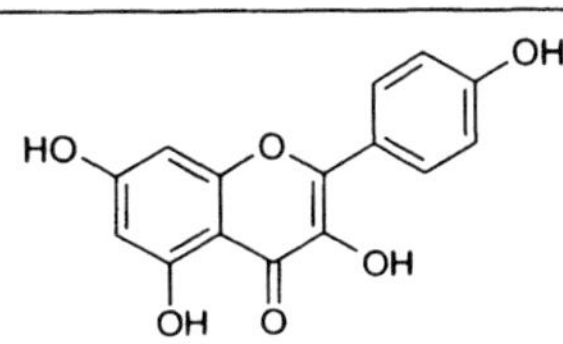	1.39 ± 0.09
B-KG	Kaempferol-3-glucoside	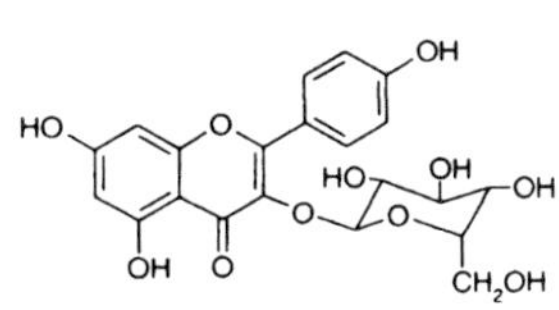	1.37 ± 0.1
B-KCG	Kaempferol-3-*p*-coumaroyl glucoside	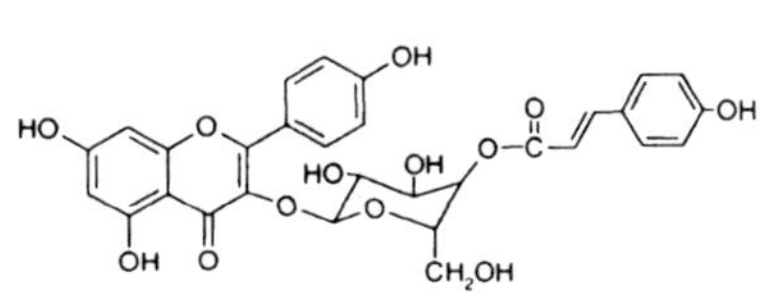	1.34 ± 0.1
B-KGR	Kaempferol-3-glucosyl rhamnoside	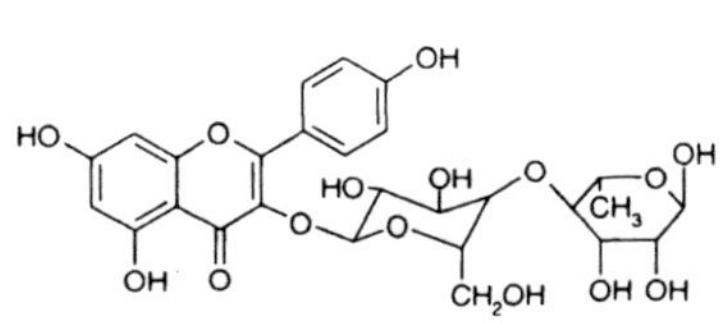	1.17 ± 0.08

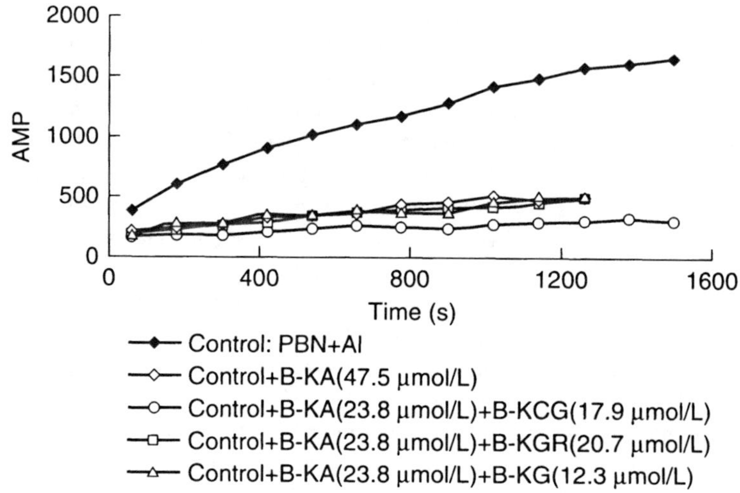

Fig. 4.7. Effects of coexisting flavonoids on the antioxidative capability of kaempferol in the *N-t*-butyl-α-phenylnitrone (PBN)-azo initiator (AI) system [electron spin resonance (ESR) assays]. Abbreviations: B-KA, kaempferol; B-KGR, kaempferol-3-glucosyl rhamnoside; B-KG, kaempferol-3-glucoside; B-KCG, kaempferol-3-*p*-coumaroyl glucoside.

results from the two methods, different antioxidative behaviors appeared to exist against etoposide phenoxyl and PBN radicals. As a whole, kaempferol compounds showed stronger capability in the Et-H_2O_2-HRP system than in the PBN-AI system when Trolox was used as a reference material. Of all flavonoids from balsam flowers, B-KCG behaved more remarkably in this aspect than the others (see Figs. 4.5 and 4.6).

The TEAC values of the flavonoids from balsam flowers were measured by the method described above and are listed in Table 4.3. Two conclusions can be drawn on the basis of these results: (i) B-KA and its derivatives, B-KG, B-KGR, and B-KCG, possess higher antioxidant potentials in aqueous solution than Trolox (TEAC = 1) or vitamin C (TEAC = 0.99). On a molar basis, their antioxidative capabilities against the $ABTS^{+\bullet}$ radicals generated in the aqueous phase are as follows (in order of decreasing effectiveness): B-KA > B-KCG > B-KG > B-KGR. (ii) Although the TEAC value of kaempferol aglycone is higher than its derivatives, the differences are small. In a certain sense, their TEAC values are nearly the same, suggesting that, in view of molecular structure, a water-soluble group such as a commonly occurring sugar or sugars attached at the 3-position and linked by an -O- bond has less effect on antioxidative potential, even though solubilities of the kaempferol derivatives in water were improved by attaching some water-soluble groups (e.g., sugars) compared with kaempferol aglycone.

Effects of Coexisting Flavonoids on Antioxidative Activity. Several experiments were conducted to determine whether the presence of other flavonoids could enhance the antioxidative activity of the flavonoid originally present. The data from ESR

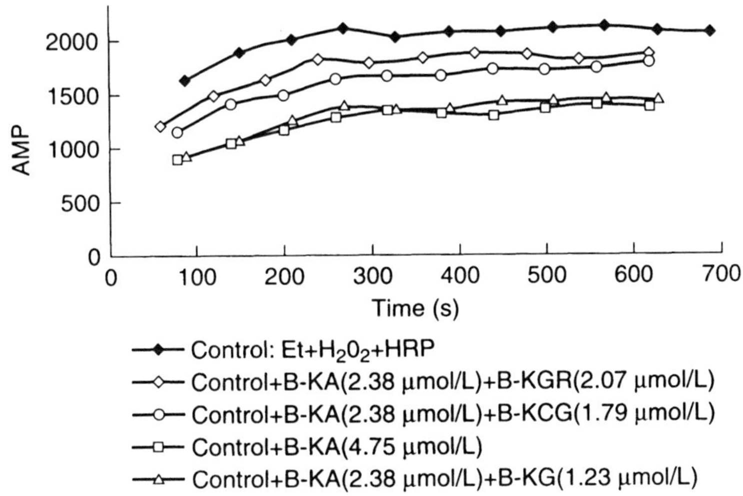

Fig. 4.8. Effects of coexisting flavonoids on the antioxidative potential of kaempferol in the etoposide-H_2O_2-horseradish peroxidase (HRP) system [electron spin resonance (ESR) assays]. Abbreviations:B-KA, kaempferol; B-KGR, kaempferol-3-glucosyl rhamnoside; B-KG, kaempferol-3-glucoside; B-KCG, kaempferol-3-*p*-coumaroyl glucoside.

assays showed that in the presence of flavonoids belonging to the same family, the antioxidant capability of kaempferol did not improve significantly in either the PBN-AI or Et-H_2O_2-HRP systems (see Figs. 4.7 and 4.8).

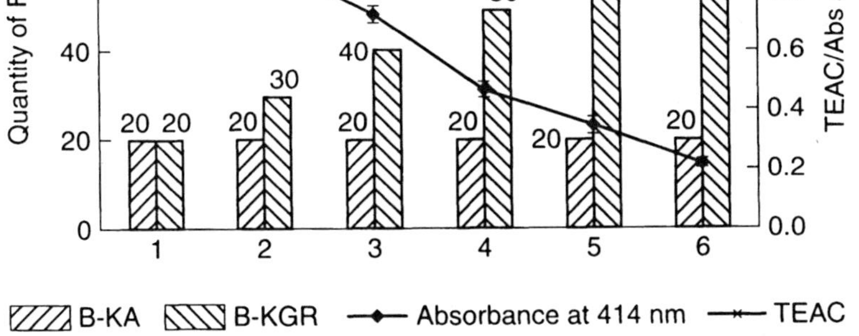

Fig. 4.9. Effect of the coexisting kaempferol-3-glucosyl rhamnoside (B-KGR) on the antioxidative potential of kaempferol (B-KA). Abbreviation: TEAC, Trolox equivalent antioxidant capacity.

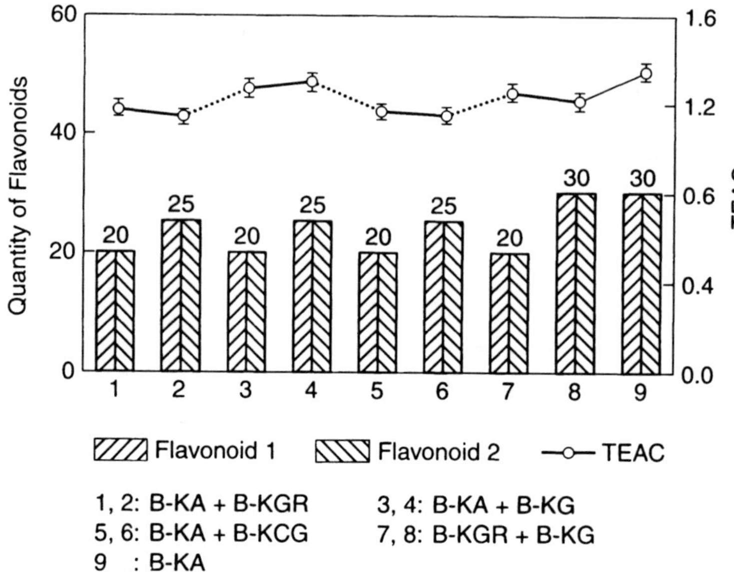

Fig. 4.10. Effect of different combinations of kaempferols on oxidative potentials. Abbreviations: TEAC, Trolox equivalent antioxidant capacity; B-KA, kaempferol; B-KGR, kaempferol-3-glucosyl rhamnoside; B-KG, kaempferol-3-glucoside; B-KCG, kaempferol-3-*p*-coumaroyl glucoside.

Moreover, the data from the UV-VIS measurement also supports the above conclusion. The results indicated that in the presence of a fixed amount of B-KA, the introduction of variable amounts of B-KGR cannot cause remarkable fluctuation of the TEAC (see Fig. 4.9), suggesting that the capability of the scavenging $ABTS^{\bullet+}$ radical remained almost the same in terms of the antioxidative potential per mole of antioxidant, although the total antioxidative capability was enhanced with the addition of another flavonoid, B-KGR (Fig. 4.9). The same conclusion was reached when different combinations of various amounts of flavonoids were tested (see Fig. 4.10) in another experiment to monitor the changes in TEAC value. As shown in Figure 4.10, the TEAC values did not appear to change significantly when the other flavonoids coexisted. To summarize, a combination of two kaempferol compounds cannot significantly improve the antioxidative potential, that is, synergistic antioxidative activity of two kaempferol compounds is not remarkable.

Conclusions

The four main flavonoids (those that are water soluble and stable in dried form) belonging to flavon-3-ol were isolated from dried balsam flowers. They include kaempferol, kaempferol-3-glucoside, kaempferol-3-glucosyl rhamnoside, and kaempferol-3-*p*-coumaroyl glucoside. The isolated kaempferol compounds demonstrated their strong antioxidative behavior *in vitro* in both the UV-VIS and ESR assays. The structural differences of these kaempferol compounds cannot affect significantly their antioxidative activities in the case of attachment of a water-soluble group at position 3. A combination of kaempferol compounds cannot significantly improve the antioxidative potential, that is, synergistic antioxidative activity of two flavonoid compounds was not observed in this study.

Acknowledgments

We express our sincere gratitude to Professor Dieter Strack and Dr. Alfred Baumert, staff of the Institute of Plant Biochemistry, Halle, Germany, for their kind assistance and help. We also acknowledge financial support from the Lee Foundation, Singapore.

References

1. Bors, W., Heller, W., Michel, C., and Stettmaier, K. (1996) Flavonoids and Polyphenols: Chemistry and Biology, in *Handbook of Antioxidants,* (Cadenas, E. and Packer, L., eds.) pp. 409–466, Marcel Dekker, New York.
2. Pincemail, J. (1995) Free Radicals and Antioxidants in Human Diseases, in *Analysis of Free Radicals in Biological Systems,* (Favier, A.E., Cadet, J., Kalyanaraman, B., Fontecavé, M., and Pierre, J.-L., eds.) pp. 83–98, Birkhauser Verlay, Basel, Switzland.
3. Pietta, P. (1998) Flavonoids in Medicinal Plants, in *Flavonoids in Health and Disease,* (Rice-Evans, C.A., and Packer, L., eds.) pp. 61–120, Marcel Dekker, New York.
4. Rice-Evans, C.A., Miller, N.J., and Paganga, G. (1997) Antioxidant Properties of Phenolic Compounds. *Trends Plant Sci. 12:* 152–159.
5. Wee, Y.C. (1992) *A Guide to Medicinal Plants*, pp. 79–80, Singapore Science Center, Singapore.
6. Markham, K.R. (1982) *Techniques of Flavonoid Identification*, Academic Press, London.
7. Harborne, J.B. (1994) *The Flavonoids: Advances in Research Since 1986*, Chapman & Hall, London.
8. Makham, K.R., and Mabry, T.J. (1975) in *The Flavonoids*, (Harborne, J.B., Mabry, T.J., and Mabry, H., eds.) pp. 45–77, Chapman & Hall, London.
9. Rice-Evans, C.A., Miller, N.J., and Paganga, G. (1996) Structure-Antioxidant Activity Relationships of Flavonoids and Phenolic Acids. *Free Radic. Biol. Med. 20*: 933–956.
10. Miller, N.J., Rice-Evans, C.A., Davies, M.J., Gopinathan, V., and Miliner, A. (1993) A Novel Method for Measuring Antioxidant Capacity and Its Application to Monitoring Status in Premature Neonates. *Clin. Sci. 84*: 407–412.
11. Niki, E. (1990) *Methods Enzymol. 186*: 100.
12. Kagan, V.E., Yalowich, J.C., Borisenko, G.G., Tyurina, Y.Y., Tyurin, V.A., Thampatty, P., and Fabrisiak, J.P. (1999) Mechanism-Based Chemopreventive Strategies Against Etoposide-Induced Acute Myeloid Leukemia: Free Radical/Antioxidant Approach. *Mol. Pharmacol. 56*: 494.

Chapter 5

Antioxidant Action of Curcumin

Thomas P.A. Devasagayam,[a] Jayashree P. Kamat,[a] and Nair Sreejayan[b]

[a]Cell Biology Division, Bhabha Atomic Research Centre, Mumbai 400 085, India
[b]Department of Physiology, College of Medicine, University of Tennessee, Memphis, TN 38163

Introduction

Turmeric (rhizome of *Curcuma longa* L., *Zingiberaceae*) is a spice used extensively to flavor various types of curries in India. Apart from its culinary properties, it is also known to have several beneficial effects and certain therapeutic uses. It is used for the treatment of liver disease, upper abdominal pain, scabies, asthma, gastric and duodenal ulcers, and is known to have skin-protective, antibacterial, antigenotoxic, anti-inflammatory, anticarcinogenic, and antiatherogenic activities (1–4). Some of these activities also have been linked to the spice's antioxidant ability in different systems (5–7). During the last two decades, the yellow pigments from turmeric, curcumin, demethoxycurcumin, and bisdemethoxycurcumin isolated from the plant have been attracting scientific interest. Among these, curcumin is the major component, constituting up to 20% of turmeric. It is also used as a dye and a food preservative. Turmeric has been used in traditional medicine for >2000 years, with its broad spectrum of biological activities ascribed to the curcuminoid content. Curcumin exhibits a variety of biological activities that include anti-inflammatory, antidiabetic, hepatoprotective, antimutagenic and antineoplastic properties (3,5). Several studies have been undertaken to evaluate the mechanism of action of curcuminoids. Most of its activities are thought to be mediated by its potent antioxidant property (8). Studies from our laboratory have shown that curcumin is a powerful scavenger of the superoxide (9) and hydroxyl radicals (10). It also protects DNA against singlet oxygen–induced strand breaks (11) and lipids from peroxidation induced by γ-radiation (12). The results obtained indicate that curcumin is a potent antioxidant. However, the mechanisms involved in relation to its possible therapeutic abilities have not been examined in detail. Curcumin, in the form of turmeric extract, has also been used extensively in skin ointments and beauty creams for its skin-protective property (2,3). However, no detailed studies have been performed on the effect of curcumin on photodamage in the skin.

Exposure of organisms to adverse pathophysiologic states causes enhanced generation of the reactive oxygen species (ROS), resulting in "oxidative stress" (13). ROS are ubiquitous in our aerobic environment; however, their excess generation has been implicated in a number of diseases including cancer, cardiovascular ailments, neural and skin disorders, arthritis, and diabetes, in addition to the aging process (14,15). Among the ROS, the hydroxyl radical ($^{\bullet}OH$), peroxyl radical ($ROO^{\bullet}$), and singlet oxygen ($^1O_2$) are the major species that induce membrane damage in cellular systems as well as in tissues (16,17).

Excess ROS generation can result from exposure to physical and chemical agents, including ionizing radiation and photosensitization. Low LET (linear energy transfer) radiations, such as γ-rays, cause their effect mainly through ROS. Further, most of the radiation-induced damage to biomolecules in aqueous media, such as those prevailing in living systems, is caused by an indirect effect, due to radiolysis of water that yields $^{\bullet}OH$, hydrogen atoms ($^{\bullet}H$), hydrated electrons (e^-_{aq}), or hydrogen peroxide (H_2O_2), for example. In the presence of oxygen, other reactive species such as the superoxide radical ($O_2^{\bullet-}$) and $^1O_2$ are also generated (18,19). Another physicochemical event, the photosensitization that occurs due to the interaction among light, sensitizer, and oxygen, is a potentially damaging event in biological systems and also generates ROS (20). This is especially true in tissues that are constantly exposed to sunlight, such as skin. Photosensitization involving a Type I process is due mainly to free radicals, whereas the Type II mechanism is predominantly a $^1O_2$ phenomenon (20,21). Lipid peroxidation, involving oxidative damage to the lipid component of the cellular membranes, is a highly damaging event. It not only drastically alters the structure and function of membranes but also generates highly toxic by-products (13,15,22). These products act as second messengers responsible for several cytotoxic events, including certain genotoxic effects, inactivation of enzymes, and activation of stress signalling pathways (22–24).

The major reactive species generated by the Type II pathway of photosensitization is $^1O_2$. It is an electronically excited species that is produced in biological systems and has the ability to damage biological molecules, including DNA. Its reaction with DNA results in single-strand breaks in addition to the formation of altered bases such as 8-hydroxydeoxyguanosine and 2,6-diamino-4-hydroxy-5-formamidopyrimidine (25–28). The biological consequences associated with these modifications in DNA are the loss of biological activity, carcinogenicity, and mutagenicity. Although the frequency of $^1O_2$-induced single-strand breaks is less than that of base modifications, the former are easier and less expensive to assess. There are a number of studies regarding $^1O_2$-quenching abilities of natural compounds, whereas there are very few studies on the ability of antioxidants to protect DNA against such damage. Anticarcinogenic and other therapeutic activities of natural compounds are correlated with their ability to protect biological molecules against $^1O_2$ and other prooxidants. Although there are a number of studies pertaining to the protective ability of established antioxidants such as vitamins C and E, as well as carotenoids such as β-carotene, there are several known more promising natural compounds that should be examined for their protective abilities. Curcumin falls into this category. Many of the antioxidants examined contain either a phenolic group or a diketone system, which is responsible for their antioxidant activity. Curcumin contains both.

The damaging effects of ionizing radiation in biological systems are mediated at least in part through oxygen free radicals (29). Curcumin has been shown to be effective in protecting against radiation-induced chromosomal aberrations *in vivo*

(30). However, there is a paucity of data on the effect of curcumin on radiation-induced lipid peroxidation.

In this study, we report that curcumin inhibited the following: (i) DNA damage induced by a potent ROS, in the form of $^1O_2$; (ii) lipid peroxidation induced by photosensitization in rat skin fractions; and (iii) peroxidation in rat liver microsomes induced by γ-radiation and the hydroxyl radical. The possible mechanisms were examined by studying the reaction of curcumin as well as its more stable metabolic product, dehydrozingerone, with different ROS using pulse radiolysis.

Materials and Methods

Materials. Curcumin and dehydrozingerone were synthesized as described (31,32). The structures were confirmed by nuclear magnetic resonance (NMR), mass spectroscopy (MS) and infrared (IR) spectroscopy in addition to elemental analysis. α-Tocopherol, β-carotene, deuterium oxide (99.8 atom%), sodium azide, agarose, methylene blue, rose Bengal, 2-thiobarbituric acid (TBA), 1,1,3,3-tetraethoxypropane, butylated hydroxytoluene, trichloroacetic acid, and superoxide dismutase were purchased from Sigma Chemical, St. Louis, MO. *tert*-Butanol was obtained from BDH Chemicals, England. Nitrous oxide used in this study was of Iolar grade from M/s Indian Oxygen. The flavonoid myricetin and polyphenol tannic acid were gifts from the late Prof. N.P. Das of the National University of Singapore, Singapore. All other chemicals used were of analytical grade from well-known manufacturers.

DNA Damage and Measurement. For the generation of $^1O_2$ in an aqueous buffer system, the endoperoxide of 3,3′-(1,4-naphthylene)dipropionate ($NDPO_2$) was prepared as described (33). Stock solutions were kept under liquid nitrogen until use. Thermal dissociation of $NDPO_2$ yields 3,3′-(1,4-naphthylene)dipropionate (NDP), $^1O_2$, and triplet molecular oxygen. Plasmid pBR322 DNA was prepared using *Escherichia coli* culture and purified by a Qiagen plasmid kit-Pack 500. The preparation contained 90–95% form I (native supercoiled form) and 5–10% form II (open circular form resulting from single-strand breaks). All of the solutions used in this study were treated with Chelex-100 (Bio-Rad Laboratories) to remove traces of metal ions present as contaminants.

To study the effect of antioxidants on single-strand breaks, 2-3 μg pBR322 DNA was incubated in a medium (final volume 100 μL) containing 40 mmol/L $NDPO_2$ in deaerated 50 mmol/L sodium phosphate buffer, pD 7.4 (= pH 7.0) in D_2O, and freshly prepared curcumin or its derivatives in ethanol (5 μL/assay), at 37°C with shaking. Separation of the different forms of DNA was performed using 0.7% agarose gels in 89 mmol/L Tris-borate/2 mmol/L EDTA buffer (pH 8.3) (34). DNA bands were stained with ethidium bromide and quantitated by scanning the resulting negatives/reverse photonegatives with a Shimadzu CD-9000 densitometer.

Preparation of Microsomes and Exposure to Radiation. Microsomes from rat liver were isolated by differential centrifugation (35). For incorporating curcumin into microsomes, 100 μL of 10 mmol/L curcumin solution in ethanol was added to the microsomal pellet, homogenized, diluted to 1.1 mL with Buffer A, and resedimented at 105,000 × *g* for 1 h. The concentration of curcumin in the microsomes was 223 μmol/L. Appropriate control microsomes were prepared using 100 μL ethanol. For examining the protective effect of curcumin against lipid peroxidation induced by •OH and other radical species generated during radiation, microsomes were subjected to γ-radiation in 5 mmol/L sodium phosphate buffer, pH 7.4, in a sealed tube in a Gamma cell (^{60}Co source). One set of samples was saturated with N_2O (by bubbling this gas for 5 min before irradiation), whereas others were not. Postirradiation incubation was carried out in air at 37°C in a shaker-water bath.

Steady-state γ-radiolysis was carried out using a ^{60}Co γ source (Bhabha Atomic Research Centre, Mumbai); the dose rate was found to be 630 Gy/h following the standard Fricke method. After incubation/irradiation, the extent of lipid peroxidation was estimated as thiobarbituric acid reactive substances (TBARS) in terms of malonaldehyde equivalents, using tetraethoxypropane as a standard (36).

Preparation of Rat Skin Fractions, Exposure to Photosensitization, and Lipid Peroxidation. The epidermal layer in the rat skin was separated essentially as described by Huang *et al.* (37), then scraped off and washed with 5 mmol/L phosphate buffered saline, pH 7.4. For isolating mitochondria and microsomes, the tissue was homogenized in 0.25 mol/L sucrose containing 1 mmol/L EDTA using a Polytron tissuemiser under cold conditions. The homogenate thus obtained was filtered through cheesecloth and centrifuged at 650 × *g* for 10 min to remove unbroken cells and nuclei. The postnuclear supernatant was again centrifuged at 10,000 × *g* for 10 min to sediment the mitochondria. The pellet thus obtained was washed three times in 0.15 mol/L Tris-HCl buffer, pH 7.4 (Buffer A) to remove sucrose and suspended in the same buffer at a concentration of 5 mg protein/mL. The postmitochondrial supernatant was centrifuged at 105,000 × *g* for 1 h in a Beckman L8-80 M ultracentrifuge to sediment microsomes. The pellet obtained was washed three times in Buffer A and resuspended at a concentration of 2.5 mg protein/mL. The protein content was determined (16). For studies using homogenate, the epidermal layer was homogenized in Buffer A, filtered through cheesecloth and diluted to a concentration of 10 mg protein/mL. Rat liver mitochondria were prepared similarly (17).

Lipid peroxidation was induced by photosensitization as described earlier (35) by exposing tissue fractions in Buffer A (final volume 3 mL) to visible light in a trap maintained at 37°C. The photosensitizers used were either methylene blue (50 μmol/L) or rose Bengal (50 μmol/L). The test compounds were dissolved in ethanol (50 μL/assay). The respective controls also contained an equal amount of ethanol. The extent of lipid peroxidation in the tissue fractions was estimated as TBARS in terms of malondialdehyde equivalents, using 1,1,3,3-tetraethoxypropane as a standard as described previously (38).

Reaction of Curcumin and Dehydrozingerone with Radicals as Analyzed by Pulse Radiolysis. The reactions of curcumin with •OH were carried out using a

N_2O-saturated mildly alkaline aqueous solution; the pH was adjusted to 7.4 with 10 mmol/L phosphate buffer. To prevent degradation of curcumin, the pH was never allowed to exceed 7.5 and the solutions were always kept under oxygen-free conditions. The spectrum showed peaks similar to those observed in a 0.1% methanol/water solution with a minor peak at 420 nm and a major peak at 350 nm. For pulse radiolysis measurements, the absorbed dose was kept to a minimum to avoid decomposition of the test compound, and the solutions were changed every pulse to minimize losses due to decomposition. Seven MeV electrons from the linear accelerator (pulse width, 50 ns; duration, 2 μs) were used and transients were detected by kinetic spectrophotometry. A typical maximum dose with 50-ns pulses was 15 Gy; for 2-μs pulses, it was 7–8 times higher. The dosimetry was performed with air-saturated KCNS solution. The kinetic spectrophotometric detection system covered the wavelength range from 250 to 800 nm. The cells with optical pathlength of 1 cm were used for these measurements.

Results

Singlet Oxygen–Induced DNA Damage and Its Prevention. Figure 5.1 presents data on DNA damage induced by $^1O_2$ and its prevention by curcumin. Single-

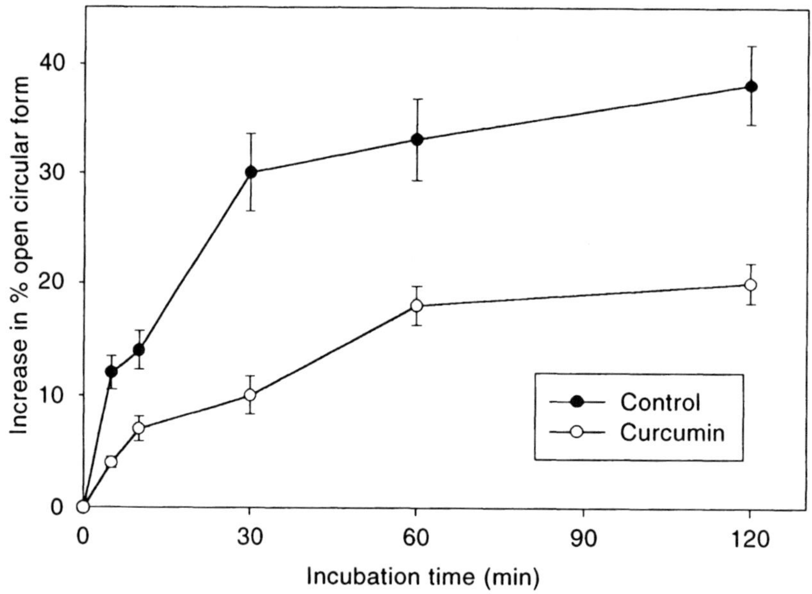

Fig. 5.1. Inhibitory effect of curcumin on singlet oxygen–induced single-strand breaks in plasmid pBR322 DNA as a function of time. Values plotted are obtained from scanning electrophorograms by scanning the reverse-negatives with a densitometer. Values are means ± SEM from four experiments. Singlet oxygen was generated by thermolysis of the endoperoxide of naphthylidene dipropionate.

strand breaks (form II) in plasmid DNA were significantly increased by incubating DNA with the thermodissociable $NDPO_2$, which generates $^1O_2$. The single-strand break formation as a function of time and its protection by curcumin were quite significant. The protection was evident from the early stages of incubation and was almost constant from 30 min until the end of incubation. This suggests that the protection afforded might be due to quenching of $^1O_2$ generated or the chemical binding of the compound to DNA, thereby making it resistant to the attack of this species.

Data on the protective ability of curcumin against the $^1O_2$-induced single-strand breaks, compared with established antioxidants, are presented in Figure 5.2. At the equimolar concentrations of 100 µmol/L, curcumin was the most effective protector, followed by the flavonoid myricetin, the polyphenol tannic acid, β-carotene, lipoic acid, and α-tocopherol. All of these antioxidants are present in mammalian tissues and/or as constituents in our normal diet.

Photosensitization-Induced Lipid Peroxidation in Rat Skin and Its Protection. Figure 5.3 presents data on lipid peroxidation in rat skin homogenate and the inhibitory

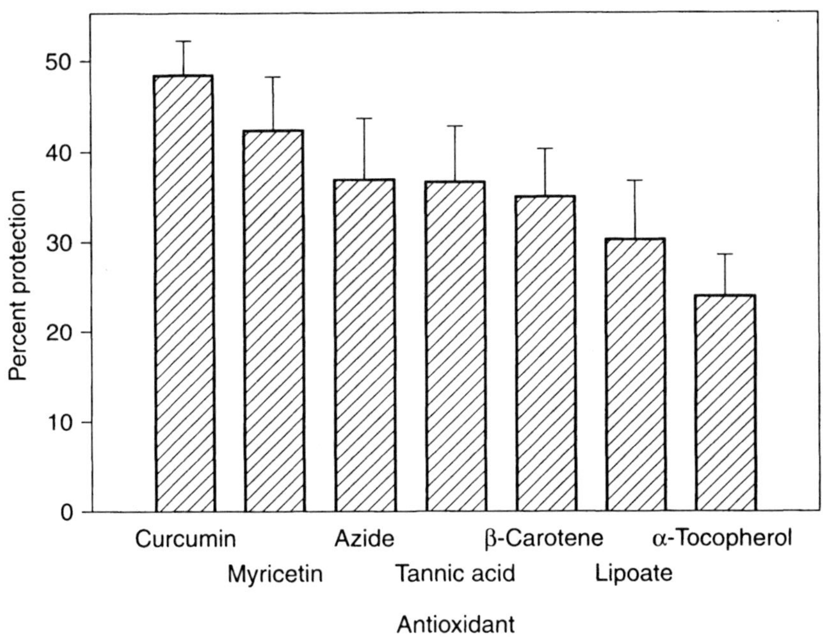

Fig. 5.2. The DNA-protecting ability of curcumin, at 100 µmol/L compared with other natural antioxidants. Curcumin and lipoate were dissolved in the minimum volume of ethanol, azide in buffer, and other antioxidants in dimethyl sulfoxide. The solvents, by themselves, did not show any significant protective abilities. Values are means ± SEM from four experiments. Singlet oxygen was generated by thermolysis of the endoperoxide of naphthylidene dipropionate.

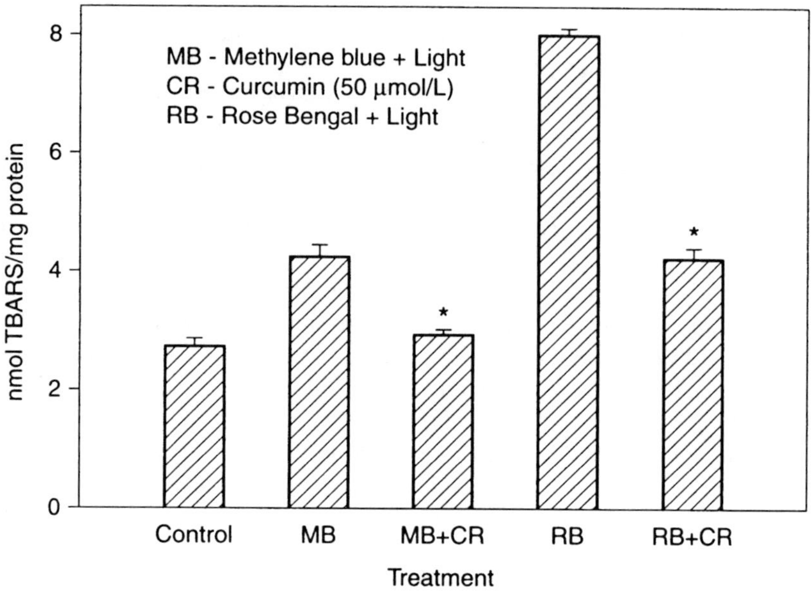

Fig. 5.3. Effect of curcumin on lipid peroxidation induced by photosensitization in rat skin homogenate. Incubations were carried out in a trap maintained at 37°C in 0.15 mol/L Tris-HCl buffer, pH 7.4, with additions as indicated. The concentrations of methylene blue, rose Bengal, and curcumin were 50 µmol/L each. Values are means ± SEM from four experiments and represent nmol TBARS as malondialdehyde equivalents/(mg protein·60 min). $^*P < 0.001$ compared with full complement of photosensitization system.

effect of curcumin. At equimolar concentrations, rose Bengal was more effective than methylene blue in inducing peroxidation. Curcumin significantly ($P < 0.01$) reduced lipid peroxidation induced by both methylene blue and rose Bengal. The extent of inhibition was greater with rose Bengal than with methylene blue. Because mitochondria are more susceptible to oxidative damage and because we observed maximum lipid peroxidation with the mitochondrial fraction, we performed subsequent experiments with this subcellular fraction. The influence of curcumin on the time course of lipid peroxidation induced by methylene blue and rose Bengal is shown in Figures 5.4 and 5.5, respectively. In both cases, the inhibition was observed from the very beginning of incubation. However, the kinetics of inhibition seemed to differ. In the case of rose Bengal–induced peroxidation, the inhibition was more pronounced in the initial stages of incubation, whereas in the case of methylene blue sensitization, the inhibition was greater during the later stage of incubation. Rose Bengal induced almost twice the amount of peroxidation compared with methylene blue. In both cases, significant protection of mitochondria by curcumin was observed against this form of oxidative damage. The extent of inhibition with methylene blue plus light seemed to

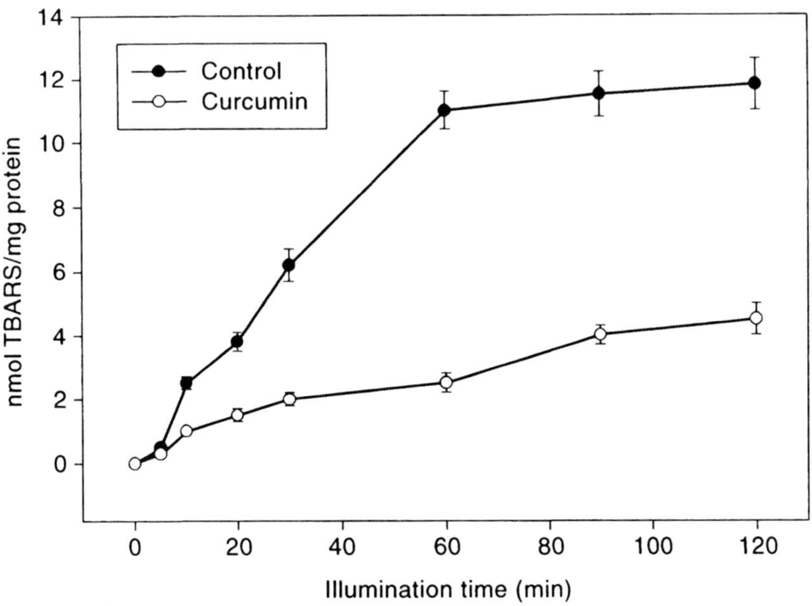

Fig. 5.4. Effect of curcumin on the time course of lipid peroxidation induced by methylene blue in rat skin mitochondria. Peroxidation was induced by exposing mitochondria (0.5 mg protein/mL) to light in the presence of oxygen, 50 μmol/L methylene blue with or without 50 μmol/L curcumin. Values are means ± SEM from three or four experiments and represent nmol TBARS as malonaldehyde equivalents/mg protein. Values were corrected for TBARS obtained at 0 min.

be greater than that of rose Bengal plus light. The concentration dependence of the inhibition of lipid peroxidation by curcumin is shown for the two systems in Figures 5.6 and 5.7, respectively. In both rose Bengal– and methylene blue–induced lipid peroxidation, the concentration dependence is very steep up to 50 μmol/L and then slows down. At 200 μmol/L, >60% inhibition was observed in both systems.

Figure 5.8 shows that curcumin is also a potent inhibitor of lipid peroxidation induced by photosensitization with methylene blue plus light in rat hepatic mitochondria. The inhibition observed was 82%.

Radiation-Induced Lipid Peroxidation in Rat Liver Microsomes and Its Inhibition by Curcumin. When rat liver microsomes were subjected to γ-irradiation doses up to 630 Gy, enhanced lipid peroxidation resulted (Fig. 5.9). The extent of peroxidation was dependent on the dose of radiation. At an absorbed dose of 600 Gy, ~6.9 nmol TBARS/mg protein was produced. When curcumin was incorporated into microsomes (23 μmol/L), peroxidation was reduced to a significant extent. The inhibition observed at 630 Gy was ~60%. Postirradiation incubation is known to cause a further increase in lipid peroxidation. Hence, microsomes exposed to γ-radiation

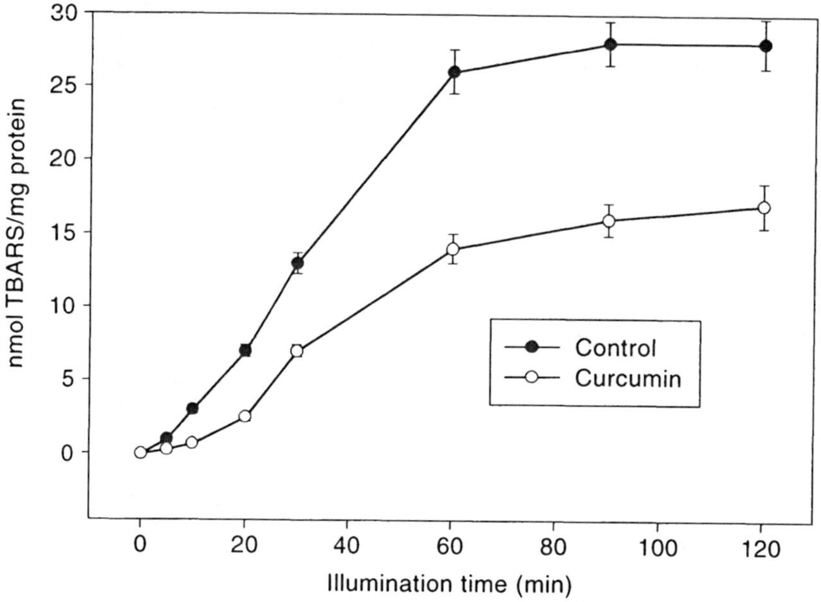

Fig. 5.5. Effect of curcumin on the time course of lipid peroxidation induced by rose Bengal in rat skin mitochondria. Peroxidation was induced by exposing mitochondria (0.5 mg protein/mL) to light in the presence of oxygen, 50 μmol/L rose Bengal with or without 50 μmol/L curcumin. Other conditions were as in Figure 5.4.

(630 Gy) were incubated for various lengths of time at 37°C. The result was in a time-dependent increase in lipid peroxidation (Fig. 10). Curcumin effectively inhibited this peroxidation induced by postirradiation incubation, the protection varying from 50 to 90%.

Studies on Pulse Radiolysis with Curcumin. The reaction of the hydroxyl radical with curcumin resulted in the formation of transient absorbing in the visible region, from 300 to 600 nm (λ_{max} 450 nm) with a simultaneous bleaching at 350 nm. An estimate of rate constant with $^{\bullet}OH$ yielded a value of 4.76×10^{10} $(mol/L)^{-1} \cdot s^{-1}$, comparable to the potent antioxidants such as α-tocopherol. The transient formed, presumably due to a phenoxyl radical, had a half-life of 780 μs.

With dehydrozingerone, a more stable metabolic product of curcumin, pulse radiolysis studies showed reaction with $^{\bullet}OH$. At pH 6.0, the protonated form reacted with $^{\bullet}OH$ with transient absorbing at 460 nm. The rate constant was 1×10^{10} $(mol/L)^{-1} \cdot s^{-1}$. At pH 10.0, the deprotonated form reacted with $^{\bullet}OH$ with a transient having absorption at 360 nm; the rate constant of the reaction was 1.1×10^{10} $(mol/L)^{-1} \cdot s^{-1}$. The transients formed were relatively long lived, with half-lives in milliseconds. Thus, the high reactivity with $^{\bullet}OH$ and the long life of the transients can explain the potent antioxidant action of dehydrozingerone. This compound also has high

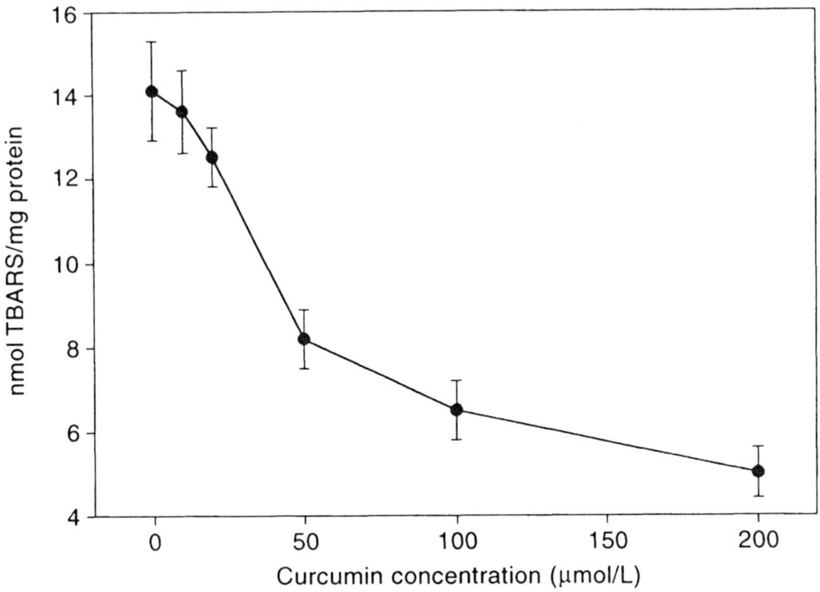

Fig. 5.6. Concentration-dependent effect of curcumin on the lipid peroxidation induced by methylene blue plus light in rat skin mitochondria. Lipid peroxidation in mitochondria was induced by exposing them (0.5 mg protein/mL) to light in the presence of oxygen and methylene blue (50 μmol/L) for 1 h. Different concentrations of curcumin were added in 50 μL ethanol. Other conditions were as in Figure 5.4.

rate constants with secondary oxidants such as $N_3^{\bullet}$, $Br^{\bullet}$, $CCl_3O_2^{\bullet}$, $NO_2^{\bullet}$ [10^8 to 10^{10} $(mol/L)^{-1}\cdot s^{-1}$]. Dehydrozingerone also has a fairly high rate constant with Trolox [8.3×10^7 $(mol/L)^{-1}\cdot s^{-1}$]; thus, it may be recycled in biological systems with the physiologically relevant analog of Trolox, α-tocopherol.

Discussion

Damage to DNA induced by oxygen-derived free radicals has been implicated in diseased states including carcinogenesis. Singlet oxygen is capable of genotoxic effects by inducing strand breaks and base alterations. This study, as well as our earlier publication (11), shows that curcumin, and to a lesser extent other natural antioxidants, significantly protects DNA against $^1O_2$. Although it has been clearly established that $^1O_2$ induces strand breaks in DNA, the exact mechanism is not clear (26,39). If we assume that the single-strand breaks result from reactions involving more than one pathway/intermediate, curcumin or its related compounds may be able to block/inhibit one or more of these to effect protection. This may also include physical and/or chemical quenching of the reactive intermediates. Although this natural compound is known to interact with $^{\bullet}OH$ and $O_2^{-\bullet}$(10,40), its reaction with $^1O_2$ has not been reported

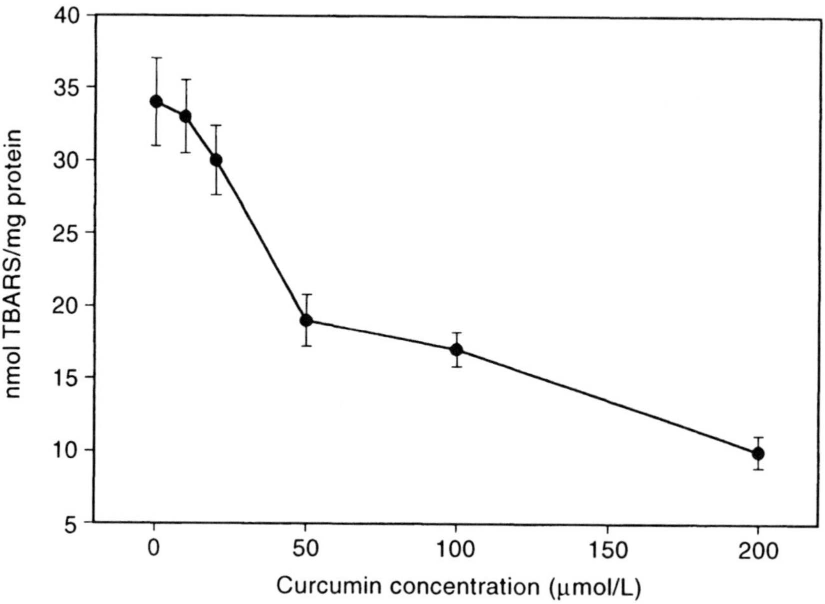

Fig. 5.7. Concentration-dependent effect of curcumin on the lipid peroxidation induced by rose Bengal plus light in rat skin mitochondria. Lipid peroxidation in mitochondria was induced by exposing them (0.5 mg protein/mL) to light in the presence of oxygen and rose Bengal (50 μmol/L) for 1 h. Different concentrations of curcumin were added in 50 μL ethanol. Other conditions were as in Figure 5.4.

to date. Turmeric contains significant amounts of curcumin and is credited with several therapeutic properties, including prevention of damage to skin exposed to sunlight (41). Because $^1O_2$ is an active component involved in photodamage (42), the mechanism of prevention of such damage by turmeric and/or curcumin may be explained in part by this study.

Turmeric, and hence its constituent curcumin, forms a component of the normal diet of people in Asian countries. There is increasing interest in the role of diet and nutrition in human health, including the pathogenesis and possible prevention of cancer (43). Animal models have shown the anticarcinogenic effects of curcumin (5,37,44–48). This study shows that curcumin protects DNA against oxidative damage induced by $^1O_2$, a ROS that has been generated *in vivo* by several reactions (20,26). Hence, our present results may explain in part the possible mechanisms behind the likely anticarcinogenic/antimutagenic properties of this antioxidant.

Light and oxygen in the presence of a photosensitizer can induce peroxidation of lipids present in biological membranes (16,17,20,35). In this study, we employed methylene blue and rose Bengal as sensitizers to induce lipid peroxidation. Photosensitization in biological systems involves Type I and Type II reactions (21,49). The former involves generation of triplet sensitizer, $O_2^{-\bullet}$ and $^\bullet OH$, whereas

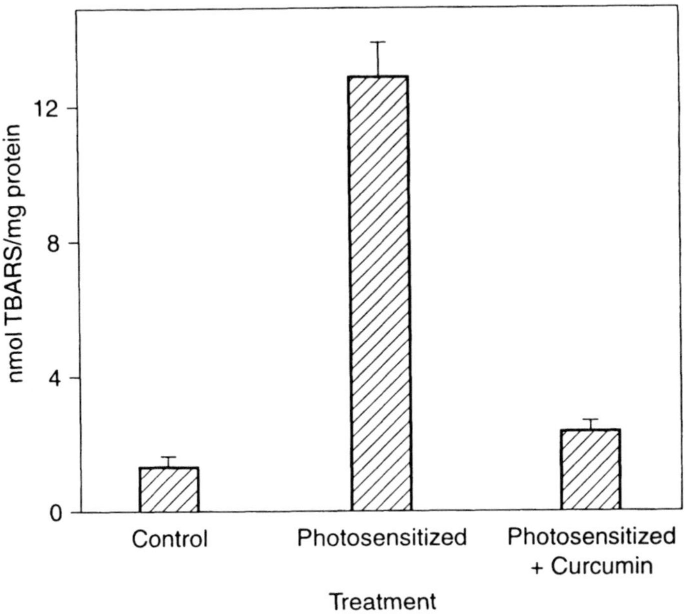

Fig. 5.8. Inhibitory effect of curcumin on photosensitization-induced lipid peroxidation in rat liver mitochondria. Lipid peroxidation in mitochondria was induced by exposing them (0.5 mg protein/mL) to light in the presence of oxygen and methylene blue (50 μmol/L) for 1 h. The concentration of added curcumin was 50 μmol/L. Other conditions were as in Figure 5.4.

the latter involves production of $^1O_2$. In simple *in vitro* systems using fatty acid micelles, rose Bengal acts predominantly *via* a Type I reaction, whereas methylene blue acts through a Type II pathway. However, in more complicated systems, such as natural biological membranes, both pathways seem to be equally important (49).

This study shows that curcumin is capable of inhibiting photosensitized lipid peroxidation induced by light, oxygen, and sensitizers (methylene blue and rose Bengal) in skin tissue fractions. Our previous studies demonstrated that curcumin is a potent inhibitor of lipid peroxidation induced by metal ions and its chelates (50) and γ-radiation (12). However, in this study, unlike the previous reports, lipid peroxidation was initiated exclusively by a photosensitization mechanism that indeed is the primary mode of oxidative damage occurring in normal skin exposed to light. Our studies show that curcumin protects rat skin fractions from such lipid peroxidation in a time- and concentration-dependent manner. Rose Bengal–induced lipid peroxidation proceeds predominantly *via* the Type I mechanism, involving the generation of triplet sensitizer, $O_2^{-\bullet}$ and $^\bullet OH$, whereas methylene blue–induced lipid peroxidation involves production of $^1O_2$. The fact that curcumin inhibits lipid peroxidation induced by both compounds suggests that curcumin may be doing so by more than one mechanism. Earlier studies have shown that curcumin can scavenge $O_2^{-\bullet}$(9).

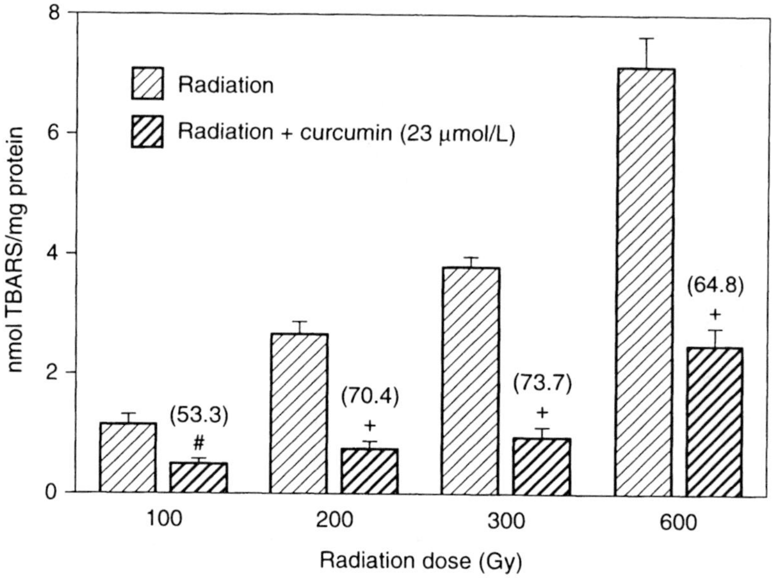

Fig. 5.9. Inhibition of radiation-induced lipid peroxidation in rat liver microsomes by curcumin.

Curcumin has been studied extensively for its antioxidant properties. The phenolic and methoxy groups on the phenyl ring and the 1,3-diketone system are important structural features that contribute to its antioxidant properties. Our earlier studies showed that the methoxy groups may not be essential for the inhibition of iron-stimulated lipid peroxidation by curcuminoids (50). Conney *et al.* (51) used similar analogs for the inhibitory effect of 12-*o*-tetradecanoyl phorbol-13-acetate–induced tumor promotion in mouse skin. Our studies revealed that the demethoxy derivatives of curcumin were poor scavengers of the superoxide anion and the nitrogen-centered free radical, 1,1-diphenyl-2 picryl-hydrazyl (9). Toda *et al.* (52) demonstrated that the methoxy groups of curcumin are essential for the inhibition of hydrogen peroxide–induced hemolysis and lipid peroxidation of erythrocytes. In this study, we found that the methoxy groups on the phenolic ring of curcumin were essential for its inhibitory effect on lipid peroxidation. The standard antioxidant α-tocopherol was more active than curcumin in inhibiting lipid peroxidation. This contrasts with the results obtained in previous studies on metal-catalyzed lipid peroxidation, in which curcumin with a 50% inhibitory value (IC_{50}) of 7.5 µmol/L was far more active than α-tocopherol (IC_{50}, 21.9 µmol/L) in inhibiting rat microsomal lipid peroxidation induced by ferric-ADP-ascorbate.

The results of this study, as well as previous observations on the structure-activity relationship of curcuminoids, led us to consider a new model. In this model, oxidant damage is induced by metal ions, the 1,3-diketone system; by functioning as a potent ligand for metal ions, this may be the structural feature most required for

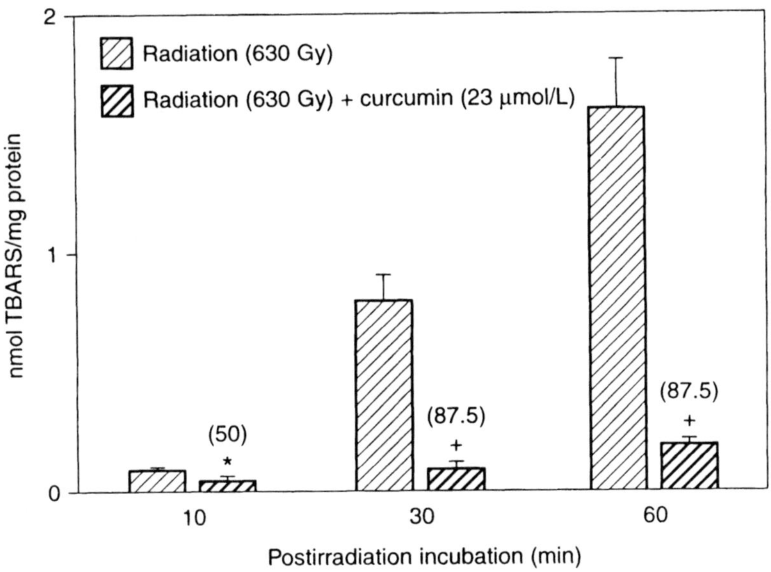

Fig. 5.10. Inhibition of postirradiation lipid peroxidation in rat liver microsomes by curcumin in aerated buffer. Microsomes were exposed to a 630-Gy dose of radiation from a ^{60}Co source.

activity. In other model systems in which scavenging of ROS is involved, the phenolic and the methoxy groups may play a dominant role.

Turmeric, and hence its constituent curcumin, forms a component of the normal diet. Turmeric is being used as a therapeutic agent in skin infections, burn injuries, and skin creams. This may be another form of activating the antioxidant defense especially of the skin, which contains endogenous and exogenous materials that can act as photosensitizers. Radiation is a major source of ROS. Low LET radiations such as γ-rays generate potent ˙OH that are capable of inducing significant tissue damage. Our earlier studies showed that three natural compounds in the form of polysaccharides from *Asparagus racemosus*, caffeine, and chlorophyllin are effective radioprotectors in membranes (53–55). They showed a significant inhibition of lipid peroxidation. Curcumin, which also has a high rate constant with this ROS, significantly inhibits lipid peroxidation induced either by γ-radiation alone or in the presence of N_2O that predominantly generates ˙OH (data not presented). An earlier study by Abraham (30) showed that curcumin was effective in protecting against chromosomal damage induced by γ-radiation *in vivo*. The ability to protect membranes against γ-radiation may explain at least in part the ability of curcumin to counter the radiation-induced damage.

Pulse radiolysis and related studies of curcumin from various laboratories (40,56) show that it is lipid soluble and hence available in membranes when needed. Most natural compounds have either phenolic or β-diketone groups, and curcumin has both. It protects DNA/membranes against $^1O_2$ and other ROS. It reacts with many oxidants, generating phenoxyl radicals that are resonance stabilized, thus neither strongly oxidizing nor reducing. It reacts with many radicals with rate constants comparable to other established antioxidants. Phenoxyl radicals of curcumin react with Trolox and ascorbate and therefore can be recycled in biological systems. Thus, curcumin may be a chain-breaking antioxidant.

Dehydrozingerone, the more stable metabolic product of curcumin, is a phenol-acting antioxidant that scavenges both chain-initiating and chain-propagating free radicals. It efficiently donates an electron to many damaging biological oxidants such as peroxyl radicals and nitrogen dioxide. The results also suggest that dehydrozingerone, like many other phenolic antioxidants, can react with primary and secondary radicals (57).

Summary

Curcumin, the major coloring compound from turmeric, has significant abilities to protect plasmid DNA against singlet oxygen; its ability is greater than that of other antioxidants. It can protect rat skin homogenate and subcellular fractions from peroxidation induced by photosensitization involving Type I and Type II pathways. Radiation and $^{\bullet}OH$-induced lipid peroxidation in rat liver microsomes were also prevented to a significant extent. Pulse radiolysis studies showed that curcumin had fairly high rate constants with oxidants; the resulting radicals were resonance-stabilized and could be recycled by reaction with other antioxidants. Our studies, taken together with other related research, show that curcumin is a potent antioxidant and that this property may explain in part its therapeutic effect, especially in relation to its anticancer and skin-protecting properties.

Acknowledgments

The authors thank Dr. K.B. Sainis, Head, Cell Biology Division, for his encouragement and support. They also wish to thank the following persons for their help or contribution to our studies in various ways : Mr. K.K. Boloor, Cell Biology Division; Dr. S.N. Guha and Dr. K. Priyadarisini, Radiation Chemistry and Chemical Dynamics Division; Dr. B.B. Singh, former Head of Radiation Biology and Biochemistry Division; Dr. M. Subramanian, Radiation Biology Division, and Dr. M.N.A. Rao, Divis Research Laboratories, Hyderabad, India.

References

1. Chopra, R.N., Chorpa, I.C., Handa, K.L., and Kapur, L.D. (1958) *Indigenous Drugs of India.* Anonymous, U.N. Dhar and Sons Pvt. Ltd., Calcutta, pp. 325–327.
2. Nadkarni, K.M. (1976) *Curcuma longa. Indian Materia Medica*, p. 414. Popular Prakashan, Bombay, India.
3. Ammon, H.P.T., and Wahl, M.A. (1990) Pharmacology of *Curcuma longa. Planta Med. 57*, 1–17.
4. Luper, S. (1999) A Review of Plants Used in the Treatment of Liver Disease: Part Two. *Altern. Med. Rev. 4*, 178–188.

5. Ruby, A.J., Kuttan, G., Babu, K.D., Rajasekharan, K.N., and Kuttan, R. (1995) Anti-Tumour and Antioxidant Activity of Natural Curcuminoids. *Cancer Lett. 94*, 83–97.
6. El Hamss, R., Analla, M., Campos-Sanchez, J., Alonso-Moraga, A., Munoz-Serrano, A., and Idaomar, M. (1999) A Dose Dependent Anti-Genotoxic Effect of Turmeric. *Mutat. Res. 446*, 135–139.
7. Ramirez-Tortosa, M.C., Mesa, M.D., Aguilera, M.C., Quiles, J.L., Baro, L., Ramirez-Tortosa, C.L., Martinez-Victoria, E., and Gil, A. (1999) Oral Administration of a Turmeric Extract Inhibits LDL Oxidation and Has Hypocholesterolemic Effects in Rabbits with Experimental Atherosclerosis. *Atherosclerosis 147*, 371–378.
8. Reddy, A.C.P., and Lokesh, B.R. (1994) Effect of Dietary Turmeric (*Curcuma longa*) on Iron-Induced Lipid Peroxidation in the Rat Liver. *Food Chem. Toxicol. 32*, 279–283.
9. Sreejayan, N., and Rao, M.N.A. (1996) Oxygen Free Radical Scavenging by Curcuminoids. *Arzneim-Forsch./Drug Res. 2*, 169–171.
10. Kunchandy, E., and Rao, M.N.A. (1989) Effect of Curcumin on Hydroxyl Radical Generation Through Fenton Reaction. *Int. J. Pharm. 57*, 173–176.
11. Subramanian, M., Sreejayan, N., Rao, M.N.A., Devasagayam, T.P.A., and Singh, B.B. (1994) Diminution of Singlet Oxygen Induced DNA Damage by Curcumin and Related Antioxidants. *Mutat. Res. 311*, 249–255.
12. Sreejayan, N., Rao, M.N.A., Priyadarsini, K.I., and Devasagayam, T.P.A. (1997) Inhibition of Radiation-Induced Lipid Peroxidation by Curcumin. *Int. J. Pharm. 151*, 127–130.
13. Sies, H. (1986) Biochemistry of Oxidative Stress. *Angew. Chem. Int. Ed. Engl. 25*, 1058–1071.
14. Kunsch, C., and Medford, R.M. (1999) Oxidative Stress as a Regulator of Gene Expression in the Vasculature. *Circ. Res. 85*, 753–766.
15. Packer, L., and Ong, A.S.H., (eds.) (1998) *Biological Oxidants and Antioxidants: Molecular Mechanisms and Health Effects*. AOCS Press, Champaign, IL.
16. Kamat, J.P., Sarma, H.D., Devasagayam, T.P.A., Nesaretnam, K., and Basiron, Y. (1997) Tocotrienols from Palm Oil as Effective Inhibitors of Protein Oxidation and Lipid Peroxidation in Rat Liver Microsomes. *Mol. Cell. Biochem. 170*, 131–138.
17. Kamat, J.P., Ghosh, A., and Devasagayam, T.P.A. (2000) Vanillin as an Antioxidant in Rat Liver Mitochondria: Inhibition of Protein Oxidation and Lipid Peroxidation Induced by Photosensitization. *Mol. Cell. Biochem. 209*, 47–53.
18. Von Sonntag, C. (1987) *The Chemical Basis of Radiation Biology*, Taylor and Francis, London.
19. Khan, A.U., and Kasha, M. (1994) Singlet Molecular Oxygen in the Haber-Weiss Reaction. *Proc. Natl. Acad. Sci. USA 91*, 12365–12367.
20. Girotti, A.W. (1990) Photodynamic Lipid Peroxidation in Biological Systems. *Photochem. Photobiol. 51*, 497–509.
21. Foote, C.S. (1991) Definition of Type I and Type II Photosensitized Oxidation. *Photochem. Photobiol. 54*, 659.
22. Esterbauer, H. (1996) Estimation of Peroxidative Damage: A Critical Review. *Pathol. Biol. 44*, 25–28.
23. Zarkovic, N., Zarkovic, K., Schauer, R.J., Stole, S., Schlab, G., Redl, H., Waeg, G., Borovic, S., Loncaric, I., Juric, G., and Hlavka, V. (1999) 4-Hydroxynonenal as a Second Messenger of Free Radical and Growth Modifying Factor. *Life Sci. 65*, 1901–1904.

24. Uchida, K., Shiraishi, M., Naito, Y., Torii, Y., Nakamura, Y., and Osawa, T. (1999) Activation of Stress Signalling Pathways by the End Product of Lipid Peroxidation—4-Hydroxy-2-nonenal Is a Potential Inducer of Intracellular Peroxide Production. *J. Biol. Chem. 274*, 2234–2242.
25. Devasagayam, T.P.A., Steenken, S., Obendorf, M.S.W., Schulz, W.A., and Sies. H. (1991) Formation of 8-Hydroxy(deoxy)guanosine and Generation of Strand Breaks at Guanine Residues in DNA by Singlet Oxygen. *Biochem. 30*, 6283–6289.
26. Epe, B. (1991) Genotoxicity of Singlet Oxygen. *Chem.-Biol. Interact. 80*, 239–260.
27. Ravanat, J.L., and Cadet. J. (1995) Reaction of Singlet Oxygen with 2′-Deoxyguanosine and DNA. Isolation and Characterization of the Main Oxidation Products. *Chem. Res. Toxicol. 8*, 379–388.
28. Agnezlima, L.F., Di Mascio, P., Napolitano, R.L., Fuchs, R.P., and Menck, C.F.M. (1999) Mutation Spectrum Induced by Singlet Oxygen in *Escherichia coli* Deficient in Exonuclease-III. *Photochem. Photobiol. 70*, 505–511.
29. Devasagayam, T.P.A., and P.C. Kesavan (1996) Radioprotective and Antioxidant Action of Caffeine: Mechanistic Considerations. *Indian J. Exp. Biol. 34*, 291–297.
30. Abraham, S.K. (1996) Anti-Genotoxic Effects in Mice After the Interaction Between Coffee and Dietary Constituents. *Food Chem. Toxicol. 34*, 15–20.
31. Pabon, H.J.J. (1964) A Synthesis of Curcumin and Related Compounds. *Recl. Trav. Chim. Pays-Bas Belg. 83*, 279–386.
32. Saldanha, L.A., and Rao, M.N.A. (1990) Oxygen Radical Scavenging Activity of Phenylbutenones and Their Correlation with Anti-Inflammatory Activity. *Arzneim-Forsch./Drug Res.*, 89–91.
33. Di Mascio, P., and Sies, H. (1989) Quantification of Singlet Oxygen Generated by Thermolysis of 3,3′-(1,4-Naphthylidene) Dipropionate. Monomal and Dimol Photoemission and the Effects of 1,4-Diazabicyclo(2,2,2)octane. *J. Am. Chem. Soc. 111*, 2909–2914.
34. Di Mascio, P., Wefers, H., Do-Thi, H.P., Lafleur M.V.M., and Sies, H. (1989) Singlet Molecular Oxygen Causes Loss of Biological Activity in Plasmid and Bacteriophage DNA and Induces Single Strand Breaks. *Biochim. Biophys. Acta 1007*, 151–157.
35. Kamat, J.P., and Devasagayam, T.P.A. (1996) Methylene Blue Plus Light-Induced Lipid Peroxidation in Rat Liver Microsomes: Inhibition by Nicotinamide (Vitamin B3) and Other Antioxidants. *Chem.-Biol. Interact. 99*, 1–16.
36. Devasagayam, T.P.A., Pushpendran, C.K., and Eapen, J. (1983) Differences in Lipid Peroxidation of Rat Liver Rough and Smooth Microsomes. *Biochim. Biophys. Acta 750*, 91–97.
37. Huang, M.T., Lysz, T., Ferraro, T., Abidi, T.F., Laskin, J.D., and Conney, A.H. (1991) Inhibitory Effects of Curcumin on *in vitro* Lipoxygenase and Cyclooxygenase Activities in Mouse Epidermis. *Cancer Res. 51*, 813–819.
38.. Sreejayan, N., and von Ritter, C. (1998) Effect of Bile Acids on Lipid Peroxidation: The Role of Iron. *Free Radic. Biol. Med. 25*, 50–56.
39. Sies, H. (1993) Damage to Plasmid DNA by Singlet Oxygen and Its Protection. *Mutat. Res. 209*, 183–191.
40. Gorman, A.A., Hamblett, V.S., Srinivasan, V.S., and Wood, P.D. (1994) Curcumin Derived Transients: A Pulse Laser and Pulse Radiolysis Study. *Photochem. Photobiol. 59*, 389–398.
41. Srimal, R.C. (1987) Curcumin. *Drugs Future 12*, 331–333.

42. Piette, J. (1991) Biological Consequences Associated with DNA Oxidation Mediated by Singlet Oxygen. *J. Photochem. Photobiol. B: Biol. 11*, 241–260.
43. Ames, B.N., Shigenaga, M.K., and Hagen, T.M. (1993) Oxidants, Antioxidants, and the Degenerative Diseases of Ageing. *Proc. Natl. Acad. Sci. USA 90*, 7915–7922.
44. Stoner, G.D., and Mukhtar, H. (1995) Polyphenols as Cancer Chemopreventive Agents. *J. Cell. Biochem. Suppl. 22*, 169–180.
45. Azuine, M.A., and Bhide, S.V. (1992) Chemopreventive Effect of Turmeric Against Stomach and Skin Tumors Induced by Chemical Carcinogens in Swiss Mice. *Nutr. Cancer 17*, 77–83.
46. Inano, H., Onoda, M., Inafuku, N., Kubota, M., Kamada, Y., Osawa, T., Kobayashi, H., and Wakabayashi, K. (1999) Chemoprevention by Curcumin During the Promotion Stage of Tumorigenesis of Mammary Gland in Rats Irradiated with Gamma-Rays. *Carcinogenesis 20*, 1011–1018.
47. Kawamori, T., Lubet, R., Steele, V.E., Kelloff, G.J., Kaskey, R.B., Rao, C.V., and Reddy, B.S. (1999) Chemopreventive Effect of Curcumin, a Naturally Occurring Anti-Inflammatory Agent, During the Promotion/Progression Stages of Colon Cancer. *Cancer Res. 59*, 597–601.
48. Khar, A., Ali, A.M., Pardhasaradhi, B.V.V., Begum, Z., and Anjum, R. (1999) Antitumor Activity of Curcumin Is Mediated Through the Induction of Apoptosis in AK-5 Tumor Cells. *FEBS Lett. 445*, 165–168.
49. Chan, H.W.S. (1977) Photosensitized Oxidation of Unsaturated Fatty Acid Methyl Esters; The Identification of Different Pathways. *J. Am. Oil Chem. Soc. 54*, 234–238.
50. Sreejayan, N., and Rao, M.N.A. (1994) Curcuminoids as Potent Inhibitors of Lipid Peroxidation. *J. Pharm. Pharmacol. 46*, 1013–1016.
51. Conney, A.H., Lysz, T., Ferraro, T., Abidi, T.F., Manchand, P.S., Laskin, J.D., and Huang, M.T. (1990) Inhibitory Effect of Curcumin and Some Related Dietary Compounds on Tumor Promotion and Arachidonic Acid Metabolism in Mouse Skin, in *Advances in Enzyme Regulation,* (Weber, G., ed.) pp. 385–396, Pergamon Press, New York.
52. Toda, S., Ohnisho, M., Kimura, M., and Nakashima, K. (1988) Action of Curcuminoids on the Hemolysis and Lipid Peroxidation of Mouse Erythrocytes Induced by Hydrogen Peroxide. *J. Ethnopharmacol. 23*, 108.
53. Kamat, J.P., Boloor, K.K., Devasagayam, T.P.A., and Venkatachalam, S.R. (2000) Radioprotective Properties of *Asparagus racemosus in vitro* in Rat Liver Mitochondria. *J. Ethnopharmacol. 71*, 425–435.
54. Kamat, J.P., Ghosh, A., and Devasagayam, T.P.A. (2000) Vanillin as an Antioxidant in Rat Liver Mitochondria: Inhibition of Protein Oxidation and Lipid Peroxidation Induced by Photosensitization. *Mol. Cell. Biochem. 209*, 47–53.
55. Kamat, J.P., Boloor, K.K., and Devasagayam, T.P.A. (2000) Chlorophyllin as an Effective Antioxidant Against Membrane Damage *in vitro* and *ex vivo*. *Biochim. Biophys. Acta 1487*, 113–127.
56. Priyadarsini, K.I. (1997) Free Radical Reactions of Curcumin in Membrane Models. *Free Radic Biol. Med. 23*, 838–843.
57. Priyadarsini, K.I., Devasagayam, T.P.A., Rao, M.N.A., and Guha, S.N. (1999). Properties of Phenoxyl Radical of Dehydrozingerone, a Probable Antioxidant. *Radiat. Phys. Chem. 54*, 551–558.

Chapter 6

Free Radical Reaction of Green Tea Polyphenols

Baolu Zhao

Institute of Biophysics, Academia Sinica, Beijing, 100101, P.R. China

Introduction

Many legends surround the origins of tea; one of them concerns the ancient Chinese emperor Shen Nong, who lived around 2700 BC. While heating some water to allay stomach pains due to overindulgence at dinner, the emperor did not notice that some leaves from a nearby shrub had dropped into the boiling water. He drank the brew and found that not only did it taste delicious but that it also caused the spontaneous disappearance of his stomach pains, thereby demonstrating the efficacy of tea for the first time.

There are two kinds of tea, green and black. Most Asian people drink green tea, whereas black tea is more popular in Western countries. Green tea is prepared with fresh leaves without fermentation. Flavonoid compounds comprise >30% of the dry weight of the green teas; the predominant form is the flavan-3-ol or catechins. Young tea leaves contain the highest catechin concentration. The leaf bud and the first leaf are especially rich in polyphenols. Black tea is prepared by fermentation of fresh tea leaves and contains one third the level of catechins present in green tea. Oxidation of the catechins results in the formation of catechin quinones, which can undergo complex condensation and coupling reactions to form theaflavins, epitheaflavic acid, and thearubigins.

A variety of clinical, pathologic events have been linked to an excessive concentration of free radicals in the body. An excess of free radicals or reactive species generated from oxygen and nitric oxide can be harmful because they attack vital cellular components such as the membrane, proteins, enzymes, and DNA, and can even kill the whole cell (1–3). If there is an imbalance in the metabolism of the free radical, which leads to a greater concentration of free radical than that scavenged, diseases such as cancer and heart disease may result (4,5). The body's inability to regulate free radical metabolism on its own may be a result of a deficiency in the antioxidants, vitamin C and vitamin E, or because the activity of the antioxidant enzymes, superoxide dismutase (SOD) and catalase, is insufficient to maintain a healthy balance. Antioxidant supplementation is therefore necessary for the body to scavenge the excessive oxygen free radicals.

Traditional herbs and natural health foods have been widely used and accepted in China for thousands of years. Although the mechanism behind the action of these products remains unclear, it is common for such herbal products to demonstrate positive clinical results in patients suffering from a variety of disorders. It is generally believed that the potent antioxidant activities of these preparations make them effective

(6–8), and an outstanding example of such a potent Chinese herb is green tea polyphenols (GTP).

Throughout history, tea has been one of the most popular beverages worldwide. Epidemiologic studies have shown that tea is beneficial to people's health by protecting the body from cancer, heart disease, and aging. It is thought to contain antitumor and antimutagenic materials. The water extract and the antioxidants isolated from green tea have been shown to inhibit the backward mutation induced by aflatoxin B1 (AFB1) and benzo(a)pyrene (BaP) in *Salmonella typhimurium*. Tea antioxidants were also found to inhibit gene mutation in V_{79} cells treated with AFB1 and BaP as well as decrease the frequency of sister chromatic exchanges and chromosome aberrations in V_{79} cells treated with AFB1 (9–12). GTP has also been shown to inhibit tumorigenesis and carcinogenesis. The anticarcinogenic action of green tea and its constituents, particularly epigallocatechin gallate (EGCG), has been studied *in vivo* in humans and animals (13–15).

This review summarizes and discusses recent studies of the scavenging effects of GTP on free radicals and the potential underlying mechanisms. It was found that tea, especially green tea, contains antioxidants, polyphenols that scavenge the pathological factors (oxygen free radicals) in different systems. GTP inhibited lipid peroxidation and changes in the biophysical properties of cell membranes, protecting V_{79} cells from the gas phase of cigarette smoke (GPCS)-induced cytotoxicity, and protecting low density lipoprotein (LDL) against lipid peroxidation. In this review, the antioxidant abilities of different green tea polyphenol components and the scavenging effects of different epimers on different free radicals were compared; measurements were made of their synergistic scavenging effects on the superoxide radical and the reducing potentials, rate constants, and quenching numbers of free radicals by GTP. From these results, the active sites and molecular mechanism were identified.

Green tea extract usually contains four types of polyphenols, i.e., (-)-epicatechin (EC), (-)-epicatechin-3-gallate (ECG), (-)-epigallocatechin (EGC), and (-)-epigallocatechin-3-gallate (EGCG) (Fig. 6.1). Because they are water soluble and easy to study, GTP mixture was used in most earlier studies (16–28).

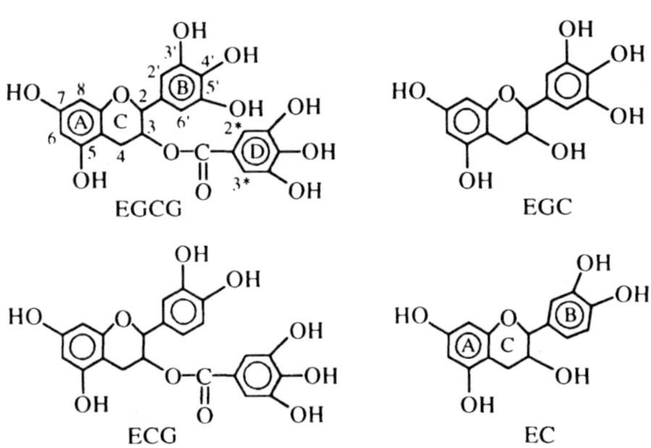

Fig. 6.1. The structures of green tea polyphenols.

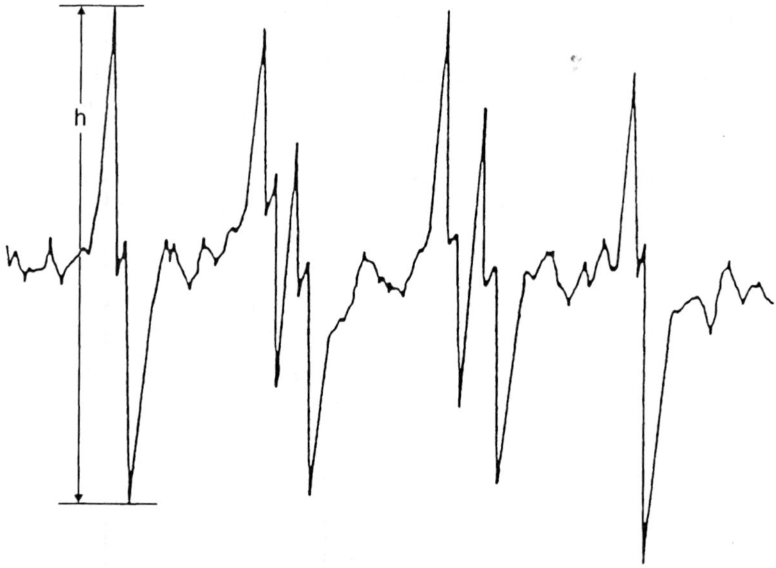

Fig. 6.2. Electron spin resonance (ESR) spectrum of the superoxide radical generated from irradiation of riboflavin (0.5 mol/L)/EDTA (50 mmol/L) system and trapped by 0.1 mol/L 5,5-dimethyl-1-pyrroline-1-oxide (DMPO). The ESR spectrum was recorded 1 min after irradiation. ESR conditions: The spectrum was recorded with a Varian E109 ESR spectrometer, X-band, 100-kHz modulation with amplitude 1 G, microwave power 10 mW, time constant 0.128 s, central magnetic field 3250 G, swept width 200 G, room temperature.

Scavenging Effect of GTP on $O_2^{-\bullet}$

We trapped $O_2^{-\bullet}$ which was generated from photoradiation of riboflavin/EDTA with 5,5-dimethyl-1-pyrroline-1-oxide (DMPO) and measured by electron spin resonance (ESR), yielding a 12-line ESR spectrum (a_N = 14.3 G, a^{β}_{H} = 11.3 G, a^{r}_{H} = 1.25 G) (Fig. 6.2). The scavenging effects of GTP and the other antioxidants, vitamin E, rosemary, curcurmin, and vitamin C, on superoxide radicals generated from the system were 72 ± 7.4, 23 ± 6.1, 23 ± 5.1, 17 ± 5.5, and 96 ± 6.4%, respectively. It was found that the scavenging effect of GTP on superoxide radicals was stronger than that of vitamin E, rosemary, and curcurmin, but weaker than that of vitamin C (16,17).

Scavenging Effect of GTP on $^{\bullet}OH$

We trapped $^{\bullet}OH$ generated from the Fenton reaction with DMPO; the ESR spectrum was measured and yielded a typical 4-line ESR spectrum with intensity 1:2:2:1 ($a_N = a_H$ = 14.9 G) (Fig. 6.3). The scavenging effects of GTP and the other antioxidants, vitamin E, rosemary, curcumin, and vitamin C, on the hydroxyl radical generated from the Fenton system were 12 ± 3.6, 35 ± 13.5, 16 ± 9.0, 69 ± 11.7 and 56 ± 5.9%,

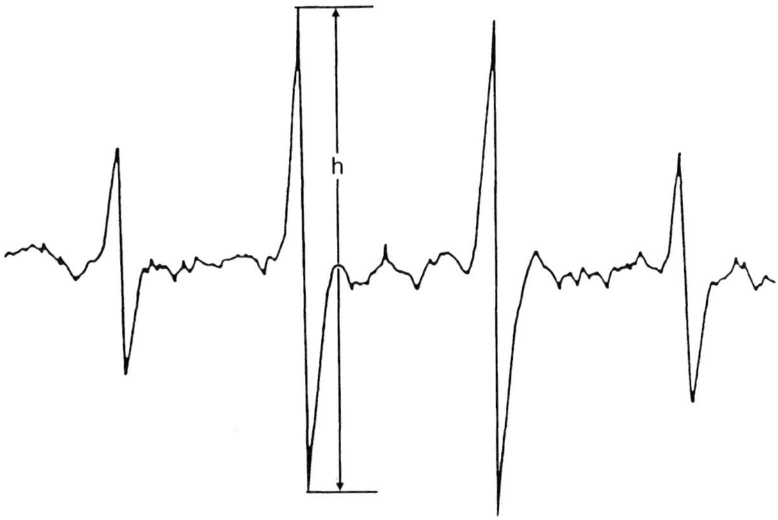

Fig. 6.3. Electron spin resonance (ESR) spectrum of the hydroxyl free radical generated from the Fenton reaction (0.1% H_2O_2 + Fe^{2+}) and trapped by 50 mmol/L 5,5-dimethyl-1-pyroline-1-oxide (DMPO). ESR conditions were as in Figure 6.2.

respectively, indicating that GTP shows a weak scavenging effect on the hydroxyl radical in the Fenton reaction (16,17).

Scavenging Effect of GTP on Oxygen Free Radicals Generated from PMA-Stimulated PMN

We compared the ESR spectra from a mixture containing 10^7 cells/mL polymorphonuclear leukocytes (PMN), 0.1 mmol/L diethylentriaminepentacid acid (DETAPAC), 100 ng/mL phorbol-1,2-myristate (PMA), 0.1 mol/L DMPO without and with 200 g/mL GTP, rosemary, curcumin, Vitamin C, and vitamin E, respectively (Fig. 6.4). It was found that GTP had the strongest scavenging effects on oxygen free radicals produced from PMA-stimulated PMN. Unlike other antioxidants, they practically eliminated all active oxygen free radicals.

It was assumed that the decrease in active oxygen radicals represented the scavenging effect of the antioxidants on oxygen free radicals, but another explanation could be that a decrease in the production of oxygen radicals was caused by an inhibitory effect of the antioxidants on the activity of PMN. To clarify this, we used spin probe oxymetry to measure the oxygen consumption during the respiratory burst of PMA-stimulated PMN with and without the antioxidants. No differences were found, which indicated that although GTP and other antioxidants could scavenge the oxygen free radicals generated from the PMA-stimulated PMN, they did not affect the activity of production of active oxygen radicals during the respiratory burst of PMN (16,17).

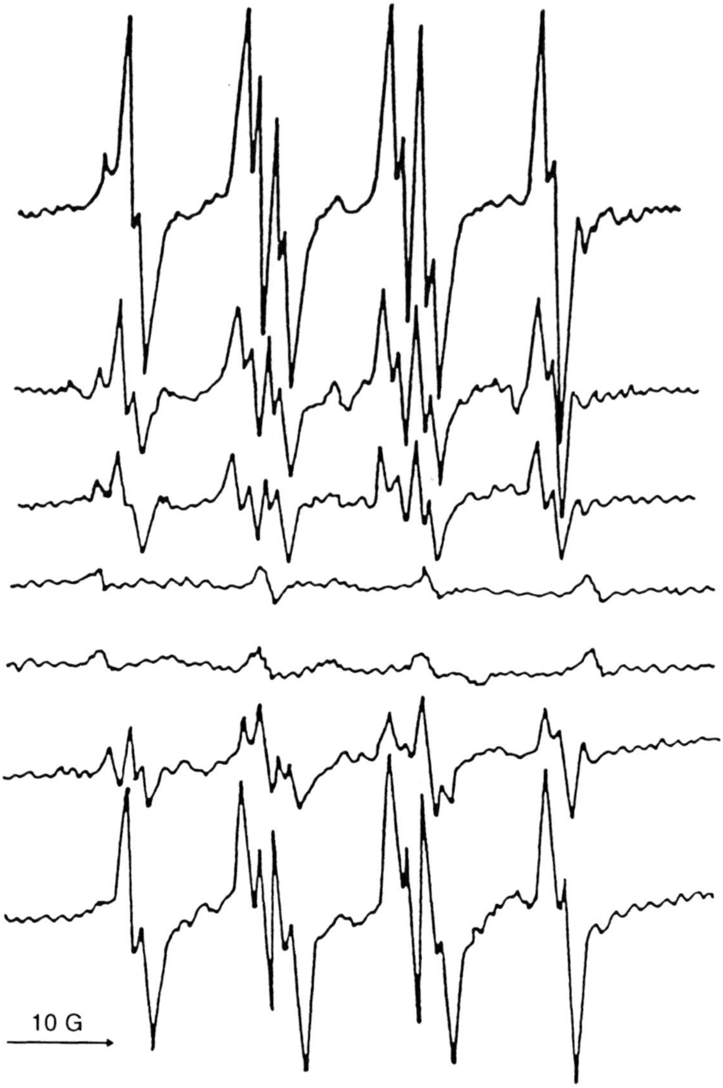

Fig. 6.4. Scavenging effects of the antioxidants on active oxygen radicals generated from respiratory burst of polymorphonuclear leukocytes (PMN): (*A*) Electron spin resonance (ESR) spectrum resulting from 1.5 × 10^7/mL PMN stimulated with 100 ng/mL phorbol-1,2-myristate (PMA) in the presence of 0.1 mmol/L diethylentriaminepentacid acid (DETAPAC) and 0.1 mol/L 5,5-dimethyl-1-pyrroline-1-oxide (DMPO) at 37°C; (*B*) conditions were the same as those for A, except that 200 mg/mL curcumin was present; (*C*) as for A, except that 200 mg/mL rosemary was present; (*D*) as for A, except that 200 mg/mL F6 was present; (*E*) as for A, except that 200 mg/mL green tea polyphenols was present; (*F*) as for A, except that 200 mg/mL vitamin C was present; (*G*) as for A, except that 200 mg/mL vitamin E was present. ESR conditions were as in Figure 6.2.

Scavenging Effect of GTP on Oxygen Free Radicals Generated from Isolated Ischemia-Reperfused Rat Heart

We used ESR to measure the free radical generation directly in ischemia-reperfused myocardium at 110K. The results showed that the isolated reperfused rat heart subjected to 30 min ischemia followed by 15 s reperfusion induced a significant increase in the production of oxygen free radicals. The concentration of oxygen free radicals in ischemic-reperfused myocardium was ~188% that in the normal myocardium. After pretreatment of the heart with 0.1 mg/mL GTP, the oxygen free radicals were reduced to ~71% ($P < 0.01$). This result indicates that the natural antioxidant GTP may protect the heart from ischemic reperfusion injury (18).

Inhibitory Effect of GTP on the Oxidant Activity of $ONOO^-$

Using the spin-trapping agent 2-methyl-2-nitrosopropane (tNB), we trapped a free radical from the reaction of dimethyl sulfoxide (DMSO) with peroxynitrite. It was identified as the $^{\bullet}CH_3$ free radical spin adduct of tNB by the analysis of its spectrum ($a_N = 17.2$ G, $A_H = 14.2$ G) (Fig. 6.5); the yield of tNB-CH_3 radical adduct was dose dependent on the concentrations of peroxynitrite and DMSO. This is a useful index for studying the oxidation properties of peroxynitrite. The scavenging effects of GTP on $^{\bullet}CH_3$ free radicals generated from the oxidation of DMSO by peroxynitrite were studied and compared with the scavenging effects of quercetin and vitamin C. Although they could all effectively inhibit the oxidation of peroxynitrite in this system, the inhibitory effect of GTP was the strongest, whereas that of vitamin C was the weakest (19).

Scavenging Effect of GTP on Lipid Free Radicals Generated from Gas-Phase Cigarette Smoke (GPCS)-Treated Microsomes

Using α-4-pyridyl-1-oxide-*N*-*t*-butylnitrone (4-POBN), we trapped the lipid free radical generated from microsomes treated with GPCS. The 2 × 3-line ESR spectrum

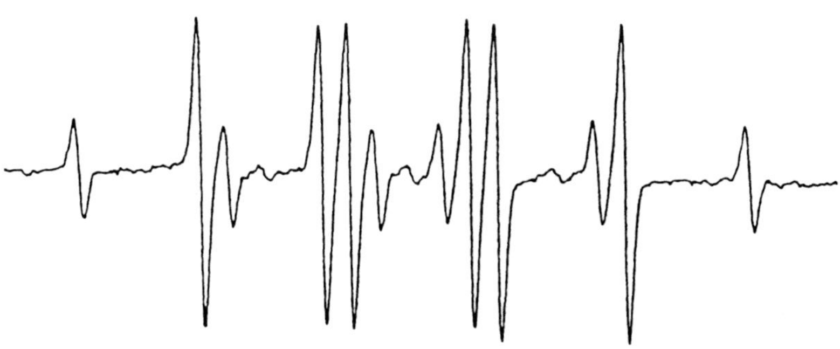

Fig. 6.5. Electron spin resonance (ESR) spectrum of the methyl free radical generated from reaction of dimethyl sulfoxide (DMSO) (1.4 mmol/L) with peroxynitrite (4.8 mmol/L) and trapped by 2-methyl-2-nitrosopropane (MNP) (80 mmol/L). ESR conditions were as in Figure 6.2.

of lipid free radical trapped by 4-POBN is shown in Fig. 6.6 (a_N = 15.5 G, a_H = 2.7 G). The scavenging effects of GTP on lipid free radicals generated from GPCS-treated microsomes were measured; GTP had a stronger inhibitory effect on lipid peroxidation (50.0 ± 4.3%) than did vitamin C (43.0 ± 9.4%) or vitamin E (30.6 ± 3.9 %) (20–25).

When the V_{79} cell suspension was incubated with GTP at 37°C for 15 min and then exposed to GPCS at the fixed flow rate for 20 s, decreased cell death and thiobarbituric acid reactive substance (TBARS) production were observed with the increased dose of GTP. The ESR spin label study with 5-doxyl indicated that GTP inhibited the changes of membrane fluidity induced by GPCS exposure in a dose-dependent manner. A lower concentration of GTP could also inhibit the increase of the conformation change of membrane proteins induced by GPCS exposure (26).

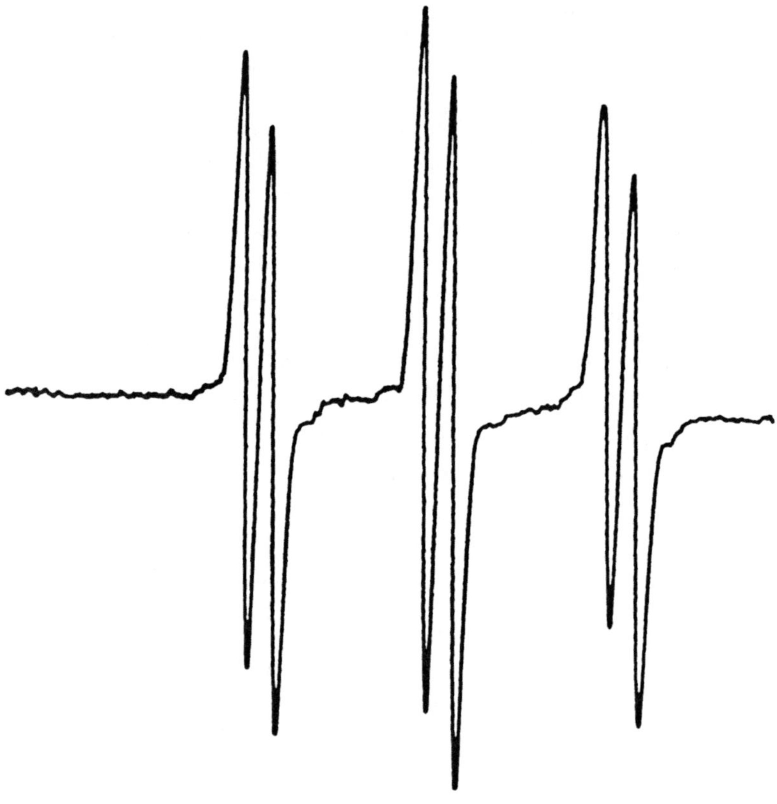

Fig. 6.6. Electron spin resonance (ESR) spectrum of lipid free radical generated from lipid peroxidation of microsomes (20 mg/mL) treated by gas-phase cigarette smoke (GPCS) and trapped by 0.2 mol/L α-4-pyridyl-1-oxide-*N*-*t*-butylnitrone (4-POBN). ESR conditions were as in Figure 6.2.

Protective Effect of GTP Against Oxidative Damage to Red Blood Cells

Tea polyphenols from black and green teas were evaluated for their antioxidant effects on normal red blood cells and β-thalassemic red blood cell membranes that were challenged with exogenous oxidations in vivo. Both black and green tea polyphenols protected red blood cells against primaquine-induced lysis and protected the whole cells and their membranes against H_2O_2-induced lipid peroxidation. At 10 mg/mL GTP, ~80% protection was reached. The mechanism underlying the effects of tea polyphenols was investigated using a chemical system generating $^{\bullet}OH$ (iron + ascorbic acid). Tea polyphenols from both black and green teas inhibited the fluctuation of $^{\bullet}OH$ generation in a concentration-dependent manner, which indicated a possibility of chelation by tea polyphenols. Spectrophotometric titration revealed that tea polyphenols could stoichiometrically bind ferric iron to form a redox-inactive Fe-GTP complex (29).

We investigated the protective effect of GTP on erythrocytes; the hydroxyl radical generated from the Fenton reaction was able to increase the concentration of TBARS and lipid peroxidation of erythrocyte membranes. GTP could protect the membranes from lipid peroxidation (30)

These results show that GTP can effectively scavenge oxygen and lipid free radicals, inhibit lipid peroxidation, and protect cell membranes in different systems. However, we do not know the antioxidant ability of different components of GTP because GTP is a mixture. Therefore, the different components of GTP were isolated and compared in different systems.

Antioxidant Properties of Different Components of GTP

We studied the reducing potentials of different components of GTP; the order of their first reducing potentials was determined to be as follows: EGCG > ECG > EGC = EC (31). EGCG had the highest reducing potential.

Jovanovic *et al.* (32) measured the rate constants of reaction of polyphenols with $O_2^{-\bullet}$. The order of the rate constants of reaction of polyphenols with $O_2^{-\bullet}$ is as follows: EGCG > ECG > EC > EGC. These results are the same as those for the reducing potential.

Salah *et al.* (33) and Rice-Evans *et al.* (34) developed a different model and obtained similar results using a Trolox equivalent antioxidant activity (TEAC) system to measure the antioxidant potential of the polyphenols in the aqueous phase. The order of their effectiveness as radical scavengers is as follows: EGCG > ECG > EGC > EC. However, when placed with a propagating lipid peroxyl radical species, EC was as effective as ECG and EGCG, whereas EGC was the least efficacious. Although the total polyphenol content of black tea extract (44.94%) was similar to that of green tea, only 6.9% by weight was comprised of catechin-gallate components and the antioxidant activity of black tea extract (3.491 ± 0.05) was very close to that of green tea (3.781 ± 0.03).

Gardner *et al.* (35) studied the quenching ability of different components of GTP on Fremys radicals (potassium nitrosodisulfonate) in water and galvinoxyl (2,6-di-*tert*-butyl-a-(3,5-di-*tert*-butyl-4-oxo-2,5,-cyctohexadien-1-ylidene)-*p*-tolyloxy) in ethanol. The quenching ability was as follows: EGCG > ECG > EC > EGC in aqueous and organic media. These results are the same as those for the reducing potentials and rate constants.

Using Fe^{2+}/Fe^{3+} to stimulate lipid peroxidation of synaptosomes, we studied the GTP inhibition of lipid peroxidation; EGCG, ECG, EGC, and EC showed different inhibitory effects on TBARS formed in the system. Preincubation of synaptosomes with EGCG, ECG, EGC, or EC before exposure to Fe^{2+}/Fe^{3+} treatment resulted in a decrease in the amount of peroxidation and was dose dependent. It was found that the 50% inhibitory concentration (IC_{50}) of EGCG, ECG, EGC, and EC was 0.1, 0.19, 0.24, and 0.35 mmol/L, respectively. Their antioxidant activities could be classified as follows: EGCG > ECG > EGC> EC (36). This result is also consistent with other findings.

The antioxidant process is dependent not only on its ability to scavenge free radicals, but also on its ability to chelate with iron (III). We therefore decided to measure the chelating ratios of the four compounds with iron (III). The ratio of EGC to iron (III) was 3:2; that of EGCG or ECG to iron (III) was 2:1, whereas that of EC to iron (III) was 3:1. This suggests that the degree of iron-chelating activity is as follows: EGC > ECG = EGCG > EC. With the exception of EGC, this result is more similar to the lipid-scavenging result with Fe^{2+}/Fe^{3+} (36).

Another characteristic that indicates antioxidant effectiveness of a compound is its ability to stabilize the semiquinone free radicals and quinones formed from the polyphenols after reaction with oxygen free radicals. Relatively stable semiquinone free radicals were produced by these compounds and measured in alkaline solution. We found that the stability of semiquinone free radicals decreased in the following order: EGCG > ECG > EC > EGC. This result is similar to that for TBARS (36,37).

Antioxidant Active Sites of EGCG, ECG, EGC, and EC

The active sites of different components of GTP must be identified to understand the mechanism behind their actions. To this end, an analysis of the ESR spectra of the semiquinone radicals formed from reaction with the oxygen radical in alkaline solution was made (36,37).

Antioxidant active sites of EGCG. The ESR spectrum of the semiquinone free radical of EGCG consisted of 12 peaks with ratio 1:1:2:2:1:1:1:1:2:2:1:1, $a_{H2} = 3.71$ G, $a_{H2'} = a_{H6'} = 0.96$ G, $a_{H3} = 0.32$ G. This indicated that its active site and reaction process may be shown in Scheme 1:

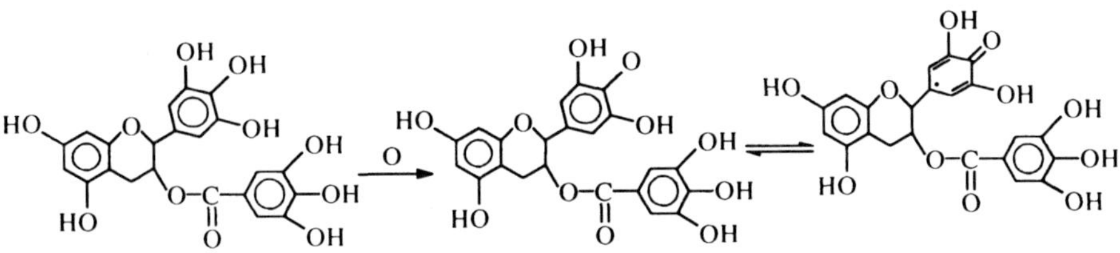

Scheme 1

Antioxidant active sites of ECG. The ESR spectrum of semiquinone free radical of ECG consisted of 6 peaks with ratio 1:1:2:2:1:1, $a_{H3} = 0.19$ G, $a_{H2*} = a_{H3*} = 1.09$ G. This indicated that its active site and reaction process may be as shown in Scheme 2:

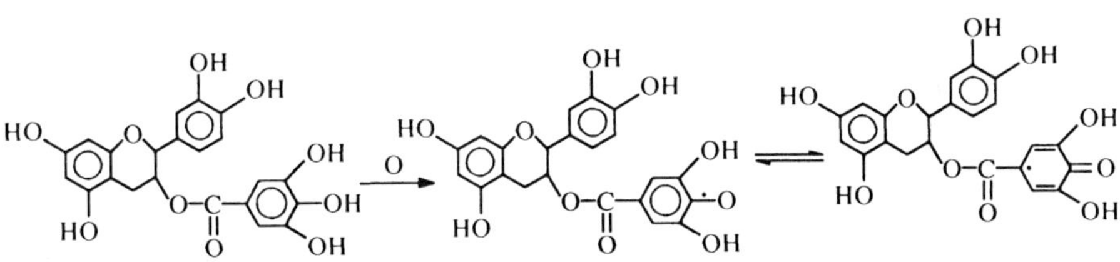

Scheme 2

Antioxidant active sites of EC. The ESR spectrum of the semiquinone free radical of EC showed that two free radicals were produced from one molecule of EC. One consisted of 14 peaks with ratio 1:1:1:2:1:1:1:1:1:1:2:1:1:1, $a_{H2'} = 0.19$ G, $a_{H2} = 0.32$ G, $a_{H5'} = 0.64$ G, $a_{H6'} = 3.39$ G. The other consisted of 8 peaks with ratio 1:1:1:1:1:1:1:1, $a_{H6} = 1.02$ G, $a_{H8} = 0.16$ G, $a_{H2} = 0.48$ G. This indicated that there were two active sites and the reaction process may be as shown in Scheme 3:

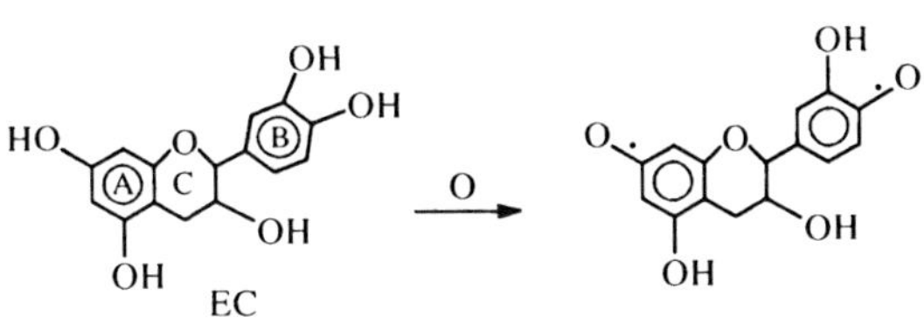

Scheme 3

Antioxidant active sites of EGC. The ESR spectrum of the semiquinone free radical of EGC was formed and stabilized 60 min after reaction in alkaline solution (6 peaks with $a_{H1} = 4.8$ G, $a_{H2'} = a_{H6'} = 0.88$ G). Before that, the spectrum varied with time (6 peaks with $a_{H6} = 1.31$ G, $a_{H4} = 0.51$ G). These differences indicated that the changes of active sites of the semiquinone free radical of EGC may be as shown in Scheme 4:

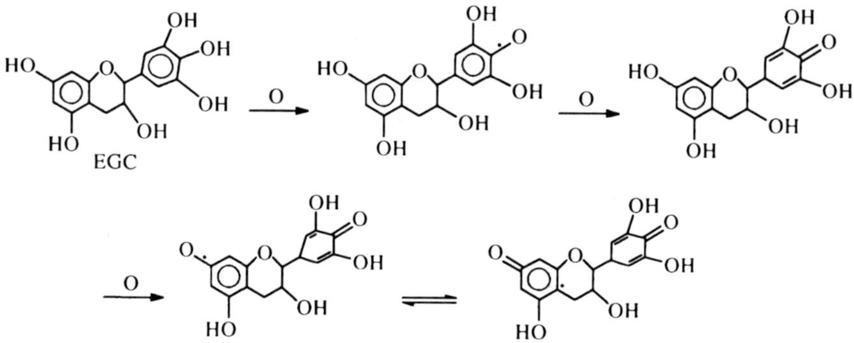

Scheme 4

These results showed that these compounds expose different antioxidant active sites during scavenging of oxygen free radicals. As a result, their protective effects on the oxidative damages caused by lipid peroxidation on synaptosomes also differed. Jovanovic *et al.* (38) also arrived at a similar conclusion from their observation using azide radical–induced oxidation of catechin.

Structure Relationship of Tea Catechins and Their Epimers

Other aspects of the relationship between the structures and activities of antioxidants that we examined were the chemical structures, including steric structure, and the free radical–scavenging activities of tea catechins (EGCG, EGC, EC) and their corresponding epimers [GCG, GC, (+)-C]. In particular, we examined the steric hindrance and stability of the catechins in relation to their abilities to scavenge both small and large free radicals. Scavenging effects were evaluated not only on superoxide anions, singlet oxygen, and the free radicals from 2,2′-azobis(2-amidinopropane)hydrochloride (AAPH) using ESR spin-trapping techniques, but also on the 1.1-diphenyl-2-picrylhydrazyl (DPPH) radical using direct ESR measurement (39).

Summary

GTP are the main polyphenols extracted from green tea, comprising ~30% of dry green tea (w/w), and they are the main source of the biological and pharmacologic functions observed. To understand the health benefits of green tea for humans, it is necessary to study the antioxidant mechanism of GTP. The mechanism includes scavenging of oxygen free radicals and lipid free radicals due to hydrogen-donating ability, delocalization of electrons and chelating metals, and synergistic effects of different components and epimers—even regulation of some antioxidant gene expression. Knowledge of the precise antioxidant active sites of different components of GTP and the different antioxidants of their epimers enables us to use them more efficiently. It also provides insight into the modifications that could be made to enhance their antioxidant effects in biological systems. But contradictory phenomena found within the different components and their apparently different antioxidant abilities in different systems must be studied further to understand the mechanism of GTP as an antioxidant in biological systems.

References

1. Simonia, N.A., and Coyle, J.T. (1996) Oxidative Stress in Neurodegenerative Diseases. *Rev. Pharmacol. Toxicol. 36*, 83–106.
2. Sohal, R.S., Amold, L.A., and Sohal, B.H. (1990) Age-Related Changes in Antioxidant Enzymes and Prooxidant Generation in Tissues of the Rate with Special Reference to Parameters in Two Insect Species. *Free Radic. Biol. Med. 10*, 495–500.
3. Zhao, B.-L., Zhang, C.-A., and Xin, W.-J. (1989) Ischemia-Reperfusion Damage of Myocardium and Active Oxygen Radicals. *Physiol. Sci. 9*, 193–196.
4. Zhao, B.-L. (1990) Oxygen Radicals and Aging. *Naure J. 13*, 511–514.
5. Chen, L.-H., Zhang,Y.-M., Zhao, B.-L., and Xin, W.-J. (1991) ESR Determination and Superoxide Dismutase Activity in Polymorphonuclear Leukocytes in Congestive Heart Failure. *Can. J. Cardiol. 8*, 756–760.
6. Ju, H.-S., Li, X.-J., Zhao, B.-L., and Xin, W.-J. (1990) The Scavenging Effect of Berbarmineon Active Oxygen Radicals in Phorbol Ester-Stimulated Human Polymorphonuclear Leukocytes. *Biochem. Pharmacol. 39*, 1673–1678.
7. Li, X.-J., Zhao, B.-L., Liu, G.-T., and Xin, W.-J. (1990) Scavenging Effects on Active Oxygen Radicals by Schizandrins with Different Structures and Configurations. *Free Radic. Biol. Med. 9*, 99–104.
8. Zhao, B.-L., Li, X.-J., and Xin, W.-J. (1990) Studies on the Effects of Schizandra on Active Oxygen Radicals by Spin Trapping Technique. *Cell Biol. Int. Rep. 14*, 95–105.
9. Katiyar, S.K., Mohan, R.R., Agarwal, R., and Mukhtar, H. (1997) Protection Against Induction of Mouse Skin Papillomas with Low and High Risk of Conversion to Malignancy by Green Tea Polyphenols. *Carcinogenesis 18*, 497–502.
10. Ley, R.D., and Reeve, V.E. (1997) Chemoprevention of ultraviolet radiation-induced skin cancer. *Environ. Health Perspect. [Suppl.] 105*, 981–984.
11. Dreosti, I.E., Wargovich, M.J., and Yang, C.S. (1997) Inhibition of Carcinogenesis by Tea: The Evidence from Experimental Studies. *Crit Rev. Food Sci. Nutr. 37*, 761–770.
12. Cheng, S.J. (1996) Study on Antimutagenicity and Anticarcinogenicity of Green Tea Epicatechins A Natural Free Radical Scavenger, in *Proceedings of the International Symposium on Natural Antioxidants Molecular Mechanisms and Health Effects* (Packer, L., Traber, M.G., and Xin, W., eds.) AOCS Press, Champaign, IL, pp. 92–99.
13. Kono, S., Ikeda, M., Tokudome, S., and Kuratsune, M. (1988) A Case Control Study of Gastric Cancer and Diet in Northern Kyushu, Japan. *Jpn. J. Cancer Res. 79*, 1067–1074.
14. Wang, Z.Y., Huang, M.-T., Ho, C.-T., Chang, R., Ma, W., Ferraro, T., Reuhl, K.R., Yang, C.S., and Conney, A.H. (1992) Inhibitory Effect of Green Tea on the Growth of Established Skin Papillomas in Mice. *Cancer Res. 52*, 6657–6665.
15. Huang, M.-T., Ho, C.-T., Wang, Z.Y., Ferraro, T., Finnegan-Olive, T., Lou. Y.-R., Mitchel, J.M., Laskin, J.D., Newmark, H., Yang, C.S., and Conney, A.H. (1992) Inhibitory Effect of Topical Application of a Green Tea Polyphenol Fraction on Tumour Initiation and Promotion in Mouse Skin. *Carcinogenesis 13*, 947–954.

16. Zhao, B.-L., Li, X.-J., Cheng, S.-J., and Xin, W.-J. (1989) The Scavenging Effects of Extract of Green Tea on Active Oxygen Radicals, in *Medical, Biochemical and Chemical Aspects of Free Radicals*, Hayaishi, Tokyo, pp. 78–85.
17. Zhao, B.-L., Li, X.-J., and Xin, W.-J. (1989) Scavenging Effects of Extracts of Green Tea and Natural Antioxidants on Active Oxygen Radicals. *Cell Biophys. 14*, 175–185.
18. Zou, X.-L.,Wan, Q., Li, M.-F., Zhao, B.-L., and Xin, W.-J. (1995) Scavenging Effect of Green Tea Polyphenols on the Oxygen Free Radicals Generated from Isolated Ischemic Reperfused Rat Myocardium. *Chin. J. Magn. Reson. 12*, 237–244.
19. Zhao, B.-L., Wang, J.-C., and Xin, W.-J. (1996) Scavenging Effect of Green Tea Polyphenols, on Peroxynitrites. *Chin. Sci. Bull. 41*, 923–927.
20. Yan, L.-J. , Zhao,B.-L., and Xin, W.-J. (1991) Experimental Studies on Some Aspects of Toxicological Effect of Gas Phase Cigarette Smoke (GPCS). *Res. Chem. Interm. 16*, 1528.
21. Yang, F.-J., Zhao, B.-L., and Xin, W.-J. (1992) Studies on Toxicological Mechanisms of Gas Phase Cigarette Smoke and Protective Effects of GTP. *Res. Chem. Interm. 17*, 3957.
22. Yang, F.-J., Shen, S.-R., Zhao, B.-L., Yang, X.-Q., and Xin, W.-J. (1992) Inhibition Effect of L-EGCG on Cigarette Smoke-Induced Damage to Rat Lung Cells. *Acta Biophys. Sin. 8*, 450–454.
23. Yang, F.-J., Zhao, B.-L., and Xin, W.-J. (1992) Toxicological Effects of Gas-Phase Cigarette Smoke on Rat Lung Cells and Protection Effects of Green Tea Polyphenols in the System. *Environ. Chem. 11*, 50–55.
24. Li, X.-J., Yan, L.-J., Zhao, B.-L., and Xin, W.-J. (1992) Studies on the Free Radical-Scavenging and the Antioxidant Effect of Green Tea Polyphenol Products (GTP). *Environ. Chem. 11*, 13–16.
25. Yang, F.-J., Zhao, B.-L., and Xin, W.-J. (1993) ESR Studies on the Effect of Green Tea Polyphenols on the Production of Lipid Free Radicals in Gas Phase Cigarette Smoke Treated Microsomes. *Acta Biophys. Sin. 8*, 468–471.
26. Zhang, S.-L., Zhao, B.-L., and Xin, W.-J. (1996) Cytotoxicity of Gas Phase Cigarette Smoke and the Protection by Green Tea Polyphenols. *Chin. J. Environ. Sci. 16*, 34–39.
27. Tijiburg, L.B., Wiseman, S.A., Meijer, G.W., and Weststrate, J.A. (1997) Effects of Green Tea, Black Tea and Dietary Lipophilic Antioxidants on LDL Oxidizability and Atherosclerosis in Hyperchlolesterolaemic Rabbits. *Atherosclerosis 135*, 37–47.
28. Luo, M., Kannar, K., Wahlqvist, M.L., and O'Brien, R.C. (1997) Inhibition of LDL Oxidation by Green Tea Extract. *Lancet 349*, 360–361.
29. Grinberg, L.N., Newmark, H., Kitrossky, N., Rahamim, E., Chevion, M., and Rachmilewitz, E.A. (1997) Protective Effects of Tea Polyphenols Against Oxidative Damage to Red Blood Cells. *Biochem. Pharmacol. 54*, 973–978.
30. Xin, W., Shi, H., Yang, F., Zhao, B.-L., and Hou, J. (1996) A Study on Effect of Green Tea Polyphenols on Lipid Free Radicals, in *Proceeding of the International Symposium on Natural Antioxidants Molecular Mechanisms and Health Effects* (Packer, L., Traber, M.G., and Xin, W., eds.) AOCS Press, Champaign, IL, pp. 56–65.
31. Yang, X.-Q., Shen, S.-R., Hou, J.-W., Zhao, B.-L., and Xin, W.-J. (1994) Mechanism of Scavenging Effects of (-)-Epigallocatechin Gallate on Active Oxygen Free Radicals. *Acta Pharm. Sin. 15*, 350–353.
32. Jovanovic, S.V., Hara,Y., and Simic, M.G. (1995) Antioxidant Potentials of Gallocatechins. A Pulse Radiolysis and Laser Photolysis Study. *J. Am. Chem. Soc. 117*, 9881–9888.

33. Salah, N., Miller, N.J., Paganga, G., Tijiburg, L., Bolwell, G.P., and Rice-Evans, C. (1995) Polyphenolic Flavanols as Scavengers of Aqueous Phase Radicals and as Chain-Breaking Antioxidants. *Arch. Biochem. Biophys. 322*, 339–346.
34. Rice-Evans, C.A., Miller, N.J., and Paganga, G. (1996) Structure-Antioxidant Activity Relationship of Flavonoids and Phenolic Acids. *Free Radic. Biol. Med. 20*, 933–956.
35. Gardner, P.T., McPhail, D.B., and Duthie, G.G. (1998) Electron Spin Resonance Spectroscopic Assessment of the Antioxidant Potential of Teas in Aqueous and Organic Media. *J. Sci. Food Agric. 76*, 257–262.
36. Guo, Q., Zhao, B.-L., Li, M.-F., Shen, S.-R., and Xin, W.-J. (1996) Studies on Protective Mechanisms of Four Components of Green Tea Polyphenols Against Lipid Peroxidation in Synaptosomes. *Biochim. Biophys. Acta l304*, 210–222.
37. Zhao, B.-L., Guo, Q., Hou, J.-W., and Xin, W.-J. (1998) Study on Oxygen Free Radical and Natural Antioxidants with ESR Spin Trapping Technique, in *Modern Applications of EPR/ESR from Biophysics to Materials Science*, (Rudowicz, C.Z., Yu, K.N., and Hiraoka, H., eds.), Springer, New York, pp. 74–82.
38. Jovanovic, S.V., Steenken, S., Simic, M.G., and Hara,Y. (1998) Antioxidant Properties of Flavonoids: Reduction Potentials and Electron Transfer Reactions of Flavonoid Radicals, in *Flavonoids in Health and Disease*, (Rice-Evans, C., Packer, L., eds.), Marcel Dekker, New York, pp. 25–35.
39. Guo, Q., Zhao, B.-L., Hou, J.-W., and Xin, W.-J. (1999) ESR Study on the Structure-Antioxidant Activity Relationship of Tea Catechins and Their Epimers. *Biochim. Biophys. Acta 1427*, 13–23.

Chapter 7

Modulation of the Peroxynitrite-Scavenging Activity of Antioxidants by Physiologic Concentrations of Bicarbonate

Matthew Whiteman,[a] Uraiwan Ketsawatsakul,[b] and Barry Halliwell[a,b]

[a]Department of Biochemistry, National University of Singapore, Singapore 119260
[b]Antioxidant Research Group, GKT School of Biomedical Sciences, London SE1 9RT

Introduction

The interaction of nitrogen monoxide ($^{\bullet}NO$) and superoxide ($O_2^{\bullet-}$) forms the cytotoxic product peroxynitrite, ($ONOO^-$), as shown in Equation 1 (1).

$$^{\bullet}NO \quad + \quad O_2^{\bullet-} \longrightarrow ONOO^- \qquad (1)$$

The rate constant for this reaction is $>10^9$ $(mol/L)^{-1}{\cdot}s^{-1}$ (2). Under physiologic conditions, $ONOO^-$ has a half-life of <1 s, and it is converted to its protonated form, peroxynitrous acid, (ONOOH), which in turn decays to generate multiple toxic products with reactivities resembling those of the nitryl cation (NO_2^+), nitrogen dioxide radical ($^{\bullet}NO_2$), and hydroxyl radical ($^{\bullet}OH$). Peroxynitrite and species derived from it can oxidize lipids, proteins, DNA, and carbohydrates (3–7). The addition of $ONOO^-$ to biological fluids leads to the depletion of ascorbate and thiols (8). One product often used as a marker of $ONOO^-$ production *in vivo*, 3-nitrotyrosine, has been detected in numerous diseases and animal models of pathologic conditions (reviewed in Refs. 9,10).

An abundant constituent of body fluids is the inorganic anion bicarbonate (HCO_3^-), present at a concentration of ~25 mmol/L in the blood plasma and 12 mmol/L in intracellular fluids (11). The HCO_3^- dissolved in plasma and the cytosol is in equilibrium with carbon dioxide (CO_2), with a normal plasma concentration of 1.3 mmol/L. Together, the HCO_3^-/CO_2 system is one of the major pH buffering systems in the blood.

Peroxynitrite has long been known to be unstable in carbonate buffers (12). Later studies suggested that bicarbonate reacted with the peroxynitrite anion ($ONOO^-$) *via* formation of the nitrosoperoxycarbonate anion ($O{=}N{-}OOCO_2^-$) (13). However, this adduct was shown more recently to be formed from the reaction of $ONOO^-$ and CO_2 (14) present in equilibrium with HCO_3^- with a rate constant of formation, $k_2 = 3 \times 10^4$ $(mol/L)^{-1}{\cdot}s^{-1}$ at 25°C and 5.8×10^4 $(mol/L)^{-1}{\cdot}s^{-1}$ at 37°C (Equation 2), one of the fastest reactions known for $ONOO^-$ (14,15).

$$ONOO^- \quad + \quad CO_2 \longrightarrow ONOOCO_2^- \qquad (2)$$

High but physiologic concentrations of bicarbonate (5–30 mmol/L) diminish the bactericidal and parasiticidal activity of $ONOO^-$ (11,16), inhibit $ONOO^-$-dependent hydroxylation and nitration of phenylalanine (17) and benzoate (18), and inhibit methionine and glutathione (GSH) oxidation (19–21). However, peroxynitrite-dependent nitrations of tyrosine, guanine, *p*-hydroxyphenylacetate, phenol, and proteins are increased by added HCO_3^- (5,19–23). Interestingly HCO_3^- inhibits low density lipoprotein (LDL) and protein oxidation induced by $ONOO^-$ but enhances LDL and protein oxidation induced by the $ONOO^-$ donor, SIN-1 (24). Therefore, the HCO_3^-/CO_2 system significantly influences the reactivity and chemistry of $ONOO^-$ toward different biomolecules.

Because of the cytotoxicity of $ONOO^-$ and its apparent formation at sites of tissue injury (9,10), there has been considerable interest in the ability of natural and synthetic antioxidants to interfere with $ONOO^-$ damage (25–27). In this paper, the effects of HCO_3^- on the ability of some important antioxidants to prevent $ONOO^-$-mediated damage were examined using two model systems, i.e., $ONOO^-$-mediated tyrosine nitration and α_1-antiproteinase (α_1-AP) inactivation. Tyrosine nitration (9,10) and α_1-AP inactivation (28,29) are observed at sites of inflammation, and $ONOO^-$ formation provides a plausible mechanism (30). Hence, it is logical to use these target molecules in assays of agents able to protect against $ONOO^-$-dependent damage.

Materials and Methods

Materials. Ascorbic acid was obtained from Calbiochem (Poole, Dorset, England). Trolox, uric acid and all other compounds, including α_1-AP (A9024) and porcine elastase (E0258) were obtained from Sigma-Aldrich (Poole, Dorset, England) and were of the highest quality available commercially.

Synthesis of Peroxynitrite. Synthesis of peroxynitrite was essentially as described in Ref. 1. Briefly, an acidic solution (0.6 mol/L HCl) of H_2O_2 (0.7 mol/L) was mixed with KNO_2 (0.6 mol/L) on ice for 1 s and the reaction quenched with ice-cold NaOH (1.2 mol/L). Residual H_2O_2 was removed by mixing with granular MnO_2 prewashed with NaOH (1.2 mol/L). The stock solution was filtered and then frozen overnight (–20°C) and the top layer of the solution collected for the experiment. Concentrations of stock $ONOO^-$ were redetermined before each experiment at 302 nm using a molar absorption coefficient of 1670 $cm^{-1}\cdot(mol/L)^{-1}$ (31). Concentrations of 200–250 mmol/L were usually obtained. Once thawed, $ONOO^-$ solutions were kept on ice for no longer than 30 min before use.

Prevention of α_1-AP Inactivation. Elastase and α_1-AP were measured essentially as described in Ref. 25. Briefly, 40 µL of α_1-AP stock solution (4 g/L) was incubated in 100 mmol/L K_2HPO_4- KH_2PO_4 buffer, pH 7.4, containing 25 mmol/L $NaHCO_3$ and various antioxidants in a water bath for 15 min at 37°C. After this time, $ONOO^-$ (500 µmol/L) was added, the samples incubated for 5 min and 2.0 mL phosphate buffer added. Residual elastase activity was measured by the addition of 100 µL elastase substrate [succinyl $(Ala)_3$ *p*-nitroanilide, SANA; 4 g/L] and the change in absorbance at

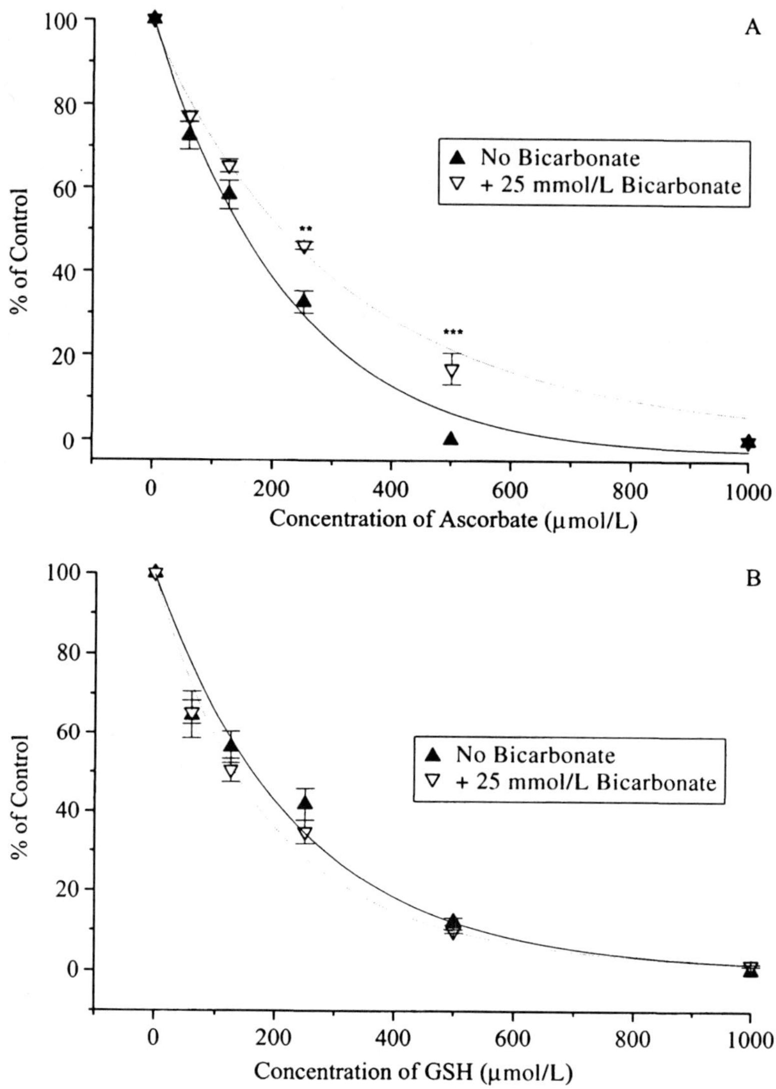

410 nm measured for 30 s. To assess the role of $ONOO^-$ decomposition products on α_1-AP activity, "decomposed" $ONOO^-$ was prepared by adding 500 μmol/L $ONOO^-$ to 100 mmol/L phosphate buffer, pH 7.4, at 37°C 5 min before the addition of α_1-AP or antioxidants (1,25).

Measurement of Tyrosine Nitration. Tyrosine nitration was measured as described in Ref. 32. Briefly, 1 mmol/L tyrosine was incubated in a solution containing 100 mmol/L K_2HPO_4-KH_2PO_4 buffer, pH 7.4, with 25 mmol/L $NaHCO_3$ and

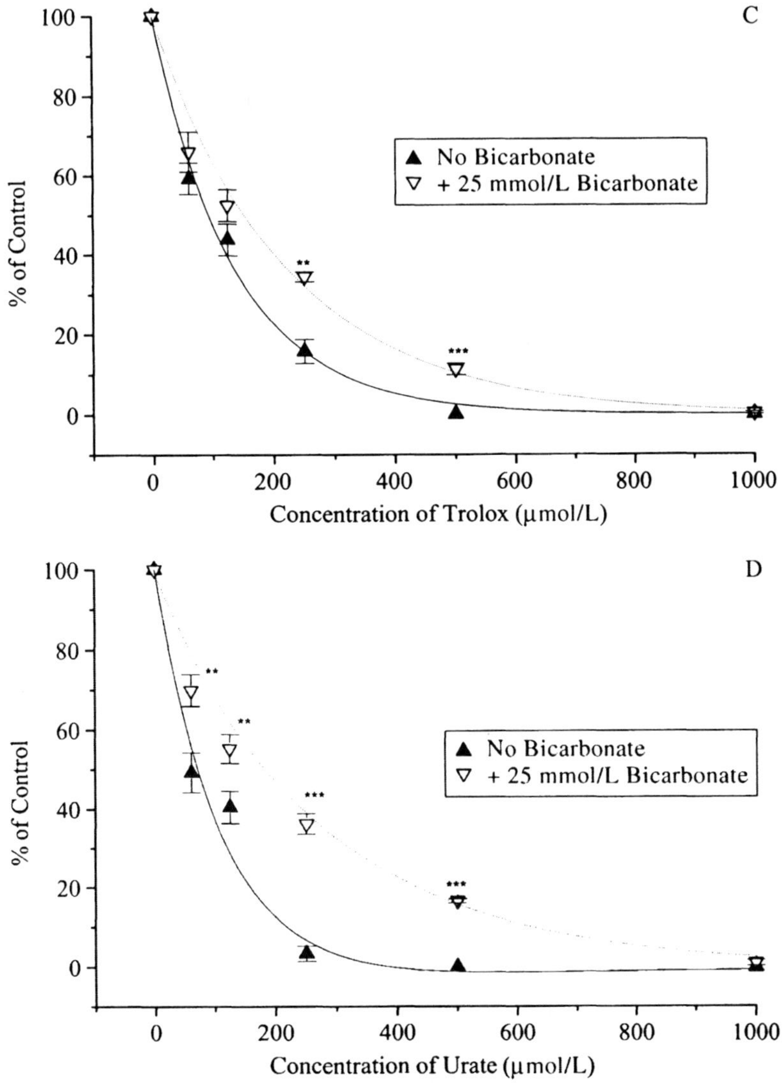

Fig. 7.1. Inhibition of tyrosine nitration by antioxidants: modulation by bicarbonate. (A) ascorbate, (B) glutathione (GSH), (C) Trolox, and (D) urate. Tyrosine (1 mmol/L) was incubated ± HCO_3^- (25 mmol/L) in phosphate buffer, pH 7.4, at 37°C for 15 min ± antioxidants (0–1 mmol/L) and $ONOO^-$ (1 mmol/L) added. 3-NO_2 tyrosine formed was measured by high-performance liquid chromatography (HPLC) as described in Materials and Methods. Data are means ± SEM of six or more independent experiments. Significance testing was performed using an independent *t*-test (Student's; 2 populations); $*P \leq 0.1$, $**P \leq 0.05$, $***P \leq 0.01$ comparing no HCO_3^- addition with HCO_3^- addition (25 mmol/L). Control = $ONOO^-$ + tyrosine in the presence or absence of HCO_3^-.

various antioxidants in a water bath for 15 mins at 37°C. Then 1 mmol/L $ONOO^-$ was added and the solutions further incubated for 15 min before high-performance liquid chromatography (HPLC) analysis. Peak area (retention time of 3.8 min) was measured and concentrations calculated from a standard curve. The detection limit for 3-NO_2 tyrosine was 0.1 µmmol/L.

Data Analysis. All graphs are plotted with mean values ± SEM. In all cases, the mean values were calculated from data taken from at least three separate experiments performed on separate days using freshly prepared reagents. When significance testing was performed, an independent *t*-test (Student's; 2 populations) was used; $*P \leq 0.1$; $**P \leq 0.05$; $***P \leq 0.01$.

Results

Inhibition of Tyrosine Nitration. When the amino acid tyrosine is exposed to $ONOO^-$ at pH 7.4, 3-nitrotyrosine is formed (1). As expected (8,25,32), the addition of 1 mmol/L $ONOO^-$ to a buffered solution of 1 mmol/L tyrosine led to the formation of 70–80 µmol/L 3-nitrotyrosine. The presence of ascorbate, GSH, Trolox or urate in the reaction mixture before $ONOO^-$ addition decreased the formation of 3-nitrotyrosine. Inclusion of 25 mmol/L bicarbonate in the reaction mixture led to a significantly higher yield of 3-nitrotyrosine, as expected (8) (95–110 µmol/L; $P < 0.01$). The presence of HCO_3^- significantly decreased the ability of ascorbate, urate and Trolox, but not that of GSH to inhibit tyrosine nitration (Fig. 7.1, A–D). Higher concentrations of these antioxidants were required in the presence of 25 mmol/L bicarbonate to achieve a similar degree of inhibition as in the absence of bicarbonate. This effect was more pronounced with urate, as previously reported (23). The addition of "decomposed" $ONOO^-$ (1) to a solution of tyrosine and bicarbonate did not result in the formation of detectable 3-nitrotyrosine (data not shown). Control experiments showed that the addition of HCO_3^- did not change the pH of the reaction mixture (data not shown).

Inactivation of α_1-AP. In agreement with previous studies (25,32), the addition of $ONOO^-$ led to substantial loss of the ability of α_1-AP to inhibit the proteolytic enzyme elastase. The inclusion of 25 mmol/L HCO_3^- in the reaction mixture resulted in a small (~10%) but significant ($P < 0.05$) decrease in the ability of $ONOO^-$ to inactivate α_1-AP. Addition of ascorbate, GSH, and Trolox to the reaction mixtures significantly protected α_1-AP from $ONOO^-$- mediated inactivation, whereas urate offered only slight protection even when tested at 1 mmol/L concentrations ($P < 0.5$), in accordance with previous results (25) (Fig. 7.2, A–D). However, in the presence of HCO_3^-, the ability of Trolox to protect α_1-AP against inactivation by $ONOO^-$ was increased (Fig. 7.2C). The protective effects of ascorbate and GSH were decreased in the presence of HCO_3^- only at 250 µmol/L and 1 mmol/L concentrations, respectively. Interestingly, in the presence of HCO_3^-, urate was able to protect α_1-AP against $ONOO^-$-mediated inactivation to a much greater extent than in the absence of HCO_3^- (Fig. 7.1D). However, protection was not complete at any of the concentrations tested.

Control experiments showed that none of the compounds tested interfered with elastase or the ability of α_1-AP to inhibit elastase or any other assay procedures used in this paper.

Discussion

Peroxynitrite-mediated oxidations are complex and involve one- and two-electron oxidation pathways involving $ONOO^-$, ONOOH and its oxidative decomposition products (1,9,10,17–24). The oxidative and nitrosative chemistry of $ONOO^-$ is significantly modified by the presence of HCO_3^-/CO_2. This rapid rate of reaction between CO_2 and $ONOO^-$ [one of the fastest known for $ONOO^-$; $k_2 = 3–5.8 \times 10^4$ $(mol/L)^{-1} \cdot s^{-1}$] (14,15) and the high normal plasma concentrations of bicarbonate and carbon dioxide in vivo (25 mmol/L and 1.3 mmol/L, respectively) make the reaction of $ONOO^-$ with HCO_3^-/CO_2 highly plausible *in vivo*. Higher levels of HCO_3^- and CO_2 could be achieved during pathologic events such as respiratory distress syndrome or ischemia-reperfusion injury (33) and probably other inflammatory conditions in which $ONOO^-$ formation has been shown to occur such as rheumatoid arthritis (reviewed in Refs. 9 and 10). The results of several investigators have suggested that HCO_3^-/CO_2 substantially modifies the reactivity of $ONOO^-$. Bicarbonate inhibits $ONOO^-$-mediated hydroxylation and nitration of phenylalanine and inhibits the oxidation of GSH and benzoate (18,20). HCO_3^- also decreases $ONOO^-$-mediated bactericidal actions (11,17). However, the effects of HCO_3^-/CO_2 are complex because enhancement of tyrosine, guanine, *p*-hydroxyphenylacetate, and protein nitration and increases in the rate of dihydrorhodamine and ABTS oxidation are observed (5,16,17,19,21–23,34). Therefore, examining the effects of antioxidants on $ONOO^-/HCO_3^-$–mediated processes was pertinent.

Bicarbonate enhanced tyrosine nitration, as previously reported (4,8). Although the direct rates of reaction between ascorbate, GSH, urate and Trolox with $ONOO^-$ may be fairly slow (35–37), these antioxidants significantly protected tyrosine from $ONOO^-$-mediated nitration. They may be reacting with nitrating species derived from $ONOO^-$/ONOOH rather than with $ONOO^-$/ONOOH themselves. Inclusion of HCO_3^- (25 mmol/L) in the reaction mixture impaired the ability of ascorbate, Trolox, and urate, but not that of GSH to inhibit $ONOO^-$-mediated tyrosine nitration at all concentrations tested. Due to their relatively high intracellular concentrations in some cells, GSH and ascorbate could be major intracellular targets for $ONOO^-$; in the extracellular milieu, however, levels are substantially lower (38). High extracellular concentrations of HCO_3^-/CO_2 could effectively outcompete these antioxidants for $ONOO^-$ in the extracellular space leading to increased nitrating ability. HCO_3^- is known to inhibit the oxidation of GSH by $ONOO^-$ (20). However, the ability of GSH to protect α_1-AP from $ONOO^-$-mediated inactivation was decreased only in the presence of HCO_3^- at high GSH concentrations (1 mmol/L) (30). Urate has been shown to react with $ONOO^-$ to form secondary species

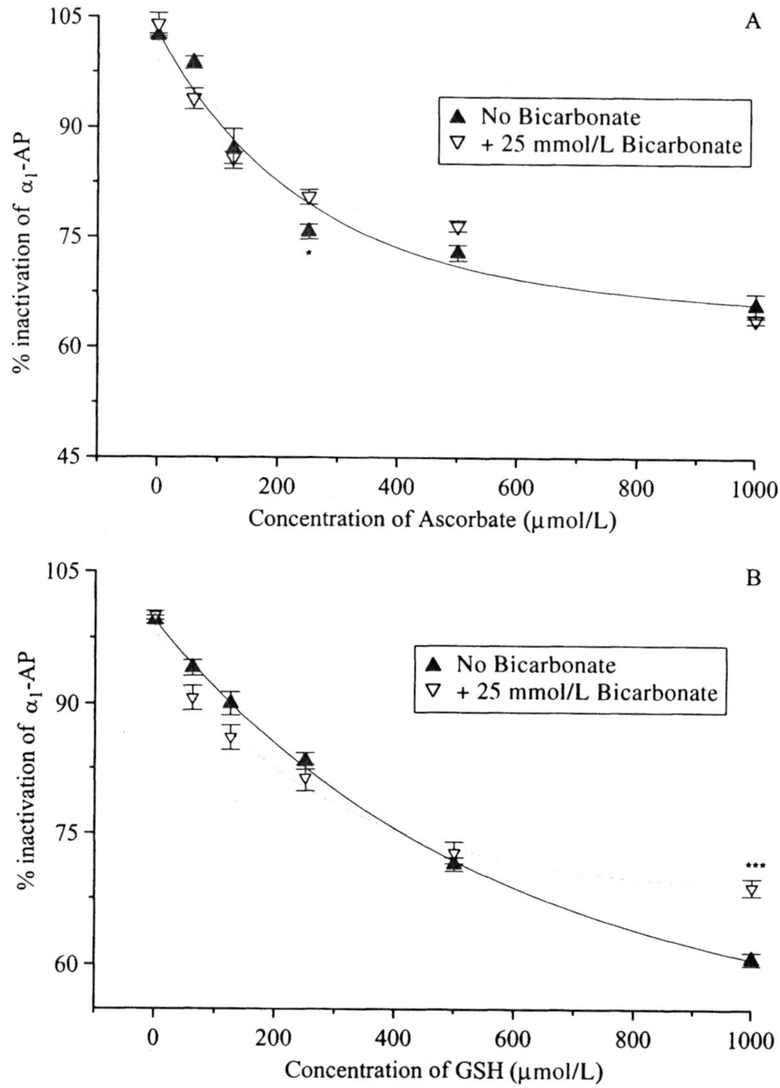

capable of inactivating α_1-AP (32) and recently to form free radical species, such as the aminocarbonyl radical, that are capable of accelerating $ONOO^-$-induced liposome and LDL oxidation [$k_2 = 4.8 \times 10^2$ $(mol/L)^{-1} \cdot s^{-1}$, pH 7.3, 37°C] (36). It is possible that HCO_3^- either quenches such α_1-AP–damaging radicals or inhibits their formation (Fig. 7.2D).

The $ONOOCO_2$ adduct is proposed to undergo either a heterolytic or homolytic cleavage at the weak peroxo O-O bond to give the strong oxidizing and nitrating species $^{\bullet}NO_2$ and $CO_3^{\bullet-}$ radicals or to give CO_3^{2-} and $^{+}NO_2$ ions (39,40). $CO_3^{\bullet-}$ is a

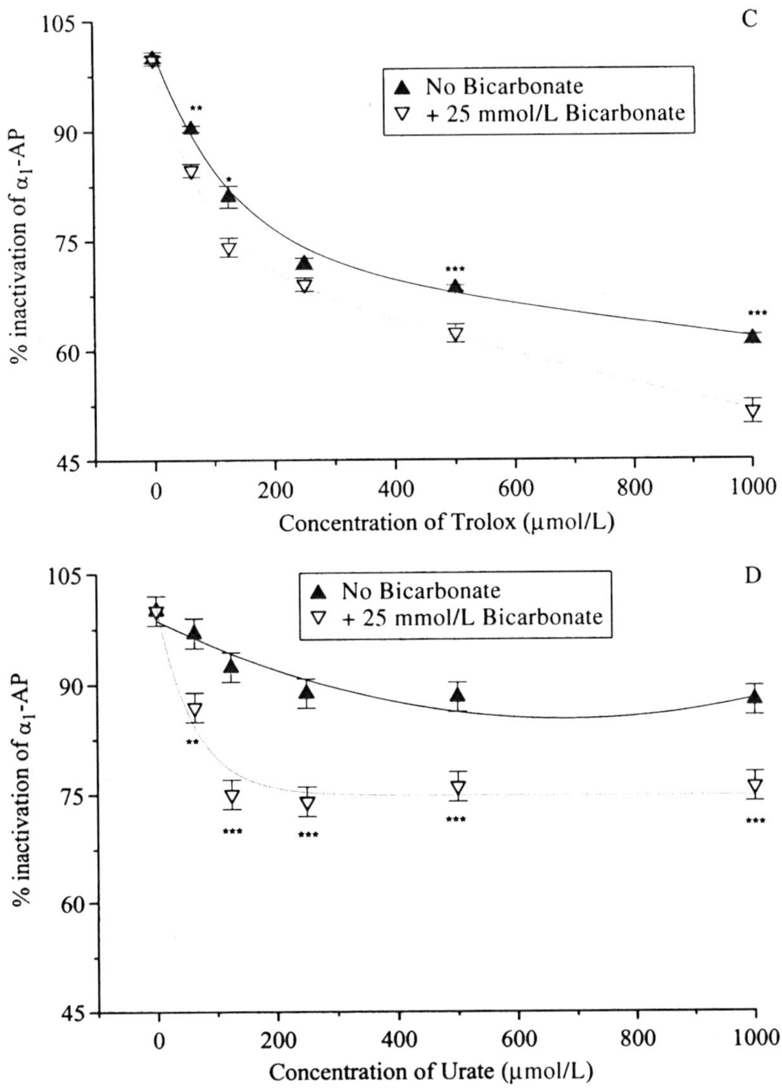

Fig. 7.2. Inhibition of $ONOO^-$-mediated α_1-antiproteinase (α_1-AP) inactivation by antioxidants: modulation by bicarbonate. (A) ascorbate, (B) glutathione (GSH), (C) Trolox, and (D) urate. α_1-AP (4 g/L) was incubated ± HCO_3^- (25 mmol/L) in phosphate buffer, pH 7.4, at 37°C for 15 min ± antioxidants (0–1 mmol/L) and $ONOO^-$ (500 μmol/L) added. Residual elastase activity was measured as described in Materials and Methods. Data are means ± SEM of six or more independent experiments. Significance testing was performed using an independent *t*-test (Student's; 2 populations); $*P \leq 0.1$, $**P \leq 0.05$, $***P \leq 0.01$ comparing no HCO_3^- addition with $NaCO_3$ addition (25 mmol/L). Control = $ONOO^-$-treated α_1-AP in the presence or absence of HCO_3^-.

strong one-electron oxidant, which may itself inactivate α_1-AP because it is known to inactivate enzymes and oxidize amino acids and proteins (41). The bactericidal potency of •OH generated extracellularly is enhanced when HCO_3^- is present in the reaction medium (16). •OH has also been shown to inactivate α_1-AP and to oxidize urate into species capable of inactivating α_1-AP (42). Formation of •OH directly from $ONOO^-$ is also possible to some extent (10,43,44). $CO_3^{\bullet-}$ reacts with various biomolecules 10^2–10^7 times more slowly than •OH, but as such, it may diffuse for longer to selectively reach and oxidize critical targets such as α_1-AP *in vivo* (41). However, whether $CO_3^{\bullet-}$ is responsible for α_1-AP inactivation must be investigated.

α_1-AP can be inactivated by $ONOO^-$ *via* the oxidation of its reactive site methionine (30). However, $ONOO^-$-mediated protein methionine oxidation is inhibited by CO_2 (19,22). Addition of HCO_3^- to the reaction media resulted in only ~10% reduction in the ability of $ONOO^-$ to inactivate α_1-AP. An additional mechanism may be *via* the oxidation of the protein's sole cysteine residue (45). Indeed, $ONOO^-$-mediated protein thiol oxidation is increased in the presence of HCO_3^- (46), and certain thiol compounds at low concentrations have been shown to aggravate $ONOO^-$-mediated inactivation of α_1-AP (32), a process enhanced by HCO_3^- (47). An alternate mechanism of α_1-AP inactivation may be *via* the nitration of one or more of the six tyrosine residues in the protein (48), a process enhanced by HCO_3^- (4,8,19,22). However, the precise mechanism of $ONOO^-$-mediated inactivation of α_1-AP in the presence of HCO_3^- is unknown; this is currently being investigated by our laboratory because $ONOO^-$ damages not only tyrosine, methionine, and cysteine residues in α_1-AP, but also many other amino acids (49).

Although local concentrations of bicarbonate (and CO_2) will ultimately determine the pathway of $ONOO^-$ decomposition formed *in vivo*, up to ~35% of the $ONOOCO_2^-$ intermediate produces reactive free radicals such as $^{\bullet}NO_2$ and $CO_3^{\bullet-}$ (40,50) that mediate nitration and oxidation reactions. Tyrosyl radicals are more effectively generated by the reaction of $ONOO^-$-derived $CO_3^{\bullet-}$ [$k = 4.5 \times 10^7$ (mol/L)$^{-1}$•s^{-1}] than by the reaction of $ONOO^-$-derived $^{\bullet}NO_2$ ($k = 10^4$–10^5) (22). The endogenous antioxidants tested here may not react quickly enough with the $ONOO^-/HCO_3^-$ adduct to prevent nitration and oxidation reactions to critical target molecules such as α_1-AP and tyrosine. Therefore, when assessing novel compounds for $ONOO^-$ scavenging abilities, experiments should be conducted in the presence of HCO_3^- to avoid misleading data.

Acknowledgments

We are grateful to the Arthritis Research Campaign (UK) and the National University of Singapore Academic Research Fund for their generous research support.

References

1. Beckman, J.S., Chen, J., Ischiropoulos, H., and Crow, J.P. (1994) Oxidative Chemistry of Peroxynitrite. *Methods Enzymol. 223*, 229–240.
2. Huie, R.E., and Padmaja, S. (1993) The Reaction of NO with Superoxide. *Free Radic. Res. Commun. 18*, 195–199.

3. Radi, R., Beckman, J.S., Bush, K.M., and Freeman, B.A. (1991) Peroxynitrite-Induced Membrane Lipid Peroxidation—The Cytotoxicity Potential of Superoxide and Nitric Oxide. *Arch. Biochem. Biophys. 288*, 481–487.
4. Ischiropoulos, H., and Al-Mehdi, A.B. (1995) Peroxynitrite-Mediated Oxidative Protein Modifications. *FEBS Lett. 364*, 279–282.
5. Yermilov, V., Yoshe, Y., Rubio, J., and Oshima, H. (1996) Effects of Carbon Dioxide/Bicarbonate on Induction of DNA Single-Strand Breaks and Formation of 8-Nitroguanine, 8-Oxoguanine and Base-Propenal Mediated by Peroxynitrite. *FEBS Lett. 399*, 67–70.
6. Spencer, J.P.E., Wong, J., Jenner, A., Aruoma, O. A., Cross, C.E., and Halliwell, B. (1996) Base Modification and Strand Breakage in Isolated Calf Thymus DNA and in DNA from Human Skin Epidermal Keratinocytes Exposed to Peroxynitrite or 3-Morpholinosydnonimine. *Chem. Res. Toxicol. 9*, 1152–1158.
7. Beckman, J.S., Beckman, T.W., Chen, J., Marshall, P.M., and Freeman, B.A. (1990) Apparent Hydroxyl Radical Production by Peroxynitrite: Implications for Endothelial Injury from Nitric Oxide and Superoxide. *Proc. Natl. Acad. Sci. USA 87*, 1620–1624.
8. Van der Vliet A., Smith, D., O'Neill, C.A., Kaur, H., Darley-Usmar, V., and Cross, C.E. (1994) Interactions of Peroxynitrite with Human Plasma and Its Constituents: Oxidative Damage and Antioxidant Depletion. *Biochem. J. 303*, 296–301.
9. Ischiropoulos, H. (1998) Biological Tyrosine Nitration: A Pathophysiological Function of Nitric Oxide and Reactive Oxygen Species. *Arch. Biochem. Biophys. 356*, 1–11.
10. Halliwell, B., Zhao, K., and Whiteman, M. (1999) Nitric Oxide and Peroxynitrite. The Ugly, the Uglier and the Not So Good. *Free Radic. Res. 31*, 651–669.
11. Zhu, L., Gunn, C., and Beckman, J.S. (1992) Bactericidal Activity of Peroxynitrite. *Arch. Biochem. Biophys. 298*, 452–457.
12. Keith, W.G., and Powell, R.E. (1969) *J. Chem. Soc. A*, 90.
13. Radi, R., Crosgrove, T.P., Beckman, B.A., and Freeman, B.A. (1993) Peroxynitrite-Induced Chemiluminescence. *Biochem. J. 290*, 51–55.
14. Lymar, S.V., and Hurst, J.K. (1995) Rapid Reaction Between Peroxynitrite Ion and Carbon Dioxide: Implications for Biological Activity. *J. Am. Chem. Soc. 117*, 8867–868.
15. Denicola, A., Freeman, B.A., Trujillo, M., and Radi, R. (1996) Peroxynitrite Reaction with Carbon Dioxide/Bicarbonate: Kinetics and Influence on Peroxynitrite-Mediated Oxidations. *Arch. Biochem. Biophys. 333*, 49–58.
16. Hurst, J.K., and Lymar, S.V. (1997) Toxicity of Peroxynitrite and Related Reactive Nitrogen Species Toward *Escherichia coli. Chem. Res. Toxicol. 10*, 802–810.
17. Van der Vliet, A., O'Neill, C.A., Halliwell, B., Cross, C.E. and Kaur, H. (1994) Aromatic Hydroxylation of Phenylalnine and Tyrosine by Peroxynitrite. *FEBS Lett. 339*, 89–92.
18. Lemercier, J.N., Padmaja, S., Cueto, R., Squadrito, G.L., Uppu, R.M., and Pryor, W.A. (1997) Carbon Dioxide Modulation of Hydroxylation and Nitration of Phenol by Peroxynitrite. *Arch. Biochem. Biophys. 345*, 160–170.
19. Bartlett, B.S., Levine, R.L., and Stadtman, E.R. (1998) Carbon Dioxide Stimulates Peroxinitrite-Medicated Nitrates of Tyrosine Residues and Inhibits Oxidation of Methionine Residues of Glutamine Synthetase: Both Modifications Mimic Effects of Adenylation. *Proc. Natl. Acad. Sci. USA 95*, 2784–2789.
20. Zhang, H., Squadrito, G.L., Uppu, R.M., Lemercier, J., Cueto, R., and Pryor, W.A. (1997) Inhibition of Peroxynitrite-Mediated Oxidation of Glutathione by Carbon Dioxide. *Arch. Biochem. Biophys. 339*, 193–189.

21. Uppu, R.M., Squadrito, G.L., and Pryor, W.A. (1996) Acceleration of Peroxynitrite Oxidations by Carbon Dioxide. *Arch. Biochem. Biophys. 327*, 335–34.
22. Tien, M., Bertlett, B., Levine, R.L., Chock, P.B., and Stadtman, E.R. (1999) Peroxynitrite-Mediated Modification of Proteins at Physiological Carbon Dioxide Concentration: pH Dependence of Carbonyl Formation, Tyrosine Nitration, and Methionine Oxidation. *Proc. Natl. Acad. Sci. USA 96*, 7809–7814.
23. Gow, A., Duran, D., Thom, S.R., and Ischiropoulos, H. (1996) Effects of Peroxynitrite-Induced Protein Modifications on Tyrosine Phosphorylation and Degradation. *FEBS Lett. 385*, 63–66.
24. Thomas, S.R., Davies, M.J., and Stocker, R. (1998) Oxidation and Antioxidation of Human Low-Density Lipoprotein and Plasma Exposed to 3-Morpholinosydnonimine and Reagent Peroxynitrite. *Chem. Res. Toxicol. 11*, 484–494.
25. Whiteman, M., and Halliwell, B. (1996) Protection Against Peroxynitrite-Dependent Tyrosine Nitration and α_1-Antiproteinase Inactivation by Ascorbic Acid: A Comparison with Other Biological Antioxidants. *Free Radic. Res. 25*, 275–283.
26. Hooper, D.C., Spitsin, S., Kean, R.B., Champion, J.M., Dickson, G.M., Chaudhry, I., and Kopowski, H. (1998) Uric Acid, a Natural Scavenger of Peroxynitrite, in Experimental Allergic Encephalomyelitis and Multiple Sclerosis. *Proc. Natl. Acad. Sci. USA 95*, 675–680.
27. Arteel, G.E., Briviba, K., and Sies, H. (1998) Protection Against Peroxynitrite. *FEBS Lett. 445*, 226–230.
28. Chidwick, K., Zhang, Z., Winyard, P.G., Farrell, A.J., and Blake, D.R. (1990) Inactivation of the Elastase Inhibitory Activity of α_1-Antityrpsin in Fresh Samples of Synovial Fluid from Patients with Rheumatoid Arthritis. *Ann. Rheum. Dis. 48*, 78–79.
29. Wong, P.S., and Travis, J. (1980) Isolation and Properties of Oxidized α_1-Proteinase Inhibitor from Human Rheumatoid Synovial Fluid. *Biochem. Biophys. Res. Commun. 93*, 1449–1454.
30. Moreno, J.J., and Pryor, W.A. (1992) Inactivation of α_1-Proteinase Inhibitor by Peroxynitrite. *Chem. Res. Toxicol. 5*, 425–431.
31. Hughes, M., and Nicklin, (1968) The Chemistry of Pernitrites. Part I. Kinetics and Decomposition of Pernitrous Acid. *J. Chem. Soc. A*, 450–452.
32. Whiteman, M., and Halliwell, B. (1997) Thiols and Disulphides Can Aggravate Peroxynitrite-Dependent Inactivation of α_1-Antiproteinase. *FEBS Lett. 414*, 497–500.
33. Levinski, N.G. (1994) in, *Harrison's Principles of Internal Medicine*, (Harrison, T.R., Isselbacher, K.J., Braunwald, E., Wilson, J.D., Martin, J.B., Farrer, A.S., and Pertersof, R.G., eds.)13th edn., pp. 253–262, McGraw-Hill, New York
34. Jourdheuil, D., Miranda, K.M., Kim, S.M., Espey, M.G., Vodovotz, Y., Laroux, S., Mai, C.T., Miles, A.M., Grisham, M.B., and Wink, D.A. (1999) The Oxidative and Nitrosative Chemistry of the Nitric Oxide Superoxide Reaction in the Presence of Bicarbonate. *Arch. Biochem. Biophys. 365*, 92–100.
35. Bartlett, D., Church, P.L., Pound, P.L., and Koppenol, W.H. (1995) The Kinetics of the Oxidation of L-Ascorbic Acid by Peroxynitrite. *Free Radic. Biol. Med. 18*, 85–92.
36. Santos, C.X.C., Edson, E.I., and Augusto, O. (1999) Uric Acid Oxidation by Peroxynitrite: Multiple Reactions, Free Radical Formation, and Amplification of Lipid Oxidation. *Arch. Biochem. Biophys. 372*, 396–294.

37. Quijano, C., Alvarez, B., Gatti, R.M., Augusto, O., and Radi, R. (1997) Pathways of Peroxynitrite Oxidation of Thiol Groups. *Biochem. J. 322*, 167–173.
38. Halliwell, B., and Gutteridge, J.M.C. (1990) The Antioxidants of Extracellular Fluids. *Arch. Biochem. Biophys. 280*, 1–8.
39. Bonini, M.G., Radi, R., Ferrer-Sueta, G., Ferreira, A.M., and Augusto, O. (1999) Direct EPR Detection of the Carbonate Radical Anion Produced from Peroxynitrite and Carbon Dioxide. *J. Biol. Chem. 274*, 10802–10806.
40. Meli, R., Nauser, T., and Koppenol, W.H. (1999) Direct Observation of Intermediates in the Reaction of Peroxynitrite with Carbon Dioxide. *Helv. Chim. Acta. 82*, 772–725.
41. Chen, S., and Hoffman, M. Z. (1973) Pulse Radioactive Studies of Sulphorous Compound in Aqueous Solution. *Radiat. Res. 56*, 40–47.
42. Aruoma, O.I., and Halliwell, B. (1989) Inactivation of α_1-Antiproteinase by Hydroxyl Radicals: The Effect of Uric Acid. *FEBS Lett. 244*, 76–80.
43. Richeson, C.E., Mulder, P., Bowry, V.W., and Ingold, K.U. (1998) The Complex Chemistry of Peroxynitrite Decomposition: New Insights. *J. Am. Chem. Soc. 120*, 7211–7219.
44. Coddington, J.W., Hurst, J.K., and Lymar, S.V. (1998) Hydroxyl Radical Formation During Peroxynitrous Acid Decomposition. *J. Am. Chem. Soc. 121*, 2438–2443.
45. Tyagi, S.C. (1991) Reversal of Inhibition of Neutrophil Elastase by Thiol Modified α_1-Proteinase Inhibitor. *J. Biol. Chem. 266*, 5279–5285.
46. Scorza, G., and Minette, M. (1998) One-Electron Oxidation Pathway of Thiols by Peroxynitrite in Biological Fluids: Bicarbonate and Ascorbate Promote the Formation of Albumin Disulphide Dimers in Human Blood Plasma. *Biochem. J. 329*, 405–413.
47. Whiteman, M., Ketsawataskul, U., and Halliwell, B. (2000) Enhancement of Thiol and Disulphide-Mediated Peroxynitrite-Dependent α_1-Antiproteinase Inactivation by Bicarbonate. *Br. J. Pharmacol. (Suppl. S) 129*, U124.
48. Miezewa, and Chan, S.K., (1987) Chemical Modification of Human α_1-Proteinase Inhibitor by Tetranitromethane. *Biochem. J. 246*, 37–42.
49. Whiteman, M. (1998) Mechanism of Oxidative Damage to Biomolecules in Rheumatoid Arthritis. Ph.D. Thesis. University of London. pp. 164–172.
50. Goldstein, S., and Czapski, G. (1998) Formation of Peroxynitrate from the Reaction of Peroxynitrite with CO_2: Evidence for Carbonate Radical Production. *J. Am. Chem. Soc. 120*, 3458–3463.

Chapter 8

Antioxidant and Prooxidant Effects of β-Carotene and Lycopene on Oxidant-Induced Damage in Hs68 Cells

Shu-Lan Yeh and Miao-Lin Hu

Department of Food Science, National Chung-Hsing University, Taichung, Taiwan ROC

Introduction

Carotenoids are a class of >600 natural pigments that are present in fruits and vegetables (1). Several carotenoids, especially β-carotene, have received tremendous research interest because they are found in high concentration in human blood (2). Epidemiologic studies have shown an inverse relationship between the intake of fruits and vegetables and the risk of several types of cancer (3); such effects of fruits and vegetables have been attributed to β-carotene (4). Both *in vitro* and animal studies have produced supportive results to this theory. Most notably, β-carotene was shown to be an effective antioxidant by scavenging certain reactive oxygen species (ROS), especially peroxyl radical and singlet oxygen, and this antioxidant activity appeared to be greatest at low oxygen tension (5,6).

However, recent clinical trials of supplemental β-carotene on the incidence and mortality of cancer and cardiovascular disease have produced disappointing results, i.e., β-carotene supplementation is either nonprotective (7) or even detrimental in smokers (8,9). Thus, the antioxidant and anticarcinogenic properties of β-carotene remain obscure and must be reexamined closely. A recent study in normal and tumor thymocytes showed that β-carotene is an antioxidant at low oxygen pressure but a prooxidant at high oxygen concentrations (10). In fact, the dependence of its antioxidant (or prooxidant) activity on oxygen pressure was noted earlier (5). β-Carotene was also shown to enhance lipid peroxidation induced by NO_2 (11). The few studies that have investigated the effects of β-carotene on DNA damage have produced conflicting results. For instance, a study in six nonsmoking and six smoking volunteers showed that a single dose of 45 mg β-carotene lowered oxidative damage to lymphocytic DNA as determined by the comet assay (12). In contrast, serum β-carotene levels were not found to be associated with the degree of DNA damage measured by the comet assay (13). It was suggested recently that some of the degradation products of β-carotene rather than β-carotene itself may be prooxidant or procarcinogenic (14). For example, in an experiment involving incubation of calf thymus DNA with rat liver microsomes treated with cytochrome P_{450}-inducing compounds, some of the degradation products of β-carotene enhanced the binding of benzo(a)pyrene to DNA, although β-carotene itself inhibits the binding (15). This observation may help explain the finding that β-carotene enhances respiratory tract cancer induced by benzo(a)pyrene in hamsters (16).

Recently, lycopene, an acyclic non-provitamin A carotenoid with 11 linearly arranged conjugated double bounds and found in relatively few foods, has received much research interest because of its potential antioxidant and antiproliferative properties (1). Lycopene has somewhat higher antioxidant activity than β-carotene. For example, lycopene is destroyed to a great extent than β-carotene in human skin irradiated with ultraviolet (UV) light (17). Other studies have shown that lycopene is more efficient than β-carotene in scavenging singlet oxygen (18) and peroxyl radicals (19) and in protecting lymphocytes against NO_2-induced membrane damage and cell death (20,21). However, contradictory findings also exist. For instance, when isolated low density lipoprotein (LDL) was enriched with various carotenoids *in vitro*, β-carotene but not lycopene (and lutin) protected against oxidation by copper ions, despite the fact that lycopene was destroyed more quickly than β-carotene (22). Similarly, in liposomes oxidized by peroxyl radicals, exogenous lycopene was destroyed more rapidly than other carotenoids including β-carotene but was least effective as an antioxidant (23). In addition, a study in healthy humans showed that dietary supplementation with β-carotene, but not lycopene (in the form of tomato juice) inhibits endothelial cell-mediated LDL oxidation (24). Interestingly, in that human study, one of the three subjects with higher serum lycopene level had elevated LDL oxidation (24). It is important to note that lycopene is structurally different from β-carotene only in its lack of the β-ionone ring (and thus devoid of vitamin A activity). Thus, the possibility that lycopene may have prooxidant activities similar to those of β-carotene cannot be ignored. The present study employed human foreskin fibroblasts (Hs68 cells) to investigate the antioxidant and prooxidant activities of β-carotene and lycopene under oxidative stress because the two compounds have rarely been compared using cell cultural systems. The oxidants used included 2,2′-azobis(2,4-dimethylvaleronitrile) (AMVN, a lipid-soluble radical generator), 2,2′-azobis(2-amidinopropane)dihydrochloride (AAPH, a water-soluble radical generator), and ferric nitrilotriacetate (Fe/NTA), a hepatic and renal carcinogen known to induce both lipid peroxidation and DNA damage (25,26).

Materials and Methods

All chemicals used were of reagent or higher grade. β-Carotene was from Sigma Chemical (St. Louis, MO). Lycopene, AAPH, AMVN, iron nitrate anhydrate, nitrilotriacetic acid (NTA), and tetrahydrofuran (THF) were from Wako Pure Chemical (Osaka, Japan). Dulbecco's modified Eagle medium (DMEM), fetal bovine serum (FBS), trypsin, penicillin, streptomycin, sodium pyruvate, and nonessential amino acids (NEAA) were from GIBCO/BRL (Rockville, MD).

Cell Culture. Hs68 cells were grown in DMEM medium containing 10% (vol/vol) FBS, 0.37% (wt/vol) $NaHCO_3$, penicillin (100 U/mL), streptomycin (100 μg/mL), 0.1 mmol/L NEAA, 1 mmol/L sodium pyruvate, and 5% CO_2 incubator at 37°C. The cells were harvested at ~90% confluence (10^6 cells/dish). The survival rate of cells was always >95% by trypan-blue assay (27).

Carotenoid Incorporation into Cells. Both the concentrations (10 and 20 μmol/L) and the method of incorporation of β-carotene and lycopene into Hs68 cells were adopted from those of Palozza *et al.* (10). A THF-carotenoid solution (5 mmol/L) was prepared freshly before each experiment. Aliquots of THF (~0.4%) or THF-carotenoid were added to Hs68 cells (~10^6 cells/dish) and incubated in 10 mL of 1X Hank's balanced salt solution buffer (HBSS), pH 7.4, at 37°C in the dark for 1 h. The cells were then washed 3 times in phosphate-buffered saline (PBS), pH 7.4, and the concentrations of β-carotene and lycopene were determined at 450 and 470 nm, respectively, after extraction in ethanol and hexane (1:2; vol/vol) as described previously (28).

Oxidative Challenge. To induce oxidative damage, carotenoid-enriched or control Hs68 cells (~10^6 cells/dish) were washed three times in PBS and incubated with an oxidant in 10 mL of 1X HBSS buffer at 37°C in the dark. AMVN was dissolved in methanol and was always included in the control experiments (at a final concentration of 5%). AAPH and Fe/NTA were dissolved in HBSS, and Fe/NTA was prepared by mixing 1 mmol/L $Fe(NO_3)_3$ with 4 mmol/L NTA just before the experiment (29). The reaction was terminated by adding butylated hydroxytoluene to a final concentration of 0.5 mmol/L.

Measurement of Lipid Peroxidation and Lactate Dehydrogenase Activity. Lipid peroxidation was measured as thiobarbituric acid-reactive substances (TBARS) released into the HBSS medium from Hs68 cells after centrifugation at 1000 × *g* for 10 min. TBARS were measured by mixing equal volumes of the supernatant with 0.7% TBA reagent and 2.5% trichloroacetic acid (30), heated at 100°C for 10 min, extracted with an equal volume (3 mL) of butanol, and measured at 515 nm excitation and 555 nm emission (31). The percentage of release of lactate dehydrogenase (LDH) was used as an index of cytotoxicity, and the activity was measured spectrophotometrically using pyruvate as substrate (32). Total LDH was measured in cell lysates obtained by treatment with 0.5% Triton X-100, and the percentage of release was determined by dividing the LDH activity in the medium by total LDH activity.

Measurement of 8-Hyroxy-2′-deoxyguanosine (8-OH-dG). DNA was isolated from Hs68 cells devoid of medium by centrifugation (10,000 × *g*, 10 min) using phenol/chloroform/isoamyl alcohol (33). An equal amount of DNA (200 μg) was then digested with nuclease P_1 and alkaline phosphatase, and the 8-OH-dG levels were analyzed by high-performance liquid chromatography (HPLC) with an electrochemical detector (Bioanalytical Systems, model LC-4C, West Lafayette, IN, USA) (34) as described previously (35). Oxidative damage was expressed as the molar ratio of 8-OH-dG to 10^5 molecules of deoxyguanosine (dG), which was calculated from the absorbance at 260 nm.

Comet Assay. The comet assay was adapted from the method of Singh *et al.* (36). After oxidant treatment, cells were suspended in low-melting-point agarose in PBS at 37°C and pipetted onto a frosted glass microscope slide precoated with a layer of 1% normal-melting-point agarose. After application of a third layer of 1% normal-melting-point agarose, the slides were immersed in cold-lysing solution (2.5 mol/L NaCl, 100 mmol/L EDTA, 10 mmol/L Tris, 1% sodium lauryl sarcosinate, 1% Triton X-100) for 1 h at 4°C. The slides were then placed in an electrophoresis tank, allowing the DNA to unwind for 15 min in the alkaline solution (300 mmol/L NaOH and 1 mmol/L EDTA). Electrophoresis was then performed at 300 mA for 20 min in the same alkaline solution at room temperature. The slides were then neutralized with 0.4 mol/L Tris-HCl buffer (pH 7.4) and stained with ethidium bromide. The image analysis was performed using the method of Collins *et al.* (37). One hundred comets on each slide were scored visually as one of five classes according to tail intensity and given a value of 0, 1, 2, 3, or 4. The total score for 100 comets ranged from 0 to 400.

Data Analysis. Values are expressed as means ± SD and analyzed using one-way analysis of variance (ANOVA) followed by Duncan's multiple range test.

Results

Lipid peroxidation. Table 8.1 shows the concentration effects of β-carotene and lycopene on oxidant-induced lipid peroxidation in Hs68 cells. In cells incubated with 1 mmol/L Fe/NTA for 2 h, enrichment with 10 and 20 μmol/L β-carotene only

TABLE 8.1 Concentration Effects of β-Carotene and Lycopene on Levels of TBARS in Hs68 Cells Incubated with an Oxidant[1,2]

	TBARS (nmol MDA equivalent/10^6 cells)[3]		
Treatment	Fe/NTA	AAPH	AMVN
Control	14.0 ± 0.9[a]	4.6 ± 1.1	4.2 ± 0.8[a]
+10 μmol/L β-carotene	12.5 ± 1.1[a]	4.0 ± 1.2	3.9 ± 0.7[a]
+20 μmol/L β-carotene	12.3 ± 0.8[a]	3.6 ± 1.1	5.7 ± 1.5[b]
+10 μmol/L lycopene	12.7 ± 0.8[a]	4.5 ± 0.8	4.4 ± 0.9[a]
+20 μmol/L lycopene	9.7 ± 0.7[b]	4.3 ± 0.9	5.9 ± 1.2[b]

[1]Cells were incubated with β-carotene or lycopene in the dark at 37°C for 1 h and then washed before incubation with 1 mmol/L Fe/NTA for 2 h or with 50 mmol/L AAPH and 50 mmol/L AMVN for 4 h.

[2]Abbreviations: TBARS, thiobarbituric acid-reactive substances; MDA, malondialdehyde; NTA, nitrilotriacetic acid; AAPH, 2,2′-azobis(2-amidinopropane)dihydrochloride; AMVN, 2,2′-azobis(2,4-dimethylvaleronitrile).

[3]Values (means ± SD of 3 experiments) in a column sharing a common letter are not significantly different ($P > 0.05$).

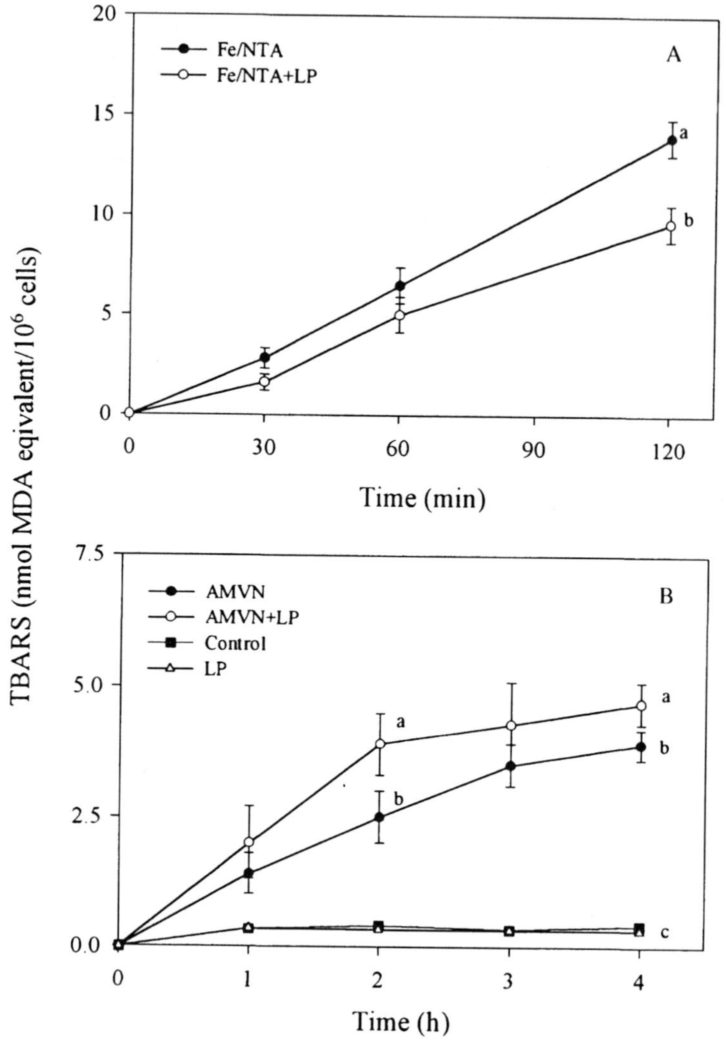

Fig. 8.1. Time course of the effects of 20 μmol/L lycopene (LP) on levels of thiobarbituric acid-reactive substances (TBARS) in Hs68 cells incubated with (A) 1 mmol/L Fe/nitrilotriacetic acid (NTA) or (B) 50 mmol/L 2,2′-azobis(2,4-dimethylvaleronitrile) (AMVN) at 37°C in the dark. Values (means ± SD of 3 experiments) at the same time points sharing a common letter are not significantly different ($P > 0.05$).

slightly ($P > 0.05$) decreased TBARS (from 14 to 12.5 and 12.3 nmol MDA/10^6 cells, respectively) and did not exhibit a concentration effect. However, 20 μmol/L lycopene significantly decreased TBARS (from 14 to 9.7 nmol MDA/10^6 cells) induced by 1 mmol/L Fe/NTA, and the effect of lycopene tended to be dose dependent. Neither β-carotene nor lycopene significantly affected lipid peroxidation during 4 h of incubation of cells with 50 mmol/L AAPH. In contrast, both lycopene and β-carotene increased TBARS released from Hs68 cells incubated with 50 mmol/L AMVN for 4 h, and TBARS released from the lycopene and β-carotene enriched cells were 40 ($P < 0.05$) and 36% ($P < 0.05$) higher than the AMVN control. The results show that lycopene was stronger than β-carotene in both antioxidant and prooxidant effects. The antioxidant and prooxidant effects of lycopene were further characterized by using 20 µmol/L lycopene to study the time course of lipid peroxidation induced by Fe/NTA and AMVN. Figure 8.1A shows a consistent inhibition of 1 mmol/L Fe/NTA-induced TBARS by lycopene during the 2-h incubation. By contrast, enrichment of cells with lycopene enhanced release of TBARS from Hs68 cells during the entire 4-h incubation with 50 mmol/L AMVN (Fig. 8.1B).

It is worth noting that β-carotene and lycopene are not stable in the presence of oxidants. Table 8.2 shows that incubation of β-carotene and lycopene with the oxidants for 1 h in the absence of cells led to the formation of malondialdehyde (MDA; measured as TBARS as described above and confirmed by HPLC with 532 nm absorption, data not shown). When incubated with 1 mmol/L Fe/NTA, β-carotene and lycopene at 20 µmol/L produced 3.04 and 3.66 µmol/L MDA, respectively, equivalent to 0.15 and 0.18 µmol/L MDA per µmol/L β-carotene or lycopene. When incubated with 50 mmol/L AMVN, β-carotene and lycopene at 20 µmol/L produced 0.20 and 0.19 µmol/L MDA, respectively, equivalent to 0.01 µmol/L MDA per µmol/L β-carotene or lycopene. These levels of MDA were subtracted from those obtained when Hs68 cells were present (data reported in Table 8.1).

DNA Damage. Although visual scoring is subjective, it shows a clear relationship to the percentage of DNA appearing in the tail, as measured by computer image analysis (36). Because DNA was damaged too extensively by 1 mmol/L Fe/NTA,

TABLE 8.2 Formation of Malondialdehyde (MDA) from β-Carotene and Lycopene Induced by Oxidants[1,2]

	MDA (µmol/L)	
Treatment	β-Carotene (20 µmol/L)	Lycopene (20 µmol/L)
Fe/NTA	3.04 ± 0.5	3.66 ± 0.34
AMVN	0.20 ± 0.10	0.19 ± 0.09

[1]β-Carotene and lycopene were dissolved in tetrahydrofuran solution and incubated for 1 h with the oxidant in the absence of cells. Values are means ± SD of 3 experiments.
[2]Abbreviations: NTA, nitrilotriacetic acid; AMVN, 2,2′-azobis(2,4-dimethylvaleronitrile).

TABLE 8.3 Effects of β-Carotene and Lycopene on DNA Damage Measured as Comet Formation in Hs68 Cells Induced by Oxidants[1,2]

	Arbitrary unit of comet assay[3]		
Treatment	Control	β-Carotene (20 μmol/L)	Lycopene (20 μmol/L)
Blank[4]	40 ± 15	—	—
Solvent control[5]	46 ± 24[a]	89 ± 33[b]	85 ± 38[b]
Fe/NTA	308 ± 46	284 ± 46	264 ± 34
AAPH	139 ± 26	133 ± 27	129 ± 26
AMVN	287 ± 119	277 ± 127	272 ± 104

[1]Cells were incubated with β-carotene or lycopene in the dark at 37°C for 1 h and then washed before incubation with 0.1 mmol/L Fe/NTA, 1 mmol/L AAPH or 1 mmol/L AMVN.
[2]Abbreviations: NTA, nitrilotriacetic acid; AAPH, 2,2′-azobis(2-amidinopropane)dihydrochloride; AMVN, 2,2′-azobis(2,4-dimethylvaleronitrile).
[3]Arbitrary unit is the total score of 100 comets ranging from 0 to 400 (each comet was scored visually as one of five classes according to tail intensity and given a value of 0, 1, 2, 3, or 4). Values (means ± SD of 3 experiments) in a row sharing a common letter are not significantly different ($P > 0.05$). Neither lycopene nor β-carotene enrichment significantly affected comet formation induced by any of the oxidants used.
[4]Blank refers to the no-solvent control, i.e., cells that were not incubated with a carotenoid or its solvent (tetrahydrofuran; THF) or with an oxidant or its solvent (water or methanol).
[5]Solvent control refers to the cells incubated with THF (solvent for lycopene and β-carotene) for 1 h at a final concentration of 0.4%. The cells were then incubated with methanol (solvent for AMVN) for 1 h at a final concentration of 5%. The solvent control and blank are not significantly different (Student's *t*-test, $P > 0.05$).

50 mmol/L AAPH, and 50 mmol/L AMVN, the cells were incubated with lower concentrations of the oxidants. Table 8.3 shows that the comet formation of most Hs68 cells treated with 1 mmol/L AAPH, 1 mmol/L AMVN, and 0.1 mmol/L Fe/NTA for 1 h was between class 0 and 2, between class 2 and 4, and between class 3 and 4, respectively. Both β-carotene and lycopene significantly elevated comet formation in the absence of an added oxidant over the solvent control and blank. Preliminary experiments show that the increased DNA damage may be caused by the autoxidized products of β-carotene and lycopene that occurred during incubation (data not shown). Neither β-carotene nor lycopene significantly affected comet formation induced by any of the three oxidants used. β-Carotene or lycopene enrichment also did not significantly affect DNA damage measured as 8-OH-dG in cells incubated for 2 h with 1 mmol/L Fe/NTA, 50 mmol/L AAPH, or 50 mmol/L AMVN (Table 8.4).

TABLE 8.4 Effects of β-Carotene and Lycopene on DNA Damage Measured as 8-OH-dG Content in Hs68 Cells Induced by Oxidants[1,2,3]

	8-OH-dG/10^5 dG		
Treatment	Control	β-Carotene (20 mol/L)	Lycopene (20 mol/L)
Control	ND	ND	—
Fe/NTA	5.8 ± 0.9	5.8 ± 1.1	4.5 ± 0.5
AAPH	6.1 ± 3.2	5.2 ± 2.3	6.3 ± 0.9
AMVN	9.1 ± 4.1	12.5 ± 5.1	7.9 ± 2.0

[1]Cells were incubated with β-carotene or lycopene in the dark at 37°C for 1 h and then washed before incubation with 1 mmol/L Fe/NTA for 2 h or with 50 mmol/L AAPH and 50 mmol/L AMVN for 4 h.
[2]Values are means ± SD of 3 experiments; ND, not detectable (<1.5 8-OH-dG/10^5 dG). Neither lycopene nor β-carotene resulted in significant differences in 8-OH-dG levels induced by any of the oxidants used.
[3]Abbreviations: 8-OH-dG, 8-hyroxy-2′-deoxyguanosine; NTA, nitrilotriacetic acid; AAPH, 2,2′-azobis(2-amidinopropane)dihydrochloride; AMVN, 2,2′-azobis(2,4-dimethylvaleronitrile).

Carotenoid Uptake and Consumption. Approximately 1–2% of the exogenous β-carotene and lycopene was incorporated into Hs68 cells after 1 h incubation at 37°C in the dark. Hs68 cells enriched with 20 μmol/L β-carotene and lycopene incorporated ~3.8 nmol lycopene/10^6 cells (or 6.3 nmol lycopene/mg protein) and 3.5 nmol β-carotene/10^6 cells (or 5.8 nmol β-carotene/mg protein), respectively. Figure 8.2 shows that oxidant incubation led to consumption of β-carotene (A) and lycopene (B) incorporated into Hs68 cells. The extent of loss of both β-carotene and lycopene by the oxidants was on the order of 50 mmol/L AMVN, 1 mmol/L Fe/NTA and 50 mmol/L AAPH. After incubation for 60 min, ~ 40% β-carotene remained in cells treated with 50 mmol/L AAPH or 1 mmol/L Fe/NTA, whereas only 10% β-carotene remained in cells incubated with 50 mmol/L AMVN (Fig. 8.2A). The loss of lycopene was faster than that of β-carotene in all three oxidants used. In cells treated with 50 mmol/L AAPH, 1 mmol/L Fe/NTA, and 50 mmol/L AMVN for 30 min, 60, 51 and 31% β-carotene remained (Fig. 8.2A) but only 46, 44 and 13% lycopene remained, respectively (Fig. 8.2B). Methanol was the solvent for AMVN and was used at a final concentration of 5%. At this level, methanol does not remove the carotenoids from the cells by a solvent effect.

Cell Morphology and Cytotoxicity. The cell morphology was markedly changed when the cells were incubated with 1 mmol/L Fe/NTA or 50 mmol/L AMVN at 37°C for 1 h, but it was not affected by 50 mmol/L AAPH for up to 4 h (data not shown). However, none of these oxidants increased cell lysis because the percentages of LDH

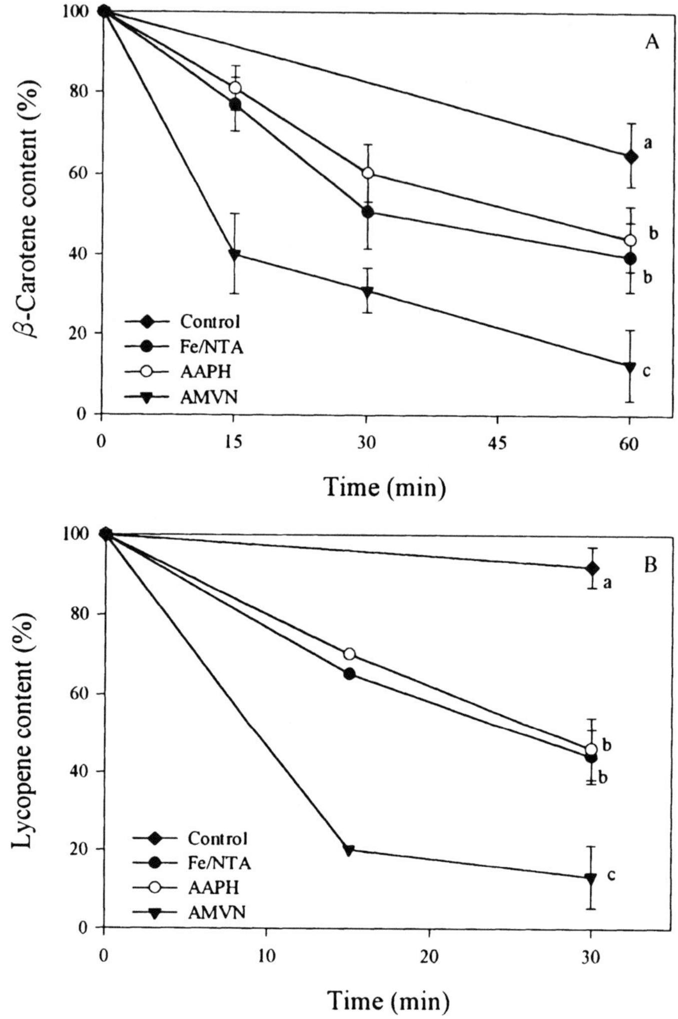

Fig. 8.2. Consumption of incorporated (A) β-carotene and (B) lycopene in Hs68 cells incubated in the dark with 1 mmol/L Fe/nitrilotriacetic acid (NTA), 50 mmol/L 2,2′-azobis(2-amidinopropane)dihydrochloride (AAPH), or 50 mmol/L 2,2′-azobis(2,4-dimethylvaleronitrile) (AMVN). Values (means of 2 experiments or means ± SD of 3 experiments) sharing a common letter are not significantly different ($P > 0.05$). The control refers to the methanol control, i.e., carotenoid-enriched cells incubated with methanol (the solvent for AMVN) at a final concentration of 5%.

released into the medium were not significantly different from that of the control (data not shown). Enrichment of the cells with either β-carotene or lycopene did not affect cell morphology (data not shown).

Discussion

Very few studies have used cell cultures to compare the antioxidant and/or prooxidant effects of β-carotene and lycopene. A recent study in normal and tumor thymocytes showed that β-carotene is an antioxidant at low oxygen pressure but a prooxidant at high oxygen concentrations (10). Our results from Hs68 cells at normal oxygen tension (under 95% air) demonstrated that lycopene and β-carotene can be either antioxidant or prooxidant depending on the type of oxidants used and that the effects of lycopene are somewhat stronger than those of β-carotene. The finding that lycopene also behaved as an prooxidant in Hs68 cells treated with AMVN is somewhat surprising because this carotenoid has been shown to be a better antioxidant than β-carotene (18–21). Thus, the two carotenoids are similar in their actions under oxidative stress. This similarity may be related to the fact that they contain the same polyene chain consisting of 11 conjugated double bonds, an important radical-scavenging structure of both compounds (6,38).

It is unclear how β-carotene and lycopene may enhance lipid peroxidation in Hs68 cells. However, two theories have been proposed to explain the possible prooxidant effects of β-carotene in smokers. One theory holds that β-carotene forms the radical cation by regenerating the vitamin E radical and that vitamin C is important in reducing the radical cation of β-carotene (39,40). It is well established that cigarette smokers have lower serum levels of vitamin C than do nonsmokers; hence, smokers may not have enough vitamin C to recycle the radical cation of β-carotene, which could damage important cellular macromolecules including DNA (39,40). However, because β-carotene is highly lipophilic and is located at the interior membrane, the water-soluble antioxidants such as vitamin C cannot efficiently reduce the carotene radicals. Thus, a second theory appears more likely, i.e., that β-carotene may react with the lipid peroxyl radical and form the radical cation, which can then be reduced by vitamin E (41,42). Vitamin C, in turn, can reduce the vitamin E radical to regenerate vitamin E and thus prevent the damaging effects of the β-carotene cation (41). In this context, it has been suggested that nutritional intervention using a combination of antioxidants, including β-carotene, vitamin E, and vitamin C, could be a rational approach to reduce cancer risk (14). The second theory may hold true for lycopene because the compound is extremely lipophilic and its reaction with lipid radicals may be confined to the hydrophobic inner core (1). In support of this theory, we showed here that the consumption of lycopene and β-carotene was much more extensive by the lipid-soluble AMVN than by the water-soluble AAPH and Fe/NTA. The carotenoid consumption by the oxidants was not due to a solvent effect (e.g., 5% methanol did not cause carotenoid loss) or to cell lysis because none of the oxidants significantly increased the percentage of LDH release (data not shown), although AMVN and Fe/NTA induced evident changes in cell morphology.

Little is known regarding the effect of β-carotene and lycopene on oxidative DNA damage *in vitro*. A recent study using the comet assay to study DNA damage in HT29 cells induced by xanthine/xanthine oxidase showed that both β-carotene and lycopene protect against DNA damage at relatively low levels (1–3 μmol/L) but rapidly lose this capacity, and in fact, may have enhanced such damage at higher concentrations (4–10 μmol/L) (43). These results are somewhat different from ours because we found no significant effects of β-carotene and lycopene on oxidant-induced DNA damage measured as comet formation. This discrepancy may have been due to several factors such as different cells, different oxidative systems, and slightly different concentrations of β-carotene and lycopene. However, our results from the 8-OH-dG assay also showed that β-carotene and lycopene did not significantly affect DNA damage induced by the three oxidants used. 8-OH-dG is a sensitive marker of DNA damage (6,33) and, unlike the comet assay, is a quantitative measure of DNA damage. As mentioned earlier (in Introduction), results from *ex vivo* studies on the effects of β-carotene on DNA damage are also mixed (12,13). Thus, whether β-carotene and lycopene affect oxidative DNA damage remains to be resolved. We found in this study that there was a slight increase in comet formation induced by both β-carotene and lycopene without oxidant treatment. This slight increase in DNA damage may be attributed to the presence of some preformed autoxidative products or the products formed during incubation (unpublished observation). In this context, we found that β-carotene and lycopene were not stable, especially when oxidants were present. MDA was detected when the carotenoids were heated (data not shown) or incubated with either Fe/NTA or AMVN (Table 8.2). The significance of this finding remains to be elaborated.

A question that may be asked is whether the concentrations used in the present *in vitro* study has any bearing *in vivo*. The mean human serum concentrations, which vary widely in different populations, range from 50 to 900 nmol/L (1). Thus, the concentrations (10–20 μmol/L) used in the present study and by others (10) seem rather high. However, it is possible that the serum lycopene concentration may be greatly increased by high intake of tomatoes and their products, which are the main dietary source of lycopene (1), and by nutritional supplements that contain lycopene. In fact, our results may have some relevance *in vivo* when comparing the levels of lycopene and β-carotene incorporated into Hs68 cells with the endogenous levels in human LDL. In the present study, ~1–2% of the 20 μmol/L carotenoids, i.e., ~3.5 nmol β-carotene/10^6 cells (or 5.8 nmol/mg protein) or 3.8 nmol lycopene/10^6 cells (or 6.3 nmol/mg protein) was incorporated into Hs68 cells in 1 h. These levels are similar to or slightly higher than the endogenous levels of β-carotene and lycopene in isolated human LDL (0.22–0.29 nmol β-carotene/mg protein and 0.37–2.0 nmol lycopene in three subjects) (22). Thus, it is possible that these cellular levels of β-carotene and lycopene are sufficient to exert antioxidant and/or prooxidant effects *in vivo*.

In summary, the present study in Hs68 cells demonstrates that both β-carotene and lycopene can be antioxidant or prooxidant depending on the types of oxidants used. Neither β-carotene nor lycopene affected DNA damage induced by Fe/NTA, AAPH, or AMVN. The similar effects of β-carotene and lycopene may be attributed to the similarity in their chemical structures. The results suggest that lycopene may not be an ideal replacement for β-carotene and that caution should be exercised in conducting clinical trials on lycopene, judging from the results of recent clinical studies on β-carotene.

References

1. Clinton, S.K. (1998) Lycopene: Chemistry, Biology, and Implications for Human Health and Disease. *Nutr. Rev. 56*, 35–51.
2. Cooper, D.A., Eldridge, A.L., and Peters, J.C. (1999) Dietary Carotenoids and Lung Cancer: A Review of Recent Research. *Nutr. Rev. 57*, 133–145.
3. Astrog, P. (1997) Food Carotenoids and Cancer Prevention: An Overview of Current Research. *Trends Food Sci. Technol. 8*, 406–413.
4. Peto, R., Doll, R., Buckley, J.D., and Sporn, M.B. (1981) Can Dietary Beta-Carotene Materially Reduce Human Cancer Rates? *Nature 290*, 201–208.
5. Burton, G.W., and Ingold, K.U. (1984) β-Carotene: An Unusual Type of Lipid Antioxidant. *Science 224*, 569–573.
6. Halliwell, B., and Gutteridge, J.M.C. (1999) *Free Radicals in Biology and Medicine*, 3rd ed., pp. 223–225, Oxford University Press, New York.
7. Hennekens, C., Buring, J., Manson, J., Stampfer, M., Rosner, B., Belanger, C., LaMotte, F., Gaziano, J., Ridker, P., Willet, W., and Peto, R. (1996) Lack of Effect of Long-Term Supplementation with Beta-Carotene on the Incidence of Malignant Neoplasms and Cardiovascular Disease. *N. Engl. J. Med. 334*, 1145–1149.
8. The Alpha-Tocopherol, Beta-Carotene Cancer Prevention Study Group (1994) The Effect of Vitamin E and Beta Carotene on the Incidence of Lung Cancer and Other Cancers in Male Smokers. *N. Engl. J. Med. 330*, 1029–1035.
9. Omenn, G.S., Goodman, G.E., Thoenquist, M.D., Balmes, J., Cullen, M.R., Glass, A., Keogh, J.P., Meyskens, F.L., Valanis, B., Williams, J.H., Jr., Barnhart, S., and Hammar, S. (1996) Effects of a Combination of Beta Carotene and Vitamin A on Lung Cancer and Cardiovascular Disease. *N. Engl. J. Med. 334*, 1150–1155.
10. Palozza P., Luberto C., Calviello G., Ricci P., and Bartoli G. M. (1997) Antioxidant and Prooxidant Role of β-Carotene in Murine Normal and Tumor Thymocytes: Effects of Oxygen Partial Pressure. *Free Radic. Biol. Med. 22*, 1065–1073.
11. Khopde, S.M., Priyadarsini, K.I., Mukherjee, T., Kulkarni, P.B., Satav, J.G., and Bhattacharya, R.K. (1998) Does β-Carotene Protect Membrane Lipids from Nitrogen Dioxide? *Free Radic. Biol. Med. 25*, 66–71.
12. Panayiotidis, M., and Collins, A.R. (1997) Ex Vivo Assessment of Lymphocyte Antioxidant Status Using the Comet Assay. *Free Radic. Res. 27*, 533–537.
13. Duthie, S.J., Ma, A., Ross, M.A., and Collins, A.R. (1996) Antioxidant Supplementation Decreases Oxidative DNA Damage in Human Lymphocytes. *Cancer Res. 56*, 1291–1295.
14. Wang, X.D., and Russell, R.M. (1999) Procarcinogenic and Anticarcinogenic Effects of β-Carotene. *Nutr. Rev. 57*, 263–272.
15. Salgo, M.G., Cueto, R., Winston, G.W., and Pryor, W.A. (1999) Beta Carotene and Its Oxidation Products Have Different Effects on Microsome Mediated Binding of Benzo(a)pyrene to DNA. *Free Radic. Biol. Med. 26*, 162–173.
16. Wolterbeek, A.P., Shoevers, E.J., Bruyntjes, J.P., Rutten, A.A., and Feron, V.J. (1995) Benzo(a)pyrene-Induced Respiratory Tract Cancer in Hamsters Fed a Diet Rich in Beta-Carotene: A Histomorphological Study. *J. Environ. Pathol. Toxicol. Oncol. 14*, 35–43.

17. Ribaya-Mercado, J.D., Garmyn, M., Gilchrest, B.A., and Russell, R.M. (1995) Skin Lycopene Is Destroyed Preferentially over β-Carotene During Ultraviolet Irradiation in Humans. *J. Nutr. 125*, 1854–1859.
18. Mascio, P.D., Kaiser, S., and Sies, H. (1989) Lycopene as the Most Efficient Biological Carotenoid Singlet Oxygen Quencher. *Arch. Biochem. Biophys. 274*, 532–538.
19. Miller, N.J., Sampson, J., Candeias, L.P., Bramley, P.M., and Rice-Evans, C.A. (1996) Antioxidant Activities of Carotenes and Xanthophylls. *FEBS Lett. 384*, 240–242.
20. Tinkler, J.H., Bohm, F., Schalch, W., and Truscott, T.G. (1994) Dietary Carotenoids Protect Human Cells from Damage. *J. Photochem. Photobiol. 26*, 253–285.
21. Bohm, F., Tinkler, J.H., and Truscott, T.G. (1995) Carotenoids Protect Against Cell Membrane Damage by Nitrogen Dioxide Radical. *Nat. Med. 1*, 98–99.
22. Romanchik, J.E., Harrison, E.H., and Morel, D.W. (1997) Addition of Lutin, Lycopene, or β-Carotene to LDL or Serum In Vitro: Effects on Carotenoid Distribution, LDL Composition, and LDL Oxidation. *J. Nutr. Biochem. 8*, 681–688.
23. Woodall, A.A., Britton, G., and Jackson, M.J. (1997) Carotenoids and Protection of Phospholipids in Solution or in Liposomes Against Oxidation by Peroxyl Radicals: Relationship Between Carotenoid Structure and Protective Ability. *Biochim. Biophys. Acta 1336*, 575–586.
24. Dugas, T.R., Morel, D.W., and Harrison, E.H. (1999) Dietary Supplementation with β-Carotene, but Not with Lycopene, Inhibits Endothelial Cell-Mediated Oxidation of Low-Density Lipoprotein. *Free Radic. Biol. Med. 26*, 1238–1244.
25. Ebina, Y., Okada, S., Hamazaki, S., Ogino F., Li, J.I., and Midorikawa, O. (1986) Nephrotoxicity and Renal Cell Carcinoma After Use of Iron- and Aluminum Nitrilotriacetate Complexes in Rats. *J. Natl. Cancer Inst. 76*, 107–113.
26. Iqbal, M., Giri, U., and Athar, M. (1995) Ferric Nitrilotriacetate (Fe-NTA) Is a Potent Hepatic Tumor Promoter and Acts Through the Generation of Oxidative Stress. *Biochem. Biophys. Res. Comm. 212*, 557–563.
27. Phillips, H.J. (1973) Dye Exclusion Tests for Cell Viability, in *Tissue Culture, Method and Applications*, (Kruse, P.F., and Patterson, M.K., eds.) pp. 406–408, Academic Press, New York.
28. Rundhaug, J.E., Pung, A., Read, C.M., and Bertram, J.S. (1988) Uptake and Metabolism of Beta-carotene and Retinal by C3H/10T1/2. *Carcinogenesis 9*,1541–1545.
29. Toyokuni, S., Uchida, K., Okamoto, K., Hatori-Hakakuri, Y., Hiai, H., and Stadtman, E. R. (1994) Formation of 4-Hydroxy-2-nonenal-Modified Protein in the Renal Proximal Tubules of Rats Treated with a Renal Carcinogen, Ferric Nitrilotriacetate. *Proc. Nat. Acad. Sci. USA 91*, 2616–2620.
30. Halliwell, B., and Gutteridge, J.M.C. (1981) Formation of a Thiobarbituric Acid-Reactive Substance from Deoxyribose in the Presence of Iron Salt. *FEBS Lett. 128*, 347–351.
31. Sano, M., Motchnik, P.A., and Tapple, A.L. (1986) Halogenated Hydrocarbon and Hydroperoxide-Induced Peroxidation in Rat Tissue Slices. *J. Free Radic. Biol. Med. 2*, 41–48.
32. Bergmeyer, H.U. (1974) Lactate Dehydrogenase Assay with Pyruvate and NADH, in *Methods of Enzymatic Analysis*, (Bergmeyer, H.U., ed.) vol. 2, pp. 574–579, Academic Press, New York.
33. Gupta, R.C. (1984) Nonrandom Binding of the Carcinogen *N*-Hydroxy-2-acetyl-aminofluorene to Repetitive Sequences of Rat Liver DNA In Vivo. *Proc. Natl. Acad. Sci. USA 81*, 6943–6947.

34. Shigenaga, M.K., Park, J.-W., Cundy, K.C., Gimeno, C.J., and Ames, B.N. (1990) In Vivo Oxidative DNA Damage: Measurement of 8-Hydroxy-2′-deoxyguanosine in DNA and Urine by High-Performance Liquid Chromatography with Electrochemical Detection. *Methods Enzymol. 186*, 521–530.
35. Hu, M.-L., and Shih, M.K. (1997) Ascorbic Acid Inhibits Lipid Peroxidation but Enhances DNA Damage in Rat Liver Nuclei Incubated with Iron Ions. *Free Radic. Res. 26*, 585–592.
36. Singh, N.P., McCoy, M.T., Tice, R.R., and Schneider, E.L.(1988) A Simple Technique for Quantitation of Low Levels of DNA Damage in Individual Cells. *Exp. Cell Res. 175*, 184–191.
37. Collins, A.R., Ai-Guo, M., and Duthie, S. J. (1995) The Kinetics of Repair of Oxidative DNA Damage (Strand Breaks and Oxidised Pyrimidines) in Human Cells. *Mutat. Res. 336*, 69–77.
38. Woodall, A.A., Lee, S., W-M., Weesie, R.J., Jackson, M.J., and Britton, G. (1997) Oxidation of Carotenoids by Free Radicals: Relationship Between Structure and Reactivity. *Biochim. Biophys. Acta 1336*, 33–42.
39. Truscott, T.G. (1996) β-Carotene and Disease: A Suggested Pro-Oxidant and Anti-Oxidant Mechanism and Speculations Concerning Its Role in Cigarette Smoking. *J. Photochem. Photobiol. 35*, 233–235.
40. Bohm, F., Edge, R., McGarvey, D.J., and Truscott, T.G. (1998) β-Carotene with Vitamins E and C Offers Synergistic Cell Protection Against NO_x. *FEBS Lett. 436*, 387–389.
41. Niki, E., Noguchi, N., Tsuchihashi, H., and Gotoh, N. (1995) Interaction Among Vitamin C, Vitamin E, and β-Carotene. *Am. J. Clin. Nutr. 62*, 1322S–1326S.
42. Mortensen, A., and Skibsted, L.H. (1998) Reactivity of β-Carotene Towards Peroxyl Radicals Studied by Laser Flash and Steady-State Photolysis. *FEBS Lett. 426*, 392–396.
43. Lowe, G.M., Booth, L.A., Young, A.J., and Bilton, R.F. (1999) Lycopene and Beta-Carotene Protect Against Oxidative Damage in HT29 Cells at Low Concentrations but Rapidly Lose This Capacity at Higher Doses. *Free Radic. Res. 30*, 141–151.

Chapter 9

Free Radical Scavenging and Antigenotoxicity: Mechanisms of Cancer Chemopreventive Effects of Plant Polysaccharides

Byung Mu Lee and Hyung Sik Kim

Division of Toxicology, College of Pharmacy, Sungkyunkwan University, Changan-ku, Chunchun-dong, Kyunggi-do, Suwon, 440-746, Korea

Introduction

Chemoprevention is a promising approach to reduce the incidence and control of human cancer by inhibiting biomarkers associated with carcinogenesis (1–3). In search of cancer chemopreventive agents, scientists have been working in various fields of cancer research. Consequently, many agents have been shown to be effective for chemoprevention of certain cancers, and other compounds are in clinical trials (4–6). For the investigation of chemopreventive agents, biomarkers have practical application because this approach is less time-consuming and less expensive. Validated biomarkers can serve as endpoints of multistage carcinogenesis and provide valuable insights into the mechanisms of carcinogenic processes (7,8).

Plant polysaccharides have been used worldwide as folk remedies, especially for chronic diseases, because their multiple biological properties include anti-inflammation, wound healing, immunomodulation, antihepatitis, antiulcer and antitumorigenic effects (9–11). Aloe polysaccharide was recently shown to exert an inhibitory effect on benzo(a)pyrene [B(a)P]-DNA adduct formation in rodent hepatocytes and animal systems (12,13). Plant polysaccharides from mushroom, *Basidiomycetes*, such as *Lentinus edodes, Ganoderma lucidum*, and from *Coriolus vesicolor* have also been shown to produce antineoplastic effects in tumor cell lines, leading to recommendations for use in cancer therapy (14,15). However, the mechanisms responsible for the chemopreventive effects of plant polysaccharide have not been demonstrated clearly.

In this paper, several plant polysaccharides were investigated comparatively for their chemopreventive effects and mechanisms of action using biomarkers such as DNA adduct formation, superoxide anion formation in phorbol myristate acetate (PMA)-induced HL-60 cells, and 8-hydroxy-2′-deoxyguanosine (8-OHdG), representing oxidative DNA damage.

Materials and Methods

Chemicals and Culture Media. [^{3}H]B(a)P (1.94×10^5 Bq/mmol), DL-ornithine hydrochloride [1-^{14}C] (7.32×10^3 Bq/mmol), and [γ-^{32}P]ATP (1.12×10^7 Bq/mmol) were purchased from Amersham (Arlington Heights, IL). DNAzol was purchased from MRC (Cincinnati, OH). Nuclease P1, Nonidet P-40, genistein, pyridoxal phosphate, poly(Glu-Tyr), Trizma base, SDS, RNase, and proteinase K were obtained from Sigma Chemical (St. Louis, MO). Mouse normal liver NCTC clone-1469 cells and human promyelocytic leukemia cells HL-60, were purchased from American Tissue Culture Collection (Manassas, VA). RPMI-1640, NCTC-115, fetal bovine serum (FBS), Dulbecco's modified Eagle's medium (DMEM), and Hanks' balanced salts solution (HBSS) were purchased from GIBCO (Grand Island, NY).

Isolation and Purification of Plant Polysaccharides. Four different plant polysaccharides were prepared from *Aloe barbadensis* Miller (APS) (Aloecorp, Harlingen, TX), *Lentinus edodes* (LPS), *Ganoderma lucidum* (GPS), and *Coriolus vesicolor* (CPS) as described previously (5). Briefly, the crude plant polysaccharide material was extracted with distilled water for 24 h at room temperature. After filtration, 70% ethanol was added to precipitate the polysaccharide, which was collected by centrifugation (15,000 × *g*, 30 min), dissolved in distilled water, dialyzed for 48 h against distilled water several times at 4°C, and lyophilized (Figs. 9.1, 9.2). The total polysaccharide content was measured by the phenol-sulfuric acid method (16). Protein content was determined by the Bradford method (17), and the sugar composition of crude polysaccharides was analyzed by high-performance liquid chromatography (HPLC) (18).

Quantification of $[^3H]$B(a)P-DNA Adduct Formation. Primary mouse hepatocytes or NCTC clone-1469 cells (1×10^7) were plated in culture flasks with 20 mL of NCTC-clone 115 medium supplemented with penicillin, streptomycin, and 10% FBS. The cells were maintained for 6 h, treated with $[^3H]$B(a)P (4 nmol/mL) in the absence (0) or presence of polysaccharides (6, 20, 60, or 180 g/mL) and incubated

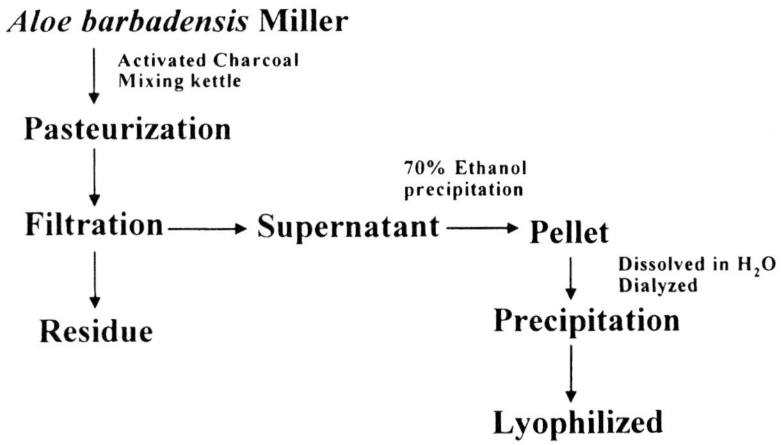

Fig. 9.1. Isolation of *Aloe* polysaccharide fraction.

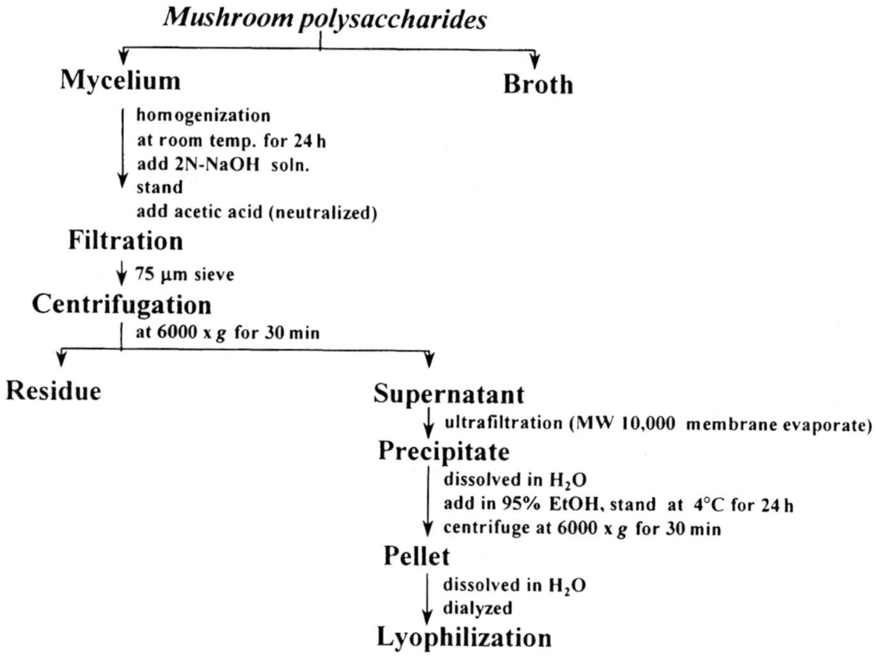

Fig. 9.2. Isolation and purification of mushroom polysaccharides.

for 12 h. After incubation, whole cells were harvested and washed twice with cold phosphate-buffered saline (PBS). The cells were resuspended in 0.1 mol/L phosphate buffer (pH 7.4). DNA was isolated from the cells by addition of DNAzol. The amount and purity of DNA were determined by ultraviolet (UV) absorbance at 260 and 280 nm (19). Radioactivity was measured by liquid scintillation counting (LKB 1215 Rackbeta, Pharmacia, Uppsala, Sweden) and expressed as pmol [^{3}H]B(a)P covalently bound/mg DNA (20).

Measurement of Superoxide Anion Formation. A modification of the method developed by Pick and Mizel (21) was used to detect the inhibition of free radical formation. HL-60 cells (1 × 10^6 cells) were plated in 96-well tissue culture flasks suspended in HBSS. Free radical formation was induced by treatment with PMA (8 mol/L), followed by addition of plant polysaccharide up to 180 g/mL simultaneously with ferricytochrome c (160 mol/L), and incubated at 37°C for 20 min. BSA was used as a blank, and superoxide dismutase (700 U) was used as a positive inhibitor. The rate of cytochrome c reduction was measured at 550 nm using 620 nm as a reference.

Measurements of Oxidative DNA Damage, 8-OHdG. In culture flasks, NCTC clone-1469 cells (1 × 10^7) were plated with 20 mL of NCTC-clone 115 medium containing 10% FBS. The cells were treated with B(a)P (4 nmol/mL) in the absence (0) or presence of polysaccharides (6, 20, 60, or 180 g/mL) and incubated for 12 h. Whole cells were harvested and washed twice with cold PBS after incubation. The cells were resuspended in 0.1 mol/L phosphate buffer (pH 7.4) and DNA was isolated as described previously (19). 8-OHdG levels as a marker of oxidative DNA damage were measured according to the method of Kasai *et al.* (22,23). Briefly, each 50 g of DNA was suspended in 50 L of 20 mmol/L sodium acetate buffer (pH 4.1) and denatured in boiling water for 10 min. The samples were digested to deoxynucleosides by incubation with 12 units of nuclease P1 at 37°C for 1 h in 40 L of 1 mol/L Tris-HCl buffer (pH 7.5). The resulting mixture was injected into HPLC equipped with both UV detector and an electrochemical detector (Waters 460, Millipore, Milford, MA); column, Supelcosil ODS (250 × 4.6 mm, 5-μm particle, Supelco, Bellefonte, PA); eluent, 10% aqueous methanol containing 12.5 mmol/L citric acid, 25 mmol/L sodium acetate, 30 mmol/L sodium hydroxide, and 10 mmol/L acetic acid; flow rate, 0.8 mL/min. The electrochemical detector (ECD) was set at 0.6 V and the level of 8-OHdG was analyzed.

Statistical Analysis. All values are expressed as means ± SD; samples were analyzed in triplicate. Statistical analysis of the data was performed using one-way analysis of variance (ANOVA) and the Bonferroni's test. *P*-values < 0.05 were considered significant.

Results

Antigenotoxic effects of plant polysaccharides on B(a)P-DNA adduct formation. Dose-dependent inhibition of [^{3}H]B(a)P-DNA adduct formation was demonstrated only with APS treatment (Fig. 9.3). APS significantly reduced [^{3}H]B(a)P-DNA adduct formation by 20–50% of the control (8.95 ± 2.13 pmol/mg DNA) at concentrations of 20–180 g/mL. On the other hand, GPS, LPS, and CPS showed no significant effect on DNA adduct formation even at the highest concentrations. In our experimental conditions, no cytotoxic effect on NCTC-clone 1469 cells was observed at the highest concentration of 180 g/mL.

Scavenging Effects of Plant Polysaccharides on Superoxide Anion. Inhibitory effects of APS, LPS, GPS, and CPS on free radical formation were investigated in PMA-induced human leukemia (HL-60) cell lines using a superoxide dismutase (SOD)-sensitive cytochrome c reduction system. In the culture system, a time-dependent increase in cellular production of free radicals was observed in HL-60 cells treated with PMA (data not shown). As shown in Table 9.1, APS and CPS showed significant scavenging effects on the free radical formation in PMA-induced HL-60 cells at 180 g/mL concentration. However, GPS and LPS had a marked but non-significant effect on PMA-induced inhibition of free radical formation.

Chemopreventive Effects of Plant Polysaccharides on 8-OHdG Formation.

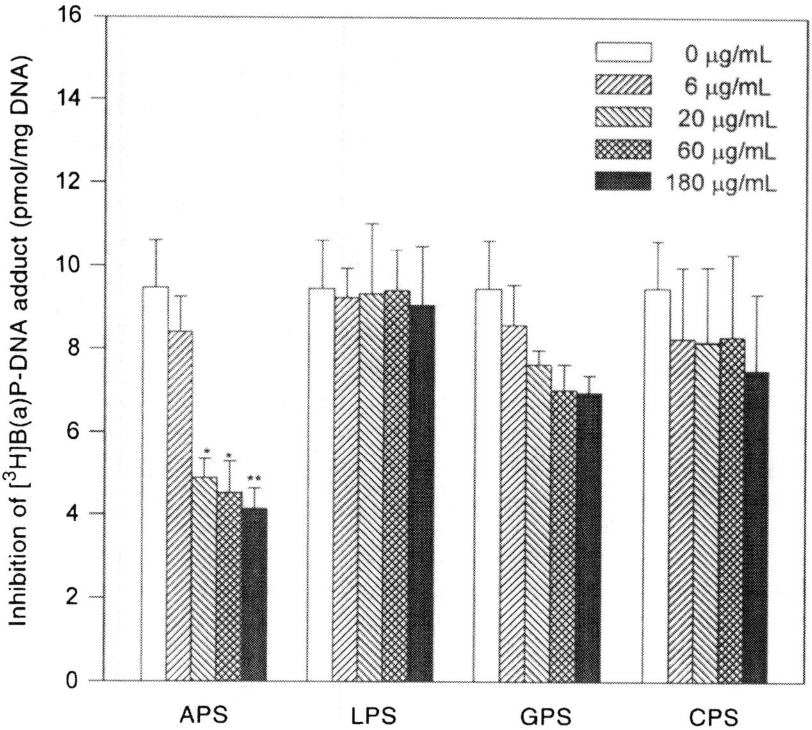

Fig. 9.3. Antigenotoxic effects of polysaccharides on [^{3}H]benzo(a)pyrene [B(a)P]-DNA adduct formation in NCTC-clone 1469 cells. The cells were incubated for 12 h in medium containing [^{3}H]B(a)P in the absence or presence of various polysaccharides. Asterisks indicate that values are significantly different from that of B(a)P alone, $*P < 0.05$ and $**P < 0.01$. Abbreviations: APS, *Aloe barbadensis* Miller; LPS, *Lentinus edodes*; GPS, *Ganoderma lucidum*; CPS, *Coriolus vesicolor.*

TABLE 9.1 Scavenging Effects of Polysaccharides on Superoxide Anion in HL-60 Cells Treated with Phorbol Myristate Acetate (PMA)[a,b]

Dose (µg/mL)	APS	LPS	GPS	CPS
0	100 ± 5.4	100 ± 5.4	1005.4	100 ± 5.4
6	92 ± 3.2	94 ± 2.3	95 ± 3.5	91 ± 1.5
20	75 ± 4.1[c]	81 ± 5.1	86 ± 4.7	79 ± 2.9
60	70 ± 6.5[c]	84 ± 5.6	79 ± 5.6	69 ± 6.1[c]
180	65 ± 2.1[c]	79 ± 2.7	81 ± 2.3	70 ± 3.2[c]

[a]The cells were treated with 80 mol/L PMA.

[b]Abbreviations: APS, *Aloe barbadensis* Miller; LPS, *Lentinus edodes*; GPS, *Ganoderma lucidum*; CPS, *Coriolus vesicolor.*

[c]Value is significantly different from control, $P < 0.05$.

TABLE 9.2 Chemopreventive Effects of Polysaccharides on Benzo(a)pyrene [B(a)P]-Induced 8-OHdG Formation in NCTC-Clone 1469 Cells[a,b]

Dose (μg/mL)	APS	LPS	GPS	CPS
0	4.25 ± 0.38	4.25 ± 0.38	4.25 ± 0.38	4.25 ± 0.38
6	3.69 ± 0.32	3.82 ± 0.21	3.73 ± 0.34	3.73 ± 0.62
20	3.52 ± 0.55	3.62 ± 0.36	3.68 ± 0.28	3.59 ± 0.55
60	3.48 ± 0.45	3.69 ± 0.44	3.59 ± 0.45	3.36 ± 0.45
180	3.13 ± 0.37[c]	3.43 ± 0.52	3.55 ± 0.35	3.02 ± 0.42[c]

[a]The cells were incubated for 24 h in medium containing B(a)P (1 μg/mL) with or without polysaccharides.
[b]Abbreviations: 8-OHdG, 8-hydroxy-2′-deoxyguanosine; APS, *Aloe barbadensis* Miller; LPS, *Lentinus edodes*; GPS, *Ganoderma lucidum*; CPS, *Coriolus vesicolor*.
[c]Value is significantly different from control, $P < 0.05$.

Inhibitory effects of APS, GPS, LPS and CPS on 8-OHdG formation are shown in Table 9.2. The background levels of 8-OHdG were 2.47 ± 0.76 residue/10^5 dG (data not shown), whereas a significant increase in 8-OHdG formation was observed in NCTC-clone 1469 cells treated with B(a)P (4.47 ± 0.76 residue/10^5 dG). APS and CPS significantly reduced 8-OHdG formation at concentrations of 180 g/mL, but LPS and CPS had no significant effect on B(a)P-induced 8-OHdG formation.

Discussion

The purpose of this study was to investigate chemopreventive potential and mechanisms of actions of plant polysaccharides widely used for folk remedies, using biomarkers expressed during multistage carcinogenesis. Our previous study indicated that APS polysaccharides exerted the greatest anticarcinogenic effect on inhibition of B(a)P-DNA adduct formation by interfering with B(a)P absorption *in vivo* (12). In that study, chemopreventive effects of four different plant polysaccharides on B(a)P-induced DNA adduct formation in NCTC-clone cells were analyzed comparatively. A dose-dependent inhibition of [^{3}H]B(a)P-DNA adduct formation was observed after APS treatment. It is possible that APS inhibits the uptake of B(a)P and subsequent binding to cellular DNA. However, enzymes such as P_{450} and glutathione *S*-transferase (GST) involved in B(a)P metabolism were not affected (data not shown), although chemopreventive mechanisms of some compounds were related to the inhibition of carcinogen activation systems or to the induction of detoxification enzymes (24). In our study, only GPS increased GST activity by 20–30% of control. The mode of action of GPS on GST activity is not clear, but the inducibility of GST by GPS appears to be related to the amount of protein present in polysaccharide-protein complexes.

There are various natural and synthetic antioxidants that possess both blocking and suppressing properties. The effect of certain fruits and vegetables containing high levels of natural antioxidants has been associated with scavenging of free radicals (25,26). Therefore, the inhibition of oxidative DNA damage induced by fruits and vegetables may serve as a basis for chemopreventive mechanisms. It has been suggested that mushroom polysaccharides possess superoxide- and hydroxy radical–scavenging activities (27). However, the mechanism of free radical scavenging by polysaccharides is still not fully understood. The protein content of polysaccharide fractions may be directly effective in free radical–scavenging activity. It is known that phenolic compounds may react with the superoxide radical by a one-electron transfer mechanism (28). APS and CPS also significantly inhibited free radical formation in PMA-induced HL-60 cells, but it is not still clear whether the mechanism of superoxide and hydroxyl radical scavenging by plant polysaccharides examined in this study is similar to that of phenolic compounds.

In conclusion, the chemopreventive potential of polysaccharides was evaluated comparatively using biomarkers associated with carcinogenic processes. Among plant polysaccharides investigated, APS was found to be the most effective in antigenotoxic and free radical–scavenging activities. These results suggest that the mechanisms underlying the activities of chemopreventive plant polysaccharides are free radical–scavenging and antigenotoxic effects.

References

1. Hong, W.K., and Sporn, M.B. (1997) Recent Advances in Chemoprevention of Cancer. *Science 278*, 1073–1077.
2. Boon, C.W., Kelloff, G.J., and Malone, W.F. (1990) Identification of Candidate Cancer Chemopreventive Agents and Their Evaluation in Animal Models and Human Clinical Trials: A Review. *Cancer Res. 50*, 2–9.
3. Bartsch, H., and Nair, J. (2000) New DNA-Based Biomarkers for Oxidative Stress and Cancer. *Eur. J. Cancer 36*, 1229–1234.
4. Wattenberg, L.W. (1985) Chemoprevention of Cancer. *Cancer Res. 45*, 1–8.
5. Sharma, S., Stutzman, J.D., Kelloff, G.J., and Steele, V.E. (1994) Screening of Potential Chemopreventive Agents Using Biochemical Markers of Carcinogenesis. *Cancer Res. 54*, 5848s–5855s.
6. Goodman, C.E. (1992) The Clinical Evaluation of Cancer Chemoprevention Agents: Defining and Contrasting Phase I, II and III Objectives. *Cancer Res. 52*, 2752s–2757s.
7. Lippman, S.M., Lee, J.S., and Lotan, R. (1990) Biomarkers as Intermediate End Points in Chemoprevention Trials. *J. Natl. Cancer Inst. 82*, 555–560.
8. Schatzkin, A., Freedman, L.S., Schiffman, M.H., and Dawsey, S.M. (1990) Validation of Intermediate End Points in Cancer Research. *J. Natl. Cancer Inst. 82*, 1746–1752.
9. Kobayashi, H., Matsuaga, K., and Fujii, M. (1993) PSK as a Chemopreventive Agent. *Cancer Epidemiol. Biomark. Prev. 2*, 271–276.
10. Sakai, R. (1989) Epidemiological Survey on Lung Cancer with Respect to Cigarette Smoking and Plant Diet. *Jpn. J. Cancer Res. 80*, 513–520.
11. Maeda, Y.Y., Takahama, S., and Yonekawa, H. (1998) Four Dominant Loci for the Vascular Responses by the Antitumor Polysaccharide, Lentinan. *Immunogenetics 47*, 159–165.
12. Kim, H.S., and Lee, B.M. (1997) Inhibition of Benzo(a)pyrene-DNA Adduct Formation by *Aloe barbadensis* Miller. *Carcinogenesis 18*, 771–776.
13. Kim, H.S., Kacew, S., and Lee, B.M. (1999) In Vitro Chemopreventive Effects of Plant Polysaccharides (*Aloe babadensis* Miller, *Lentinus edodes*, *Ganoderma lucidum*, and *Coriolus vesicolor*). *Carcinogenesis 20*, 1637–1640.

14. Wang, H.X., Liu, W.K., Ng, T.B., Ooi, V.E., and Chang, S.T. (1995) Immunomodulatory and Antitumor Activities of a Polysaccharide-Peptide Complex from a Mycelial Culture of *Tricholoma* sp., a Local Edible Mushroom. *Life Sci. 57*, 269–281.
15. Kobayashi, H., Matsunaga, K., and Oguchi, Y. (1995) Antimetastatic Effects of PSK (Keratin), a Protein-Bound Polysaccharide Obtained from Basidomycetes: An Overview. *Cancer Epidemiol. Biomark. Prev. 4*, 273–281.
16. Dubois, M., Gilles, K.K., Hamilton, J.K., Rebers, P.A., and Smith, F. (1956) Colorimetric Methods for Determination of Sugars and Related Substances. *Anal. Chem. 28*, 350–356.
17. Bradford, M.M. (1976) A Rapid and Sensitive Method for Quantitation of Microgram Quantities of Protein Utilizing the Principles of Dye Binding. *Anal. Biochem. 72*, 248–256.
18. Sturgen, G.J. (1990) Monosaccharides, in *Methods in Plant Biochemistry*, vol. 2, pp. 1–37, Academic Press, New York.
19. Kaizuka, H., and Takahashi, K. (1983) High-Performance Liquid Chromatographic System for a Wide Range of Naturally Occurring Glycosides. *J. Chromatogr. 258*, 135–146.
20. Choi, M.J., Lee, J.W., and Lee, B.M. (1996) Comparative Assessment of DNA Adduct Formation, *Salmonella* Mutagenicity, and Chromosome Aberration Assay as Short-Term Tests for DNA Damage. *J. Toxicol. Environ. Health 49*, 271–284.
21. Pick, E., and Mizel, D.C. (1981) Rapid Microassays for the Measurement of Superoxide and Hydrogen Peroxide Production by Macrophages in Culture Using an Automatic Enzyme Immunoassay Reader. *J. Immunol. Methods 46*, 211–226.
22. Kasai, H., Crain, P.F., Kuchino, Y., Nishimura, S., Ootsuyama, A., and Tanooka, H. (1986) Formation of 8-Hydroxyguanine Moiety in Cellular DNA by Agents Producing Oxygen Radicals and Evidence for Its Repair. *Carcinogenesis 7*, 1849–1851.
23. Kim, K.B., and Lee, B.M. (1997) Oxidative Stress to DNA, Protein, and Antioxidant Enzymes (Superoxide Dismutase and Catalase) in Rats Treated with Benzo(a)pyrene. *Cancer Lett. 113*, 205–212.
24. Davidson, N.E., Egner, P.A., and Kensler, T.W. (1990) Transcriptional Control of Glutathione *S*-Transferase Gene Expression by the Chemopreventive Agent 5-(2-Pyrazinyl)-4-methyl-1,2-dithiol-3-thione(oltipraze) in Rat Liver. *Cancer Res. 50*, 2251–2258.
25. Katiyar, S.K., and Mukhtar, H. (1997) Tea Antioxidants in Cancer Chemoprevention. *J. Cell Biochem.* (Suppl.) *27*, 59–67.
26. Shi, H., Hiramatsu, M., Komatsu, M., and Kayama, T. (1996) Antioxidant Property of *Fructus momordicae* Extract. *Biochem. Mol. Biol. Int. 40*, 1111–1121.
27. Liu, F., Ooi, V.E., and Chang, S.F. (1998) Free Radical Scavenging Activities of Mushroom Polysaccharide Extracts. *Life Sci. 60*, 763–771.
28. Wang, P.F., Kang, J.H., Zheng, R.L., Yang, Z.H., Lu, J.F., Gao, J.J., and Jia, Z.J. (1996) Scavenging Effects of Phenylpropanoid Glycosides from *Pedicularis* on Superoxide Anion and Hydroxyl Radical by the Spin Trapping Method (95)02255-4. *Biochem. Pharmacol. 51*, 687–691.

Chapter 10

Efficacy of Natural and Synthetic Antioxidants in RBD Palm Olein by Differential Scanning Calorimetry

C.P. Tan,[a] Y.B. Che Man,[a] J. Selamat,[b] and M.S.A. Yusoff[c]

[a]Department of Food Technology and [b]Department of Food Science, Faculty of Food Science and Biotechnology, Universiti Putra Malaysia, 43400 UPM Serdang, Selangor D.E., Malaysia
[c]Malaysian Palm Oil Board (MPOB), No. 6 Persiaran Institusi, Bandar Baru Bangi, 43000 Kajang, Selangor D.E., Malaysia

Introduction

The importance of vegetable oils as valuable commodities in world trade and for human nutrition is well recognized. Vegetable oil quality and stability are the main factors that influence its acceptability and market value. These characteristics can be physical, such as color, viscosity, or crystal structure, as well as those involving a chemical change, such as oxidation, hydrolysis, polymerization, or a change in flavor (1). Thus, maintenance of oil quality acceptable to the consumer is an important function of quality control in the oils and fats industry. One of the major deteriorative reactions that markedly affect oil quality is lipid oxidation (2). It may reduce the flavor and nutritive value of fats, oils, and lipid-containing products. For these reasons, a number of methods have been developed for evaluating the oxidative stability of edible oils. Basically, the analytical methods can be divided into two major groups, i.e., those measuring either the consumption of oxygen or oxidizing material or detecting the hydroperoxide products, and those measuring secondary oxidation products such as aldehydes, ketones, dimers, and polymers. A performance evaluation of the oil product in a frying application is also conducted occasionally to assess the oxidative stability of the oil (3). However, this effort is time-consuming and labor intensive. Therefore, oil and food processors are always seeking rapid methods with which to assess the stability of oils and fats (4).

Today, preference is given to various accelerated stability tests. Because oxidation is the major cause of oil degradation (5), most of the accelerated tests are designed to speed up the oxidation process by exposing oil samples to elevated temperatures in the presence of excess amounts of air or oxygen. Historically, the Schaal Oven Test (SOT) and the Active Oxygen Method (AOM) have been the most widely used (3). However, the SOT requires a large sample and a relatively long time period (4–8 d) to complete; the AOM is both time-consuming and expensive to run because of the requirement of repeated titration to determine peroxide value of an oil (3,6). Many objective instrumental and chemical methods have been proposed over the years to evaluate the quality and stability of edible oils. Currently, oxidative stability of oils and fats can be determined automatically by two commercially available instruments, the Rancimat from Brinkmann Instrument (Westbury, NY) and the Oxidative Stability Instrument from Omnion (Rockland, MA) (6). These methods monitor the volatile organic acids, which develop in thermally oxidized oil. Volatiles from the heated oil are trapped in deionized water, and their presence increases the electroconductivity of the water. The oxidative stability index (OSI) for a specific oil at a selected temperature is defined as the point of maximum change of rate of oxidation. A disadvantage of OSI is that fat-containing foods are difficult to test directly (3). Application of thermal analysis as a rapid oil stability test has been studied by several researchers. Cross (7) and Hassel (8) used differential scanning calorimetry (DSC) at isothermal modes with oxygen purge to measure the stability of oils. The end point of DSC was taken as the time at which a rapid exothermic reaction of oil and oxygen occurred. Hassel's results showed that oil samples that might require 14 d via AOM were evaluated in <4 h by DSC (8).

Synthetic as well as natural antioxidants are organic molecules; they can delay the development or progress of lipid oxidation. They are added to fats, oils, and foods containing fats to inhibit the development of off-flavors arising from the oxidation of unsaturated fatty acids (9). Such an inhibition mechanism leads to an increase in the antioxidant induction period, thus leading to a longer shelf life of packaged fatty food. Synthetic compounds such as butylated hydroxyanisole (BHA), butylated hydroxy-toluene (BHT), mono-tertiary butylhydroquinone (TBHQ), propyl-3,4,5-trihydroxy-benzoate, nordihydroquaiaretic acid, thiodipropionic acid, dilauryl thiodipropionate, and 1,2-dihydrox-6-ethoxy-2,2,4-trimethyl quinoline, or ethoxyquin are incorporated into edible oils to overcome the lipid oxidation (1). In recent years, antioxidants have been recognized for their health-promoting qualities (10). Therefore, much of interest has been devoted to preparing antioxidants from natural sources by extraction, purification, and isolation (11). Two methods are available for the inhibition of lipid oxidation of edible oils, i.e., the protection of indigenous antioxidants present and the promotion of new antioxidants produced *in situ* (12). Continued interest in natural compounds by consumers showed that they are just as concerned about their health as they are about the quality of the foods they consume. Many plants, spices, and herbs, including teas, cereals, oilseeds, sage, rosemary, and clove contain natural antioxidants (12,13).

As mentioned earlier, determining the time point at which edible oils reach their critical levels of oxidative deterioration is a challenging task. A rapid method for judging the relative stability of oxidative degradation would be of great importance to the edible oils industry, as well as for the selection of a suitable antioxidant and its optimum concentration in relation to the oil's stability. Therefore, the present study was designed to evaluate the efficacy of synthetic and natural antioxidants at different concentrations in preventing the oxidative degradation of refined, bleached, and deodorized (RBD) palm olein using the DSC technique.

Materials and Methods

Materials. RBD palm olein (without additives) was obtained from a local refinery [Ngo Chew Hong Oils and Fats (M) Sdn. Bhd., Semenyeh, Malaysia]. Tenox BHT and TBHQ were from Eastman Chemical Company (Kingsport, TN). BHA and α-tocopherol (TOCO) were purchased from Sigma Chemical (St. Louis, MO). Oleoresin rosemary (RE) (Herbalox Brand, Type O) and sage extract (SE) (Herbalox Seasoning, Type S-O) were gifts from Kalsec (Kalamazoo, MI). The appropriate amounts of synthetic (50–200 mg/kg) and natural (50–2000 mg/kg) antioxidants were added into RBD palm olein. Each sample was thoroughly mixed to ensure complete dispersion of the antioxidants. All chemicals and solvents used were of analytical grade unless otherwise mentioned.

Initial Oil Quality Analyses. The American Oil Chemists' Society (AOCS) methods (14) were used for determining the initial oil quality in terms of free fatty acid content (Method Cd 5a-40), iodine value (Method Cd 1b-87), peroxide value (Method Cd 8b-90), and anisidine value (Method Cd 18-90). The fatty acid composition of RBD palm olein was analyzed by capillary gas chromatography (GC). GC analysis was performed as described previously for edible oils (15).

DSC Analysis. The oxidative stability of oil was determined by a Perkin-Elmer differential scanning calorimeter DSC-7 (Norwalk, CT). The equipment was calibrated with pure indium, and the baseline was obtained with an empty open aluminum pan, which was used as the reference. Oil samples of 5.0 ± 0.5 mg were weighed in the pan and placed in the sample chamber. The isothermal temperature was programmed at 150°C, and purified oxygen (99.8%) was passed through the sample enclosure at 50 mL/min. The onset time (T_o) of the oxidation reaction

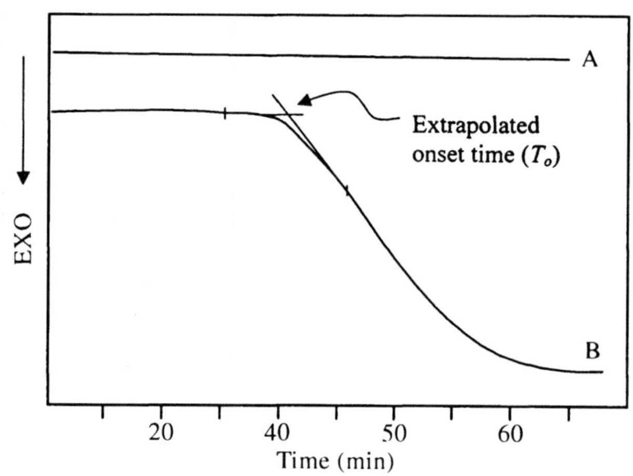

Fig. 10.1. Differential scanning calorimetric oxidation curve of refined, bleached, and deodorized palm olein without antioxidant. (A) isothermal curve at 150°C with nitrogen (99.999%) flowing at 50 mL/min; (B) isothermal curve at 150°C with oxygen (99.8%) flowing at 50 mL/min.

corresponded closely to the intersection of the extrapolated baseline and the tangent line (leading edge) of the exotherm (Fig. 10.1). This parameter was calculated with the 7 Series/UNIX DSC software library (16).

Statistical Analysis. The analytical data were analyzed using SAS software (Cary, NC); Duncan's multiple range test was used to compare differences among means. Significance was defined at $P < 0.01$. The SAS REG and RSREG procedures were conducted on T_0 and antioxidant levels (17). These procedures were used to fit simple linear and second-order polynomial equations to the results. From the best-fit equations, the standard deviations of the slopes, the intercepts of regression lines, and their correlation of determination were calculated.

Results and Discussion

The initial characteristics of RBD palm olein used in this study indicated that the oil was of good quality, as shown by its initial low peroxide value (0.82 ± 0.06 meq/kg), free fatty acid content (0.10 ± 0.01%), and anisidine value (1.33 ± 0.15). The iodine value (56.55 ± 0.32 g of I_2/100 g oil) and fatty acid composition of RBD palm olein were within the range for Malaysian palm olein.

Because lipid oxidation is accelerated at higher temperature, our research was aimed at determining the induction period for oxidation of RBD palm olein at high temperature appropriate for heating operations (e.g. frying, roasting, and microwave heating). The oxidation process in edible oil is primarily an exothermic reaction. This process can be reduced by antioxidant components, which prevent the attachment of

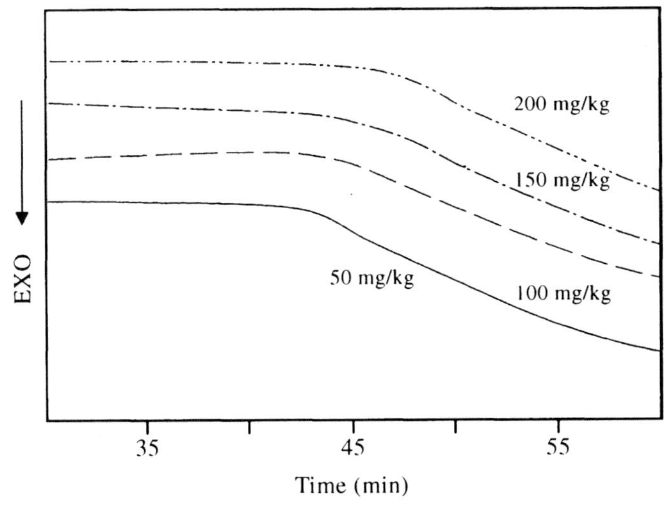

Fig. 10.2. Differential scanning calorimetric oxidation curves of refined, bleached, and deodorized palm olein with butylated hydroxyanisole (BHA) at various concentrations.

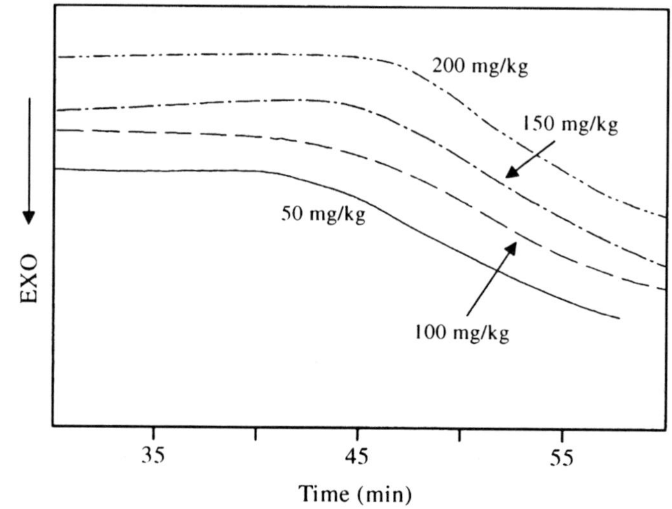

Fig. 10.3. Differential scanning calorimetric oxidation curves of refined, bleached, and deodorized palm olein with butylated hydroxytoluene (BHT) at various concentrations.

oxygen to an unsaturated fatty acid molecule, thus delaying the oxidation process in edible oil. The exothermic oxidation reactions produce traces such as those shown in Figure 10.1B. No exothermic peak (i.e., no oxidation reaction) was detected when the oil sample was scanned under nitrogen conditions (Fig. 10.1A). The extrapolated

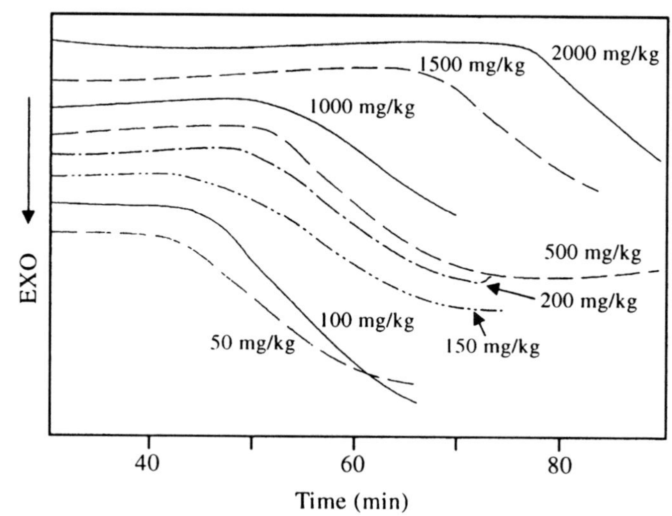

Fig. 10.4. Differential scanning calorimetric oxidation curves of refined, bleached, and deodorized palm olein with oleoresin rosemary (RE) at various concentrations.

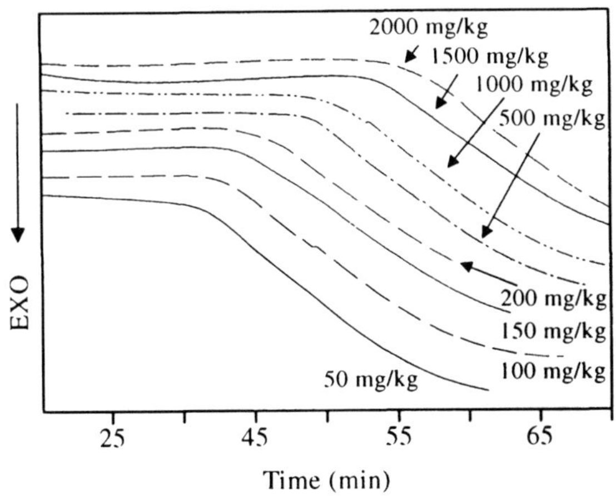

Fig. 10.5. Differential scanning calorimetric oxidation curves of refined, bleached, and deodorized palm olein with sage extract (SE) at various concentrations.

onset time (T_o) was taken as a measure of the relative stability of the oil toward oxidation. Figures 10.2–7 show examples of stacked DSC oxidation curves of RBD palm olein with the addition of various antioxidants at four or eight different levels. Because the chemical composition of the RBD palm olein was identical, oil systems containing higher amounts of antioxidant would have a longer extent of T_o. The T_o

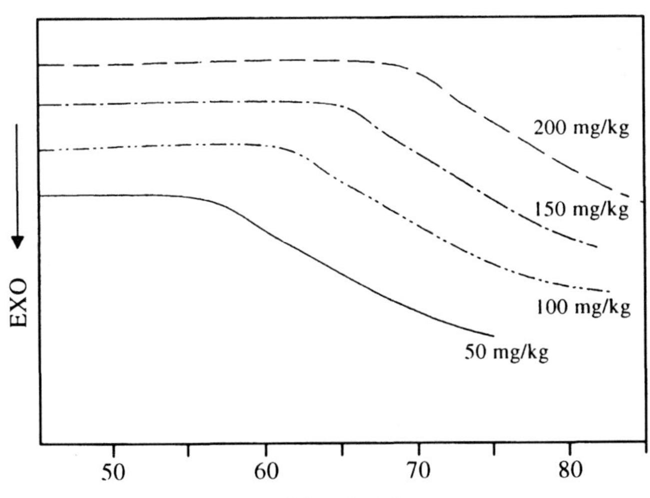

Fig. 10.6. Differential scanning calorimetric oxidation curves of refined, bleached, and deodorized palm olein with mono-tertiary butylhydroquinone (TBHQ) at various concentrations.

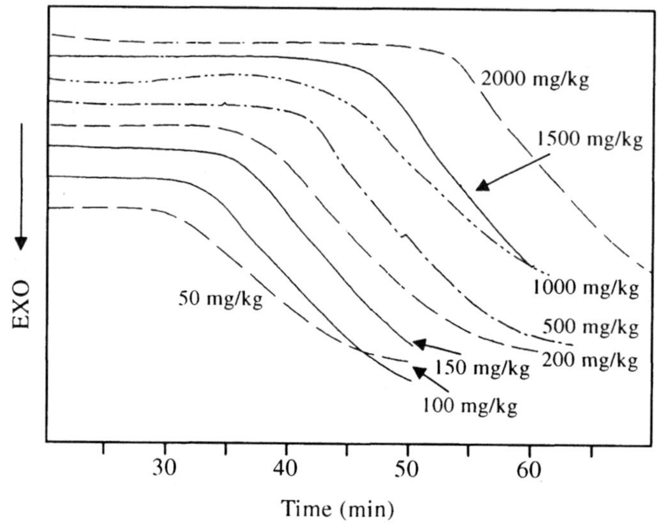

Fig. 10.7. Differential scanning calorimetric oxidation curves of refined, bleached, and deodorized palm olein with α-tocopherol (TOCO) at various concentrations.

of control RBD palm olein without any antioxidants was only 40.31 ± 0.15 min. The DSC oxidation data of each RBD palm olein with different antioxidants additions at four or eight levels are summarized in Table 10.1. For all antioxidants, the T_0 were significantly ($P < 0.01$) increased as the concentrations of antioxidants increased. Therefore, the results of this study indicated that increasing the amount of antioxidant significantly ($P < 0.01$) improved the oxidative stability of RBD palm olein. In general, these results also indicated that TBHQ was the most effective ($P < 0.01$) antioxidant in retarding the oxidation reaction in RBD palm olein. On the other hand, RE showed the greatest antioxidant activity among the natural antioxidants used in this study. Judging from the T_0 values, the order of activity found for antioxidants in RBD palm olein was TBHQ > RE > BHA ≈ BHT ≈ TOCO > SE, although some variation from this order was found, depending on the antioxidant concentration.

Because some synthetic antioxidants such as BHA, have been found to be toxic to experimental animals (18), natural compounds isolated from plant sources began to receive more attention as sources of safe antioxidants (19). Many plant extracts have been found to contain chemicals that have inhibitory activity against lipid oxidation. Rosemary and sage extracts are two potential natural antioxidants that could replace or lower the amount of synthetic antioxidants. They may be added as a natural antioxidant to foodstuffs in which slight flavor changes are not found objectionable by the consumer (9). In view of this fact, the results of this study suggest that RE and SE could replace those synthetic antioxidants, which have been questioned as a result of their possible undesirable side effects.

TABLE 10.1 Effects of Various Antioxidants on DSC Onset Time (T_o) Values of Refined, Bleached, and Deodorized Palm Olein[a,b]

Concentration (mg/kg)	DSC onset time (T_o) (min) BHA	BHT	RE	SE	TBHQ	TOCO
50	$42.52 \pm 0.33^{d}_{B}$	$42.45 \pm 0.07^{d}_{B}$	$42.66 \pm 0.33^{h}_{B}$	$41.08 \pm 0.29^{h}_{C}$	$55.59 \pm 0.36^{d}_{A}$	$40.58 \pm 0.26^{h}_{C}$
100	$43.57 \pm 0.20^{c}_{C}$	$43.78 \pm 0.15^{c}_{C}$	$45.71 \pm 0.27^{g}_{B}$	$42.58 \pm 0.09^{g}_{C}$	$61.11 \pm 0.41^{c}_{A}$	$42.56 \pm 0.20^{g}_{C}$
150	$45.23 \pm 0.30^{b}_{C}$	$45.69 \pm 0.30^{b}_{C}$	$47.55 \pm 0.20^{f}_{B}$	$44.32 \pm 0.15^{f}_{D}$	$64.93 \pm 0.45^{b}_{A}$	$45.10 \pm 0.41^{f}_{C}$
200	$46.61 \pm 0.12^{a}_{C}$	$46.93 \pm 0.38^{a}_{C}$	$50.32 \pm 0.36^{e}_{B}$	$45.73 \pm 0.42^{e}_{D}$	$68.59 \pm 0.19^{a}_{A}$	$46.81 \pm 0.31^{e}_{C}$
500			$51.26 \pm 0.14^{d}_{A}$	$48.64 \pm 0.24^{d}_{B}$		$51.10 \pm 0.32^{d}_{A}$
1000			$53.44 \pm 0.26^{c}_{A}$	$50.76 \pm 0.25^{c}_{B}$		$52.99 \pm 0.17^{c}_{A}$
1500			$67.18 \pm 0.24^{b}_{A}$	$53.23 \pm 0.12^{b}_{C}$		$56.73 \pm 0.31^{b}_{B}$
2000			$76.58 \pm 0.12^{a}_{A}$	$55.90 \pm 0.43^{a}_{C}$		$62.72 \pm 0.20^{a}_{B}$

[a]Each value in the table represents the mean ± SD of four analyses from two replications. Means within each column with different superscripts are significantly ($P < 0.01$) different. Means within each row with different subscripts are significantly ($P < 0.01$) different.

[b]Abbreviations: DSC, differential scanning calorimetry; BHA, butylated hydroxyanisole; BHT, butylated hydroxytoluene; RE, rosemary extract; SE, sage extract; TBHQ, mono-tertiary butylhydroquinone; TOCO, α-tocopherol.

The relationship between T_0 values and different levels of antioxidants was further subjected to linear and second-order (quadratic) polynomial regression analyses (Table 10.2). Generally, the results of the present study indicated that the coefficients of determination (R^2) for linear regression were > 0.88. For quadratic regression, the R^2 values were > 0.94. However, for all antioxidants, the statistical analysis of each equation showed a more linear (high F ratio value, $P < 0.001$) than quadratic (low F ratio value, $P < 0.05$) influence on the relationship between the T_0 value and different levels of antioxidants. The high correlation found between T_0 values and different levels of various antioxidants suggests that DSC can be recommended as an appropriate method for assessing the antioxidant activity in RBD palm olein.

Summary

The palm oil industry is concerned with the stability of its final products for use and under long storage conditions. One of the major phenomena leading to such problems is the lipid oxidation of unsaturated fatty acids. In this study, we attempted to establish a relationship between the various synthetic and natural antioxidants in RBD palm olein system and its oxidative stability. On the basis of the data presented, the onset time T_0 was delayed by increasing the antioxidant concentration. Therefore, it was concluded that the DSC method provided a quick way for determining the efficacy of antioxidants in maintaining the oxidative stability of RBD palm olein. The technique used in this study may also be applied to other edible oil systems or lipid-containing products, as well as to the selection of an appropriate antioxidant (or combination of antioxidants) and its optimum level in various edible oils. The DSC method is simple, safe, and rapid, and is appropriate for routine analysis in the oils and fats industry.

Acknowledgment

This research work was supported by the Universiti Putra Malaysia, under IRPA Project 03-02-04-003.

References

1. Smouse, T.H. (1995) in *Methods to Assess Quality and Stability of Oils and Fat-Containing Foods*, (Warner, K., and Eskin, N.A.M., eds.) pp. 17–36, AOCS Press, Champaign, IL.
2. Alexander, J.C. (1978) Biological Effects Due to Changes in Fats During Heating. *J. Am. Oil Chem. Soc. 55*, 711–717.
3. Wan, P.J. (1995) in *Methods to Assess Quality and Stability of Oils and Fat-Containing Foods*, (Warner, K., and Eskin, N.A.M., eds.) pp. 17–36, AOCS Press, Champaign, IL.
4. Hill, S.E., and Perkins, E.G. (1995) Determination of Oxidative Stability of Soybean Oil with the Oxidative Stability Instrument: Operation Parameter Effects. *J. Am. Oil Chem. Soc. 72*, 741–743.

TABLE 10.2 Relationship Between DSC Onset Time (T_o) Values and Different Levels of Antioxidants in Refined, Bleached, and Deodorized Palm Olein

Antioxidant	DSC onset time (T_o) vs. antioxidant level			
	Regression equation (Linear regression)[a]	Correlation of determination, R^2	Regression equation (Second-order polynomial regression)[b]	Correlation of determination, R^2
BHA	$y = 40.5841 + 0.0306x$	0.9807	—[c]	—[c]
BHT	$y = 40.5366 + 0.0329x$	0.9848	$y = 40.3613 + 0.0399x - 3.5\text{E-}05x^2$	0.9887
RE	$y = 43.1105 + 0.0158x$	0.9418	$y = 43.9971 + 0.0103x + 2.9\text{E-}06x^2$	0.9496
SE	$y = 42.5102 + 0.0073x$	0.9131	$y = 41.5288 + 0.0134x - 3.3\text{E-}06x^2$	0.9568
TBHQ	$y = 44.9233 + 0.1318x$	0.8883	$y = 41.3612 + 0.2743x - 7.1\text{E-}04x^2$	0.9791
TOCO	$y = 42.4928 + 0.0103x$	0.9328	$y = 41.6933 + 0.0152x - 2.7\text{E-}06x^2$	0.9477

[a]Significance at 0.001 level ($P < 0.001$).
[b]Significance at 0.05 level ($P < 0.05$).
[c]The quadratic equation was not statistically significant ($P > 0.05$).
Abbreviations: see Table 10.1.

5. Paul, S., and Mittal, G.S. (1997) Regulation the Use of Degraded Oil/Fat in Deep-Fat/Oil Food Frying. *Crit. Rev. Food Sci. Nutr. 37*, 635–662.
6. Akoh, C.C. (1994) Oxidative Stability of Fat Substitutes and Vegetable Oils by the Oxidative Stability Index Method. *J. Am. Oil Chem. Soc. 71*, 211–216.
7. Cross, C.K. (1970) Oil Stability: A DSC Alternative for the Active Oxygen Method. *J. Am. Oil Chem. Soc. 47*, 229–230.
8. Hassel, R.L. (1976) Thermal Analysis: An Alternative Method of Measuring Oil Stability. *J. Am. Oil Chem. Soc. 53*, 179–181.
9. Che Man, Y.B., and Tan, C.P. (1999) Effects of Natural and Synthetic Antioxidants on Changes in Refined, Bleached, and Deodorized Palm Olein During Deep-Fat Frying of Potato Chips. *J. Am. Oil Chem. Soc. 76*, 331–339.
10. Houlihan, C.M., and Ho, C.T. (1985) in *Flavor Chemistry of Fats and Oils*, (Min, D.B., and Smouse, T.H.,eds.) p. 117, American Oil Chemists' Society, Champaign, IL.
11. Economou, K.D., Oreopoulou, V., and Thomopoulos, C.D. (1991) Antioxidant Activity of Some Plant Extracts of the Family Labiatae. *J. Am. Oil Chem. Soc. 68*, 109–113.
12. Six, P. (1994) Current Research in Natural Food Antioxidants. *INFORM 5*, 679–688.
13. Valenzuela, A., and Nieto, S. (1996) Synthetic and Natural Antioxidants: Food Quality Protectors. *Grasas Aceites 47*, 186–196.
14. Firestone, D. (1995) *Official Methods and Recommended Practices of the American Oil Chemists' Society*, 4th edn., AOCS Press, Champaign, IL.
15. Tan, C.P., and Che Man, Y.B. (1999) Differential Scanning Calorimetric Analysis for Monitoring the Oxidation of Heated Oils. *Food Chem. 67*, 177–184.
16. Anonymous (1995) *7 Series/UNIX DSC7 User's Guide*, Version 4.0, Perkin Elmer Corporation, Norwalk, CT.
17. Anonymous (1989) *Statistical Analysis System User's Guide: Basic Statistics*, SAS Institute, Cary, NC.
18. Food, S.M., Hook, J.B., and Bond, J.T. (1980) The Effects of Butylated Hydroxyanisole and Butylated Hydroxytoluene on Renal Function in the Rat, II. Effects on Organic Acid and Base Transport. *Food Cosmet. Toxicol. 18*, 21–26.
19. Frankel, E.N., Huang, S.W., Aeschbach, R., and Prior, E. (1996) Antioxidant Activity of a Rosemary Extract and Its Constituents, Carnosic Acid, Carnosol, and Rosmarinic Acid, in Bulk Oil and Oil-in-Water Emulsion. *J. Agric. Food Chem. 44*, 131–135.

Chapter 11

Modulation of Apoptosis by Superoxide Radical

Marie-Véronique Clément,[a] Jeya Kumar Ramalingam,[a] and Shazib Pervaiz[b]

[a]Oncology Research Institute, National University Medical Institutes and
[b]Department of Physiology, National University of Singapore, Singapore 119260

Introduction

Production of ROI (reactive oxygen intermediates) has been thought for a long time to have an adverse effect on the physiology and survival of a cell. There is now a growing body of evidence to suggest that ROI, such as $O_2^{\bullet-}$ and H_2O_2, may influence the growth of mammalian cells *in vitro*. A tight balance between signals that trigger cells to proliferate and stimuli that drive cells to activate the cell suicide program maintains homeostatic functioning in invertebrate and highly complex mammalian systems. Dysregulation of one or the other could then herald the beginning of a pathologic process, as evidenced by the increased rate of cell death in diseases such as Alzheimer's, and contrarily, enhanced proliferation and defective death signaling as seen in tumorigenesis. Because of the diverse physiologic effects of ROI, in particular as mediators of cell death and survival, it is worthwhile to decipher how ROI influence the response of cells to signals that activate cell death pathway(s).

On the bases of morphologic and pathologic criteria, cell death is currently subdivided into two categories, necrosis (accidental cell death) and apoptosis (programmed cell death) (1). Aside from the phenotypic features that separate apoptotic cell death from necrotic cell death, apoptosis is an active process that involves activation of the caspase family of proteases. Activation of one or the other caspase members triggers a cascade of events culminating in specific morphologic and biochemical changes, leading to cell death *via* proteolytic degradation of a number of cellular proteins (2–4). In contrast, necrotic cell death is a passive process, which results in disruption of the cell membrane and death of the cell without a series of programmed events. Apoptotic cell death results either from developmentally controlled activation of endogenous execution programs (5) or *via* transduction of death signals triggered by a variety of exogenous stimuli. Potential exogenous inducers of apoptosis range from growth factor withdrawal to ligand- or antibody-mediated engagement of specific cell surface receptors [reviewed in (6)] to anticancer drugs (7–10).

Using antibodies to the CD95 receptor or anticancer drugs as triggers of apoptosis, we show that an increased intracellular level of $O_2^{\bullet-}$ regulates cell response to apoptosis. Moreover, our results suggest that the small-GTP–binding protein Rac1 may be involved in the regulation of the response of tumor cells to apoptosis through its role in the intracellular production of $O_2^{\bullet-}$. Finally, we demonstrate that

H_2O_2-induced apoptosis is mediated by reduction of the intracellular milieu, as opposed to oxidation detected at necrotic concentrations (≥1 mmol/L) of H_2O_2.

Discussion

Superoxide Anion Regulates Cell Response to Apoptotic Triggers

In 1996, we demonstrated that $O_2^{\bullet-}$ is a natural inhibitor of Fas (CD95)-mediated cell death (11). In that report, an increased intracellular level of $O_2^{\bullet-}$ was achieved using one of the best- characterized inhibitors of the Cu/Zn superoxide dismutase (Cu/Zn SOD), namely, diethyldithiocarbamate (DDC). Preincubation of the human melanoma cell line M14 expressing a chimeric TNF-CD95 receptor with 1 mmol/L DDC for 1 h significantly increased intracellular $O_2^{\bullet-}$. In addition, oxidative stress induced by inhibition of SOD and the resultant increase in $O_2^{\bullet-}$ strongly inhibited CD95-mediated apoptosis. These data were further supported by observations that resistance to CD95-mediated death induced by DDC was abolished by the antioxidant, *N*-acetylcysteine, and the $O_2^{\bullet-}$ scavenger, tiron. In light of these findings, we argued strongly in favor of a regulatory role of intracellular $O_2^{\bullet-}$ during death receptor–mediated apoptosis.

It is now well accepted that most anticancer agents kill tumor cells by apoptosis (7–10). Hence, we set out to investigate whether the inhibition of cell death by increased intracellular $O_2^{\bullet-}$ is restricted to the CD95 system or whether it could also be a mechanism underlying tumor cell response to drug-induced apoptosis. To do so, the intracellular $O_2^{\bullet-}$ level was manipulated by overexpressing or repressing the expression of cytoplasmic Cu/Zn SOD protein *in vivo* using a tetracycline-inducible expression system. This allowed the same clone to be analyzed in the presence or absence of tetracycline. M14 cells, tailored to overexpress or suppress Cu/Zn SOD, showed a direct relationship between intracellular levels of Cu/Zn SOD and $O_2^{\bullet-}$ and cell sensitivity to anticancer drug–induced apoptosis. Overexpression of Cu/Zn SOD

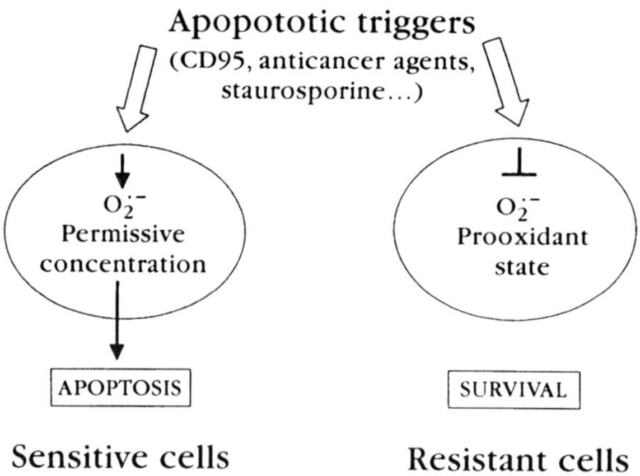

Fig. 11.1. Regulation of cell sensitivity to apoptotic triggers by $O_2^{\bullet-}$.

enhanced cell sensitivity to etoposide, daunorubicine, and pMC540. Conversely, a decrease in intracellular Cu/Zn SOD in tumor cells inhibited apoptosis induced by the same anticancer drugs. The role of intracellular $O_2^{\bullet -}$ in regulating tumor cell sensitivity thus appears not to be exclusive for CD95-signaling–dependent apoptosis, but may be common to a variety of anticancer drugs known to induce cell death by activation of the apoptotic machinery (12). Taken together, these data demonstrate that manipulation of intracellular $O_2^{\bullet -}$ concentration influences sensitivity of cells to apoptosis. In light of these findings, we suggest a scenario in which sensitive cells have a permissive $O_2^{\bullet -}$ concentration, which enhances sensitivity to apoptotic triggers and conversely, a prooxidant state, which inhibits apoptotic execution, thereby rendering cells resistant to death signals (Fig. 11.1).

The Small-GTP–Binding Protein Rac1 and Cell Response to Apoptotic Triggers

The metabolic pathways leading to the generation of ROI are best characterized in phagocytic cells. In these cells, $O_2^{\bullet -}$ is generated by the β-nicotinamide adenine dinucleotide phosphate (NADPH)-oxidase complex (13,14). In nonphagocytic cells, the proteins responsible for producing $O_2^{\bullet -}$ and other ROI are less well defined, but could well function in a manner similar to the phagocyte NADPH-oxidase complex. Indeed, it has recently been shown that, similar to the phagocyte oxidant generating system, the production of ROI in nonphagocytic cells is regulated by the small guanosine triphosphate (GTP)-binding protein Rac1 (15–24). Rac1 is one of the downstream targets of the oncogene ras, whose overexpression and mutations have been described in ~30% of all human tumors (25–27). Interestingly, a mitogenic signal triggered by Ras in a fibroblast cell line was shown to be mediated by the intracellular production of $O_2^{\bullet -}$ lending support to the hypothesis that $O_2^{\bullet -}$ acts as an important proliferative signal in tumor cells (28). Stimulated by these findings, we hypothesized that in addition to triggering proliferation, an oncogenic mutation of Ras could also result in inhibition of the apoptotic pathway brought about by Ras-mediated $O_2^{\bullet -}$ production. Thus, increased proliferation coupled with inhibition of the cell death pathway could be an ideal combination, resulting in an abnormal accumulation of cells and tumorigenesis. Indeed, using the T24 bladder carcinoma cell line, which overexpresses Ras (29) and is resistant to a variety of apoptotic triggers, we showed that a decrease in intracellular $O_2^{\bullet -}$ concentration could enhance tumor cell sensitivity to apoptosis. In this set of experiments, apoptosis was induced by anti-CD95, and reduction in intracellular $O_2^{\bullet -}$ concentration was obtained using an oxidase inhibitor, diphenyleneiodonium (DPI), or two protein kinase C inhibitors, Bis-indolmaleimide (BIM) and staurosporine. Our results showed that T24 cells could be sensitized to CD95-mediated apoptosis by decreasing intracellular $O_2^{\bullet -}$. Contrarily, an increase in intracellular $O_2^{\bullet -}$ achieved by DDC-induced inhibition of Cu/Zn SOD resulted in enhanced survival after triggering with anti-CD95. Similar results were obtained when T24 cells were transiently transfected with a dominant negative form of the Rac protein, RacV12N17. Intracellular $O_2^{\bullet -}$ dropped and caspase activity, a marker of apoptosis, increased after

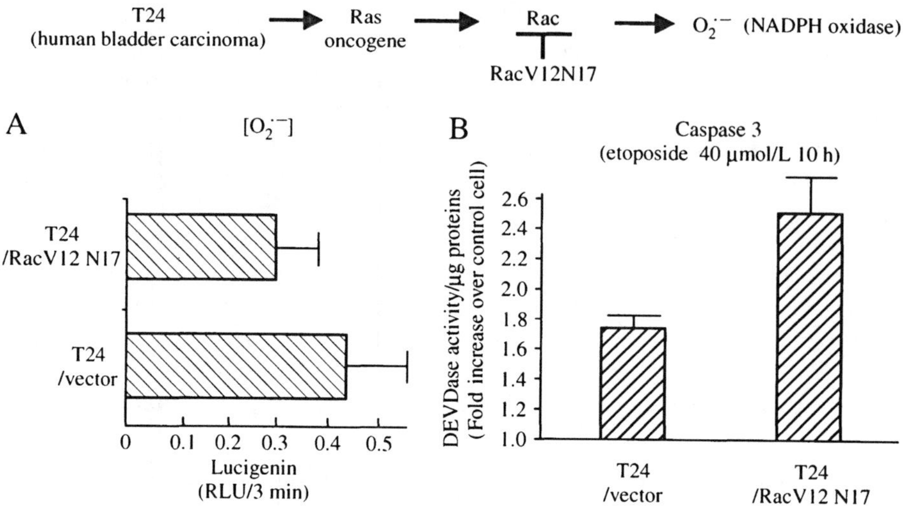

Fig. 11.2. Inhibition of caspase 3 activity in T24 cells is associated with Ras-mediated intracellular $O_2^{\bullet-}$ production through a Rac-dependent pathway. T24 cells (from ATCC) were transiently transfected with an empty pIRES1hyg vector (T24/pIRES), or the same vector encoding a dominant negative form of Rac1 (T24/pIRES RacN17). Transient transfection was performed using the SuperFect Transfection Reagents from QIAGEN Gmbh (Germany). T24 cells (2.5 × 10^5) were plated in a 6-well plate. Transfection was performed according to vendor's instruction using 5 µg of DNA and 20 µL of SuperFect Transfection Reagent. To monitor transfection efficiency, cells used in the experiment were also transfected with the pIRES vector encoding the yellow-green variant of the wild-type GFP protein, the EYFP protein. After 48 h of incubation, EYFP-expressing cells were analyzed by flow cytometry using an emission wavelength of 525 nm after excitation at 513 nm. An average of 25–30% transfection efficiency was regularly achieved using the conditions described above. (*A*) 48 h post-transfection intracellular $O_2^{\bullet-}$ level was measured and is represented as relative light units (RLU)/3 min; (*B*) DEVDase activity induced with 40 mmol/L etoposide for 10 h was measured. DEVDase activity per µg of protein is shown as fold increase over transfected cells incubated for the same period of time without etoposide (Fold increase over control cells) ± SD for two experiments done in duplicate. 1X represents no caspase activity.

activation of the apoptotic pathway with etoposide (11) (Fig. 11.2). These results led us to conclude that the intracellular level of $O_2^{\bullet-}$ in tumor cells could be one critical regulator of tumor cell response to apoptosis, irrespective of the trigger, and may play a role in tumorigenesis.

Oxidative vs. Reductive Stress-Induced Apoptosis

After establishing that a mild oxidative stress could inhibit induction of apoptosis, we wanted to explain these findings in the light of the age-old dogma in free radical biology that production of radical oxygen intermediates or oxidative stress induces apoptosis. It is well accepted (and has been confirmed in our work) that H_2O_2 induces both apoptotic and necrotic cell death (30). However, in contradiction to the oxidative stress hypothesis, we demonstrated that apoptosis induced by H_2O_2 was associated with a decrease in intracellular $O_2^{\bullet-}$ concentration and acidification of the intracellular milieu, suggesting a trend toward reduction rather than oxidation of the intracellular environment. Thus, similar to apoptosis induced in the absence of ROI, a relatively reduced (decreased $O_2^{\bullet-}$ concentration and low pH) intracellular state mediates H_2O_2-induced apoptotic cell death. In contrast, cell death triggered by H_2O_2 concentrations that induce an overwhelming oxidative stress, as measured by a dramatic drop in the total intracellular glutathione content, is of a necrotic nature (30).

These results show that although an overwhelming increase in intracellular ROI (oxidative stress) provides a direct effector mechanism for necrotic cell death, a mild increase that favors reduction of the intracellular milieu (reduced state) is conducive for apoptotic execution. These observations suggest that a decrease in $O_2^{\bullet-}$ concentration, coupled with an increase in intracellular H^+ ion concentration (reduced intracellular milieu), may represent a common mechanism for triggering apoptosis by stimuli that either induce generation of low levels of H_2O_2 or directly inhibit intracellular $O_2^{\bullet-}$ production. We therefore propose to refer to the mechanism of apoptosis induced by such stimuli as "reductive stress" as opposed to "oxidative stress," which should be reserved for the production of intracellular ROI that induce necrotic as opposed to apoptotic cell death [for review see (31)].

Summary

In summary, our findings underscore the importance of distinguishing between the role of ROI in necrotic vs. apoptotic cell death. Although ROI provide a direct effector mechanism for necrotic cell death, they seem rather to function as regulators of cell sensitivity to apoptosis. To survive, all cells depend on a constant repression of their intrinsic suicide program by signals from surrounding cells and the extracellular matrix. An important effect of extracellular survival signals may therefore be to maintain a critical cellular redox equilibrium, based, at least in part, on adequate intracellular $O_2^{\bullet-}$production (31).

References

1. Wyllie, A.H. (1981) in *Cell Death in Biology and Pathology*, (Bowen, I.D., and Lockshin, R.A., eds.), pp. 9–34, Chapman & Hall, London.
2. Earnshaw, W.C., Martins, L.M., and Kaufmann, S.H. (1999)Mammalian Caspases: Structure, Activation, Substrates, and Functions During Apoptosis. *Annu. Rev. Biochem. 68*, 383–424.
3. Martin, S.J., and Green, D.R. (1995) Protease Activation During Apoptosis: Death by a Thousand Cuts? *Cell 82*, 349–352.
4. Fraser, A., and Evan, G. (1996) A Licence to Kill. *Cell 85*, 781–784.
5. Shearwin-Whyatt, L.M., and Kumar, S. (1999) Caspases in Developmental Cell Death. *IUBMB Life 48*, 143–150.

6. Schneider, P., and Tschopp, J. (2000) Apoptosis Induced by Death Receptors. *Pharm. Acta Helv. 74*, 281–286.
7. Eastman, A. (1990) Activation of Programmed Cell Death by Anticancer Agents: Cisplatin as a Model System. *Cancer Cells (Cold Spring Harbor) 2*, 275–280.
8. Dive, C., Evans, C.A., and Whetton, A.D. (1992) Induction of Apoptosis—New Targets for Cancer Chemotherapy. *Semin. Cancer Biol. 3*, 417–427.
9. Gibb, R.K., Taylor, D.D., Wan, T., O'Connor, D.M., Doering, D.L., and Gercel-Taylor, C. (1997) Apoptosis as a Measure of Chemosensitivity to Cisplatin and Taxol Therapy in Ovarian Cancer Cell Lines. *Gynecol. Oncol. 65*, 13–22.
10. Benjamin, C.W., Hiebsch, R. R., and Jones, D.A. (1998) Caspase Activation in MCF7 Cells Responding to Etoposide Treatment. *Mol. Pharmacol. 53*, 446–450.
11. Clément, M.-V., and Stamenkovic, I. (1996) Superoxide Anion Is a Natural Inhibitor of Fas-Mediated Cell Death. *EMBO J. 15*, 216–225.
12. Pervaiz, S., Ramalingam, J.K., Hirpara, J.L., and Clément, M.-V. (1999) Superoxide Anion Inhibits Drug-Induced Tumor Cell Death. *FEBS Lett. 459*, 343–348.
13. Babior, B.M. (1999) NADPH Oxidase: An Update. *Blood 93*, 1464–1476.
14. DeLeo, F.R., and Quinn, M.T. (1996) Assembly of the Phagocyte NADPH Oxidase: Molecular Interaction of Oxidase Proteins. *J. Leukoc. Biol. 60*, 677–691.
15. Abo, A., Pick, E., Hall, A., Totty, N., Teahan, C.G., and Segal, A.W. (1991) Activation of the NADPH Oxidase Involves the Small GTP-Binding Protein p21rac1. *Nature 353*, 668–670.
16. Bokoch, G.M. (1994) Regulation of the Human Neutrophil NADPH Oxidase by the Rac GTP-Binding Proteins. *Curr. Opin. Cell Biol. 6*, 212–218.
17. Dagher, M.C., Fuchs, A., Bourmeyster, N., Jouan, A., and Vignais, P.V. (1995) Small G Proteins and the Neutrophil NADPH Oxidase. *Biochimie 77*, 651–660.
18. Irani, K., Xia, Y., Zweier, J.L., Sollott, S.J., Der, C.J., Fearon, E.R., Sundaresan, M., Finkel, T., and Goldschmidt-Clermont, P.J. (1997) Mitogenic Signaling Mediated by Oxidants in Ras-Transformed Fibroblasts. *Science 275*, 1649–1652.
19. Irani, K., and Goldschmidt-Clermont, P.J. (1998) Ras, Superoxide and Signal Transduction. *Biochem. Pharmacol. 55*, 1339–1346.
20. Kreck, M.L., Uhlinger, D.J., Tyagi, S.R., Inge, K.L., and Lambeth, J.D. (1994) Participation of the Small Molecular Weight GTP-Binding Protein Rac1 in Cell-Free Activation and Assembly of the Respiratory Burst Oxidase. Inhibition by a Carboxyl-Terminal Rac Peptide, *J. Biol. Chem. 269*, 4161–4168.
21. Kreck, M.L., Freeman, J.L., Abo, A., and Lambeth, J.D. (1996) Membrane Association of Rac Is Required for High Activity of the Respiratory Burst Oxidase. *Biochemistry 35*, 15683–15692.
22. Moore, K.A., Sethi, R., Doanes, A.M., Johnson, T.M., Pracyk, J.B., Kirby, M., Irani, K., Goldschmidt-Clermont, P.J., and Finkel, T. (1997) Rac1 Is Required for Cell Proliferation and G2/M Progression. *Biochem. J. 326*, 17–20.
23. Pracyk, J.B., Tanaka, K., Hegland, D.D., Kim, K.S., Sethi, R., Rovira, I.I., Blazina, D.R., Lee, L., Bruder, J.T., Kovesdi, I., Goldshmidt-Clermont, P.J., Irani, K., and Finkel, T. (1998) A Requirement for the Rac1 GTPase in the Signal Transduction Pathway Leading to Cardiac Myocyte Hypertrophy. *J. Clin. Investig. 102*, 929–937.
24. Sundaresan, M., Yu, Z.X., Ferrans, V.J., Sulciner, D.J., Gutkind, J.S., Irani, K., Goldschmidt-Clermont, P.J., and Finkel, T. (1996) Regulation of Reactive-Oxygen-Species Generation in Fibroblasts by Rac1. *Biochem. J. 318*, 379–382.

25. Bos, J.L. (1988) The Ras Gene Family and Human Carcinogenesis. *Mutat. Res. 195*, 255–271.
26. Downward, J. (1990) The Ras Superfamily of Small GTP-Binding Proteins. *Trends Biochem. Sci. 15*, 469–472.
27. Downward, J. (1998) Signal Transduction. New Exchange, New Target. *Nature 396*, 416–417.
28. Irani, K., Xia, Y., Zweier, J.L., Sollott, S.J., Der, C.J., Fearson, E.R., Sundaresan, M., Finkel, T., and Goldshmidt-Clermont, P.J. (1997) Mitogenic Signaling Mediated by Oxidants in Ras-Transformed Fibroblasts. *Science 275*, 1649–1652.
29. Senger, D.R., Perruzzi, C.A., and Ali, I.U. (1988) T24 Human Bladder Carcinoma Cells with Activated Ha-Ras Protooncogene: Nontumorigenic Cells Susceptible to Malignant Transformation with Carcinogen. *Proc. Natl. Acad. Sci. USA 85*, 5107–5111.
30. Clément, M.-V., Ponton, A., and Pervaiz, S. (1998) Apoptosis Induced by Hydrogen Peroxide Is Mediated by Decreased Superoxide Anion Concentration and Reduction of Intracellular Milieu. *FEBS Lett. 440*, 3–8.
31. Clément, M.-V., and Pervaiz, S. (1999) Reactive Oxygen Intermediates Regulate Cellular Response to Apoptotic Stimuli: An Hypothesis. *Free Radic. Res. 30*, 247–252.

Chapter 12

Aerobic Glycolysis by Proliferating Cells—A Protective Strategy Against Reactive Oxygen Species

K. Brand, U. Aulwurm, U. Hermfisse, E. Greiner, B. Hamm-Kuenzelmann, D. Philipp, and R. Netzker

Institute of Biochemistry, University of Erlangen-Nuremberg, 91054 Erlangen, Germany

Introduction

The phenomenon of aerobic glycolysis in tumor cells, first described by Otto Warburg as early as 1924 (1), is one of the fundamental problems of tumor biochemistry that is not yet fully understood. Intense investigations of a variety of cancer cells confirmed the high rate of lactate production from glucose despite the presence of oxygen and mitochondria (2–8). However, aerobic glycolysis is not a unique feature of tumor cells because is also found in nontransformed proliferating cells when sufficient glucose is available (9–13). Increases in glycolytic enzyme capacities can account, at least in part, for aerobic glycolysis (14,15), yet the reason for the transition of proliferating cells from an oxidative glucose metabolism to aerobic glycolysis remains to be elucidated. In particular, it is still unclear why tumor cells and normal proliferating cells meet their enhanced energy requirements from glycolysis even though this pathway is far less effective in ATP production than glucose oxidation.

Primary cultures of rat thymocytes provide a useful cell cycle system with which to study the changes in energy metabolism as cells undergo a transition from the resting to the proliferating state.

The rates of glycolytic and oxidative glucose degradation by resting unstimulated as well as by mitogen-stimulated proliferating rat thymocytes have been quantified to calculate the ATP yields from both pathways. The results indicate that aerobic glycolysis in proliferating thymocytes supplies the enhanced energy demand during the S phase and cell division. We hypothesize that this transition to enhanced nonoxidative glycolytic glucose degradation serves as a means to minimize the production of reactive oxygen species (ROS) during the critical phases of enhanced biosyntheses and cell division.

Materials and Methods

The materials and methods employed are described or referred to in Refs. 15–17.

Results and Discussion

ATP Production from Glucose Metabolism by Resting and Proliferating Thymocytes

The rate of glucose consumption by proliferating cells is 19-fold higher than that by nonstimulated resting cells. More importantly, an alteration of partly oxidative to almost completely glycolytic glucose degradation to lactate occurs during the transition from the resting to the proliferating state (Table 12.1).

The amount of [U-^{14}C]glucose recovered in $^{14}CO_2$ during the incubation by stimulated and nonstimulated thymocytes, which is indicative of the rate of complete glucose oxidation, is almost the same (6.6 vs. 8.4 μmol). This finding suggests that the enhanced energy demand for increased biosynthesis and cell division during proliferation is met solely by glycolysis.

Calculations of the ATP yields reveal that 86% of total ATP in the proliferating cells is produced by glycolytic glucose breakdown to pyruvate and lactate and only 14% by oxidation to CO_2 and *vice versa* in resting cells (Table 12.1). Aerobic glycolysis renders growing cells less dependent on oxygen and thereby improves their survival in a hypoxic environment (6).

Our finding that aerobic glycolysis meets the enhanced ATP demand of proliferating thymocytes leads to the of question of why, despite lower energy yields, proliferating cells maintain a high glycolytic rate even under aerobic conditions and in the presence of intact mitochondria. A prerequisite for this is a high catalytic capacity of glycolytic enzymes in the cells during the S phase of the cell cycle. In previous experiments

TABLE 12.1 ATP Yield in Resting and Proliferating Rat Thymocytes from Glycolytic and Oxidative Glucose Metabolism[a,b]

[U-^{14}C]Glucose recovered in	Resting thymocytes [μmol/(h·10^{10} cells)]		Proliferating thymocytes [μmol/(h·10^{10} cells)]	
Lactate	19 ± 2.8		700 ± 46.7	
Pyruvate	1.5 ± 0.15		20.8 ± 2.2	
$^{14}CO_2$	8.4 ± 0.8		6.6 ± 0.7	
ATP produced from		(%)		(%)
Glycolysis	41	12	1442	86
Oxidation	302	88	238	14
Total ATP yield	344	100	1680	100

[a]*Source:* Ref. 16.
[b]Proliferation of cultured thymocytes was achieved by concanavalin A (Con A; 10 μg/mL) and interleukin-2 (10 U/mL). Nonstimulated resting and Con A-stimulated proliferating cells, harvested after 48 h of culture, were incubated at a cell density between 1 and 5 × 10^8 with 4 mmol/L [U-^{14}C]labeled glucose for 60–129 min at 37°C. Values are means ± SEM and are expressed in μmol/(h•10^{10}cells) for 14 separate experiments. The calculation of ATP is based on the production of 2 mol ATP/mol glycolitically degraded glucose and 36 mol ATP/mol oxidatively degraded glucose [3 mol ATP/mol NADH and 2 mol ATP/mol FADH2 oxidized; a decrease in these ratios resulting from a proton leak (24) was not considered in this calculation].

(14,15) we showed that the V_{max} activities of these enzymes increased after stimulation of thymocytes with concanavalin A (Con A; 10 μg/mL) and interleukin (IL)-2 (10 U/mL) during the G1 phase and peaked with a 8- to 10-fold induction at the S phase (44–48 h of culture). In the absence of glucose in the culture medium, induction of the glycolytic enzymes and hence cell division did not occur (15,18). We hypothesize that the reduction of mitochondrial glucose oxidation and transition to aerobic glycolysis is a means to protect the cells against ROS during the critical phases of enhanced biosynthesis and cell division.

Measurements of Reactive Oxygen Production

To test this hypothesis, we measured the production of ROS in glucose-containing incubations using resting and proliferating thymocytes. Con A–stimulated and –nonstimulated thymocytes were harvested after 46 h of culture. Resting thymocytes, cultured without Con A, show a marked phorbol 12-myristate 13-acetate

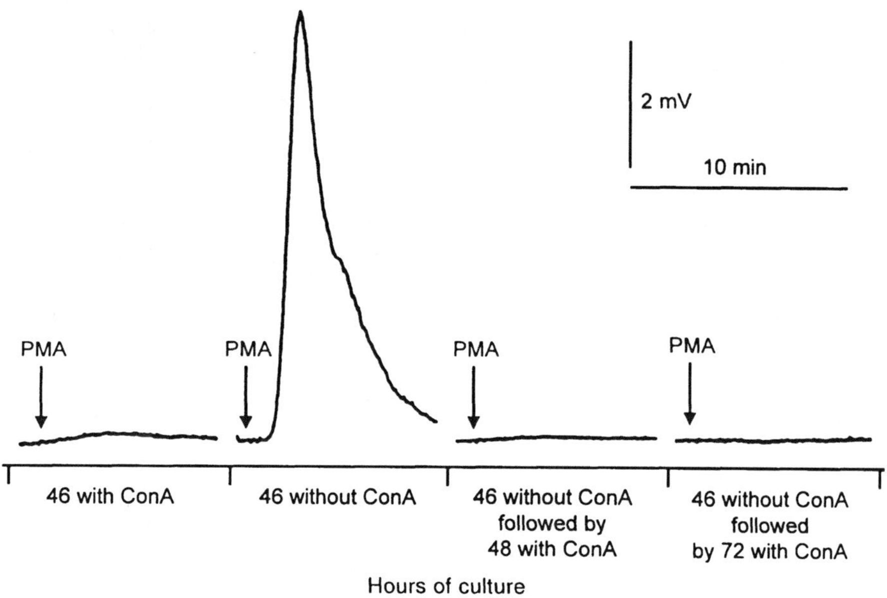

Fig. 12.1. Phorbol 12-myristate 13-acetate (PMA)-initiated luminol chemiluminescence of rat thymocytes—comparison between proliferating [cultured with concanavalin A (Con A)] and nonproliferating (cultured without Con A) cells. The incubations (total volume of 1 mL) contained 2×10^7 cells each, 4 mmol/L glucose, and 170 μmol/L luminol in phosphate-buffered saline, pH 7.4, with 0.02% EDTA. Luminol chemiluminescence as a measure of peroxide anion release was initiated by the addition of 2 μg/mL PMA and 1 μg/mL calcium ionophor A23187. Photon emission rate at 37°C from one assay vial is plotted on the vertical axis in mV and traced for 10 min by continuous recording with a chromato-integrator. One representative experiment of 9 is shown. The nonproliferating cells were recultured for 48 and 72 h with Con A. *Source*: Ref. 16.

(PMA)-initiated luminol chemiluminescence indicative of the formation of peroxide anions (Fig. 12.1). In contrast, with Con A–stimulated thymocytes (S-phase cells), virtually no chemiluminescence response could be observed. To test whether this phenomenon is indeed correlated with proliferation, thymocytes cultured for 46 h without Con A were then stimulated by the addition of Con A to enter the cell cycle and to divide. The marked chemiluminescence response observed with the nonstimulated cells vanished when the cells were assayed again for chemiluminescence 48 or 72 h after the addition of Con A to the cultures (Fig. 12.1). The origin of ROS could be shown to be the site of complex III of the mitochondrial respiratory chain (16).

In addition to the PMA-initiated luminol chemiluminescence, 2′,7′-dichlorofluorescein (DCF) fluorescence measurements at various phases of the cell cycle were also performed. DCF fluorescence is indicative of intracellular hydrogen peroxide,

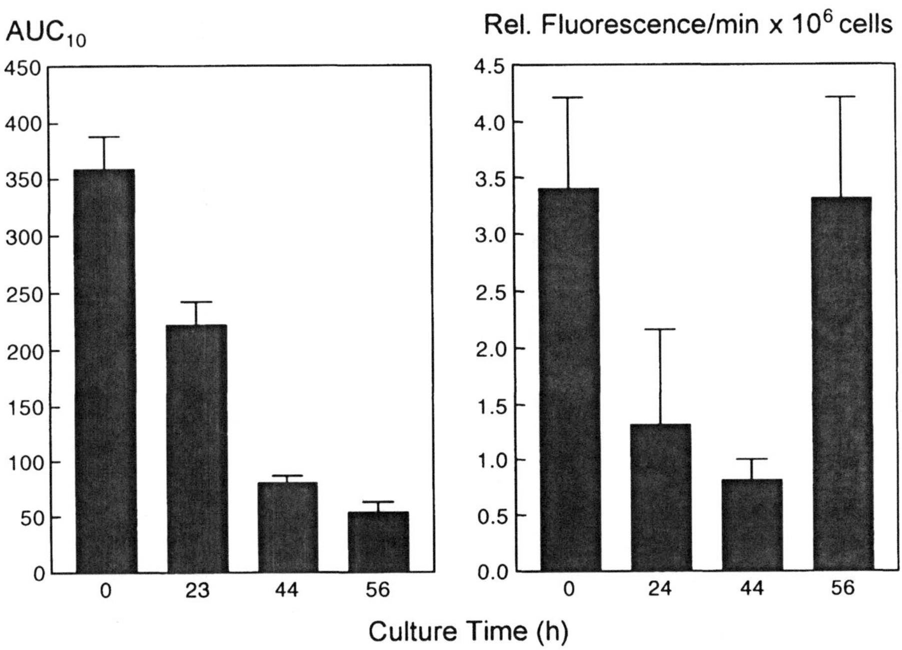

Fig. 12.2. Phorbol 12-myristate 13-acetate (PMA)-initiated luminol chemiluminescence (left) and 2′,7′-dichlorofluorescein (DCF) fluorescence (right) of rat thymocytes at various phases of the cell cycle. Chemiluminescence was measured as described in the legend of Fig. 12.1. The integrated photon emission intensities at 37°C for 10 min from one assay (of 3) are plotted on the vertical axis as the area under the curve $(AUC)_{10}$. DCF fluorescence was measured in incubations with a total volume of 2 mL in 10-mm precision quartz cuvettes (Hellma), containing 2×10^6 cells each, 10 µmol/L 2′,7′-dichlorodihydrofluorescein-diacetate (DCFH-DA), and HEPES-buffered saline (HBS), pH 7.4. After a preincubation of 30 min, the fluorescence rate was recorded for an additional 20 min on a chromato-integrator. The resulting kinetics of the slopes from 40 to 50 min were used for calculation. One representative experiment of three is shown.

whereas luminol chemiluminescence measures both the intra- and extracellular hydrogen peroxide concentration in the incubations. With both measurements (Fig. 12.2), a decrease of peroxide production was found when cells proceeded from the resting state (nonstimulated) to the S phase (44 h after stimulation). DCF fluorescence increased again after mitosis (68 h). The observed marked reduction of ROS during the S phase of the cell cycle supports the concept of aerobic glycolysis as a means to protect the cells against oxidative stress.

Redox-Regulated Expression of Glycolytic Enzymes via *Stimulatory Protein 1 (Sp1)*

Hydrogen peroxide has been shown to decrease the binding efficiency of the transcription factor Sp1 to its DNA consensus sequence (17,19,20). From the reported increase of ROS formation after glucose depletion in 44-h cultures (18), it was expected

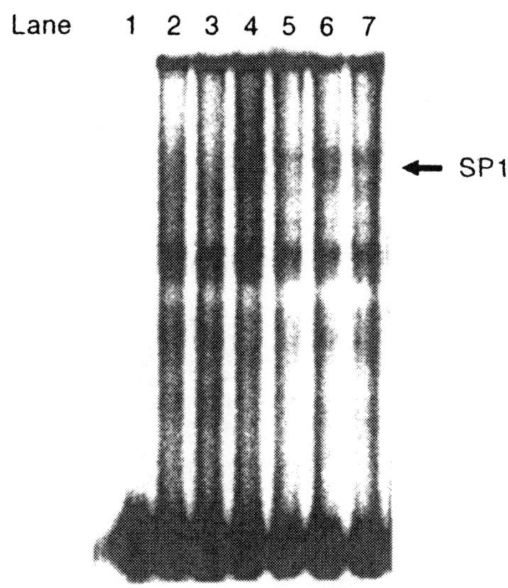

Fig. 12.3. Binding efficiency of stimulatory protein 1 (Spl) to its consensus sequence. Electrophoretic mobility shift assays were performed using a fragment of the aldolase AH1 promoter that spans from 201 to 86 and contains two GC-boxes. The following nuclear extracts were used:

Lane I Control: no nuclear extract

	Culture time (h)	Anti-Spl	Glucose (mmol/L)
Lane 2	0	–	–
Lane 3	0	+	–
Lane 4	44	–	10
Lane 5	44	+	10
Lane 6	44	–	1.2
Lane 7	44	+	1.2

Source: Ref. 19.

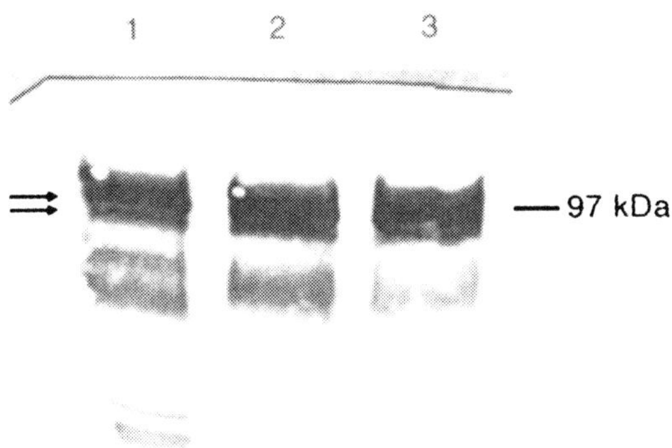

Fig. 12.4. Immunoblot of stimulatory protein 1 (Spl) with nuclear extracts from rat thymocytes. Immunoblot of nuclear extracts from nonstimulated (lane 1) and concanavalin A (Con A)- and interleukin (IL)-2–stimulated rat thymocytes cultured for 46 h with glucose in concentrations of 10 mmol/L (lane 2) and 1.2 mmol/L (lane 3), respectively, are shown. Nuclear protein (25 μg) was loaded on each lane. The proteins were detected with a polyclonal antibody against Spl. The upper and lower arrows indicate the phosphorylated and dephosphorylated forms of Spl, respectively. *Source*: Ref. 18.

that Sp1 binding to DNA would be affected. To verify this, electrophoretic mobility shift assays were conducted with an aldolase promoter fragment containing two GC-boxes (Fig. 12.3) and nuclear extracts from nonstimulated (lanes 2 and 3) and stimulated rat thymocytes cultured for 44 h in media with 10 mmol/L glucose (lanes 4 and 5) initially or 1.2 mmol/L glucose (lanes 6 and 7). At the initially low glucose concentration, Sp1 binding (lane 6) is markedly reduced compared with that at high glucose concentration (lane 4). This is most likely due to an oxidative alteration of the cysteine-rich zinc-finger motif of Sp1 (21 and references therein). The incubations underlying lanes 3, 5, and 7 also contained antibodies to Sp1, which reduced the binding intensity to DNA as shown in lanes 5 and 7. Analogous results were obtained also with a fragment of the pyruvate kinase M2 promoter (data not shown). From Western-blot analyses (Fig. 12.4), it can be deduced that the cellular concentration of Sp1 is equal in cells cultured with either 1.2 or 10 mmol/L glucose. This indicates constitutive expression of Sp1 and excludes proteolytic degradation in the glucose-depleted cells.

Pyruvate Generated by Aerobic Glycolysis Is an Effective ROS Scavenger

The results presented in Figures 12.1 and 12.2 suggest that either generation of ROS is abolished in cells during proliferation, or ROS are effectively scavenged by antioxidants. Because an almost equal amount of glucose was found to be oxidized in both resting and proliferating cells (Table 12.1), the potential for ROS production is nearly identical in both cells. Lactate is the main end product of aerobic glycolysis, but the rate of pyruvate formation is significantly increased as well (Table 12.1). Because the antioxidative function of pyruvate is well documented in the literature (22,23), the lack of ROS production by proliferating thymocytes with enhanced glycolytic activity is likely due to the effective scavenging of ROS by pyruvate. To address this question,

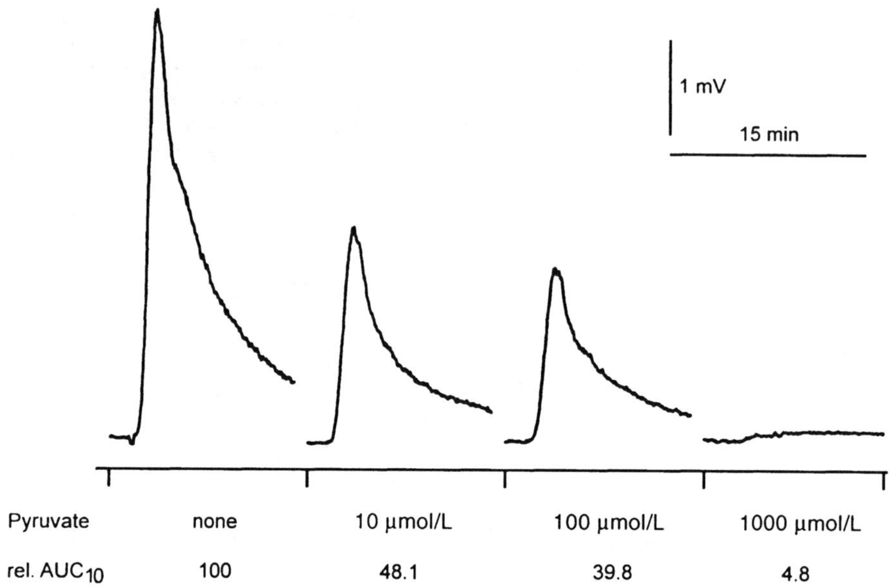

Fig. 12.5. Effect of pyruvate on phorbol 12-myristate 13-acetate (PMA)-primed luminol chemiluminescence of nonproliferating rat thymocytes. The incubation conditions, initiation, and measurement of chemiluminescence are described in the legend to Figure 12.1. In each experiment, 2×10^7 cells were preincubated with Na-pyruvate at the indicated concentration for 10 min. Chemiluminescence was recorded continuously for 15 min, and the total light emission was quantified by integration. For each analysis, the area under the curve $(AUC)_{10}$ was related to the control without pyruvate (set to 100). Traces of one representative experiment of three are shown. *Source*: Ref. 16.

nonproliferating cells were incubated with physiologically relevant concentrations of pyruvate in the luminol-chemiluminescence assays. Pyruvate indeed suppressed the PMA-induced chemiluminescence very effectively (Fig. 12.5). These results suggest that the transition to aerobic glycolysis by proliferating cells results in two cooperative effects: (i) generation of antioxidative pyruvate and (ii) prevention of excessive ROS production by diminishing oxidative glucose metabolism (Table 12.1).

Summary

Our previous studies with primary cultures of rat thymocytes revealed that glucose is essential for glycolytic enzyme induction and proliferation. Due to the sensitivity of Sp1 to redox changes with respect to its DNA binding, gene expression of glycolytic enzymes is markedly suppressed. As a consequence, cell division does not occur. The transition from glycolytic glucose degradation to lactate during the late G1 and S phases of the cell cycle is the only means for the cell to produce ATP without utilization of oxygen. Wherever oxygen reacts with iron-containing proteins, e.g., complexes of the mitochondrial respiratory chain, ROS such as superoxide and peroxide anions can be generated. The interaction of ROS with cellular macromolecules (DNA, proteins) and lipids under steady-state conditions can lead to oxidative damage, if the antioxidant defense is not fully efficient. Our data indicate that the long-known, yet still unexplained transition to aerobic glycolysis by proliferating cells is a simple, ingenious, yet effective strategy to minimize the exposure of proliferating cells to ROS. This is achieved not only by limiting the production of ROS, but also by supplying sufficient pyruvate to strengthen the cellular antioxidant system.

Acknowledgments

This work was supported by Deutsche Forschungsgemeinschaft Grant BR 612/15 and by Wilhelm Sander-Stiftung Grant 88.031.

References

1. Warburg, O., Poesener, K., and Negelein, E. (1924) Über den Stoffwechsel der Carcinomzelle. (About the Metabolism of Carcinoma Cells) *Biochem. Z. 152*, 309–344.
2. Warburg, O. (1929) Ist die aerobe Glykolyse spezifisch für die Tumoren? (Is Aerobic Glycolysis Specific for Tumors?) *Biochem. Z. 204*, 482–483.
3. Crabtree, H.G. (1929) Observations on the Carbohydrate Metabolism of Tumours. *Biochem. J. 23*, 536–545.
4. Racker, E. (1976) Why Do Tumor Cells Have a High Aerobic Glycolysis? *J. Cell Physiol. 89*, 697–700.
5. Burk, D., Woods, M., and Hunter, J. (1967) On the Significance of Glycolysis for Cancer Growth, with Special Reference to Morris Rat Hepatomas. *J. Natl. Cancer Inst. 38*, 839–863.
6. Eigenbrodt, E., and Glossmann, H. (1980) Glycolysis—One of the Keys to Cancer? *Trends Pharmacol. Sci. 1*, 240–245.
7. Eigenbrodt, E. (1985) in *Biochemical and Molecular Aspects of Selected Cancers*, (Gerbracht, U., Mazurek, S., Presek, P., and Friis, R., eds.) vol. 2, pp. 311–385, Academic Press, New York.
8. Brand, K., Leibold, W., Luppa, P., Schoerner, C., and Schulz, A. (1986) Metabolic Alterations Associated with Proliferation of Mitogen-Activated Lymphocytes and of Lymphoblastoid Cell Lines: Evaluation of Glucose and Glutamine Metabolism. *Immunobiology 173*, 23–34.
9. Krebs, H.A. (1972) The Pasteur Effect and the Relations Between Respiration and Fermentation. *Essays Biochem. 8*, 1–34.
10. Wang, T., Marquardt, C., and Foker, J. (1976) Aerobic Glycolysis During Lymphocyte Proliferation. *Nature 261*, 702–705.
11. Brand, K. (1985) Glutamine and Glucose Metabolism During Thymocyte Proliferation. Pathways of Glutamine and Glutamate Metabolism. *Biochem. J. 228*, 353–361.
12. Tollefsbol, T.O., and Cohen, H.J. (1985) Culture Kinetics of Glycolytic Enzyme Induction, Glucose Utilization, and Thymidine Incorporation of Extended-Exposure Phytohemagglutinin-Stimulated Human Lymphocytes. *J. Cell Physiol. 122*, 98–104.
13. Dröge, W., Roth, S., Altmann, A., and Mihm, S. (1987) Regulation of T-Cell Functions by L-Lactate. *Cell. Immunol. 108*, 405–416.

14. Brand, K., Aichinger, S., Forster, S,, Kupper, S., Neumann, B., Nürnberg, W., and Ohrisch, G. (1988) Cell-Cycle-Related Metabolic and Enzymatic Events in Proliferating Rat Thymocytes. *Eur. J. Biochem. 172*, 695–702.
15. Greiner, E.F., Guppy, M., and Brand, K. (1994) Glucose Is Essential for Proliferation and the Glycolytic Enzyme Induction That Provokes a Transition to Glycolytic Energy Production. *J. Biol. Chem. 269*, 31484–31490.
16. Brand, K., and Hermfisse, U. (1997) Aerobic Glycolysis by Proliferating Cells: A Protective Strategy Against Reactive Oxygen Species. *FASEB J. 11*, 388–395.
17. Schäfer, D., Hamm-Künzelmann, B., Hermfisse, U., and Brand, K. (1996) Differences in DNA-Binding Efficiency of Sp1 to Aldolase and Pyruvate Kinase Promoter Correlate with Altered Redox States in Resting and Proliferating Rat Thymocytes. *FEBS Lett. 391*, 35–38.
18. Aulwurm, U.R., and Brand, K.A. (2000) Increased Formation of Reactive Oxygen Species Due to Glucose Depletion in Primary Cultures of Rat Thymocytes Inhibits Proliferation. *Eur. J. Biochem., 267*, 5693–5698.
19. Ammendola, R., Mesuraca, M., Russo, T., and Cimino, F. (1994) The DNA-Binding Efficiency of Sp1 Is Affected by Redox Changes. *Eur. J. Biochem. 225*, 483–489.
20. Hamm-Künzelmann, B., Schäfer, D., Weigert, C., and Brand, K. (1997) Redox-Regulated Expression of Glycolytic Enzymes in Resting and Proliferating Rat Thymocytes. *FEBS Lett. 403*, 87–90.
21. Wu, X., Bishopric, N.H., Discher, D.J., Murphy, B.J., and Webster, K.A. (1995) Physical and Functional Sensitivity of Zinc Finger Transcription Factors to Redox Change. *Mol. Cell. Biol. 16*, 1035–1046.
22. Andrae, U., Singh, J., and Ziegler-Skylakakis, K. (1985) Pyruvate and Related Alpha-Ketoacids Protect Mammalian Cells in Culture Against Hydrogen Peroxide-Induced Cytotoxicity. *Toxicol. Lett. 28*, 93–98.
23. O'Donnell-Tormey, J., Nathan, C.F., Lanks, K., DeBoer, C.J., and De La Harpe, J. (1987) Secretion of Pyruvate—An Antioxidant Defense of Mammalian Cells. *J. Exp. Med. 165*, 500–514.
24. Brand, M.D. (1990) The Proton Leak Across the Mitochondrial Inner Membrane. *Biochim. Biophys. Acta 1018*, 128–133.

Chapter 13

Saponin from *Schefflera odorata* as Potential Modulator of the Cell-Signaling Pathways

Gloria de Castro-Bernas and Ma. Cristina R. Ramos

College of Science and Research Center for the Natural Sciences, University of Santo Tomas, Manila, Philippines

Introduction

Once initiated by extracellular signaling agents, pathways involved in the transduction of biological signals within the cells directly affect different kinds of cytoplasmic machinery or lead to the cell nucleus where activities ultimately result in such diverse responses as proliferation, differentiation, and apoptosis (1). These are all biologic events in multicellular organisms that are particularly relevant to neoplasia (cancer) and development among others. These cellular responses can be modulated either intracellularly or extracellularly. Intracellular agents are those produced inside the cell that are capable of initiating other transduction pathways to proceed. Extracellular agents are the ones found in the environment or outside the cell. These extracellular agents can be chemical compounds derived from natural products. In this study, saponin isolated from the leaves of an indigenous Philippine ornamental plant, *Schefflera odorata*, was used as an external agent to determine its potential signal-transducing properties.

Saponins are plant-derived compounds named for their characteristic foaming action in aqueous solution. They are glycosides of either triterpene or steroids (Fig. 13.1). The sugar moiety differs with the kind, number, and nature of the glycosidic linkage (2). The amphipathic property of saponins makes them biologically active compounds. Several saponins have shown anti-inflammatory, antitumoral, antiviral, antifungal,

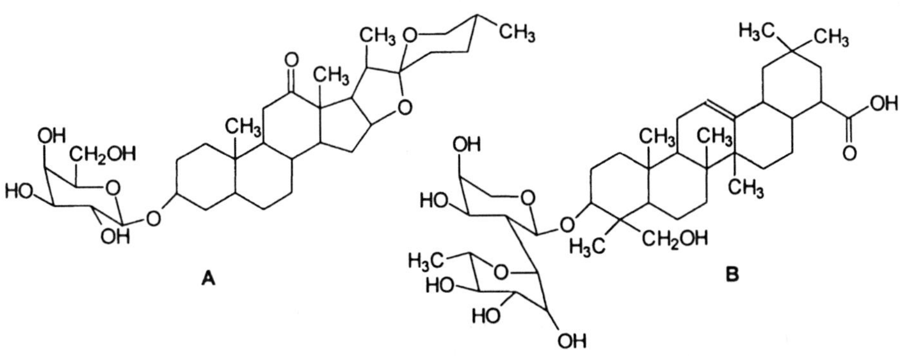

Fig. 13.1. Sample of (*A*) steroidal and (*B*) terpenoidal saponin.

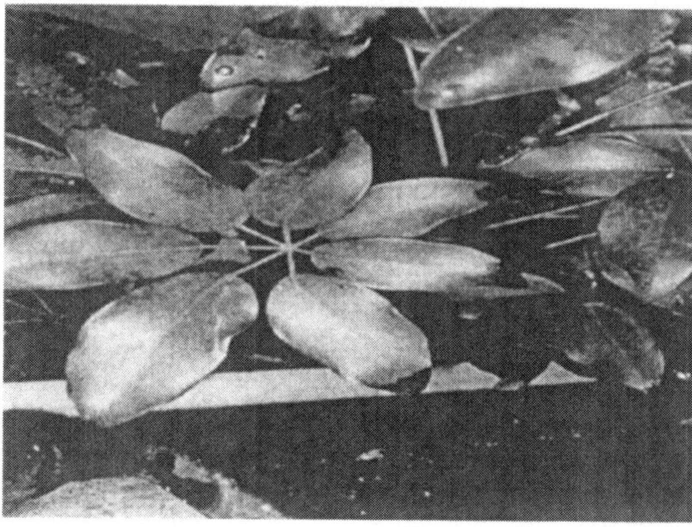

Fig. 13 .2. *Schefflera odorata.*

immunomodulating, antithrombotic, cardiovascular, spermicidal, and molluscidal activities (3). Saponins present in the diet have expectorant and antibiotic properties; they can reduce plasma cholesterol concentration in the blood and may induce bile acid adsorption to dietary fibers (4). Saponins from *Quillaja saponaria* have been found to induce higher level of antibodies and increased production of both interferon (IFN)-δ and interleukin (IL)-4 (5). They can act as transducers by binding to receptors. Interactions with receptors initiate a complex series of intracellular reactions.

Schefflera odorata, known as Lima-lima, is a locally grown plant (Fig. 13.2). It is a glaborous plant with a smooth vine reaching 2–6 m in height. The leaves are compound with 5–6 leaflets having long stalks, all of which originate from the tip of the main petiole, which is longer than the leaflets (6).

Initial studies on *S. odorata* revealed that the saponins constitute the major bioactive compound identified in the leaves and roots of the plant. The median lethal dose (LD_{50}) of the leaf and root decoction was found to be 4.00 and 3.25 g/kg body, respectively. Butanol extracts from both leaves and roots were not directly cytotoxic to a number of established cancer cell lines (7), nor were they mutagenic. Thus, to investigate the possible mechanism for its purported biological activity, this study aims to determine how the saponins from the leaf extract of *S. odorata* can modulate cell signaling pathways. Here, we address questions such as the nature of the effect of the extract on the activation of phosphotyrosine kinases and mitogen-activated protein kinase (MAPK) and on DNA synthesis of airway smooth muscle (ASM) cells. Could the extract induce differentiation and apoptosis on the human lung adenocarcinoma cell line (A549)? Because saponins from diverse sources exhibit immunomodulatory (8) and free radical–scavenging activities, this study also examined these properties of the leaf extract.

Materials and Methods

Materials. General chemicals were from Sigma (St. Louis, MO, USA). [^{3}H] thymidine and [^{32}P] ATP were from Amersham International (Buckinghamshire, England). All cell culture media and reagents, DNAzol and NyCo Prep were from Gibco Life Techniques (Grand Island, New York, USA). Enzyme-linked immunosorbent assay (ELISA) kits for IL-1 and TNF-α release were purchased from Boehringer-Mannheim–Roche Diagnostics (Indianapolis, IN, USA). The A549 cell line was a gift from Dr. Robert Hay of American Type Culture Collection. Xanthine oxidase (XOD, 1 U/mg from cow's milk) was obtained from Boehringer Mannheim (Indianapolis, IN, USA). Hypoxanthine, the spin trap 5,5-dimethyl-1-pyrroline-*N*-oxide (DMPO), diethyleneamine-N,N,N',N",N"-pentaacetic acid (DTPA) were from Labotec (Tokyo, Japan).

Cell Culture. The preparation of the primary cultures of guinea pig airway smooth muscle (ASM) cells was achieved as described previously (9). The cells were maintained in Dulbecco's modified Eagle's medium (DMEM) containing 10% fetal calf serum (FCS) and 10% donor horse serum (DHS); cells were passaged twice, using trypsin before experimentation. Cells were grown to confluence on 24- or 6-well plates and routinely used at passage number 3 or 4 after the initial preparation. Their identity was confirmed to be smooth muscle by the presence of α-actin using a smooth muscle–specific mouse (anti-β-actin) monoclonal antibody (mAb) (9).

Preparation of Sample. Solutions of varying concentrations (μg/mL) of the butanol extract from the leaves of *S. odorata* were prepared. A stock solution was prepared initially by dissolving 1 g of the extract in 1 mL dimethyl sulfoxide. Dilutions of the stock solutions in RPMI 1640 were done. All solutions were then filter sterilized.

SDS-PAGE and Western Blotting. ASM cells in 6-well plates placed in 0.1% FCS and 0.1% DHS DMEM were stimulated with leaf extract for 15 min at 37°C. FCS was added to a final concentration of 10% and incubated for another 20 min. The cells were then lysed in 0.5 mL boiling sample buffer [0.125 mol/L Tris/HCl, pH 6.7, 0.5 mmol/L $Na_2P_2O_7$, 0.25 mmol/L EDTA, 2.5% glycerol, 0.5% sodium dodecylsulfate (SDS), 25 mmol/L dithiothreitol (DTT)]. The cell lysates were subjected to 10% SDS-PAGE, transferred to nitrocellulose sheets, and subsequently blocked with 3% bovine serum albumin (BSA) in Tween-Tris buffered saline (T-TBS) overnight. The nitrocellulose sheet was then probed with a horse radish peroxidase (HRP)-linked antiphosphotyrosine antibody (1:10,000 dilution) in 1% BSA T-TBS for 1 h. The blot was then washed four times with T-TBS. Immunoreactive bands were finally detected with an enhanced chemiluminescence (ECL) detection kit.

SDS/PAGE Mobility Shift. ASM cells in 6-well plates placed in DMEM (0.1% FCS, 0.1% DHS) were incubated with the leaf extract for 15 min at 37°C. Fetal calf serum (10%) was added to stimulate the cells and incubated for another 10 min. The cells were then lysed in 0.5 mL boiling sample buffer. The cell lysates were subjected to 10% SDS-PAGE, transferred to nitrocellulose sheet, and blocked in 3% BSA in T-TBS for 1 h. The nitrocellulose was probed with primary mAb against MAPK (1:5000 dilution) overnight. The nitrocellulose sheet was then washed four times with T-TBS, incubated with HRP-linked anti-mouse antibody for 1 h, and subsequently washed with four times T-TBS. Immunoreactive bands were detected with an ECL detection kit. Activation was indicated by the formation of a shift blot.

MAPK Peptide Assay. ASM cells in 6-well plates placed in 0.1% FCS and 0.1% DHS for 24 h were stimulated with the extract for 15 min. FCS was then added and incubated for 10 min. The reaction was stopped by adding 0.5 mL of ice-cold MAPK lysis buffer [10 mmol/L Trizma base, 150 mmol/L NaCl, 2 mmol/L ethylene glycol tetraacetic acid, 25 mmol/L DTT, 1 mmol/L sodium orthovandate, 1 mmol/L phenylmethylsulfonyl fluoride (PMSF), 10 µg/mL leupeptin, and 10 µg/mL aprotinin, pH 7.4]. Cell lysate (15 µL) was transferred into an Eppendorf tube and 10 µL of substrate (a special peptide that can be phosphorylated by MAPK) was added to each tube. [^{32}P]-ATP (37,000 Bq/ tube) was added and the tubes were then incubated for 20 min at 30°C. Stop solution was added to each tube. The solution in each tube was spotted onto binding paper; the paper was then washed twice with 1% acetic acid and then with distilled water. The degree of phosphorylation was measured in terms of radioactivity, using the scintillation counting machine.

Thymidine Incorporation Assay. ASM cells in 24-well plates having 70-80% confluence were placed in DMEM (0.1% FCS, 0.1% DHS) for 24 h to make the cells quiescent. After 24 h, the medium was replaced with DMEM containing leaf extract of *S. odorata* and/or stimulant. FCS (10%) was used to stimulate DNA synthesis. The cells were then incubated for another 20 h. [^{3}H]-Thymidine (9.250 Bq/0.25 × 10^6 cells) was added to the wells and incubated for another 5 h. The reaction was terminated by washing in 1 mL iced-cooled phosphate-buffered saline (PBS), pH 7.4. The supernatant was removed and the cells were washed three times with 1 mL of 10% trichloroacetic acid. Nuclear material was then dissolved in 0.25 mL of 0.1% (SDS) and 0.3 mol/L sodium hydroxide (NaOH). DNA synthesis was then determined by quantifying [^{3}H]-thymidine incorporated using the liquid scintillation counter.

Treatment of A549 Cell Line for Differentiation Assay. A549 cells were grown in Leighton tubes until semiconfluent; the cells were then exposed overnight to 50 and 100 µg/mL concentrations of the leaf extract.

Immunocytochemistry. The slides in the Leighton tubes in which the cells grew were washed with PBS and fixed with 4% buffered formalin for 5 min, 1% formalin in PBS for 10 min, 5 min in a –10°C methanol, and in ice-cold acetone/methanol mixture (50:50) for 2 min. Antigen was gathered through enzyme digestion with 0.1% freshly prepared trypsin for 3-5 min at 37°C and then rinsed thoroughly with water.

The slides were washed three times with PBS for 5 min each time. The new specific antigens were blocked with 10% normal goat serum, nonfat powdered milk and BSA. They were then washed with PBS twice. The fixed cells were exposed to a cytokeratin (CK4) mAb, incubated for 1–2 h, and then washed three times with PBS. The slides were then exposed to a secondary antibody labeled with the enzyme, HRP, incubated at room temperature for 30 min, and washed with PBS three times. They were exposed to aminoethyl carbazole (AEC)-HRP for 30 min at room temperature, then washed three times with PBS. Chromogen AEC/DAB (Diamino benzidine) was added for 30 min at room temperature, then washed three times with PBS. Chromogen AEC/DAB was added for 5 min at room temperature and rinsed thoroughly with water.

DNA Fragmentation Assay. Cell suspension (1 mL) was inoculated onto 12-well plates and grown overnight to allow the cells to adhere. After 24 h, the medium was removed and replaced with RPMI 1640 without serum and antibiotics. The cells were then incubated with the leaf extract of *Schefflera odorata* for 24 h. The concentrations of *S. odorata* used were 20, 100, and 150 µg/mL. After incubation, the cells were harvested by trypsinization and treated with DNAzol to isolate the DNA. The isolated DNA was then subjected to electrophoresis using 1% agarose gel in TBE (Tris-borate-ethylene-diamine tetracetic acid) buffer for 1 h at 100 V. The gel was then stained with ethidium bromide, washed with deionized water, and photographed under ultraviolet (UV) illumination.

Isolation of Mononuclear Cells. Fresh human blood (100 mL) was collected into tubes containing heparin. The blood was then diluted with an equal volume of 0.9% NaCl solution. Diluted blood (6 mL) was carefully layered with 3 mL of NyCo Prep solution and centrifuged at 800 × *g* for 20 min at room temperature. After 20 min, the mononuclear cells formed a distinct band at the interface between the sample layer and the NyCo Prep solution. The cells were then removed from the interface using a Pasteur pipette without disturbing the upper layer. The cells were then washed with PBS and resuspended in RPMI with 10% FCS.

Induction of IL-1 and TNF-α Release from the Mononuclear Cells. Mononuclear cells (1 mL), with a cell density of 1×10^6 cells/mL, were placed in each well of a 12-well tissue culture plate. The cells were incubated in the absence and presence of increasing concentrations of the leaf extract of *S. odorata* (20, 40, 50, 100, and 150 µg/mL) and 10 µg/mL of lipopolysaccharide (LPS) in duplicate for 24 h at 37°C, 5% CO_2. After 24 h, the supernatants were collected and dialyzed against PBS.

Quantitative Determination of IL-1 by ELISA Method. Standard solutions or samples (20 µL) were pipetted into the wells of the streptavidin-coated microtiter plate (MTP). To each of these wells, 200 µL of the immunoreagent (anti-IL-1-POD + anti-IL-1-biotin) was added, covered with an adhesive foil, and incubated for 2 h at room temperature. After 2 h, the incubation buffer was removed by suction and the wells were washed three times with 300 µL of washing buffer. Then 200 µL of the substrate solution (tetramethyl benzidine solution [TMB]) was placed into each wells, covered with an adhesive cover foil, and incubated in the dark for 20 min. The reaction was stopped by the addition of 50 μL of stop solution (H_2SO_4), and the absorbance was read at 490 nm (reference wavelength 600 nm) against a blank.

Quantitative Determination of TNF-α by ELISA Method. Standard solutions or samples (20 μL) were pipetted into the wells of streptavidin-coated MTP. To each of these wells, 200 μL of the immunoreagent (anti-TNF-α-POD + antiTNF-α-biotin) was added. The plate was then covered with an adhesive foil and incubated for 4 h under constant shaking. The incubating buffer was then removed and the wells were then washed with the washing buffer three times; then 200 μL of TMB was added and incubated for another 20 min. The addition of 50 μL stop solution halted the reaction. Absorbance was measured at 490 nm (reference wavelength 600 nm).

Determination of Hydroxyl Radical–Scavenging Activity. Mixing H_2O_2 and iron (III) salt generated hydroxyl radicals. The reaction mixture was prepared by mixing 20 μL of 0.092 mol/L DMPO, 75 μL of 1 mmol/L H_2O_2, 75 μL of 0.01 mol/L $FeSO_4$, and 50 μL of leaf extract (dissolved in deionized water). This mixture was then transferred into a flat cell (200 μL). Exactly 40 s after mixing, electron spin resonance (ESR) spectra of the spin adduct, DMPO·OH was measured by a Free Radical Monitor.

Determination of Superoxide Radical–Scavenging Activity. Superoxide anion was generated by the hypoxanthine (HPX)-XOD system. All solutions were dissolved in PBS, 50 μL of 1 mol/L MHPX, 35 μL of 5.5 mmol/L DTPA, and 50 μL of the sample solution; 15 μL of 9.2 mol/L DMPO and 50 μL of 0.4 unit/mL XOD were mixed and transferred into the flat cell. Exactly 40 s after mixing, the ESR spectra of DMPO-OO-spin adduct were analyzed.

Results and Discussion

Effect of S. odorata on Phosphotyrosine Kinases. Phosphotyrosine kinases are extracellular enzymes that are activated by phosphorylation. Phosphorylation of these enzymes on the cell surface plays an important role in the control of cell growth and proliferation induced by growth factors and oncogenes (10). In this study, airway smooth muscle (ASM) cells were used to study the effect of the leaf extract on its propagation. Propagation of ASM cells is a characteristic of asthma (11). The activation of phosphotyrosine kinases was stimulated by FCS as demonstrated in Figure 13.3. The formation of bands corresponds to all phosphorylated proteins. Increased concentration of the leaf extract showed increased inhibition of band formation at 205, 112, and 42 kDa. Disappearance of these bands means that some proteins were not phosphorylated, suggesting that some enzymes responsible for phosphorylation were not activated. Inhibition of band formation implies that the leaf extract could inhibit the propagation of these cells.

Stimulation of phosphotyrosine kinase could lead to the activation of several enzymes, one of which is MAPK.

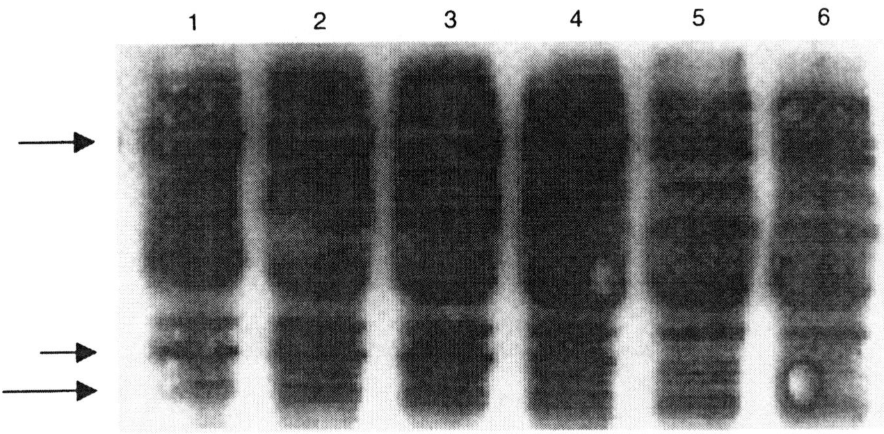

Fig. 13.3. Effect of leaf extract on the activation of phosphotyrosine kinase in airway smooth muscle (ASM) cells. Immunoblot demonstrating the fetal calf serum (FCS)-induced activation of phosphotyrosine kinase and the effect of the leaf extract. Lane 1, control cells; lane 2, 10% FCS; lane 3, FCS + 50 µg/mL leaf extract; lane 4, FCS + 100 (g/mL leaf extract; lane 5, FCS + 150 µg/mL leaf extract; lane 6, FCS + 200 µg/mL leaf extract. This is a representative result of an experiment done on three separate cell preparations.

Effect of S. odorata on MAPK Activation. The MAPK cascade is the major signaling system by which cells transduce extracellular cues into intracellular responses (12). The effect of the leaf extract on the activation of the MAPK cascade was determined by two methods, SDS-PAGE mobility shift and MAPK peptide assay (Fig. 13.4). The activation of MAPK as stimulated by FCS is indicated by its retarded mobility upon SDS-PAGE. This shift in mobility is caused by its phosphorylation by an upstream enzyme (13). The shift in mobility is not observed in ASM cells treated with 100 µg/mL leaf extract; for ASM cells treated with 200 µg/mL leaf extract, no band

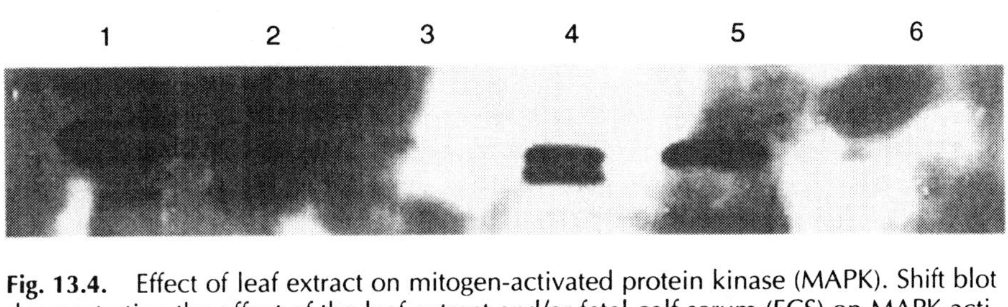

Fig. 13.4. Effect of leaf extract on mitogen-activated protein kinase (MAPK). Shift blot demonstrating the effect of the leaf extract and/or fetal calf serum (FCS) on MAPK activation. Lane 1, control cells; lane 2, 100 µg/mL leaf extract; lane 3, 200 µg/mL leaf extract; lane 4, 10% FCS; lane 5, FCS + 100 µg/mL leaf extract; lane 6, FCS + 200 µg/mL leaf extract.

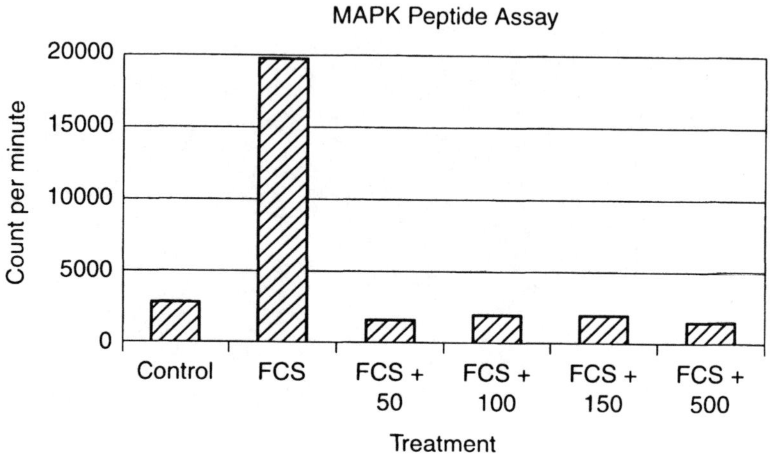

Fig. 13.5. Bar graph showing the inhibition of mitogen-activated protein kinase (MAPK) activation by the leaf extract. Ten percent fetal calf serum (FCS) was used to stimulate MAPK activation. The concentration of leaf extract is expressed in μg/mL. Cpm indicated for each concentration represents the mean of three replicates for each trial.

was formed at all. The result in the MAPK mobility shift blot was further confirmed by another assay, the MAPK peptide assay. In this assay, a special peptide is incubated with the cell lysate. If the MAPK in the cell lysate is activated, it will phosphorylate its substrate (peptide), and the amount of phosphorylation is indicated as radioactivity (cpm). The results are shown in Figure 13.5. The figure shows that FCS induced the activation of MAPK as indicated in the increased amount of radioactivity. However, when ASM cells were treated with the leaf extract in combination with FCS, the activation of MAPK was inhibited.

Effect of S. odorata on DNA Synthesis. Because the activation of MAPK is affected by the leaf extract, there is a high probability that leaf extract can also the affect the DNA of the nucleus. This was determined by the incorporation of tritiated thymidine during DNA synthesis. Fetal calf serum (10%) stimulates DNA synthesis in ASM cells as indicated by an increase in the amount of [^{3}H] thymidine incorporated (see Figure 13.6). When ASM cells were treated with FCS in combination with the leaf extract, the incorporation of [^{3}H]-thymidine into DNA was inhibited (Fig. 13.6). Fifty percent of DNA synthesis inhibition was observed at 100 μg/mL and almost 100% inhibition was observed at 200 μg/mL.

Induction of Differentiation in A549 Cell Line by S. odorata. A549 cells treated with the leaf extract of *S. odorata* at concentrations of 50 and 100 μg/mL for 24 h exhibited distinct expression of CK4, which was greater than that seen when treated with 10% FCS alone. CK4, an intermediate filament marker of epithelial differentiation, is

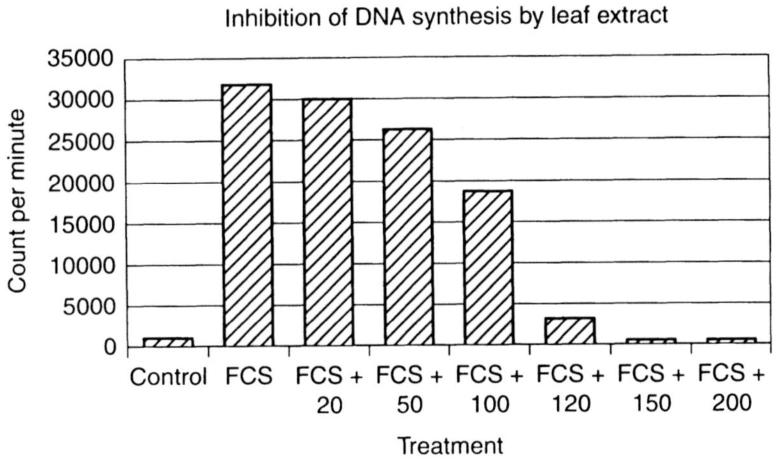

Fig. 13.6. Bar graph showing the inhibition of DNA synthesis by the leaf extract. Ten percent fetal calf serum (FCS) was used to stimulate MAPK activation. The concentration of leaf extract is expressed in µg/mL. Cpm indicated for each concentration represents the mean of three replicates for each trial.

shown as red-stained cells. Maximum expression of CK4 was observed in almost 80% of the cells treated with 50 µg/mL of leaf extract (Figures 13.7-13.10). Interestingly, reduced expression was observed in cells treated with 100 µg/mL leaf extract (Figure 13.11).

DNA Fragmentation Induced by S. odorata. Activation of the phosphatases/kinases has been implicated in internucleosomal fragmentation, leading to apoptosis (14). The DNA fragmentation pattern of A549 (cell density used is 1×10^6 cells/mL) incubated with 20 and 100 µg/mL for 24 h is shown in Figure 13.12.

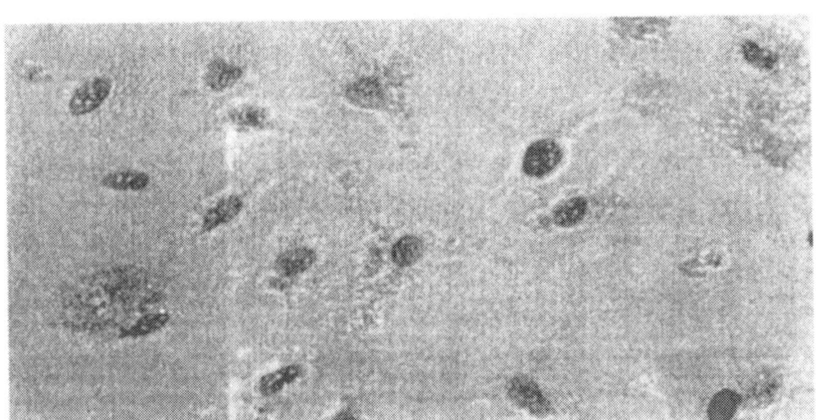

Fig. 13.7. Untreated A549 cells grown in serum-free RPMI and incubated for 24 h.

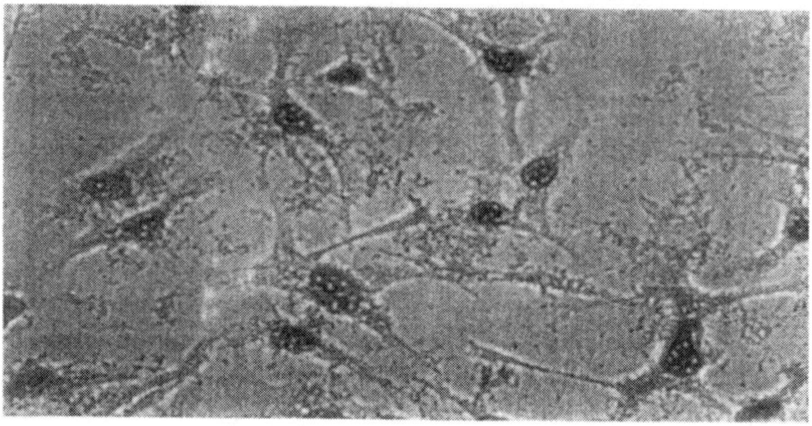

Fig. 13.8. Untreated A549 cells grown in serum-supplemented (10% fetal calf serum) RPMI and incubated for 24 h.

Immunomodulating Activity of S. odorata. LPS is a cell wall polymer from gram-negative bacteria that stimulates the release of cytokines such as IL-1 and TNF-α (15). This observation is consistent with the result of the assays shown in Figures 13.13 and 13.14. In the case of IL-1, when the cells are treated in the absence and presence of increasing concentrations of the leaf extract, there was an increase in the release of IL-1 in a dose-related manner (Figure 13.13). This increase in the release of IL-1 as induced by the leaf extract is comparable to the activity of LPS. Figure 13.14 shows the release of TNF-α from the mononuclear cells when stimulated by the leaf extract. The leaf extract of *S. odorata* at 150 μg/mL stimulated

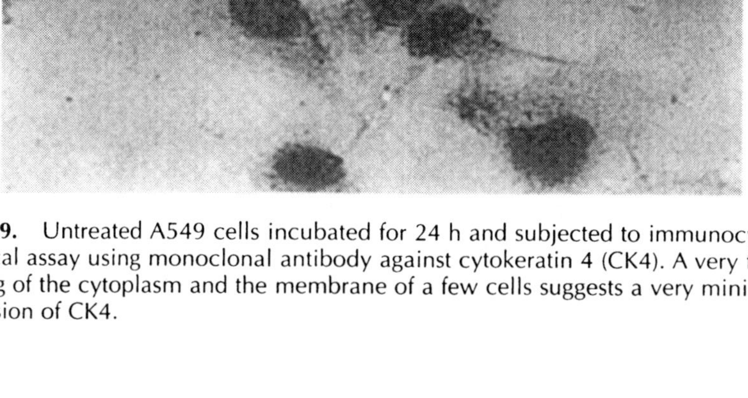

Fig. 13.9. Untreated A549 cells incubated for 24 h and subjected to immunocytochemical assay using monoclonal antibody against cytokeratin 4 (CK4). A very faint staining of the cytoplasm and the membrane of a few cells suggests a very minimal expression of CK4.

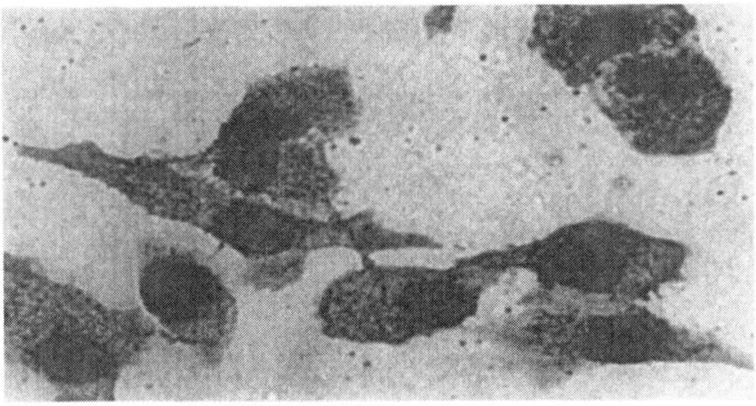

Fig. 13.10. A549 cells treated with 50 μg/mL leaf extract and subjected to immunocytochemical assay using monoclonal antibody against cytokeratin 4 (CK4). Distinct red stains in the cytoplasm and in the cell membrane, characteristic of CK4 expression, were observed in >80% of the cell population.

a release of TNF-α that was much higher than that of the negative control. However, the activity of the leaf extract is not comparable to that of LPS.

The results from these two assays indicate that *S. odorata* has a unique way of modulating the immune system by the release of IL-1. IL-1 is credited with several biological activities. It plays an important role in the activation of the cells of the im-

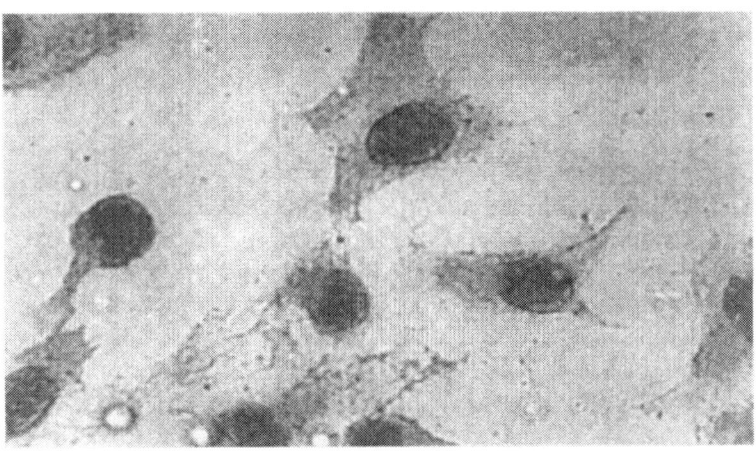

Fig. 13.11. A549 cells treated with 100 μg/mL leaf extract and subjected to immunocytochemical assay using monoclonal antibody against cytokeratin 4 (CK4). Slight staining in a few cells is indicative of CK4 expression. Changes in the morphology of the cells were evident.

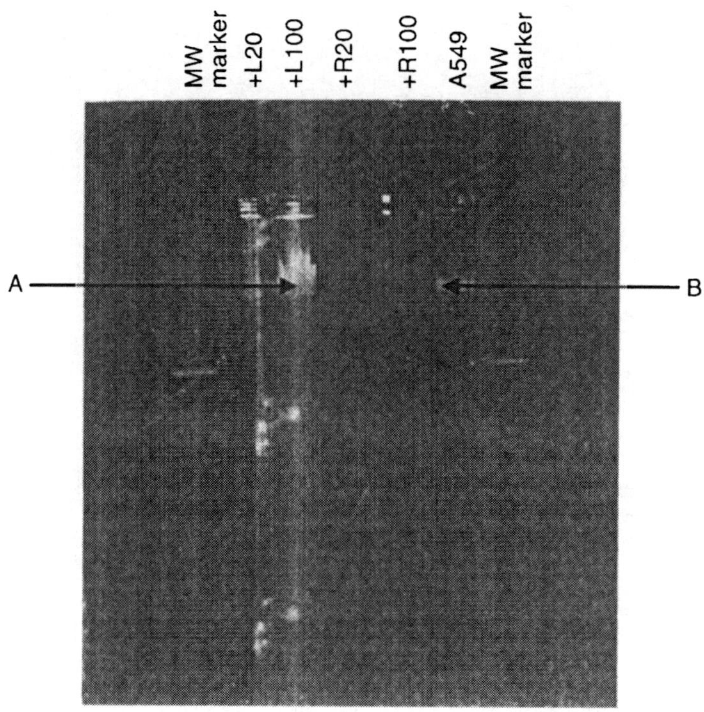

Fig. 13.12. DNA fragmentation pattern of A549 cells inoculated with 20 and 100 μg/mL of the leaf extract for 24 h. Fragmented A549 DNA isolated from cells treated with 100 μg/mL leaf extract (*A*) shows a pronounced tailing compared with the DNA from untreated A549 cells (*B*).

mune system. It acts on macrophages and monocytes, triggering its own production and the production of other cytokines and growth factors. It also induces the cytotoxic and tumoricidal activity of mononuclear cells (16).

Free Radical–Scavenging Activity of S. odorata. The leaf extract was investigated for its hydroxyl- and superoxide radical–scavenging activity. Hydroxyl radicals were generated by mixing hydrogen peroxide and iron salt. This reaction is known as the Fenton reaction. Figure 13.15 shows that the leaf extract of *S. odorata* trapped or scavenged the hydroxyl radicals produced in a dose-related manner. This indicates that the saponins from the leaf extract can scavenge hydroxyl radicals.

The superoxide anion radical was generated by the HPX-XOD system. Figure 13.16 shows that the leaf extract also has superoxide radical scavenging activity. However, the activity does not seem to be concentration dependent. The ability of the leaf extract from *S. odorata* to break free radical chain reactions may be attributed to its rich saponin content. By trapping free radicals, saponins are able to protect biomolecules from uncontrolled oxidation reactions.

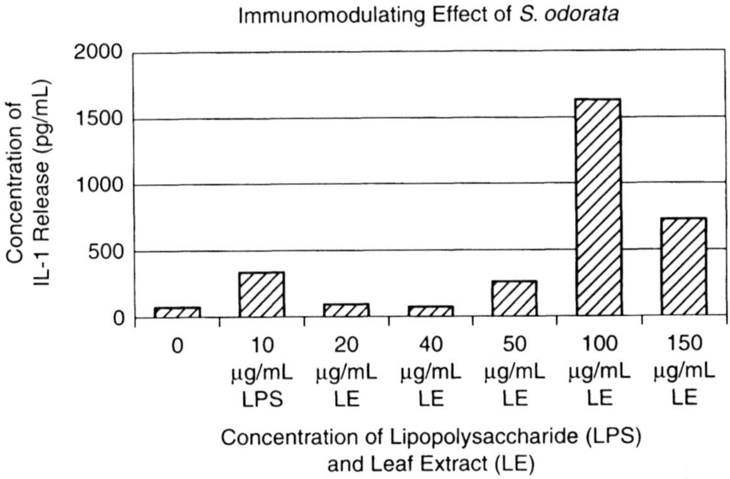

Fig. 13.13. *S. odorata*–induced release of interleukin (IL)-1 from the mononulcear cells. The concentration of IL-1 released (expressed in pg/mL) represents the mean of three replicates.

Hydroxyl radicals are the most reactive free radical species, capable of direct oxidative damage to macromolecules, including DNA, protein, and lipid membranes (13). Although the superoxide anion free radical has been implicated as the active species that causes oxidative damage to red blood cells, the body is protected from the harmful effects of the radical by elimination (17).

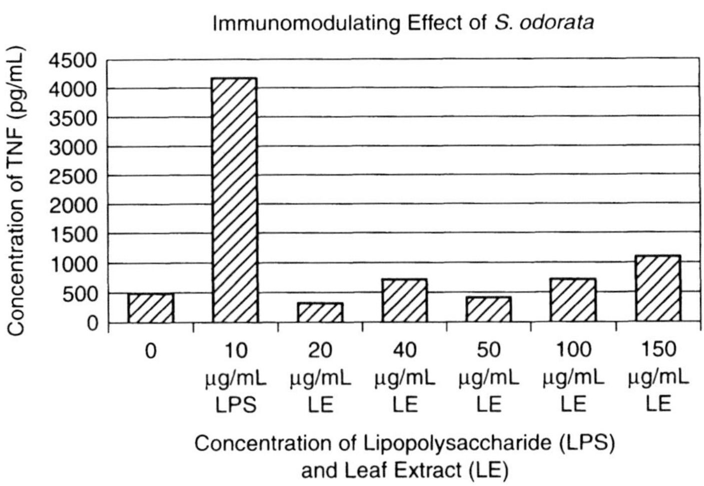

Fig. 13.14. Tumor necrosis factor (TNF)-α release from the mononuclear cells. The concentration of TNF-α released (expressed in pg/mL) represents the mean of three replicates.

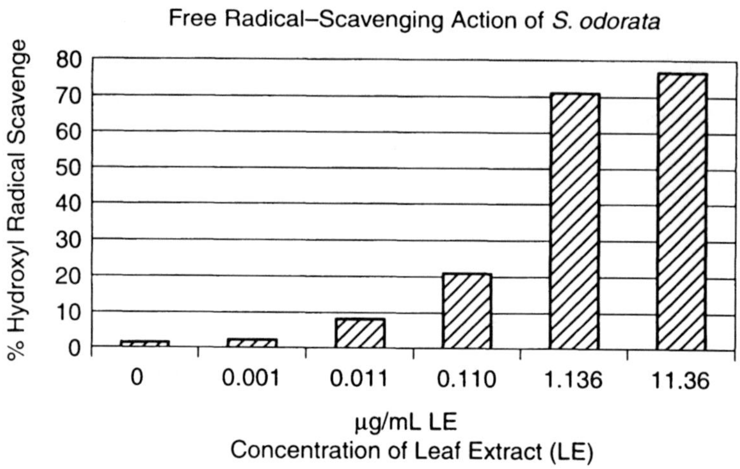

Fig. 13.15. Dose response of the leaf extract of *S. odorata* on 5,5-dimethyl-1-pyrroline-*N*-oxide (DMPO)-OH spin adducts. The values for % hydroxyl free radical scavenge are means, $n = 6$.

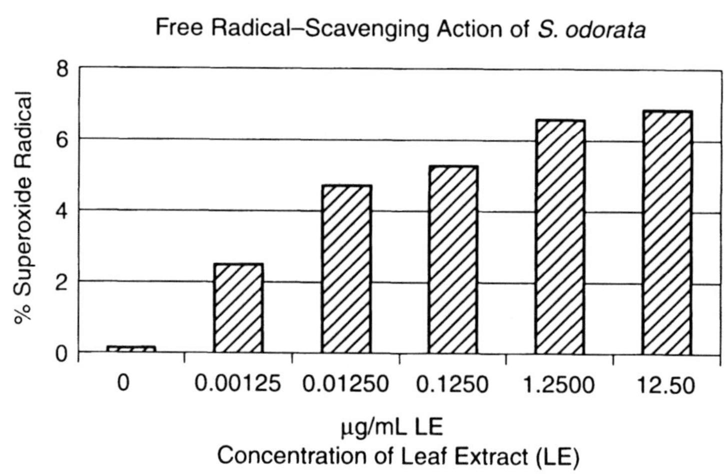

Fig. 13.16. Dose response of the leaf extract of *S. odorata* on 5,5-dimethyl-1-pyrroline-*N*-oxide (DMPO)-O^- spin adducts. The values of the superoxide free radical scavenge are means, $n = 6$.

Summary

This study shows that saponins from the leaf extract of *S. odorata* can serve as modulators of the cell signaling pathway. The leaf extract acts as an extracellular signal to switch off extracellular enzymes that are required for the proliferation of ASM cells. The signal can then be transmitted into the nucleus, which in turn promotes

DNA fragmentation of A549 lung cancer cell lines, suggesting that *S. odorata* can induce A549 cells to undergo programmed cell death. At present, this approach has gained wide acceptability by most cancer scientists working in the area of drug development for cancer.

Recent experiments have also revealed the potential immunomodulating property of the leaf extract. Monocytes incubated with the leaf extract gave a dose-dependent release of Il-1 but not TNF-α. The ESR technique showed that the leaf extract could quench hydroxyl free radicals, suggesting its antioxidant property.

Acknowledgments

The authors thank the Philippine Council for Health Research and Development (PCHRD) for the research fellowship grant; Dr. Nigel Pyne, Department of Pharmacology, University of Strathclyde, Scotland for the training in signal transduction experiments; the British Council for the travel grant; and Dr. Robert Hay of ATTC for kindly providing the cell lines.

References

1. Heldin, C.H., and Purton, M., eds. (1996) *Signal Transduction,* 1st edn., pp. 1–15, Chapman and Hall, London.
2. Basu, N., and Rastogi, R.P. (1976) Triterpenoid Saponins and Sapogenins. *Phytochemistry 6*, 1249–1270.
3. Bader, G, Plohmann, B., Hiller, K., and Franz, G. (1996) Cytotoxicity of Triterpenoid Saponins. *Pharmazie 51*, 414–417.
4. Maharaj, I.K., Froh, K.J., and Campbell, J.B. (1986) Immune Responses of Mice to Inactivated Rabies Vaccine Administered Orally: Potentiation by *Quillaja* saponin. *Can. J. Microbiol. 32*, 414–420.
5. Sjolander, A., van't Land, B., and Bengtsson, K.L. (1997) Iscoms Containing Purified *Quillaja* Saponins Upregulate both Th1-Like Immune Responses. *Cell. Immunol. 177*, 68–76.
6. Quisumbing, E. (1978) *Medicinal Plants of the Philippines*, JMC Press, Manila, Philippines.
7. Sarau, J.K. (1997) Preliminary Screening of Cytotoxic Activity of *Raphanus sativus* L. Seeds and *Schefflera odorata* B. Leaves and Roots on Human-Derived Cancer Cell Lines. M.S. Thesis, University of Santo Tomas, Manila, pp. 97–114.
8. Behboudi, S. , Morein, B., Eriksson-Villacres, M., *In Vivo* and *In Vitro* Induction of Il-6 by *Quillaja saponaria* Molina Triterpenoid Formulations. *Cytokines 9*, 682–687.
9. Pyne, S., and Pyne , N.J. (1993) Bradykinin Stimulates Phospholipase D in Primary Cultures of Guinea Pig Tracheal Smooth Muscle. *Biochem. Pharmacol. 45*, 593–603.
10. Guan, K.L. (1994)The Mitogen Activated Protein Kinase Signal Transduction Pathway from the Cell Surface to the Nucleus. *Cell Signalling 6*, 581–589.
11. Johnson, P., Ra, C.L., Armour, C., Carey, C., and Black, J.L. (1995) Heparin and pge2 Inhibit DNA Synthesis in Human Airway Smooth Muscle Cells in Culture, Abstract 2, 0094L.
12. Caro, E. and Mahadevan, L. (1995) Parallel Signal Processing Among Mammalian

MAPKs. *Trends Biochem. Sci. 20*, 117–121.

13. Pyne, S. Chapman, J., Steele, L., and Pyne, N. (1996) Sphingomyelin-Derived Lipids Differently Regulated Kinase 2 (ERK-2) and c-Jun N-Terminal Kinase (JNK) Signal Cascades in Airway Smooth Muscle. *Eur. J. Biochem. 237*, 819–826.
14. Hockenberry, D.M., Oltval, Z., Yin, X., Miliman, C., and Korsmeyer, S.J. (1993) Bcl-2 Functions in an Antioxidant Pathway to Prevent Apoptosis. *Cell 75*, 241–251
15. Lichtman, S.N., Wang, J., Scwab, J.H., and Lemasters, J. (1994) Comparison of Peptidoglycan-Polysaccharide and Lipopolysaccharide Stimulation of Kupffer Cells to Produce Tumor Necrosis Factor and Interleukin-1. *Hepatology 19*, 1013–1022.
16. Roitt, I., Brostoff, J., and Male, D. (1989) *Immunology*, 2nd edn., pp. 9.11–9.11, Gower Medical Publishing, London.
17. Hodgson, E., and Guthrie, F. (1980) *Biochemical Toxicology*, pp. 345–356, Blackwell Science, Cambridge.

Chapter 14

Accelerated Cellular Senescence and Altered Response to Nitric Oxide (NO) in Glucose-6-Phosphate Dehydrogenase (G6PD)-Deficient Human Fibroblasts

Hung-yao Ho,[a] Mei-ling Cheng,[a] and Daniel Tsun-yee Chiu[a,b]

[a]School of Medical Technology, Chang Gung University, Kwei-san, Tao-yuan, Taiwan
[b]Graduate Institute of Basic Medical Sciences & School of Medical Technology, Chang Gung University, Kwei-san, Tao-yuan, Taiwan

Introduction

Glucose-6-phosphate dehydrogenase (G6PD), the key regulatory enzyme in the hexose monophosphate shunt (HMS), catalyzes the oxidation of glucose-6-phosphate (G6P) to 6-phosphogluconolactone and the production of reducing equivalents in the form of NADPH to meet the cellular needs for reductive biosynthesis and maintenance of the cellular redox status. The importance of G6PD is illustrated by clinical manifestations of its deficiency. G6PD deficiency, a common enzymopathy affecting >200 million people worldwide, can cause neonatal jaundice, drug- or infection-induced hemolytic crisis, favism, and, less commonly, nonspherocytic hemolytic anemia (1–3). The hemolytic nature of all of these syndromes is attributed to the inability of G6PD-deficient erythrocytes under oxidative stress to maintain NADPH in its reduced form. This subsequently causes oxidation of cellular components and eventual removal of the damaged cells from circulation (4,5). Most studies of G6PD have explored the pathophysiology of G6PD-deficient erythrocytes and the molecular characterization of different G6PD variants. In contrast, the chronic effects of G6PD deficiency on cells other than erythrocytes remain largely unknown.

The long-term effect of redox imbalance is the accumulation of oxidative damage, which has been implicated as a causative factor of cellular senescence. Reactive oxygen species (ROS) produced during metabolism may cause cumulative damages, provoking senescence (6–9). This view is supported by studies with *Drosophila* strains overexpressing Cu/Zn superoxide dismutase and/or catalase, in which significantly extended mean and maximum life spans were observed (10,11), and studies in which exogenous SOD1 expression in motor neurons of *Drosophila* increased the organism's normal life span by up to 40% (12). Because G6PD is indispensable to maintenance of the cellular redox balance and detoxification of ROS (13), it is likely that the G6PD activity regulates cell growth, and any change related to it alters the course of cellular senescence.

In addition to the cumulative effect of oxidative damage, cellular redox status can modulate growth and survival signals (14–16). For example, tumor necrosis factor (TNF)-α–induced apoptosis is inhibited by treatment with *N*-acetyl cysteine (17); mitogenic effects of PDGF can be blocked by antioxidants (18). As a result of diminished G6PD activity in the deficient cells, the redox balance is likely to shift toward the formation of more ROS, which may lead to altered responses to growth factors or other signaling molecules.

Although the complete picture of the roles of G6PD in nucleated cells is not yet available, the findings of our laboratory and those of others are beginning to shed light on this. It is the goal of this chapter to summarize some of these developments.

Materials and Methods

Cell Culture, Plasmid Construction, Retroviral Packaging, and Infection. The G6PD-deficient human foreskin fibroblast, designated HFF1 and HFF2, and its normal counterpart, designated HFF3, were isolated and maintained as previously described (19). HFF1 and HFF2 were identified to carry the Taiwan-Hakka ($G6PD^{1376T}$) and Gaohe ($G6PD^{95G}$) variants of the G6PD gene, respectively (20–22). The cell strain GM01150, GM01869, GM01163, and GM01870, the fibroblasts derived from human skin, were acquired from NIGMS Human Genetic Mutant Cell Repository of Coriell Institute for Medical Research (CIMR) (Camden, NJ). The cell strains GM01163 and GM01870 carry the 563 C→T Mediterranean mutation in their *G6PD* gene. The cells were cultured in Dulbecco's modified Eagle's medium (DMEM) supplemented with 10% fetal calf serum (FCS), 100 U/mL penicillin, 100 U/mL streptomycin, and 0.25 g/L amphotericin at 37°C in a humidified atmosphere of 5% CO_2. The cells were fed every other day and passaged at a ratio of 1:6 before the cultures were confluent. The cell number was determined by cell counting. The number of population doublings is defined as $\log_2 N/N_0$, where N is the cell number at the time of harvesting and N_0 is the cell number at the time of seeding. Population doubling level (PDL) refers to the cumulative number of population doublings that cells have undergone since their isolation from primary culture.

For cultures receiving NO treatment, ~2×10^5 cells were seeded on d –1 (i.e., 24 h before drug treatment) and treated with indicated concentrations of sodium nitroprusside (SNP; Calbiochem, San Diego, CA) on d 0. The cell number and the extent of apoptosis were quantified on subsequent days.

The retroviral vectors, pLXIN, pLEIN, pLGIN, and pLKGIN, were constructed as mentioned elsewhere (19). Retroviral packaging and infection were done as previously described (19,23).

Senescence-Associated β-Galactosidase (SA-β-Gal) Staining and Glucose-6-Phosphate Dehydrogenase (G6PD) Activity Assay. Cells were stained for SA-β-Gal activity as previously described (24). In brief, they were washed in phosphate-buffered saline (PBS), fixed for 3 min at room temperature in 2% formaldehyde/0.2%

glutaraldehyde, washed, and then incubated at 37°C with fresh stain solution [0.1% (wt/vol) 5-bromo-4-chloro-3-indolyl-β-D-galactosidase (X-Gal)/40 mmol/L citric acid/sodium phosphate (pH 6)/5 mmol/L potassium ferrocyanide/5 mmol/L potassium ferricyanide/150 mmol/L NaCl/ 2 mmol/L $MgCl_2$]. Staining was evident in 2–4 h and maximal in 12–16 h. The number of SA-β-Gal positive cells was counted.

G6PD activity was measured spectrophotometrically at 340 nm by the reduction of $NADP^+$ in the presence of glucose-6-phosphate as described (19,25).

Detection of ROS by Dichlorofluorescin (H_2DCF) Staining. Formation of ROS in cells was detected by monitoring the fluorescence of dichlorofluorescein (DCF), the oxidation product of H_2DCF (26). The cells were loaded with 10 mmol/L dichlorofluorescein diacetate (H_2DCFDA) for 5 min at 37°C. After treatment, they were immediately refed with fresh medium and observed under a fluorescent microscope.

Flow Cytometric Analysis of Apoptotic Cells. Cells were rinsed with ice-cold PBS, trypsinized, and resuspended in 0.3 mL PBS. They were then fixed and permeabilized by addition of 0.7 mL ethanol. After a brief wash, the cells were gently resuspended in 1 mL propidium iodide (PI) stain solution [40 µg/mL propidium iodide (Sigma Chemical, St. Louis, MO), 100 µg/mL RNase A, and 0.5% Triton X-100 in PBS] and incubated at room temperature for 30 min before analysis on a FACSCAN flow cytometer (Becton Dickinson, San Jose, CA). The sub-G_1 fraction is considered as the apoptotic cells and taken as a measure of the extent of apoptosis. The sub-G_1 phase was quantified using Modfit software (Becton Dickinson).

Statistical Analysis. Results are expressed as means ± SEM. Data were analyzed by two-way analysis of variance (ANOVA). When necessary, *t*-test, Tukey's test, or Dunnett's test was used to compare the mean values of groups. *P*-values < 0.05 were considered significant.

Early Onset of Growth Cessation and Senescence in G6PD-Deficient Cells

Retarded Growth and Shortened Life span in G6PD-Deficient Cells. Study of growth kinetics showed strikingly different growth patterns for G6PD-deficient (HFF1) and normal (HFF3) human foreskin fibroblasts. Our G6PD-deficient HFF1 cells were derived from an individual carrying the 1376 G→T transversion, which changes the corresponding amino acid from arginine to leucine and causes a marked reduction in G6PD activity (20–22). At early passages (PDL 5–13), the HFF1 cells grew with nearly the same doubling time (23.8 ± 1.6 h, n = 10) as the normal cells (Fig. 14.1A). However, after PDL 30, these cells grew at an increasingly retarded rate; the averaged doubling time increased from 38.2 ± 4.3 h (n = 10) at PDL 30–38 to 68.6 ± 11.0 h (n =10) at PDL 50–58. In contrast, the doubling time of HFF3 cells remained essentially the same from PDL 5 to PDL 58. It is only after PDL 60 that the HFF3 began growing at a slower pace. When growth histories of HFF1 and HFF3 cells were inspected, the former cell strain ceased to grow at PDL 63 ± 2.5, whereas

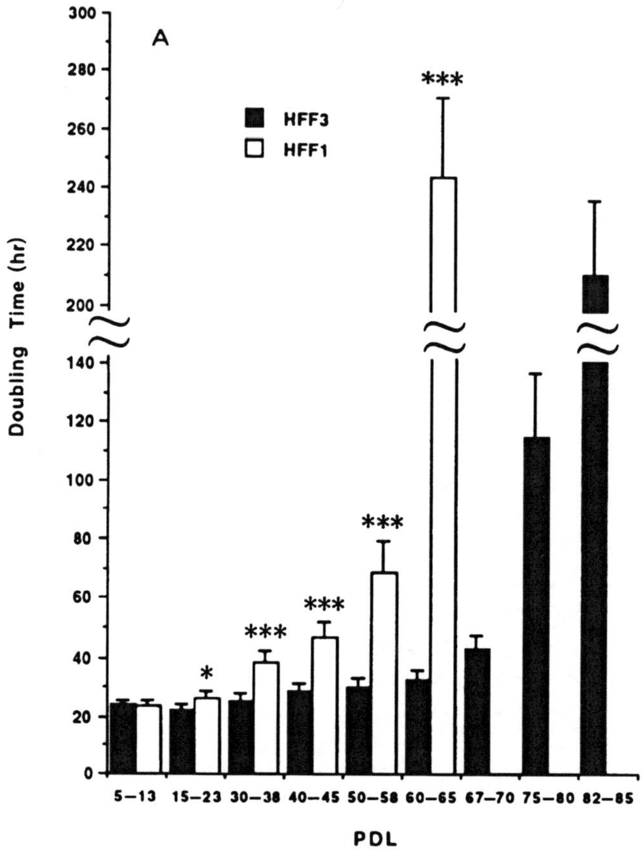

Fig. 14.1. Effects of glucose-6-phosphate dehydrogenase (G6PD) deficiency on human foreskin fibroblasts (HFF). (A) The averaged doubling times of normal HFF3 cells and G6PD-deficient HFF1 cells at different population doubling levels (PDL) are shown. Because HFF1 cells ceased to grow after PDL 63, the PDL 60–65 bar of HFF1 represents the doubling time of HFF1 cells from PDL 60 to 63. Results are expressed as means ± SEM, $n = 10$ experiments. *$P < 0.05$ vs. HFF3; ***$P < 0.001$ vs. HFF3.

the latter did so after ~20 more population doublings (Fig. 14.1B). Consistent with the greatly reduced replicative potential in HFF1 cells, their rate of [H^3] thymidine incorporation dropped significantly upon passage from PDL 6 to PDL 55.

It is likely that the retarded growth and the shortened replicative life span are general characteristics of G6PD-deficient cells. Another cell strain, HFF2, which had G6PD activity between those of HFF1 and HFF3, exhibited intermediate growth kinetics. Furthermore, analysis of several cell strains from CIMR with varying levels of G6PD activity revealed a similar trend (Table 14.1). The lower the G6PD activity in the cells, the greater their tendency to undergo growth arrest.

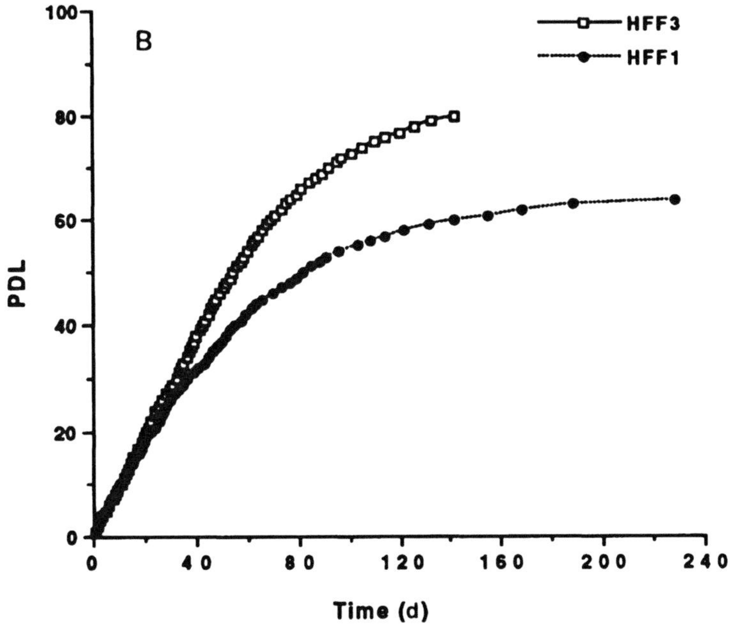

Fig. 14.1. *(continued)* (B) The growth history of HFF1 cells and HFF3 cells. A representative experiment is shown here. *Source*: Ref. 19.

Inverse Correlation Between Doubling Time and G6PD Activity. When the correlation between G6PD activity and retarded growth was examined, a progressive loss of G6PD activity during the continual passage was observed. The G6PD activity in HFF1 cells was reduced by >50% upon passage to PDL 60, whereas the corresponding change in HFF3 cells was slight. This phenomenon was not restricted to our cells because similar observations were made on cell strains from CIMR (Table 14.1). An inverse correlation existed between the doubling times of HFF1 and HFF3 (up to PDL 60) and their G6PD activities. This is consistent with the notion that cells with higher G6PD activity also have greater replicative potential.

G6PD Deficiency Predisposed the Cells to Premature Senescence. Cellular senescence was originally defined by the observation that primary fibroblasts have finite proliferative capacity (27). In addition to the shortened life span of HFF1 cells, several lines of evidence suggest that the early growth arrest of G6PD-deficient cells is phenotypically indistinguishable from cellular senescence. Flow cytometric analyses showed that the premature growth cessation of HFF1 cells was accompanied by a cell cycle arrest in G_1 phase. This arrest state was different from quiescence induced by serum deprivation because the addition of medium supplemented with 20% serum did not stimulate the growth of G6PD-deficient cells once they ceased prolif-

TABLE 14.1 Retarded Growth of Glucose-6-Phosphate (G6PD)-Deficient Cell Strains[a]

	Doubling time (h) G6PD activity (U/mg protein in cell lysate)			
	Cell strain			
	GM01150	GM01869	GM01163	GM01870
PDL 15	68.87 ± 5.43	73.94 ± 1.88	64.68 ± 3.82	75.52 ± 6.67
	(0.265 ± 0.079)	(0.293 ± 0.095)	(0.125 ± 0.026)[b,c]	(0.110 ±0.051)[b,c]
PDL 21	68.10 ± 4.88	68.55 ± 8.24	102.79 ± 18.04[d]	110.88 ± 5.54[e]
	(0.260 ± 0.025)	(0.322 ± 0.095)	(0.120 ± 0.067)[b,c]	(0.101 ± 0.070)[b,c]
PDL 27	74.32 ± 12.26	74.11 ± 8.21	166.32 ± 10.85[e]	179.98 ± 14.09[e]
	(0.263 ± 0.041)	(0.318 ± 0.080)	(0.086 ± 0.027)[b,c]	(0.071 ± 0.054)[b,c]

[a]The doubling times of normal (GM01150 and GM01869) and G6PD-deficient (GM01163 and GM01870) cell strains at different population doubling levels (PDL) are tabulated. Results are the means ± SEM, $n = 5$ determinations. [d]$P < 0.01$, [e]$P < 0.001$ vs. GM01150 and GM01869, respectively, at the corresponding PDL. The G6PD activity of cells at the corresponding passage is given means ± SEM ($n = 5$) in the parenthesis. [b]$P < 0.05$ vs. GM01150 at the corresponding PDL; [c]$P < 0.01$ vs. GM01869 at the corresponding PDL.

erating. Despite their proliferative incompetence, these cells could be kept alive in culture for at least 2 mo.

Morphology is another important property for judging the senescence of human fibroblasts. Senescent cells are enlarged, flattened, and have an increased ratio of cytoplasm to nucleus. Some HFF1 cells showed the senescent morphology at PDL 22, and by PDL 60, nearly all of the cells were senescent (Fig. 14.2). In contrast, the HFF3 cells did not show such morphology even at passages up to PDL 60. Moreover, the HFF1 cells displayed lower saturation density than the HFF3 cells. SA-β-Gal activity staining was also taken as another senescence biomarker (24) (Fig. 14.2). Neither HFF1 nor HFF3 cells showed any staining at an early passage (PDL 12). An increase in the percentage of SA-β-Gal positive HFF1 cells from <8% at PDL 22 to >95% at PDL 60 was noted. Most of the cells classified morphologically as senescent cells were SA-β-Gal positive. Meanwhile, the majority of HFF3 cells remained SA-β-Gal negative at PDL 52, and only a few cells (<5%) were stained positive at PDL 60.

Apart from morphological changes, Western blots revealed that the G6PD-deficient HFF1 cells displayed changes normally associated with senescence in levels of $p16^{INK4a}$, $p21^{CIP1}$, and p53 ~20 doublings earlier than the HFF3 cells (28). Simultaneous induction of $p16^{INK4a}$ and p53 specifically characterizes the G_1 arrest in senescent cells (29–35). By these criteria, G6PD deficiency is considered to cause accelerated senescence of HFF1 cells.

Reversion of Senescent Phenotypes by Ectopic Expression of G6PD. The HFF1 cells were infected with G6PD-expressing retroviral vectors, LGIN and

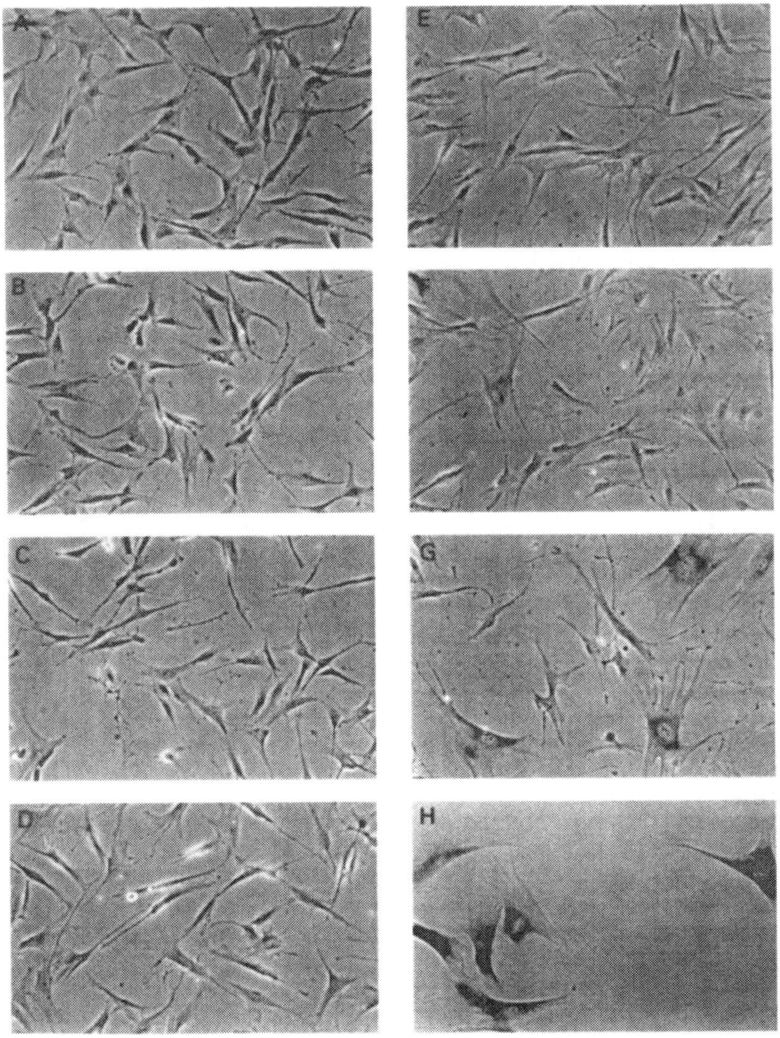

Fig. 14.2. Senescence-associated-β-galactosidase (SA-β-Gal) staining of human foreskin fibroblast HFF1 and HFF3 cells. The HFF3 (A–D) and HFF1 (E–H) cells at population doubling levels (PDL) 12 (A, E), 22 (B, F), 52 (C, G), and 60 (D, H) were stained for SA-β-Gal activity, which was manifested as a blue coloration of cytoplasm. The representative photographs shown here were taken from one of six experiments (original magnification: X100). *Source*: Ref. 19.

LKGIN, to test the effects of G6PD replenishment. The G6PD activities of progeny lines derived from transduction with LGIN or LKGIN at PDL 8, 23, and 50, were elevated 10-fold compared with those infected with the control vector LEIN. On close inspection of the morphology and growth properties of these lines, we found that infection of HFF1 cultures with LEIN did not alter their doubling times, irrespective of the PDL at which infections were carried out (Table 14.2). All six lines arising from infection with LEIN (at PDL 8, 23 or 50) stopped proliferating when they approached the growth limit of uninfected HFF1 cells (~PDL 63). These cultures comprised mainly large, flattened cells with strong SA-β-Gal staining. On the contrary, transduction with either LGIN or LKGIN significantly reduced the doubling times (Table 14.2). The life spans of lines originating from infection with LGIN (or LKGIN) at PDL 50 and PDL 23 exceeded that of LEIN (or uninfected) control by ~5 and 7 population doublings, respectively. Those derived from infection at PDL 8 carried on their growth to PDL 82, ~20 doublings beyond the mean life span of the control. Morphological changes also accompanied the life span extension. A majority of cells derived from infection with LGIN (97 ± 2%; n = 3) or LKGIN (98 ± 2%; n = 3) at PDL 8 remained negative for SA-β-Gal staining at PDL 60 (Table 14.2). It appeared that the number of SA-β-Gal positive cells was related to the passage at which infection was initially performed. Less than 10% of cells in cultures arising from infection with either LGIN or LKGIN at PDL 23 showed pos-

TABLE 14.2 Ectopic Glucose-6-Phosphate Dehydrogenase (G6PD) Expression Prevented Growth Retardation and Premature Senescence in Human Foreskin Fibroblast HFF1 Cells[a]

Doubling time of LEIN-, LGIN-, and LKGIN-transduced lines at different population doubling levels (PDL) (h) (Senescence-associated-β-galactosidase (SA-β-Gal) positive cells counted at PDL 60 [%])				
Transduction of HFF1 cells at PDL	Doubling time measured at PDL	LEIN	LGIN	LKGIN
8	25–30	35.20 ± 3.88	29.83 ± 2.32[b]	30.42 ± 3.62[b]
	40–45	56.00 ± 3.31	36.25 ± 2.00[c]	37.38 ± 3.75[c]
	60	193.38 ± 20.33	44.25 ± 4.42[c]	44.38 ± 4.51[c]
		(95.4 ± 4.0)	(3.0 ± 2.0)	(2.0 ± 2.0)
	80	ND	158.25 ± 21.00	145.25 ± 22.30
23	40–45	46.34 ± 7.56	31.68 ± 3.21[d]	31.68 ± 5.98[d]
	60	211.25 ± 31.10	66.75 ± 13.69[c]	61.25 ± 8.93[c]
		(98.6 ± 3.8)	(5.2 ± 2.0)	(6.4 ± 2.0)
50	60	183.50 ± 38.40	74.40 ± 18.64[c]	74.40 ± 9.34[c]
		(96.8 ± 3.4)	(35.0 ± 4.0)	(30.0 ± 4.0)

[a]The HFF1 cells were infected with control (LEIN), or G6PD-expressing retroviral vectors (LGIN and LKGIN) at PDL 8, 23, or 50 to generate progeny lines. Six lines were derived for each vector at each PDL. The doubling times of these lines at various PDL were determined, and are tabulated as shown. Results are expressed as averaged doubling time ± SEM of six transduced lines. [b]$P < 0.05$ vs. LEIN, [d]$P < 0.01$ vs. LEIN, [c]$P < 0.001$ vs. LEIN at the corresponding PDL. In addition, these lines were stained for SA-β-Gal activity, and the percentage of blue cells was quantified. Results are means ± SEM, n = 3 determinations; ND, not determined.

itive staining, whereas 35 ± 4% of LGIN-transduced cells (or 30 ± 4% of LKGIN) did so when infection was carried out at PDL 50. Most of these latter SA-β-Gal positive cells exhibited paler staining. Apart from the SA-β-Gal marker, ectopic G6PD expression had profound effects on other morphological characteristics. The LGIN- or LKGIN-transduced cells, which had been derived from infection at PDL 8, displayed slender, spindle-shaped morphology at passage up to PDL 60. Meanwhile, the cultures of those lines derived from infection at later passages consisted of a mixture of spindle-shaped cells, flattened cells, and cells with extended processes. Apparently, the greater the PDL of HFF1 at which the LGIN- or LKGIN-transduced lines were derived, the larger the proportion of flattened cells. These data clearly show that ectopic expression of G6PD prevents the growth retardation and early onset of senescence in HFF1 cells, especially when the G6PD is reintroduced at early passages. This also indicates unequivocally that G6PD status *per se* modulates cell growth and senescence.

Increased Oxidative Stress Accounts for Premature Senescence in G6PD-Deficient Fibroblasts. One hypothesis for the cause of cellular senescence is that the progressive shortening of telomeres triggers the senescence checkpoint mechanism, the so-called Hayflick limit, in human diploid cells (36). Analysis of the size distribution of terminal restriction fragments (TRF) revealed no significant differences in the rates of telomere shortening and loss of total amount of telomeric DNA between HFF1 and HFF3 cells (19). This suggests that the premature onset of senescence in G6PD-deficient cells is not associated with accelerated shortening of telomeres. This also implies that signals other than telomere loss trigger the senescence program in G6PD-deficient cells.

The accumulation of oxidative damage of macromolecules, in particular DNA, may act as one such signal, which ultimately leads to senescence (37). As a major source of stress in cellular milieu, ROS are generated by normal cellular metabolic activities such as oxidative respiration, and are known to cause damage to organelles and cellular macromolecules. To deal with the oxidative stress, cells possess a battery of antioxidants, which include enzymes such as superoxide dismutase, catalase, and glutathione peroxidase, and such low-molecular-weight components as glutathione, ascorbic acid, and α-tocopherol. G6PD provides the ultimate reducing power for many of these antioxidant pathways. A deficiency in G6PD activity is associated with a lowered $NADPH/NADP^+$ ratio, and hence an abatement of antioxidant defense in our HFF1 cells. Consistent with this, increased oxidative stress, as shown by DCF fluorescence, was observed in HFF1 cells (Fig. 14.3). Experiments with dihydrorhodamine 123 gave similar results. In addition, the extent of oxidative stress was greater at a later passage in G6PD-deficient cells (Fig. 14.3). This may well be related to the significant reduction of G6PD activity during their serial propagation in culture. Furthermore, the importance of G6PD in antioxidant defense was demonstrated by the effect of ectopic G6PD expression on the production of ROS in HFF1 cells, i.e., transduction of HFF1 cells with LGIN and LKGIN, but not the parental vector LXIN, greatly reduced the level of DCF fluorescence (Fig. 14.3).

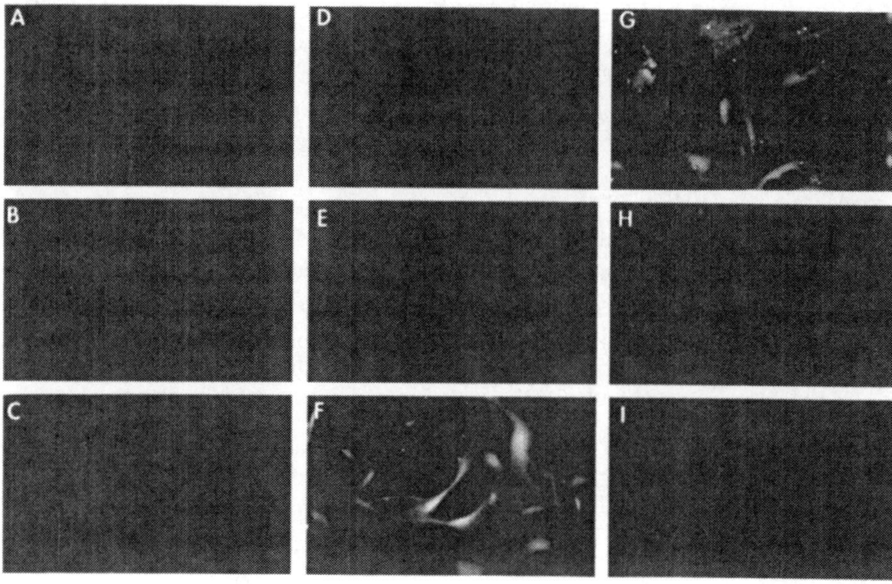

Fig. 14.3. Dichlorofluorescin diacetate (H_2DCF) staining for reactive oxygen species (ROS) in human foreskin fibroblast HFF1, HFF3, and the HFF1 cells overexpressing glucose-6-phosphate dehydrogenase (G6PD). The normal HFF3 (A–C) and G6PD-deficient HFF1 (D–F) cells at population doubling levels (PDL) 8 (A, D), 22 (B, E), and 52 (C, F) were analyzed for generation of ROS. One of six experiments is shown here (original magnification: X100). In addition, HFF1 cells were infected with the parental control virus LXIN (G), or the G6PD-expressing viruses LGIN (H) or LKGIN (I) at PDL 50, and analyzed for ROS generation after two population doublings following infection. Infection and the subsequent DCF staining were repeated at least three times. *Source*: Ref. 19.

Increased oxidative stress, but not the accelerated loss of telomeric repeats suggests that the former may be causally related to the premature senescence in G6PD-deficient cells. This also has important implications for understanding of senescence biology. Apparently, telomere shortening is not the sole factor that can elicit the senescence program. A phenotype suggestive of senescence can be induced by constitutive activation of the Ras pathway (32,34,38), or by exposure of cell cultures to DNA-demethylating drugs, ceramide, inhibitors of histone deacetylation, and oxidants (39–44). Moreover, cell fusion studies support the existence of multiple potential pathways that implement the senescence program (45). It can be envisaged that senescence is not simply a passive consequence of the mitotic clock, but exists as an active mechanism to respond to a variety of cellular stresses. In this respect, the limited replicative life span may reflect the accumulated cellular burden that occurs during the continuous growth of cells.

Increased oxidative stress and reduced antioxidant capacity in HFF1 cells may foster a rapid accumulation of macromolecular damage, resulting in the onset of premature senescence. Consistent with the cumulative nature of such cellular burden, expression of G6PD in the young HFF1 cells rather than the late-passage cells could extend the life span to that attained by HFF3 cells. It is conceivable that the expression of G6PD at an earlier passage can prevent the build-up of oxidative damage to a critical level, which would otherwise drive the cells toward senescence. The late-passage cells, which are already laden with cellular damage as well as an increased rate of oxidative attack, are less effectively rescued from premature senescence. The involvement of an antioxidant in controlling the onset of senescence is not unprecedented. Expression of SOD1 alone, or together with catalase, is able to extend the life span of *Drosophila* (10–12). In this way, G6PD is another antioxidant enzyme added to the growing list of molecules associated with cellular aging.

Altered Cellular Response to Signaling Molecule in G6PD-Deficient Cells

Exogenous Nitric Oxide (NO) Donor Evoked Different Responses in Normal and G6PD-Deficient Human Fibroblasts. Redox homeostasis is undoubtedly critical to numerous physiologic processes, such as enzyme regulation, modulation of transcriptional factors, DNA synthesis, cell cycle regulation, and apoptosis (46,47). A change in intracellular milieu toward an oxidizing environment in G6PD-deficient cells likely alters the cellular responses to growth factors and other signaling molecules. The normal (HFF3) and G6PD-deficient (HFF1) cells showed entirely different growth patterns upon exposure to the NO donor, SNP. At concentrations ranging from 10 to 50 mmol/L, SNP enhanced the growth of HFF3 cells in a dose-dependent manner (Fig. 14.4A), whereas it caused the death of HFF1 cells (Figs. 4B and 5B), which displayed the morphological features typical of apoptosis. Appearance of cells with low DNA stainability (sub-G_1 fraction) in cell populations has been considered to be a marker of apoptosis (48). The level of apoptosis in HFF1 cells significantly increased on d 3 after SNP addition. Treatment with 50 and 100 μmol/L of SNP for 7 d resulted in ~35.12 ± 4.12 and 53.06 ± 5.07% apoptosis, respectively (Fig. 14.5B). Moreover, addition of SNP to HFF1 cells caused a significant increase in the percentage of terminal dUTP nick-end labeling (TUNEL)-positive cells in a dose-dependent manner (49).

It is likely that NO released from SNP mediates the observed biological effect of SNP. Cotreatment of HFF1 (or HFF3 cells) with hemoglobin or freshly prepared erythrocytes, both of which are well-known NO scavengers, effectively inhibited the biological effect of SNP. Furthermore, potassium ferrocyanide [$K_4Fe(CN)_6$] or potassium ferricyanide [$K_3Fe(CN)_6$], which are analogs of SNP but devoid of NO generation, did not mimic the effects of SNP.

Replenishment of G6PD Changed Biological Response of HFF1 Cells to NO from Apoptosis to Growth Stimulation. To test the possibility that G6PD alone was responsible for different biological responses of fibroblasts to NO, we studied the effect of NO on LGIN- and LKGIN-infected HFF1 cells. The addition of SNP caused a decrease in cell number of cells transduced with LEIN vector, whereas it

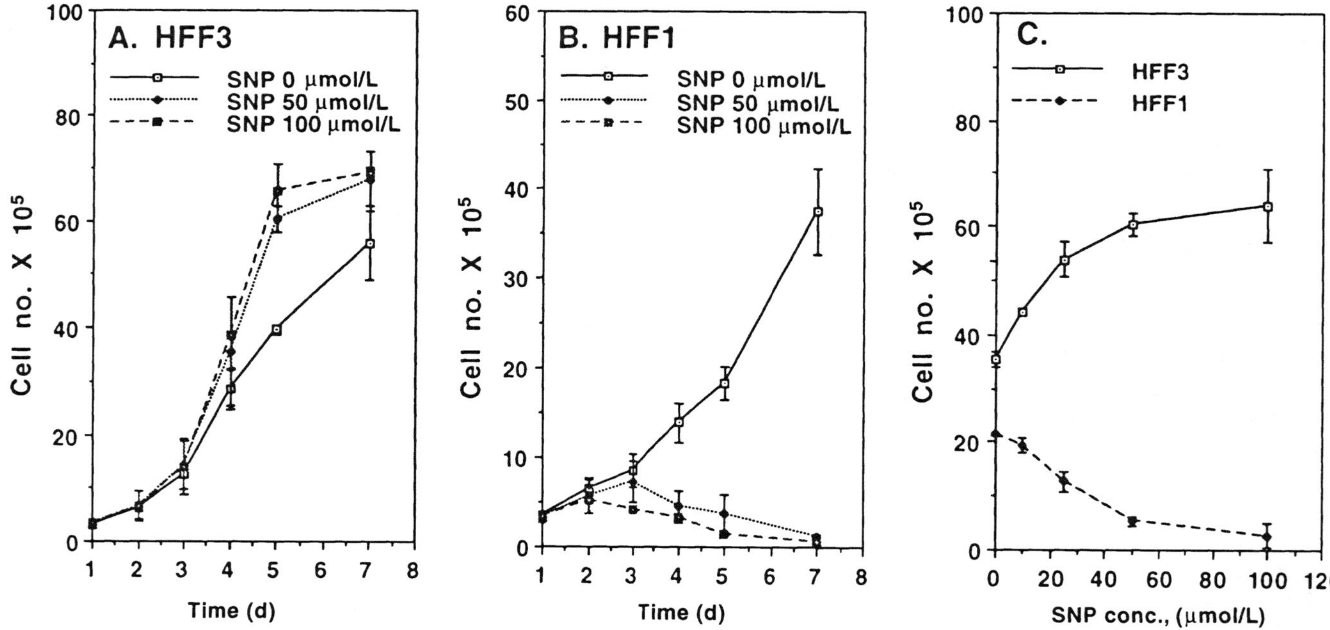

Fig. 14.4. Effects of sodium nitroprusside (SNP) on growth kinetics of normal human foreskin fibroblasts HFF3 and glucose-6-phosphate dehydrogenase (G6PD)-deficient HFF1. Twenty-four hours before SNP addition (i.e., d –1), ~2 $\times 10^5$ HFF3 (A) or HFF1 (B) cells were seeded, and treated with 0, 50, and 100 µmol/L SNP on d 0. Cell number was determined at daily intervals. (C). Effects of SNP on HFF3 and HFF1 cells showed dose dependence. HFF3 or HFF1 cells (~2 $\times 10^5$) were treated with indicated concentrations of SNP, and cell number was determined 5 d after treatment. Results are expressed as means ± SEM, n = 5 experiments. *Source*: Ref. 49.

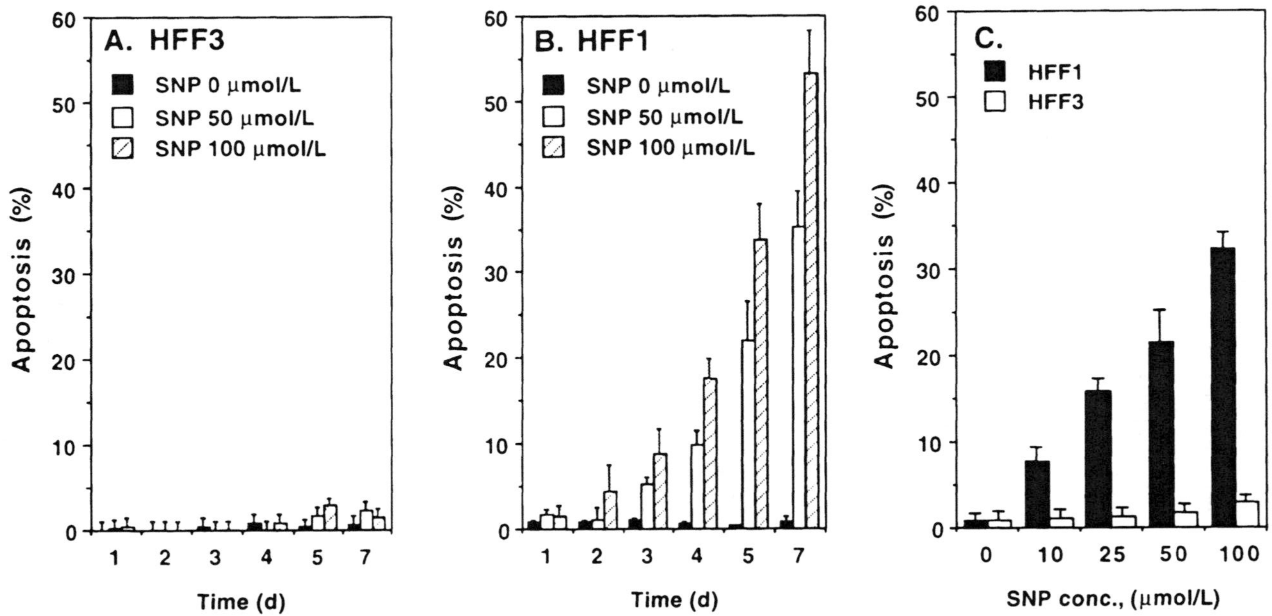

Fig. 14.5. Sodium nitroprusside (SNP)-induced apoptosis in glucose-6-phosphate dehydrogenase (GGPD)-deficient fibroblasts HHF1 cells. HFF3 (A) and HFF1 (B) cells were treated as described in Fig. 14.4 The extent of apoptosis was measured by propidium iodide (PI) staining and flow cytometric analysis. (A) and (B) show temporal course of SNP induced apoptosis. (C) SNPinduced apoptosis of HFF1 cells in a dose-dependent manner. The level of apoptosis in HFF1 and HFF3 cells incubated with indicated concentrations of SNP was determined 5 d after treatment. The data are presented as means ± SEM, $n = 5$ experiments. *Source*: Ref. 49.

stimulated growth of LGIN and LKGIN transductants (49). This suggests that the G6PD status, and probably the redox balance, determines the cellular responses to NO, i.e., a reducing cellular environment in HFF3 cells favors proliferation, whereas a more oxidizing environment predisposes HFF1 cells to apoptosis. Consistent with this, addition of Trolox, a potent antioxidant of lipid peroxidation, could protect the G6PD-deficient cells from SNP-induced apoptosis. Taken together, these findings reiterate the importance of G6PD in modulation of redox homeostasis and cell physiology.

Summary

We have described some of the recent developments in the study of glucose-6-phosphate dehydrogenase (G6PD) deficiency. In particular, the chronic effect of G6PD deficiency on cell growth and cellular senescence was discussed in depth. Additionally, the alteration in the cellular response to a signaling molecule, NO, in G6PD-deficient cells was depicted. To some extent, our data challenge the long-standing idea that G6PD deficiency affects only the erythrocytes, which are unable to maintain an adequate NADPH level during oxidative stress. Clinically, this manifests as neonatal jaundice, drug- or infection-induced hemolytic crisis, favism, and, less commonly, nonspherocytic hemolytic anemia. Now, we demonstrate that the effect of G6PD deficiency is not restricted to erythrocytes. Although the effect may not be as severe as in erythrocytes, deficiency in G6PD activity still affects the physiology of nucleated cells. To date, there remain some unresolved issues, i.e., does the reduced proliferative potential associated with G6PD deficiency impair the turnover of parenchyma cells in the affected individuals? If so, does this, together with increased oxidative damage, undermine the normal physiologic functions of various tissues? Are G6PD-deficient individuals susceptible to diseases other than the hematological disorders? With respect to this latter question, G6PD appears to have subtle functions in other aspects of health. Our preliminary study indicated that G6PD deficiency predisposes the affected subjects to higher risk of hypertension. Moreover, granulocytes isolated from G6PD-deficient individuals are impaired in their bactericidal activity (50). Studies, including those of an epidemiologic nature, are ongoing in our laboratory to clarify the role of G6PD in human health.

Acknowledgments

The work described in this chapter is supported by grants from Chang Gung University (CMRP 1024) and National Science Council of Taiwan (NSC 89-2314-B182-101).

References

1. Luzzatto, L., and Battistuzzi, G. (1985) Glucose-6-phosphate Dehydrogenase. *Adv. Hum. Genet. 14*, 217–229.
2. Beutler, E. (1990) The Genetics of Glucose-6-phosphate Dehydrogenase Deficiency. *Semin. in Hematology 27*, 137–164.

3. Beutler, E. (1991) Glucose-6-phosphate Dehydrogenase Deficiency. *New Engl. J. Med. 324*,169–174.
4. Scott, M.D., Zuo, L., Lubin, B.H., and Chiu, D.T.Y. (1991) NADPH, not Glutathione, Status Modulates Oxidant Sensitivity in Normal and Glucose-6-phosphate Dehydrogenase-Deficient Erythrocytes. *Blood 77*, 2059–2064.
5. Liu, T.Z., Lin, T.F., Hung, I.J., Wei, J.S., and Chiu, D.T.Y. (1994) Enhanced Susceptibility of Erythrocytes Deficient in Glucose-6-phosphate Dehydrogenase to Alloxan/Glutathione-Induced Decrease in Red Cell Deformability. *Life Sci. 55*, 55–60.
6. Johnson, F.B., Sinclair, D.A., and Guarente, L. (1999) Molecular Biology of Aging. *Cell 96*, 291–302.
7. Beckman, K.B., and Ames, B.N. (1997) in *Oxidative Stress, and the Molecular Biology of Antioxidant Defenses*, (Scandalios, J.G., ed.) pp. 201–272, Cold Spring Harbor Laboratory Press, New York.
8. Levine, R.L., and Stadtman, E.R. (1996) in *Handbook of the Biology of Aging*, (Schneider, E.L., and Rowe, J.W., eds.) pp. 184–197, Academic Press, New York.
9. Randerath, K., Randerath, E., and Filburn, C. (1996) in *Handbook of the Biology of Aging*, (Schneider, E.L., and Rowe, J.W., eds.) pp. 198–214, Academic Press, New York.
10. Orr, W.C., and Sohal, R.S. (1994) Extension of Life-Span by Overexpression of Superoxide Dismutase and Catalase in *Drosophila melanogaster*. *Science 263*, 1128–1130.
11. Sun, J.T., and Tower, J. (1999) FLP-Recombinase-Mediated Induction of Cu/Zn Superoxide Dismutase Transgene Expression Can Extend the Life Span of Adult *Drosophila melanogaster* Flies. *Mol. Cell. Biol. 19*, 216–228.
12. Parkes, T.L., Elia, A.J., Dickinson, D., Hilliker, A.J., Philips, J.P., and Boulianne, G.L. (1998) Extension of *Drosophila* Lifespan by Overexpression of Human SOD1 in Motor Neurons. *Nat. Genet. 19*, 171–174.
13. Pandolfi, P.P., Sonati, F., Rivi, R., Mason, P., Grosveld, F., and Luzzatto, L. (1995) Targeted Disruption of the Housekeeping Gene Encoding Glucose-6-phosphate Dehydrogenase (G6PD): G6PD Is Dispensable for Pentose Synthesis but Essential for Defense Against Oxidative Stress. *EMBO J. 14*, 5209–5215.
14. Halliwell, B., and Gutteridge, J.M.C. (1999) in *Free Radicals in Biology and Medicine*, pp. 246–350, Oxford University Press, New York.
15. Wolin, M.S., and Mohazzab H.K.M. (1997) in *Oxidative Stress, and the Molecular Biology of Antioxidant Defenses*, (Scandalios, J.G., ed.) pp. 21–48, Cold Spring Harbor Laboratory Press, New York.
16. Fuchs, D., Baier-Bitterlich, G., Wede, I., and Wachter, H. (1997) in *Oxidative Stress, and the Molecular Biology of Antioxidant Defenses*, (Scandalios, J.G., ed.) pp. 139–168, Cold Spring Harbor Laboratory Press, New York.
17. Zimmerman, R. J., Marafino, B. J., Chan, A., Landre, P., and Winkelhake, J. L. (1989) The Role of Oxidant Injury in Tumor Cell Sensitivity to Recombinant Human Necrosis Factor *In Vivo*. Implications for Mechanisms of Action. *J. Immunol. 142*, 1405–1409.
18. Sundaresan, M., Yu, Z.X., Ferrans, V.J., Irani, K. and Finkel, T. (1995) Requirement for Generation of H_2O_2 for Platelet-Derived Growth Factor Signal Transduction. *Science 270*, 296–299.
19. Ho, H.Y., Cheng, M.L., Liang, C.M., Lu, F.J., Chou, Y.H., Stern, A., and Chiu, D.T.Y. (2000) Enhanced Oxidative Stress and Accelerated Cellular Senescence in Glucxose-6-phosphate Dehydrogenase (G6PD)-Deficient Human Fibroblasts. *Free Radic. Biol. Med. 29*, 156–169.

20. Chiu, D.T.Y., Zuo, L., Chen, E., Chao, L., Louie, E., Lubin, B., Liu, T.Z., and Du, C.S. (1991) Two Commonly Occurring Nucleotide Base Substitutions in Chinese G6PD Variants. *Biochem. Biophys. Res. Commun. 180*, 988–993.
21. Chiu, D.T.Y., Zuo, L., Chao, L., Chen, E., Louie, E., Lubin, B., Liu, T.Z., and Du, C.S. (1993) Molecular Characterization of Glucose-6-phosphate Dehydrogenase Deficiency in Patients of Chinese Descent and Identification of New Base Substitution in the Human G6PD Gene. *Blood 81*, 2150–2154.
22. Stevans, D.J., Wanachiwanawin, W., Mason, P.J., Vulliamy, T.J., and Luzzatto, L. (1990) G6PD Canton a Common Deficient Variant in South East Asia Caused by a 459 Arg→Leu Mutation. *Nucleic Acids Res. 18*, 7190.
23. Pear, W. (1996) in *Current Protocols in Molecular Biology*, (Ausubel, F.M., Brent, R., Kingston, R.E., Moore, D.D., Seidman, J.G., and Struhl, K., eds.) pp. 9.11.1–9.11.18, Greene Publishing Associates and Wiley-Interscience, New York.
24. Dimri, G.P., Lee, X., Basile, G., Acosta, M., Scott, G., Roskelley, C., Medrano, E.E., Linskens, M., Rubelj, I., Pereira-Smith, O., Peacocke, M., and Campisi, J. (1995) A Biomarker That Identifies Senescent Human Cells in Culture and in Aging Skin *In Vivo*. *Proc. Natl. Acad. Sci. USA 92*, 9363–9367.
25. Bautista, J.M., Mason, P.J., and Luzzatto, L. (1992) Purification and Properties of Human Glucose-6-phosphate Dehydrogenase Made in *E. coli*. *Biochem. Biophys. Acta 119*, 74–80.
26. Royall, J.A., and Ischiropoulos, H. (1993) Evaluation of 2′,7′-Dichloro-fluorescin and Dihydrorhodamine 123 as Fluorescent Probes for Intracellular H_2O_2 in Cultured Endothelial Cells. *Arch. Biochem. Biophys. 302*, 348–355.
27. Hayflick, L., and Moorhead, P.S. (1961) The Serial Cultivation of Human Diploid Cell Strains. *Exp. Cell Res. 25*, 585–621.
28. Ho, H.Y. (2000) Oxidative Stress and Senescence: A Model Based on the Study of the Glucose-6-phosphate Dehydrogenase (G6PD)-Deficient Cells, pp. 49–50, Ph.D. Thesis, National Defense Medical Centre, Taiwan.
29. Chang, Z.F. (1997) Regulatory Mechanisms of Replication Growth Limits in Cellular Senescence. *J. Formos. Med. Assoc. 96*, 784–791.
30. Stein, G.H., Drullinger, L.F., Soulard, A., and Dulic, V. (1999) Differential Roles for Cyclin-Dependent Kinase Inhibitors p21 and p16 in the Mechanisms of Senescence and Differentiation in Human Fibroblasts. *Mol. Cell. Biol. 19*, 2109–2117.
31. Alcorta, D.A., Xiong, Y., Phelps, D., Hannon, G., Beach, D., and Barrett, J.C. (1996) Involvement of the Cyclin-Dependent Kinase Inhibitor p16 (INK4a) in Replicative Senescence of Normal Human Fibroblasts. *Proc. Natl. Acad. Sci. USA 93*, 13742–13747.
32. Serrano, M., Lin, A.W., McCurrach, M.E., Beach, D., and Lowe, S.W. (1997) Oncogenic *ras* Provokes Premature Cell Senescence Associated with Accumulation of p53 and $p16^{INK4a}$. *Cell 88*, 593–602.
33. Afshari, C.A., Vojta, P.J., Annab, L.A., Futreal, P.A., Willard, T.B., and Barrett, J.C. (1993) Investigation of the Role of G_1/S Cell Cycle Mediators in Cellular Senescence. *Exp. Cell Res. 209*, 231–237.
34. Lin, A.W., Barradas, M., Stone, J.C., Aelst, L., Serrano, M., and Lowe, S.W. (1998) Premature Senescence Involving p53 and p16 Is Activated in Response to Constitutive MEK/MAPK Mitogenic Signaling. *Genes Dev. 12*, 3008–3019.
35. Sugrue, M.M., Shin, D.Y., Lee, S.W., and Aaronson, S.A. (1997) Wild-Type p53 Triggers a Rapid Senescence Program in Human Tumor Cells Lacking Functional p53. *Proc. Natl. Acad. Sci. USA 94*, 9648–9653.

36. Wright, W.E., and Shay, J.W. (1995) Time, Telomeres and Tumours: Is Cellular Senescence More than an Anticancer Mechanism? *Trends Cell Biol. 5*, 293–297.
37. Gilchrest, B.A., and Bohr, V.A. (1997) Aging Processes, DNA Damage, and Repair. *FASEB J. 11*, 322–330.
38. Zhu, J., Woods, D., McMahon, M., and Bishop, M. (1998) Senescence of Human Fibroblasts Induced by Oncogenic Raf. *Genes Dev. 12*, 2997–3007.
39. Holliday, R. (1986) Strong Effects of 5-Azacytidine on the *In Vitro* Lifespan of Human Fibroblasts. *Exp. Cell Res. 166*, 543–552.
40. Fairweather, D.S., Fox, M., and Margison, G.P. (1987) The *In Vitro* Lifespan of MRC-5 Cells Is Shortened by 5-Azacytidine-Induced Demethylation. *Exp. Cell Res. 168*, 153–159.
41. Venable, M.E., Lee, J.Y., Smyth, M.J., Bielawska, A., and Obeid, L.M. (1995) Role of Ceramide in Cellular Senescence. *J. Biol. Chem. 270*, 30701–30708.
42. Ogryzko, V.V., Hirai, T.H., Russanova, V.R., Barbie, D.A., and Howard, B.H. (1996) Human Fibroblast Commitment to a Senescence-Like State in Response to Histone Deacetylase Inhibitors Is Cell Cycle Dependent. *Mol. Cell. Biol. 16*, 5210–5218.
43. Chen, Q., and Ames, B.N. (1994) Senescence-Like Growth Arrest Induced by Hydrogen Peroxide in Human Diploid Fibroblast F65 Cells. *Proc. Natl. Acad. Sci. USA 91*, 4130–4134.
44. Chen, Q., Fischer, A., Reagan, J.D., Yan, L.J., and Ames, B.N. (1995) Oxidative DNA Damage and Senescence of Human Diploid Fibroblast Cells. *Proc. Natl. Acad. Sci. USA 92*, 4337–4341.
45. Vojta, P. J., and Barrett, J. C. (1995) Genetic Analysis of Cellular Senescence. *Biochim. Biophys. Acta 1242*, 29–41.
46. Powis, G., Briehl, M., and Oblong, J. (1995) Redox Signalling and the Control of Cell Growth and Death. *Pharmacol. Ther. 68*, 149–173.
47. Arrigo, A. P. (1999) Gene Expression and the Thiol Redox State. *Free Radic. Biol. Med. 27*, 936–944.
48. Nicoletti, I., Migliorati, G., Pagliacci, M.C., Grignani, F., and Riccardi, C. (1991) A Rapid and Simple Method for Measuring Thymocyte Apoptosis by Propidium Iodide. *J. Immunol. Methods 139*, 271–279.
49. Cheng, M.L., Ho, H.Y., Liang, C.M., Chou, Y.H., Stern, A., Lu, F.J., and Chiu, D.T.Y. (2000) Cellular Glucose-6-phosphate Dehydrogenase Status Modulates the Effects of Nitric Oxide (NO) on Human Foreskin Fibroblasts. *FEBS Lett. 475*, 257–262.
50. Tsai, K.J., Hung, I.J., Chow, C.K., Stern, A., Chao, S.S., and Chiu, D.T.Y. (1998) Impaired Production of Nitric Oxide, Superoxide, and Hydrogen Peroxide in Glucose-6-phosphate Dehydrogenase-Deficient Granulocytes. *FEBS Lett. 436*, 411–414.

Chapter 15

Increase of Mitochondrial Mass and Mitochondrial DNA Content as a Response to Oxidative Stress of Human Cells Harboring Mitochondrial DNA Mutation

Yau-Huei Wei, Cheng-Feng Lee, Chun-Yi Liu, Hsin-Chen Lee, Yi-Shing Ma, and Cheng-Yoong Pang

Department of Biochemistry and Center for Cellular and Molecular Biology, National Yang-Ming University, Taipei 112, Taiwan

Introduction

In the past decade, an increasing number of human diseases have been associated with or caused by mutations in mitochondrial DNA (mtDNA) (1–5). Among them, A3243G point mutation is associated with ~80% of patients with mitochondrial encephalopathy, myopathy, lactic acidosis, and stroke-like episodes (MELAS) syndrome (3), and large-scale deletions frequently occur in the affected tissues of patients with mitochondrial myopathies such as chronic progressive external ophthalmoplegia (CPEO) and Kearns-Sayre syndromes (1,6–8). It has been demonstrated that A3243G mutation and large-scale deletions significantly affect mitochondrial gene expression (9,10) and result in defects in the respiratory chain. Impairment of mitochondrial electron transport may increase the production of the reactive oxygen species (ROS) and free radicals in the mitochondria (11–13). Indeed, it was found that the tissues or cultured cells containing mutant mtDNA(s) were subjected to higher endogenous oxidative stress and inflicted with more severe oxidative damage due to a defect of the electron transport system (14,15). It has been documented that patients with mitochondrial diseases exhibit premature aging (16) and their clinical symptoms generally worsen with time (17–19). This age-related progression of the disease is quite similar to the natural course of some neurodegenerative diseases (20,21). In the past few years, ROS and oxidative stress have been shown to stimulate the expression of growth-related genes such as *c-fos* and *c-jun* (22). Hydrogen peroxide (H_2O_2) is thought to play a role in the communication between mitochondria and the nucleus in coordinating gene expression in mammalian cells (23,24). These observations have led us to hypothesize that the mitochondrial function is subject to change in response to enhanced oxidative stress in human cells harboring the mtDNA mutation (25,26). To test this hypothesis, we employed the cytoplasmic transfer technique (27,28) to construct a series of cybrids harboring different proportions of mtDNA with the A3243G mutation or 4977-bp deletion by fusing enucleated fibroblasts of two patients with MELAS and CPEO syndromes, respectively, with an osteosarcoma cell line that is devoid of mtDNA (termed ρ^o cells). We examined the growth kinetics of the cybrids that harbor different proportions of the mutant mtDNA. The intracellular levels of the reduced glutathione (GSH)/oxidized glutathione (GSSG) ratio and lipid peroxides of the cybrids were determined to assess the oxidative stress of the cybrids. To assess mitochondrial response to oxidative stress, we determined the mitochondrial mass by flow cytometry and measured the relative content of mtDNA by slot-blot analysis in the cybrids treated with and without H_2O_2 (26). The results showed that cybrids harboring mutated mtDNA had higher amounts of mitochondria and mitochondrial genome, which were further increased by oxidative stress elicited by the treatment with H_2O_2 at a sublethal level.

Materials and Methods

Cell Culture. We established primary cultures of fibroblasts from the skin biopsies of a patient with MELAS syndrome and another with CPEO. The cells were maintained at 37°C in Dulbecco's modified Eagle medium (DMEM) supplemented with 5% fetal bovine serum (FBS), 100 μg/mL pyruvate and 50 μg/mL uridine in humidified 5% CO_2/95% air. A mtDNA-less human cell line (ρ^o cell) was established by treatment of the osteosarcoma 143B TK^- cells with 50 ng/mL ethidium bromide for 3 mo (27). The ρ^o cells were used to fuse with the fibroblasts, which had been enucleated by treatment with 10 μg/mL of cytochalasin B according to King and Attardi (28). Cybrids were selected in a medium containing 100 μg/mL 5-bromo 2′-deoxyuridine and were subcloned in DMEM supplemented with 5% FBS, 100 μg/mL pyruvate, and 50 μg/mL uridine. To study oxidative stress, the cybrids harboring mtDNA with 4977-bp deletion or A3243G mutation were cultured in the above medium containing H_2O_2 at a final concentration of 180 or 200 μmol/L for different periods of time. Cell number was counted in duplicate by use of a hemocytometer.

Cell viability assay. Lactate dehydrogenase (LDH) release was used as an index of cell viability. Usually, 1×10^4 cybrids were seeded onto a 12-well culture plate and were grown to confluence at 37°C for 36 h. After treatment with H_2O_2 for 48 h, the culture medium was aspirated and stored at 4°C. The remaining cells on the well were disintegrated with a lysis buffer (81.3 mmol/L Tris-HCl, 203.3 mmol/L NaCl, and 0.5% Triton X-100, pH 7.2) at 25°C for 20 min. The levels of LDH activity in the culture medium and cell lysate were then determined spectrophotometrically by monitoring the decrease of the absorbance of NADH at 340 nm (29). The cell viability was calculated as the ratio between the LDH activity of the cell lysate and total LDH activity.

Cytochrome c Oxidase Activity Stain. This stain employed the capability of a functional cytochrome *c* oxidase complex to oxidize 3,3′-diaminobenzidine (DAB) to yield an insoluble brown deposit. In brief, $\sim 1.0 \times 10^5$ cells were washed with SP buffer (7.5% sucrose in 0.05 mol/L phosphate buffer, pH 7.2) before incubation with cytochrome *c* (1 g/L in the SP buffer) for 20 min at 37°C. After being washed, the cells were resuspended in the DAB solution (2.7 g/L DAB in the SP buffer) and incubated for 3 h at 37°C. After incubation, cells were washed three times before being subjected to microscopic examination (30).

Determination of Mitochondrial Mass. Mitochondrial mass was determined by staining the cybrids with the fluorescent dye 10-*n*-nonyl-acridine orange (NAO; Molecular Probes, Eugene, OR), which specifically binds to cardiolipin at the inner membrane of mitochondria independently of membrane potential ($\Delta \Psi_m$) (31,32). Cells were trypsinized and resuspended in 0.5 mL phosphate-buffered saline (PBS, pH 7.3) containing 4 μmol/L NAO. After incubation for 10 min at 25°C in the dark, cybrids were transferred immediately to a tube on ice for fluorographic analysis by flow cytometry.

Determination of Intracellular Level of Reactive Oxygen Species. The intracellular level of reactive oxygen species (ROS) was determined by staining the cybrids with the fluorescent dye DCFH-diacetate. Cells were trypsinized and resuspended in 0.5 mL PBS (pH 7.3) containing 80 μmol/L DCFH-diacetate. After incubation for 30 min at 37°C in the dark, cybrids were immediately transferred to a tube on ice for fluorographic analysis by flow cytometry.

Flow Cytometric Analysis. We performed all flow cytometric analyses wih the use of a FACScan flow cytometer (Becton Dickinson, Bedford, MA) equipped with a 488-nm argon laser (26). Forward and side scatters were used to establish size gates and exclude cellular debris from the analysis. The excitation wavelength was set at 488 nm. The wavelength of 530 nm was chosen for detection of green fluorescence and 585 nm for red fluorescence; the intensities of emitted fluorescence were collected on FL1 and FL2 channels, respectively. Generally, a total of 20,000 cells were analyzed in each experiment. Data were collected and analyzed using the Cell Quest software (Becton Dickinson). Relative change in the fluorescence intensity was measured as the ratio between the mean fluorescence intensity of the treated cells and that of the control cells (26).

Analysis of mtDNA Mutation. Total cellular DNA was prepared from each of the cybrids by the method developed in this laboratory (33). The proportions of mtDNA with the A3243G mutation and 4977-bp deletion in the cybrids were quantified by polymerase chain reaction (PCR)-restriction fragment length polymorphism (RFLP) (34) and Southern hybridization (35), respectively, as described previously.

Determination of the Relative Content of mtDNA. The relative content of the cybrid was determined by slot-blot analysis using the α-[^{32}P]dCTP-labeled D-loop sequence (np16455-1462) of human mtDNA as the probe. DNA (~1 μg) was denatured in 0.4 N NaOH and 10 mmol/L EDTA at 100°C for 10 min and then transferred onto a piece of Hybond-N$^+$ nylon membrane. Hybridization and washing were done essentially according to the conditions described above, except that a probe for the 28S rRNA gene was also included to determine the amount of nuclear DNA in each sample. The intensities of the DNA species representing the mitochondrial genome and nuclear DNA (28S rRNA gene) on the blot were measured on a phosphorimager.

Determination of Lipid Peroxides by High-Performance Liquid Chromatography (HPLC). The content of lipid peroxides in the cybrid was measured as malondialdehyde (MDA) according to the method described by Wong *et al.* (36). Cybrids (~5.0×10^5) were resuspended in 25 μL PBS with 100 μmol/L deferoxamine (DFAM) on ice and transferred to a 1.5-mL Eppendorf vial. To the suspension, 375 μL of 0.44 mol/L phosphoric acid and 125 μL of 42 mmol/L thiobarbituric acid (TBA) solution were added, and the final volume was adjusted to 750 μL with distilled water. The vial was capped and boiled at 95°C for 1 h and then immediately cooled in an ice-water bath. An aliquot of 0.25 mL of each boiled sample was delivered to a new vial and was then neutralized with 0.25 mL of 1 N NaOH in methanol. The neutralized solution was centrifuged at 9500 × *g* for 5 min to remove denatured proteins. An aliquot of 25 μL of the supernatant was injected into a C_{18} column (5-μm particle, 4.6 × 200 mm, Waters Associates, Milford, MA). Before injection of the samples, the column was pre-equilibrated in a stepwise manner by 80 and 40% (vol/vol) methanol each for 30 min and then eluted with a mobile phase consisting of methanol and 50 mmol/L potassium phosphate buffer (pH 6.8; 4:6, vol/vol). The flow rate of the mobile phase was 1.0 mL/min, and the fluorescence of the eluate was monitored with a fluorescence detector (excitation wavelength, 525 nm; emission wavelength, 550 nm). The area under each fluorescence peak of the adduct of MDA and TBA was determined, and the lipid peroxide content of each sample was calculated from a standard curve constructed by using 1,1,3,3-tetraethoxy-propane as standard.

Determination of Reduced and Oxidized Glutathione. The concentrations of reduced glutathione (GSH) and oxidized glutathione (GSSG) in the cybrids were determined by a recycling assay as described previously (37).

Protein Determination. The cell lysate or enriched mitochondrial fraction from subcellular fractionation was suspended in the solution of 0.1 N NaOH, 1% deoxycholate and kept for the determination of protein by a modified Lowry method (38).

Results

Retarded Growth of Cybrids Harboring Mutant mtDNA. We first examined the growth kinetics of the cybrids harboring the A3243G mtDNA mutation. The results showed that the cybrids harboring high proportions of mtDNA with the A3243G mutation or 4977-bp deletion grew more slowly than the control cybrid in the presence or absence of H_2O_2 (Table 15.1). The growth was dramatically retarded by the addition of H_2O_2 for all of the cybrids harboring 0–85% of 4977 bp–deleted mtDNA. By contrast, the growth of the cybrid harboring the A3243G mtDNA mutation was only slightly retarded by the treatment with 180 μmol/L H_2O_2. The population doubling time was 19.5 h for the cybrids containing 75% mtDNA with 4977-bp deletion, and was 15.6 h for the control cybrids grown in the DMEM supplemented with 5% FBS, 100 μg/mL pyruvate, and 50 μg/mL uridine (Table 15.1).

TABLE 15.1 Comparison of the Doubling Time of Various Cybrids Before and After H_2O_2 Treatment

Cybrids	Types of mtDNA mutation	Proportion of the mutant mtDNA	Doubling time[a] (h)	
			$-H_2O_2$	$+H_2O_2$
Lu 02	A3243G point mutation	Undetectable	17.4 ± 0.1	22.2 ± 0.1[d]
Lu 04		80 ±1.1	19.8 ± 0.7	22.5 ± 0.7[d]
Lu 03		88 ± 2.5	22.2 ± 0.1[b]	25.3 ± 0.3[c,d]
1-3-16	4977-bp deletion	Undetectable	15.6 ± 0.9	19.9 ± 0.7[d]
14-6		17.1 ± 1.7	16.7 ± 0.4	21.6 ± 0.9[d]
51-18		56.3 ±4.1	17.1 ± 2.1[b]	22.9 ± 0.0[c,d]
1-3-51		75.6 ± 3.5	19.5 ± 0.2[b]	30.7 ± 4.1[c,d]
51-10		85.4 ± 2.2	20.8 ± 0.8[b]	32.3 ± 4.1[c,d]

[a]Doubling time = $(T_1 - T_0) \times \log 2/(\log N_1 - \log N_0)$; data are expressed as means ± SEM.
[b]$P < 0.05$ vs. control cybrids without H_2O_2 treatment.
[c]$P < 0.05$ vs. control cybrids with 180 μmol/L H_2O_2 treatment.
[d]$P < 0.05$ between 180 μmol/L H_2O_2-treated and untreated cybrid lines.

A3243G mtDNA Mutation Resulted in the Loss of Cytochrome c Oxidase Activity. Activity staining revealed that cytochrome *c* oxidase was almost undetectable in the cybrids harboring >90% of mtDNA with the A3243G mutation (Fig. 15.1).

Increase of Lipid Peroxides in Cybrids Harboring Mutant mtDNAs. As indicated by the level of MDA in the cell lysate, the content of lipid peroxides of the cybrid was significantly increased in the cybrids harboring high proportions of mtDNA with either the A3243G mutation or 4977-bp deletion. The average specific MDA content of the cybrids harboring >90% mtDNA with A3243G mutation (3.5 ± 0.5 nmol/mg) was higher than that of the control cybrids (2.2 ± 0.5 nmol/mg).

Enhanced Oxidative Stress in Cybrids Harboring Mutant mtDNAs. Compared with the control, the cybrids containing >90% of mtDNA with A3243G mutation or >56% of mtDNA with 4977-bp deletion had a significantly lower GSH/GSSG ratio, indicating enhanced oxidative stress (Table 15.2).

Increase in the Content of mtDNA in the Cybrids Harboring Mutant mtDNA. We found that the content of mtDNA in the cybrids harboring A3243G mutation was 20–25 % higher than that in the control cybrids. The relative content of mtDNA was also increased significantly in the cybrids that contained <60% of 4977 bp–deleted mtDNA. By contrast, the mtDNA content was slightly decreased in the cybrids harboring >70% of mtDNA with the 4977-bp deletion (Fig. 15.2).

Increase of Mitochondrial Mass of the Cybrids Harboring Mutant mtDNA. By NAO staining of the mitochondrial membrane, we found that the mitochondrial mass

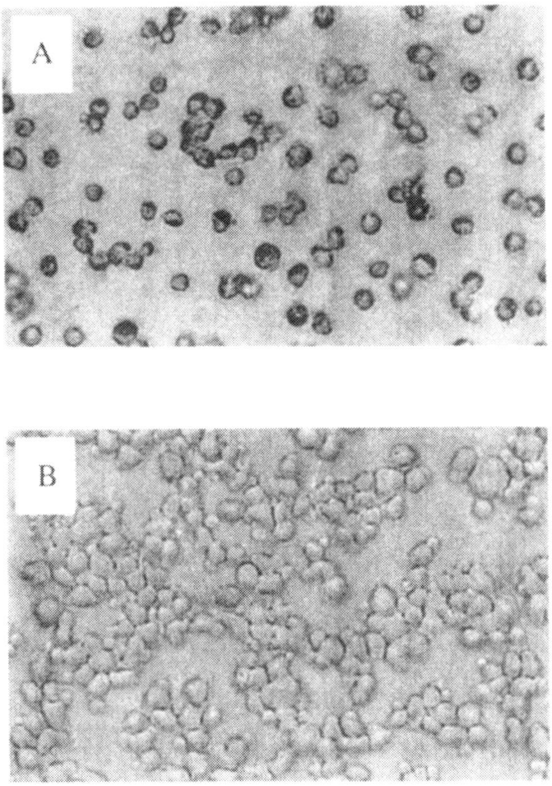

Fig. 15.1. Activity staining of cytochrome *c* oxidase. Cybrids harboring an undetectable level of the A3243G mtDNA mutation (A) and cybrids containing >90% of mtDNA with the A3243G mutation (B) were incubated with 3,3′-diaminobenzidine and cytochrome *c*. Insoluble brown deposits were formed in the presence of functional cytochrome *c* oxidase.

of the cybrids was increased with the proportion of mtDNA with either A3243G mutation or 4977-bp deletion (Fig. 15.3). It is noteworthy that the mitochondrial mass in each of the cybrids harboring >70% of mtDNA with A3243G mutation was significantly less than that in the cybrids containing 0–85% of mtDNA with the 4977-bp deletion.

TABLE 15.2 Comparison of Oxidative Stress in the Cybrids Harboring Different Proportions of Mutated mtDNA

Types of mtDNA mutation	Proportion of the mutant mtDNA	GSH/GSSG ratio[a]
A3243G point mutation	Undetectable	4.6 ± 0.3
	>90%	2.2 ± 0.1
4977-bp deletion	Undetectable	16.5 ± 3.6
	17.1 ± 1.7	16.6 ± 0.6
	56.3 ± 4.1	13.7 ± 1.4
	85.4 ± 2.2	12.5 ± 0.4

[a]The reduced glutathione (GSH)/oxidized glutathione (GSSG) ratio is used as an index of oxidative stress.

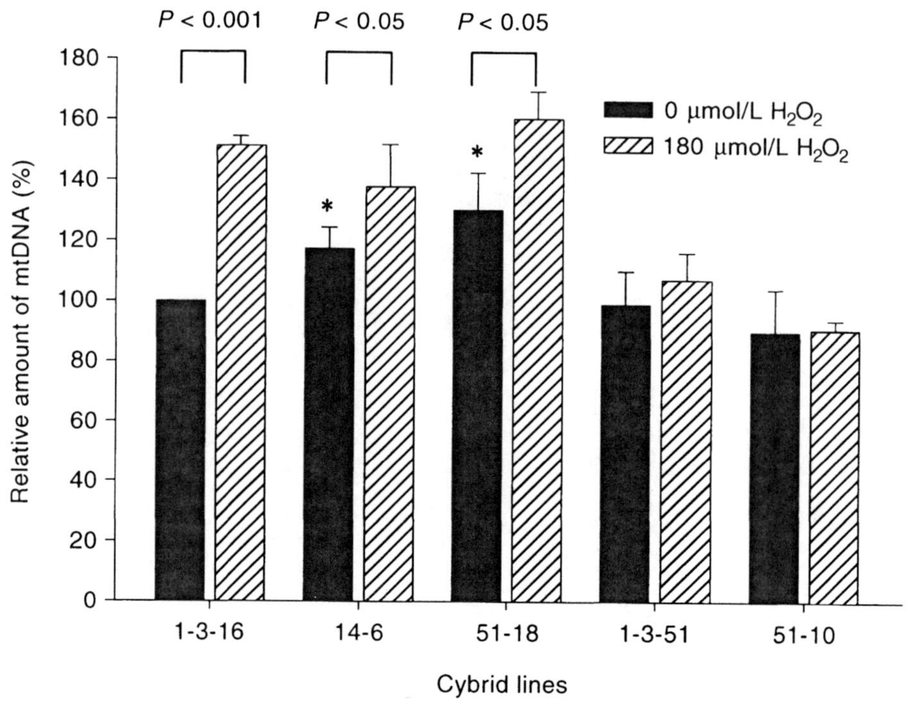

Fig. 15.2. The relative amounts of mtDNA in different cybrids with and without treatment of 180 μmol/L H_2O_2 for 48 h. The total cellular DNA was probed with the labeled DNA of the mitochondrial D-loop region (np 16445-1462) and with the labeled DNA of the nuclear 28S rRNA gene. Each bar represents the mean ± SD of the results obtained for the indicated cybrid by three determinations. The intensity ratio of the mtDNA/28S rRNA gene of the wild type (control) cybrid was taken as 100% for the determination of the relative amount of mtDNA in various mutant cybrids. *Indicates significant difference in the relative amount of mtDNA between untreated cybrids 14-6 and 51-18 and untreated cybrid 1-3-16, $P < 0.005$.

Response of Cybrids to Oxidative Stress Treatment. To assess the effect of H_2O_2 on the cybrids, we measured the mitochondrial mass of each of the cybrids by staining with the fluorescent dye NAO. We found that after treatment with H_2O_2 for 48 h, the relative NAO fluorescence intensity of the treated cybrid was increased significantly compared with that of the untreated cybrids (Fig. 15.3). The viability of the cybrid harboring either A3243G mutation or 4977-bp deletion was only slightly affected by H_2O_2 below 200 μmol/L (Fig. 15.4). These results indicate that the oxidative stress induced by addition of a sublethal dose of H_2O_2 can lead to a further increase of mitochondrial mass in the cybrids harboring mtDNA with either A3243G or 4977-bp deletion.

On the other hand, we employed slot-blot analysis to determine the mtDNA content of the cybrids harboring the 4977 bp–deleted mtDNA with and without treatment

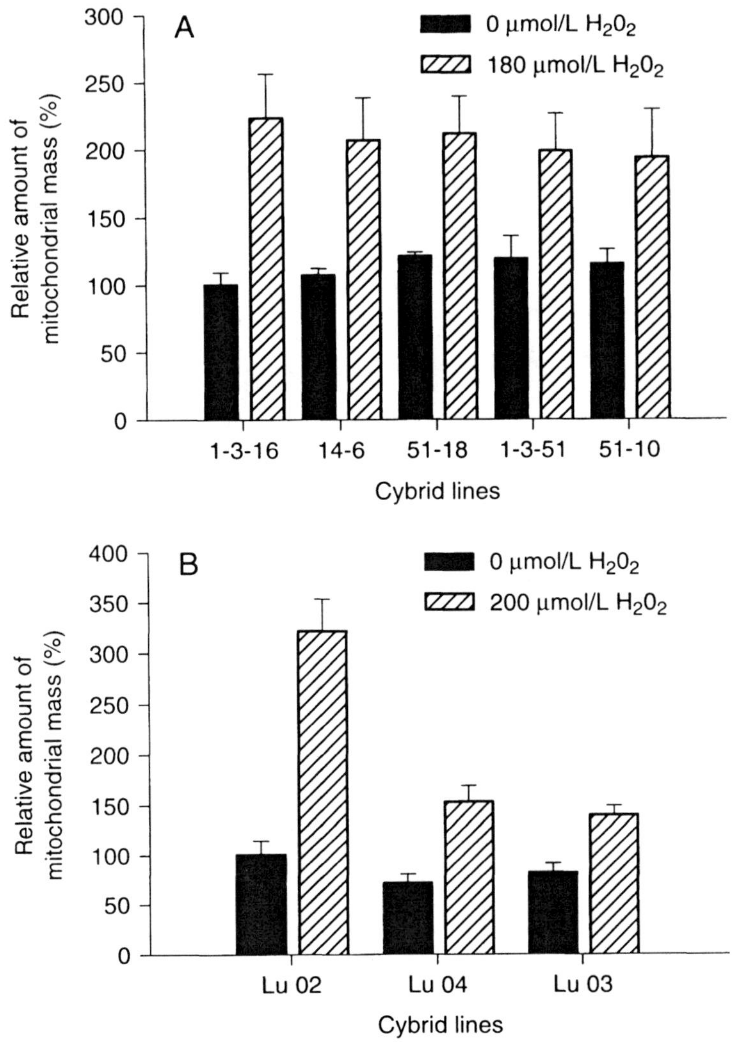

Fig. 15.3. Increase of mitochondrial mass induced by H_2O_2 treatment in the cybrids harboring different proportions of mutated mtDNA. The cybrids containing mtDNA with 4977-bp deletion (A) and with A3243G mutation (B) were subjected to staining with 10-*n*-nonyl-acridine orange (NAO) after treatment with 180 and 200 μmol/L H_2O_2, respectively, for 48 h. Each bar represents the mean ± SD of the results obtained from six (panel A) and three (panel B) determinations. The NAO fluorescence intensity of the wild type (control) cybrid was taken as 100% for the determination of mitochondrial mass of various mutant cybrids. The results showed that the mitochondrial mass was significantly increased by H_2O_2 treatment in each of the cybrid clones.

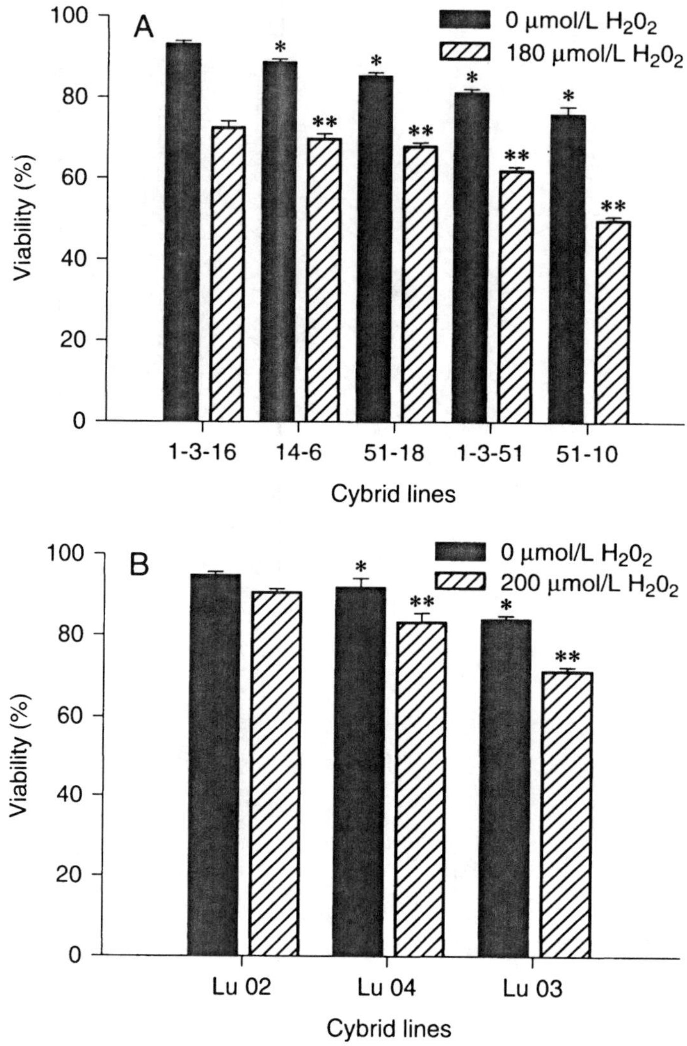

Fig. 15.4. Effect of H_2O_2 treatment on the viability of cybrids. The viability of the cybrids harboring different proportions of 4977 bp–deleted mtDNA (A) and A3243G mutated mtDNA (B) was assessed by lactate dehydrogenase (LDH) release after treatment with 180 or 200 μmol/L H_2O_2. Each bar represents the mean ± SD of the results obtained from three determinations. *Indicates significant difference ($P < 0.001$) in the viability between untreated mutant cybrids and untreated control cybrid line 1-3-16; **indicates significant difference ($P < 0.05$) in the viability between treated mutant cybrids and treated control cybrid lines.

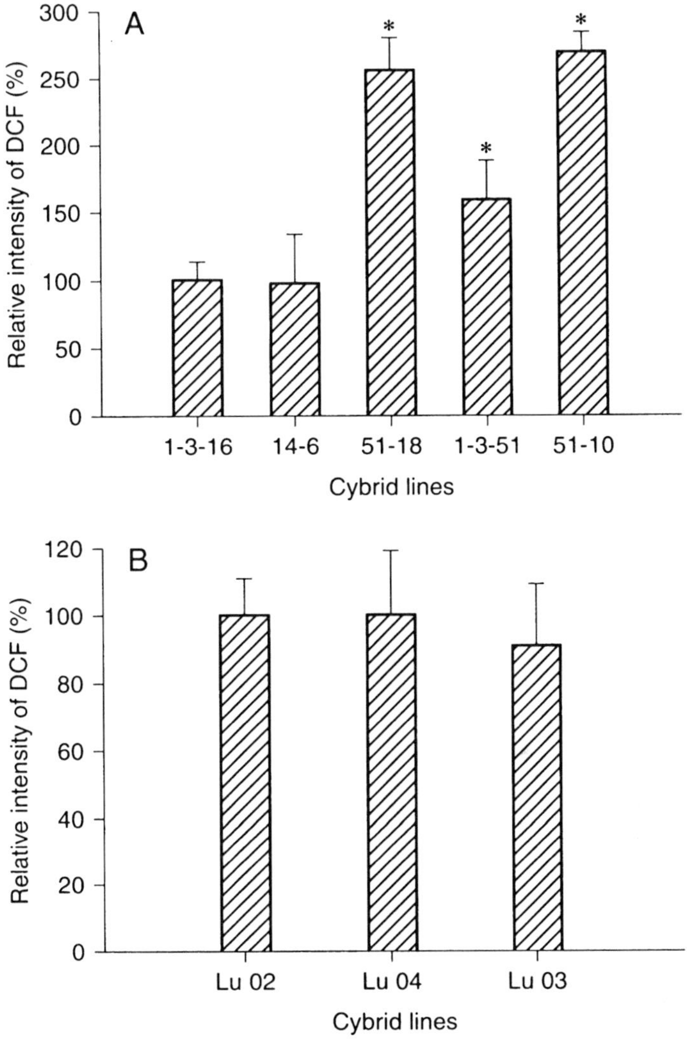

Fig. 15.5. Relative amount of intracellular reactive oxygen species (ROS) of the cybrids harboring different proportions of mutated mtDNA. Cybrids harboring 4977 bp–deleted mtDNA (A) and A3243G mutated mtDNA (B) were subjected to flow cytometry after staining with DCFH-diacetate. Each bar represents the mean ± SD of the results obtained from three determinations. The DCF fluorescence intensity of the wild type (control) cybrid was taken as 100% for the determination of intracellular concentration of superoxide anions and H_2O_2 of various mutant cybrids. *Indicates significant difference ($P < 0.05$) in intracellular levels of ROS between mutant cybrids and cybrid line 1-3-16 in panel A.

of 180 mmol/L H_2O_2. The results showed that the relative content of mtDNA in the cybrids harboring mtDNA with 4977-bp deletion was higher than that in the control cybrids (Fig. 15.2). This increase of mtDNA content is consistent with the observation of the increase of mitochondrial mass in the H_2O_2-treated cells as revealed by the aforementioned NAO staining.

Increased Production of Intracellular ROS in the Cybrids Harboring Mutant mtDNA. By flow cytometric analysis of the cybrids staining with DCFH-diacetate, we found that the intracellular levels of ROS in the cybrids harboring a high level of 4977 bp–deleted mtDNA were significantly higher than that of the control cybrid or the cybrid harboring a low level (17%) of 4977 bp–deleted mtDNA (Fig. 15.5). However, no significant increase in the intracellular levels of ROS was found in the cybrids harboring mtDNA with A3243G mutation.

Discussion

In this study, a series of cybrids harboring varying proportions of mtDNA with A3243G mutation and 4977-bp deletion were constructed for the studies of relationship between genotype and phenotype. We first showed that the cybrids harboring a high level of mtDNA with either point mutation or large-scale deletion exhibited retarded growth (Table 15.1). Although a wide spectrum of mtDNA mutations has been associated with mitochondrial diseases (3–5,39,40), the pathogenesis of these diseases has remained elusive. The A3243G transition and large-scale deletions of mtDNA are associated with most of the patients with the MELAS and CPEO syndromes, respectively (5–12). It is now established that the cells harboring the mutant mtDNA(s) are defective in mitochondrial respiratory functions; an alteration in intracellular GSH/GSSG and $NADH^+$/ NAD^+ ratios is expected. Impairment of the respiratory chain leads to an increase of electron leak through the mitochondrial inner membrane as a result of inefficient NADH oxidation and deregulation of oxygen metabolism in the mitochondria (41). A deleterious consequence of the electron leak from the impaired respiratory enzyme system is the partial reduction of molecular oxygen to form superoxide anions and other ROS in mitochondria (41,42). Indeed, the cytochrome *c* oxidase activity was almost completely diminished in the cybrids containing >90% of mtDNA with A3243G mutation (Fig. 15.1). Moreover, several groups of investigators have clearly demonstrated that defective respiratory chain function in drug-treated cells or aged human and animal tissues results in increased levels of superoxide anion and H_2O_2 (43–45). We showed previously that the oxidative stress and oxidative damage of the mitochondria and the cell as a whole are enhanced by mtDNA mutation (25). We also demonstrated previously that the electron transport activities of the respiratory enzymes examined all decreased with the increase of the proportion of the 4977 bp–deleted mtDNA (46). These results strongly indicate an energy deficit in the cybrids harboring the mutant mtDNA, and are consistent with the previous findings that the rate of oxygen consumption is decreased in tissue cells containing mutant mtDNA (13–15). In light of the earlier observations that oxidative stress and oxidative damages are enhanced in the aged human and animal tissues, we further investigated intracellular levels of ROS and lipid peroxides of the cybrids. The results showed that the levels of ROS and lipid peroxides in the cybrids containing a high proportion of the 4977 bp–deleted mtDNA were significantly higher compared with those of the control cybrids (Fig. 15.5 and Ref. 46). In line with this observation, we found that the GSH/GSSG ratio was significantly decreased in the cybrids containing high levels of mtDNA with either A3243G mutation or 4977-bp deletion (Table 15.2). These results clearly indicate that the mutant mtDNA–containing cybrids were subjected to higher oxidative stress and suffered more severe oxidative damage.

Because we found that the mutant cybrids contained higher levels of oxidized glutathione (GSSG), we employed them for the study of mitochondrial response to

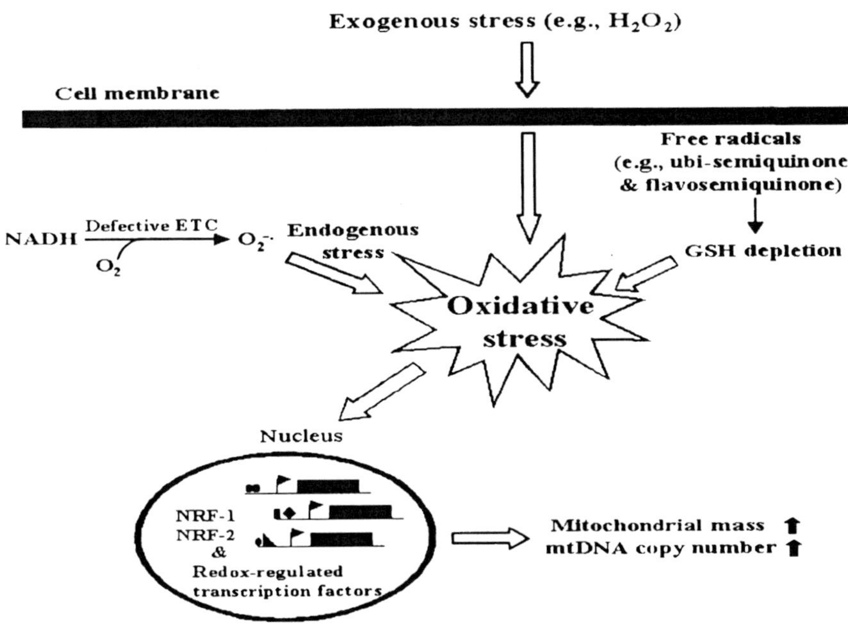

Fig. 15.6. Possible molecular mechanism underlying the oxidative stress–elicited increase of mitochondrial mass and mtDNA copy number in human cells. Oxidative stress caused by overproduction of superoxide anions in defective electron transport chain (ETC), glutathione depletion or by exogenous source of reactive oxygen species (ROS) (e.g., H_2O_2) may be sensed by the nucleus *via* certain specific signaling pathway(s). Some redox-sensitive transcription factors or DNA binding proteins related to mtDNA replication and/or mitochondrial biogenesis may be up-regulated by elevated oxidative stress. This redox-relay mechanism may play a role in the communication between the nucleus and mitochondria in coping with the endogenous and exogenous oxidative stress.

oxidative stress. We demonstrated by flow cytometry that the cybrids harboring mtDNA with 4977-bp deletion contained higher levels of mitochondrial mass and mitochondrial genome (Figs. 15.2 and 15.3). In a separate set of experiments, we noted that cybrids that harbor higher proportions of the A3243G mutant mtDNA released lactate to the culture medium at a much higher rate than did the cybrids containing low or no mutant mtDNA (data not shown). This implies that the mutant mtDNA–containing cybrids obtain their energy mainly through anaerobic glycolysis as a result of impaired respiratory function. Although these mutant cybrids can survive without too much difficulty in a rich medium such as the DMEM supplemented with 5 or 10% FBS, pyruvate, and uridine, the mutant mtDNA–containing cybrids were found to respond poorly to exogenous challenge such as H_2O_2 treatment. We believe that redox therapy for patients with mitochondrial encephalomyopathies may partially relieve the oxidative stress and alleviate oxidative damage to various cellular constituents induced by the relatively high level of mtDNA with oxidative modification and/or mutation in the affected tissues.

The data obtained in this study led us to conclude that increases of mitochondrial mass and mtDNA are the molecular events associated with enhanced oxidative stress in human cells with a defective electron transport chain caused by mtDNA deletion (Fig. 15.6). This may also explain, at least in part, the well-documented pathological manifestation of the overproliferation of abnormal mitochondria in ragged-red fibers in muscle of patients with mitochondrial myopathy or encephalomyopathies.

Acknowledgments

This work was supported by a grant (NSC89-2316-B010-012) from the National Science Council and an Institutional Excellence Research Grant to National Yang-Ming University on Genome-Based Biomedical Research for the 21st Century (89B-FA22-2-4), Ministry of Education, Republic of China. The authors are grateful for the assistance of Dr. Edward K. Wang in the procurement of the skin biopsies of the patient used in this study. One of the authors, Yau-Huei Wei, would like to express his sincere appreciation for the generous support of the National Science Council and National Health Research Institutes of the Republic of China in the course of this study.

References

1. Holt, I., Harding, A.E., and Morgan-Hughes, J.A. (1988) Deletions of Muscle Mitochondrial DNA in Patients with Mitochondrial Myopathies. *Nature 331*, 717–719.
2. Wallace, D.C., Singh, G., Lott, M.T., Hodge, A., Schurr, T.G., Lezza, A.M.S., Elasa, L., II, and Nikoskelainen, E.K. (1988) Mitochondrial DNA Mutation Associated with Leber's Hereditary Optic Neuropathy. *Science 242*, 1427–1430.
3. Goto, Y., Nonaka, I., and Horai, S. (1990) A Mutation in the $tRNA^{Leu(UUR)}$ Gene Associated with the MELAS Subgroup of Mitochondrial Encephalomyopathies. *Nature 348*, 651–653.
4. Wallace, D.C. (1992) Diseases of the Mitochondrial DNA. *Annu. Rev. Biochem. 61*, 1175–1212.

5. Lestienne, P., and Bataille, N. (1994) Mitochondrial DNA Alterations and Genetic Diseases: A Review. *Biomed. Pharmacother. 48*, 199–214.
6. Zeviani, M., Moraes, C.T., DiMauro, S., Nakase, H., Bonilla, E., Schon, E., and Rawland, L.P. (1988) Deletions of Mitochondrial DNA in Kearns-Sayre Syndrome. *Neurology 38*, 1339–1346.
7. Zeviani, M., Servidei, S., Gellera, C., Bertini, E., DiMauro, S., and DiDonato, S. (1989) An Autosomal Dominant Disorder with Multiple Deletions of Mitochondrial DNA Starting at the D-Loop Region. *Nature 339*, 309–311.
8. Larsson, N.-G., and Clayton, D.A. (1995) Molecular Genetic Aspects of Human Mitochondrial Disorders. *Annu. Rev. Genet. 29*, 151–178.
9. Hayashi, J., Ohta, S., Kikuchi, A., Takemitsu, M., Goto, Y., and Nonaka, I. (1991) Introduction of Disease-Related Mitochondrial DNA Deletions into HeLa Cells Lacking Mitochondrial DNA Results in Mitochondrial Dysfunction. *Proc. Natl. Acad. Sci. USA 88*, 10614–10618.
10. King, M.P., Koga, Y., Davidson, M., and Schon, E.A. (1992) Defects in Mitochondrial Proteins and Respiratory Chain Activity Segregate with the $tRNA^{Leu(UUR)}$ Mutation Associated with Mitochondrial Myopathy, Encephalopathy, Lactic Acidosis, and Strokelike Episodes. *Mol. Cell. Biol. 12*, 480–490.
11. Piccolo, G., Banfi, P., Azan, G., Rizzuto, R., Sandona, D., and Bellomo, G. (1991) Biological Markers of Oxidative Stress in Mitochondrial Myopathies with Progressive External Ophthalmoplegia. *J. Neurol. Sci. 105*, 57–60.
12. Pitkänen, S., and Robinson, B.H. (1996) Mitochondrial Complex I Deficiency Leads to Increased Production of Superoxide Radicals and Induction of Superoxide Dismutase. *J. Clin. Investig. 98*, 345–351.
13. Luo, X., Pitkänen, S., Kassovska-Bartinova, S., Robinson, B.H., and Lehotay, D.C. (1997) Excessive Formation of Hydroxyl Radicals and Aldehydic Lipid Peroxidation Products in Cultured Skin Fibroblasts from Patients with Complex I Deficiency. *J. Clin. Investig. 99*, 2877–2822.
14. Mitsui, T., Kawai, H., Nagasawa, M., Kunishige, M., Akaike, M., Kimura, Y., and Saito, S. (1996) Oxidative Damage to Skeletal Muscle DNA from Patients with Mitochondrial Encephalomyopathies. *J. Neurol. Sci. 139*, 111–116.
15. Esposito, L.A., Melov, S., Panvo, A., Cottrell, B.A., and Wallace, D.C. (1999) Mitochondrial Disease in Mouse Results in Increased Oxidative Stress. *Proc. Natl. Acad. Sci. USA 96*, 4820–4825.
16. Katsumata, K., Hayakawa, M., Tanaka, M., Sugiyama, S., and Ozawa, T. (1994) Fragmentation of Human Heart Mitochondrial DNA Associated with Premature Aging. *Biochem. Biophys. Res. Commun. 202*, 102–110.
17. Larson, N.-G., Holme, E., Kristiansson, B., Oldfors, A., and Tulinius, M. (1990) Progressive Increase of the Mutated Mitochondrial DNA Fraction in Kearns-Sayre Syndrome. *Pediatr. Res. 28*, 131–136.
18. Feigenbaum, A., Chitayat, D., Robinson, B., MacGregor, D., Myint, T., Arbus, G., and Nowaczyk, J.M. (1996) The Expanding Clinical Phenotype of the $tRNA^{Leu(UUR)}$ $A \rightarrow G$ Mutation at np 3243 of Mitochondrial DNA: Diabetes Embryopathy Associated with Mitochondrial Cytopathy. *Am. J. Med. Genet. 62*, 404–409.
19. Wallace, D.C. (1999) Mitochondrial Diseases in Man and Mouse. *Science 283*, 1482–1488.
20. Ikebe, S., Tanaka, M., and Ozawa, T. (1995) Point Mutations of Mitochondrial Genorne in Parkinson's Disease. *Mol. Brain Res. 28*, 281–295.

21. Swerdlow, R.H., Parks, J.K., Cassarino, D.S., Trimmer, P.A., Currie, L.J., Dougherty, J., Bridges, W.-S., Bennett, J.P., Jr., Wooten, G.F., and Parker, W.D. (1998) Matrilineal Inheritance of Complex I Dysfunction in a Multigenerational Parkinson's Disease Family. *Ann. Neurol. 44*, 873–881.
22. Allen, R.G., and Tresini, M. (2000) Oxidative Stress and Gene Regulation. *Free Radic. Biol. Med. 28*, 463–499.
23. Poyton, R.O., and McEwen, J.E. (1996) Crosstalk Between Nuclear and Mitochondrial Genomes. *Annu. Rev. Biochem. 65*, 563–607.
24. Suzuki, H., Kumagai, T., Goto, A., and Sugiura, T. (1998) Increase in Intracellular Hydrogen Peroxide and Upregulation of a Nuclear Respiratory Gene Evoked by Impairment of Mitochondrial Electron Transfer in Human Cells. *Biochem. Biophys. Res. Commun. 249*, 542–545.
25. Wei, Y.H. (1998) Oxidative Stress and Mitochondrial DNA Mutations in Human Aging. *Proc. Soc. Exp. Biol. Med. 217*, 53–63.
26. Lee, H.C., Yin, P.H., Lu, C.Y., Chi, C.W., and Wei, Y.H. (2000) Increase of Mitochondria and Mitochondrial DNA in Response to Oxidative Stress in Human Cells. *Biochem. J. 348*, 425–432.
27. King, M.P., and Attardi, G. (1988) Injection of Mitochondria into Human Cells Leads to a Rapid Replacement of the Endogenous Mitochondrial DNA. *Cell 52*, 811–819.
28. King, M P., and Attardi, G. (1989) Human Cells Lacking mtDNA Repopulation with Exogenous Mitochondria by Complementation. *Science 246*, 500–503.
29. Vassault, A. (1983) Lactate Dehydrogenase, in *Methods of Enzymatic Analysis* (Bergmeyer, H. U., ed.) 3rd ed., pp. 118–126, Verlag Chemie GmbH, Weinheim.
30. Pang, C Y. (1998) Molecular Epidemiological and Cellular Biological Studies of Mitochondrial Diseases in Taiwan, Ph.D. Thesis, Institute of Biochemistry, National Yang-Ming University, Taipei.
31. Petit, J M., Maftah, A., Ratinaud, M H., and Julien, R. (1992) 10-*n*-Nonyl Acridine Orange Interacts with Cardiolipin and Allows the Quantification of this Phospholipid in Isolated Mitochondria. *Eur. J. Biochem. 209*, 267–273.
32. Maftah, A., Petit, J M., Ratinaud, M.H., and Julien, R. (1989) 10-*n*-Nonyl Acridine Orange: A Fluorescent Probe Which Stains Mitochondria Independently of Their Energetic State. *Biochem. Biophys. Res. Commun. 164*, 185–190.
33. Shih, K D., Yen, T C., Pang, C Y., and Wei, Y H. (1991) Mitochondrial DNA Mutation in a Chinese Family with Myoclonic Epilepsy and Ragged-Red Fibers Disease. *Biochem. Biophys. Res. Commun. 174*, 1109–1116.
34. Huang, C.C., Chen, R.S., Chen, C.M., Wang, H.S., Lee, C.C., Pang, C.Y., Hsu, H.S., Lee, H.C., and Wei, Y.H. (1994) MELAS Syndrome with Mitochondrial $tRNA^{Leu(UUR)}$ Gene Mutation in a Chinese Family. *J. Neurol. Neurosurg. Psychiatry 57*, 586–589.
35. Wang, E.K., Kao, K.P., Hsieh, R.H., Lu, C.Y., Pang, C.Y., and Wei, Y.H. (1998) Large Scale Mitochondrial DNA Deletions in Patients with CPEO Syndrome in Taiwan. *J. Biochem. Mol. Biol. Biophys. 1*, 165–170.
36. Wong, S.H.Y., Knight, J.A., Hopfer, S.M., Zaharia, O., Leach, C.N., and Sunderman, F.W. (1987) Lipoperoxides in Plasma as Measured by Liquid-Chromatographic Separation of Malondialdehyde-Thiobarbituric Acid Adduct. *Clin. Chem. 33*, 214–220.
37. Anderson, M.E. (1985) Recycling Assay for Glutathione. *Methods Enzymol. 113*, 548–555.
38. Lowry, O.H., Rosebrough, N., Farr, A.L., and Randall, R. J. (1951) Protein Measurement with the Folin Phenol Reagent. *J. Biol. Chem. 193*, 265–275.

39. Grossman, L.I., and Shoubridge, E.A. (1996) Mitochondrial Genetics and Human Disease. *BioEssays 18*, 983–991.
40. Giulivi, C., Boveris, A., and Cadenas, E. (1995) Hydroxyl Radical Generation During Mitochondrial Electron Transfer and the Formation of 8-Hydroxydeoxyguanosine in Mitochondrial DNA. *Arch. Biochem. Biophys. 316*, 909–916.
41. Sohal, R.S. (1993) Aging, Cytochrome Oxidase Activity, and Hydrogen Peroxide Release by Mitochondria. *Free Radic. Biol. Med. 14*, 583–5 88.
42. Muscari, C., Frascaro, M., Guarneri, C., and Caldarera, C. (1990) Mitochondrial Function and Superoxide Generation from Submitochondrial Particles of Aged Rat Hearts. *Biochim. Biophys. Acta 1015*, 200–204.
43. Ku, H.H., Brunk, U.T., and Sohal, R.S. (1993) Relationship Between Mitochondrial Superoxide and Hydrogen Peroxide Production and Longevity of Mammalian Species. *Free Radic. Biol. Med. 15*, 621–627.
44. Sohal, R.S., Agarwal, S., and Sohal, B.H. (1995) Oxidative Stress and Aging in the Mongolian Gerbil *(Meriones unguiculatus). Mech. Ageing Dev. 81*, 15–25.
45. Nagley, P., Zhang, C., Martinus, R.D., Vaillant, F., and Linnane, A.W. (1992) Mitochondrial DNA Mutation and Human Aging: Molecular Biology, Bioenergetics, and Redox Therapy, in *Mitochondrial DNA in Human Pathology* (DiMauro, S., and Wallace, D.C., eds.) pp. 137–157, Raven Press, New York.
46. Wei, Y.H., Lee, C.F., Lee, H.C., Ma, Y.S. Wang, C.W., Lu, C.Y., and Pang, C.Y. (2001) Increase of Mitochondrial Mass and Mitochondrial Genome in Association with Enhanced Oxidative Stress in Human Cells Harboring 4,977 bp–deleted Mitochondrial DNA. *Ann. N.Y. Acad. Sci., 928,* 97–112.

Chapter 16

MAP Kinase Activation and Environmental Stress

Lars-Oliver Klotz, Darius P. Buchczyk, and Helmut Sies

Institut für Physiologische Chemie I, Heinrich-Heine-Universität Düsseldorf, Germany

Introduction: MAP Kinases

It has become widely accepted that environmental stresses elicit cellular reactions, ranging from adaptive responses to toxicity. Mitogen-activated protein kinases (MAPK) have been studied as players in such cellular responses, regulating transcription factor activities and the balance between cellular survival and apoptotic cell death.

The major MAPK (for reviews, see Refs. 1–3) are activated by upstream-kinases by dual (Thr- and Tyr-) phosphorylation of a Thr-X-Tyr-motif (see Table 16.1); they are "proline-directed" Ser/Thr-kinases that in turn phosphorylate their substrates on Ser- or Thr-residues at positions defined by the direct C-terminal attachment of proline. In addition to the classical mitogen-activated protein kinases [the extracellular-signal-regulated kinases (ERK) 1 and 2], which are activated by mitogenic stimuli such as growth factors, the MAPK group comprises those kinases that can be activated by stress: One subgroup, termed p38, with four members of apparent molecular weights between 38 and 43 kDa (4) and one, the c-Jun-N-terminal kinases (JNK), that consists of 10 isoforms with molecular weights between 46 and 57 kDa that are derived from three genes, jnk-1 through jnk-3, and generated by alternative splicing (5). These three MAPK subfamilies not only share similarities in their way of activation but also in the way the upstream events leading to their activation are organized, i.e., they are activated by more or less specific MAPK kinases (MKK; for terminology, see Table 16.1) which, in turn, are phosphorylated and activated by MKK kinases (MKKK). Further upstream of these three-kinase modules, small GTP-binding proteins such as Ras may be found. Among the substrates of activated MAPK are transcription factors such as Elk1, Sap, c-Jun, or ATF2 (Table 16.1). Upon phosphorylation by MAPK, these factors are activated and lead to the expression of proteins constituting the leucine-zipper transcription factor AP-1, e.g., c-Jun and c-Fos, *via* the c-jun-track (JNK→ c-Jun → c-jun expression; or JNK/p38 → ATF2 → c-jun expression) or the c-fos-track [ERK/p38 → Elk-1 → c-fos expression; or ERK/p38 → MAPKAP-K(1/2)/CREBkinase → CREB → c-fos expression] (2,3,6). As a consequence of activation of AP-1, the expression of genes with functional AP-1 elements (also termed *t*etradecanoyl-phorbol acetate-*r*esponsive *e*lements, TRE, because of their ability to be activated by this phorbol ester) in their promoter regions, such as heme oxygenase-1 (7,8) and matrix metalloproteinase-1 (9), may be induced.

TABLE 16.1 Terminology of MAPK and MKK[a,b]

	Aliases	Selected substrates	Comments (Hugo Nomenclature)[c]
MAPK			
ERK		Connexin 43, CPSII, cPLA2, Elk-1 Sap-1, MAPKAP-K1, cyclin D1	• -T-E-Y- Phosphorylation motif
ERK1	MAPK1, $p44^{MAPK}$		(MAPK3)
ERK2	MAPK2, $p42^{MAPK}$		(MAPK1)
JNK		c-Jun, ATF-2, Elk-1, Sap-l	• -T-P-Y- Phosphorylation motif
JNK1	SAPK1c; SAPKγ		Four splice variants (MAPK8)
JNK2	SAPK1a; SAPKα		Four splice variants (MAPK9)
JNK3	SAPK1b; SAPKβ		Two splice variants (MAPK10)
p38		MAPKAP-K2, ATF-2, Elk-1, SAP-1, MEF-2C, CHOP/Gadd153, $cPLA_2$	• -T-G-Y- Phosphorylation motif
p38α	SAPK2a; CSBP; RK		(MAPK14)
p38β	SAPK2b		(MAPK11)
p38γ	SAPK3; ERK6		(MAPK12)
p38δ	SAPK4		(MAPK13)
Further MAPK			
ERK3	$p97^{MAPK}$	?	-S-E-G- Phosphorylation motif (MAPK6)
ERK4	$p63^{MAPK}$	?	-S-E-G- Phosphorylation motif (MAPK4)
ERK5	BMK1	c-Myc; MEF-2C	-T-E-Y- Phosphorylation motif (MAPK7)
MKK			
MKK1	MEK1; MAPKK1	ERK1/2	(MAP2K1)
MKK2	MEK2; MAPKK2	ERK1/2	(MAP2K2)
MKK3	MEK3; SKK2; SAPKK2	p38α,γ,δ	(MAP2K3)
MKK4	JNKK; SKK1; SEK1; SAPKK1	JNK1–3; p38α,δ	(MAP2K4)
MKK5	MEK5	ERK5	(MAP2K5)
MKK6	MEK6; SKK3; SAPKK3	p38α–δ	(MAP2K6)
MKK7	JNKK2; SKK4; SAPKK4	JNK1–3; p38δ	(MAP2K7)

[a]*Sources:* Refs. 44,45.
[b]Abbreviations: ATF, activating transcription factor; BMK, big MAP kinase; CHOP, CCAAT/enhancer binding protein-homologous protein; $cPLA_2$, cytosolic phospholipase A_2; CPSII, carbamoyl phosphate synthetase II; CSBP, cytokine-suppressive anti-inflammatory drug binding protein; ERK, extracellular regulated kinase; Gadd, growth arrest and DNA damage; JNK, c-Jun-N-terminal kinase; JNKK, JNK kinase; MAPK, mitogen-activated protein kinase; MAPKAP-K, MAPK-activated protein kinase; MEF, myocyte enhancer factor; MEK, MAPK/ERK kinase; MKK, MAP kinase kinase; RK, reactivating kinase; Sap, stress-activated protein; SAPK, stress-activated protein kinase; SKK = SAPKK, SAPK kinase.
[c]MAPK and MKK nomenclature as recommended by The Human Genome Organization (Hugo). The recommendations can be found at http://www.gene.ucl.ac.uk/users/hester/prkm.html.

In 1995, Xia *et al.* (10) proposed a crucial role of p38 and JNK as proapoptotic stimuli in PC12 cells, whereas activation of ERK1/2 seemed to be antiapoptotic. This model of an increased JNK/p38 to ERK activity ratio as a stimulus toward apoptosis has since become widely accepted and verified, but has also been proven not to be valid under all circumstances. One such case is apoptosis induced by irradiation of cells with visible light in the presence of the sensitizer hypericin (11), i.e., inhibition of activation of JNK and p38 by this so-called photodynamic treatment using pharmacologic inhibitors or by overexpression of either dominant-negative upstream regulators or the dominant-positive form of a regulating phosphatase, MAPK phosphatase-1 (MKP-1), sensitized the treated HeLa cells toward the treatment. In yet another system (12), the opposite seems to be true, i.e., p38 and JNK are activated in murine leukemic lymphoblasts upon photodynamic treatment employing the sensitizing phthalocyanine Pc4, and pharmacologic inhibition of p38 inhibited apoptosis. In summary, the role of MAP kinases in stress-induced apoptosis is not completely resolved.

In addition to the role of MAP kinases in the regulation of transcription factors, other proteins are phosphorylated by activated MAPK as well. Two examples are as follows: (i) carbamoyl phosphate synthetase II (13,14), the enzyme catalyzing the initial, rate-limiting step in pyrimidine biosynthesis, which is phosphorylated by ERK1/2 (leading to a conformational change that enhances activation by phosphoribosyl pyrophosphate and blocks feedback-inhibition by UTP); and (ii) the interaction of JNK with p53 (15,16). The first exemplifies the role ERKs may play in proliferation and preparation for DNA synthesis, and the second demonstrates the significance of JNKs in the regulation of apoptotic responses.

Activation of MAP Kinases by Environmental Stimuli and Oxidative Stress

Ultraviolet (UV) radiation is among the stressful environmental stimuli leading to MAPK activation. It has traditionally been divided into defined regions of wavelengths, such as UVA (320–400 nm), UVB (280–320 nm), and UVC at wavelengths <280 nm. Physiologically, the last-mentioned is of the least importance because the stratospheric ozone layer hinders UVC from reaching the earth´s surface. Of the three regions, UVA is the one that penetrates skin most deeply, reaching subepidermal layers (17,18). UVA was shown to play a role not only in the context of damage to biomolecules and cells (19,20), but also to be capable of inducing more complex responses such as the induction of genes and the activation of signaling pathways including those that depend on MAP kinases.

Treatment of primary human skin fibroblasts with UVA leads to a rapid and transient activation of p38 and JNK, but not the ERK1/2 MAP kinases (21,22). These effects are mediated by an electronically excited form of molecular oxygen that is generated by irradiation of cellular photosensitizers, singlet oxygen ($^1O_2$), as suggested from experiments using $^1O_2$ scavengers such as azide ions or imidazole (21,22).

In line with this, only p38 and JNK are activated significantly by $^1O_2$ generated chemically or photochemically (22). From experiments with $^1O_2$ generating systems, it is known that activation of p38 and JNK MAP kinases requires the intracellular generation of $^1O_2$ (22). Although photochemical generation of $^1O_2$ by irradiation of cells in the presence of the lipophilic dye Rose Bengal leads to activation of the mentioned kinases, the immobilization of rose Bengal on agarose and thus the extracellular generation of $^1O_2$ prevents this activation. Similarly, the light-independent chemical generation of $^1O_2$ by thermodecomposition of the membrane permeant 1,4-endoperoxide of N,N′-di(2,3-dihydroxypropyl)-1,4-naphthalene dipropionamide leads to p38 and JNK activation, different from the thermodecomposition of the ionic derivative, the 1,4-endoperoxide of sodium 3,3′-(1,4-naphthylidene) dipropionate, which has no effect on MAPK. An identical pattern of MAPK activation (p38 and JNK but not ERK1/2) results from treatment of HaCaT keratinocytes with 5-aminolevulinic acid (ALA), followed by irradiation with red light (23); this so-called ALA-photodynamic treatment relies upon the cellular synthesis of photosensitizing porphyrins from ALA. Activation of p38 is also found in human melanoma cells undergoing ALA-PDT (23). Interestingly, the activation of p38 by UVA can be seen at much lower doses after pretreatment of skin cells with ALA.

Different from UVA and $^1O_2$, oxidative stress induced by treatment with the redox cycler menadione leads to activation of ERK1/2 (24); two other reactive oxygen species, hydrogen peroxide and peroxynitrite (a potent oxidative and nitrating species formed in a diffusion-limited reaction of nitrogen monoxide and superoxide), do activate all three major MAPK subfamilies, including ERK1/2 (25–27), suggesting that the MAPK activation pattern elicited by oxidant treatment is selective as to the nature of the respective oxidant. Activation of JNK by H_2O_2 in HeLa cells is mediated at least in part by the activation of MKK4, as was shown by employing expression of a dominant-negative form of MKK4 (26). Activation of MAP kinases by

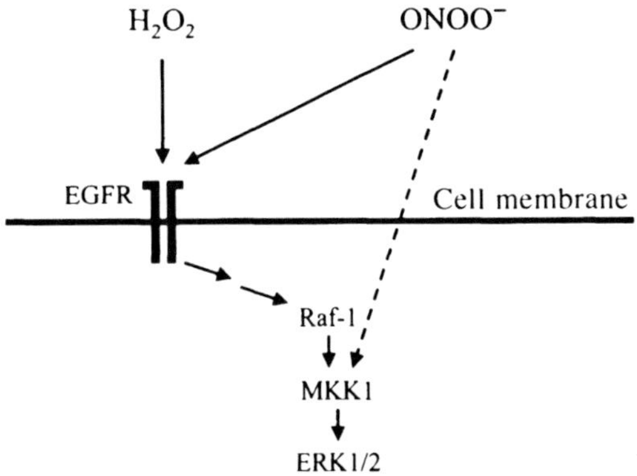

Fig. 16.1. Activation of extracellular signal–regulated kinases (ERK)1/2 by hydrogen peroxide and peroxynitrite (26,28). Both oxidants activate the epidermal growth factor receptor (EGFR), Raf-1 kinase and MKK1. However, although the activation of ERK1/2 by H_2O_2 is inhibited by pharmacologic blockade of any upstream kinase (EGFR kinase, Raf-1 or MKK1), MKK1 is sufficient for peroxynitrite-induced activation of ERK, which appears to be independent of EGFR or Raf-1 and mediated by induced autophosphorylation of MKK1 (see text).

hydrogen peroxide in HeLa cells is accompanied by apoptosis (26). Although pharmacologic inhibition of p38 does not influence the apoptotic response toward H_2O_2, inhibition of MKK1, a kinase directly upstream of ERK1/2, leads to increased apoptosis, pointing to an antiapoptotic role of ERK1/2 in the cellular response to H_2O_2. The activation of ERK by H_2O_2 was further shown to be mediated by EGF receptor (EGFR) activation and the consecutive activation of the MKK1/2 kinase, Raf-1, in rat lung myofibroblasts (Fig. 16.1). Peroxynitrite was also shown to activate EGFR, Raf-1, and MKK1, but activation of ERK1/2 was demonstrated to be dependent solely on MKK1, not EGFR or Raf (28). Different from the above-mentioned findings in HeLa cells (26), pharmacologic inhibition of MKK1 decreased (27) toxicity of both peroxynitrite and H_2O_2 in rat myofibroblasts (28). Thus, it seems inappropriate to generalize the findings by Xia *et al.* (10) on the antiapoptotic properties of ERK.

In summary, the activation of MAP kinases by different oxidative stresses may occur *via* different mechanisms and result in different responses, also varying with the cell type tested.

On the Mechanism of MAPK Activation by Oxidative Stress

Three mechanisms for the oxidant-induced activation of a kinase regulated by phosphorylation may be imagined as follows (Fig. 16.2): (i) The indirect targeting of the kinase by inactivation of a regulating phosphatase; (ii) the direct oxidation resulting in activation of the kinase; and (iii) the activation by activation of upstream events. There are examples in the literature for all three mechanisms.

In 1996, Knebel *et al.* (29) and Cavigelli *et al.* (30) introduced a new and now somewhat classical aspect into the discussion concerning which could be the cellular integrating point that leads to activation of signaling pathways by noxae such as UV, oxidants, or arsenite. Knebel *et al.* (29) showed that receptor tyrosine kinases (RTK) are activated (phosphorylated) by inhibition of a phosphatase activity upon treatment with UV (A, B, or C), hydrogen peroxide, or iodoacetamide and that phosphatase

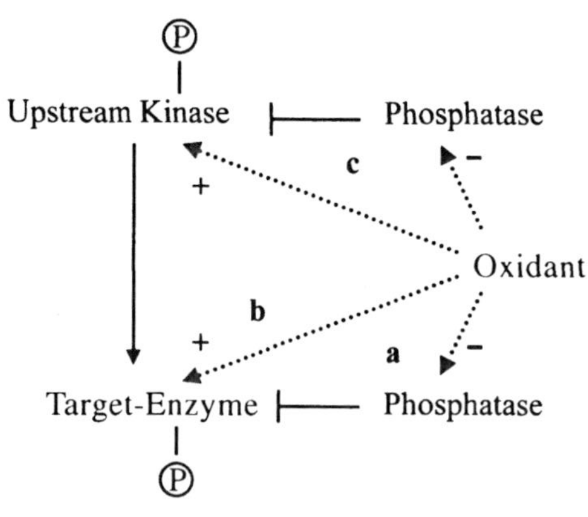

Fig. 16.2. Possible mechanisms of activation of a phosphorylation-regulated kinase by oxidants. The kinase (target enzyme) may be activated indirectly by inactivating a regulating phosphatase leading to a net activation (**a**). An oxidant may also act on a kinase directly (**b**), leading to autophosphorylation, e.g., facilitated by conformational changes. Third (**c**), activation of the target enzyme may also be achieved by activation of an upstream kinase by either of the above-mentioned mechanisms.

activity, i.e., dephosphorylation and inactivation of RTK, is restored upon the addition of thiol regenerating agents, if not inhibited irreversibly by iodoacetamide. Further, H_2O_2 has been pointed out not only to inactivate membrane-bound phosphatases (29) but also to diminish cytosolic general protein tyrosine phosphatase activity in mouse fibroblasts (31). Cavigelli and co-workers (30) found that the activation of JNK by sodium arsenite, which is reactive toward thiols (especially vicinal dithiols), is by inactivating a JNK phosphatase.

All protein tyrosine phosphatases known to date rely on the presence of a cysteine in their active site; it serves as a nucleophile, accepting the phosphate moiety of the phosphatase substrate and forming an intermediate phosphocysteine (32). An oxidation of this cysteine residue, e.g., by hydrogen peroxide or by singlet oxygen formed during UVA irradiation, would lead to the inactivation of the phosphatase, concomitantly allowing kinase activities to become predominant.

A mechanism different from the above and corresponding to (**b**) and (**c**) in Figure 16.2 has been shown to apply for peroxynitrite-induced activation of ERK1/2 (28), which was mediated by the activation of an upstream kinase, MKK1. MKK1, in turn, was directly able to be activated by peroxynitrite, apparently by induced autophosphorylation, which was likely due to biochemical modification (such as tyrosine nitration) and conformational changes of MKK1 after treatment with the oxidant.

A further example for activation of a signaling pathway by an oxidant that does not rely solely on the oxidative inactivation of a phosphatase is the peroxynitrite-induced activation of Akt (protein kinase B, see below).

Beyond MAPK: Activation of Akt (Protein Kinase B) by Oxidative Stress

A stress-responsive pathway closely linked to the ERK pathway is the antiapoptotic phosphoinositide 3-kinase (PI3K)/Akt (synonymous to protein kinase B, PKB) pathway, which also emanates from receptor tyrosine kinases and is Ras-dependent for activation. Further, Akt has recently been shown to be capable of inactivating the MKK1/2 kinase Raf by phosphorylation (33,34). The PI3K/Akt pathway has been implicated in the antiapoptotic and proliferative cellular response to growth factors such as platelet-derived growth factor (PDGF), epidermal growth factor (EGF), but also in the response to stressful stimuli such as heat shock or hydrogen peroxide (for review, see Ref. 35). PI3K has been shown to be upstream of Akt and regulate Akt activity by generating 3′-phosphorylated phosphoinositides that reside in the cell membrane and lead to binding of Akt′s pleckstrin homology domain, concomitant with a transfer of Akt to the cell membrane. This relocalization of Akt renders it accessible to regulating kinases (35,36), resulting in the phosphorylation of Akt at Thr-308 and Ser-473, which have been shown to trigger the activation of Akt. PI3 kinases, in turn, are activated by the binding of their regulatory p85 subunit to tyrosine-phosphorylated (activated) receptor-tyrosine kinases *via* an SH (Src homology)-2 domain.

Akt has been shown to be activated by oxidants such as hydrogen peroxide (38–41), by certain NO donors (42), and peroxynitrite, either added to the cells as a bolus of authentic peroxynitrite or generated *in situ* from SIN-1 (43). EGFR plays a primary role in mediating Akt activation by hydrogen peroxide because activation was blocked in the presence of specific inhibitors of EGFR phosphorylation (41). Activation by peroxynitrite in primary human skin fibroblasts is mediated by PI-3 kinase and emanates mainly from PDGF receptors that are tyrosine phosphorylated upon treatment. As a consequence, downstream targets of Akt, such as glycogen synthase kinase-3 (GSK-3), are phosphorylated (43). Further, prior peroxynitrite treatment renders cells refractory to subsequent Akt activation by growth factors (43), indicating that phosphatase inhibition (as discussed above) cannot be the sole mechanism responsible for activation of the kinase. If the inhibition of a regulating phosphatase by peroxynitrite were responsible for the increased Akt phosphorylation, then phosphorylation would not be expected to be inhibited by peroxynitrite pretreatment; rather, it would be expected to be enhanced due to the loss of negative regulation.

Summary

Environmental stimuli such as UV radiation and a variety of reactive oxygen species lead to the activation of MAP kinases and related signaling molecules. Exposure results in different MAPK activation patterns depending on the type of stressful stimulus and the type of cell employed. The role of MAPK activation by UV or reactive oxygen species in apoptosis and cellular survival is not completely understood; to date, there is also no explanation for the differential activations of kinases by reactive oxygen species. However, in mechanisms leading to UV- and oxidant-induced MAPK- or Akt-activations, the ligand-independent activation of membrane receptor tyrosine kinases appears to play a central role.

Acknowledgment

The authors' work was supported by Deutsche Forschungsgemeinschaft (Bonn, Germany), SFB 503/B1. Helmut Sies is a Fellow of the National Foundation for Cancer Research (NFCR), Bethesda, MD, USA.

References

1. Whitmarsh, A.J., and Davis, R.J. (1996) Transcription Factor AP-1 Regulation by Mitogen-Activated Protein Kinase Signal Transduction Pathways. *J. Mol. Med. 74*, 589–607.
2. Karin, M., Liu Z.G., and Zandi, E. (1997) AP-1 Function and Regulation. *Curr. Opin. Cell Biol. 9*, 240–246.
3. Karin, M. (1995) The Regulation of AP-1 Activity by Mitogen-Activated Protein Kinases. *J. Biol. Chem. 270*, 16483–16486.
4. Ono, K., and Han, J. (2000) The p38 Signal Transduction Pathway—Activation and Function. *Cell. Signalling 12*, 1–13.

5. Gupta, S., Barrett, T., Whitmarsh, A.J., Cavanagh, J., Sluss, H.K., Derijard, B., and Davis, R.J. (1996) Selective Interaction of JNK Protein Kinase Isoforms with Transcription Factors. *EMBO J. 15*, 2760–2770.
6. Iordanov, M., Bender, K., Ade, T., Schmid, W., Sachsenmaier, C., Engel, K., Gaestel, M., Rahmsdorf, H.J., and Herrlich, P. (1997) CREB Is Activated by UVC Through a P38/HOG-1-Dependent Protein Kinase. *EMBO J. 16*, 1009–1022.
7. Lavrovsky, Y., Schwartzman, M.L., Levere, R.D., Kappas, A., and Abraham, N.G. (1994) Identification of Binding Sites for Transcription factors NF-κB and AP-2 in the Promoter Region of the Human Heme Oxygenase 1 Gene. *Proc. Natl. Acad. Sci. USA 91*, 5987–5991.
8. Elbirt, K.K., Whitmarsh, A.J., Davis, R.J., and Bonkovsky, H.L. (1998) Mechanism of Sodium Arsenite-Mediated Induction of Heme Oxygenase-1 in Hepatoma Cells. Role of Mitogen-Activated Protein Kinases. *J. Biol. Chem. 273*, 8922–8931.
9. Angel, P., Imagawa, M., Chiu, R., Stein, B., Imbra, R.J., Rahmsdorf, H.J., Jonat, C., Herrlich, P., and Karin, M. (1987) Phorbol Ester-Inducible Genes Contain a Common *cis* Element Recognized by a TPA-Modulated *trans*-Acting Factor. *Cell 49*, 729–739.
10. Xia, Z., Dickens, M., Raingeaud, J., Davis, R.J., and Greenberg, M.E. (1995) Opposing Effects of ERK and JNK-p38 MAP Kinases on Apoptosis. *Science 270*, 1326–1331.
11. Assefa, Z., Vantieghem, A., Declercq, W., Vandenabeele, P., Vandenheede, J.R., Merlevede, W., de Witte, P., and Agostinis, P. (1999) The Activation of the c-Jun N-Terminal Kinase and p38 Mitogen-Activated Protein Kinase Signaling Pathways Protects HeLa Cells from Apoptosis Following Photodynamic Therapy with Hypericin. *J. Biol. Chem. 274*, 8788–8796.
12. Xue, L.Y., He, J., and Oleinick, N.L. (1999) Promotion of Photodynamic Therapy-Induced Apoptosis by Stress Kinases. *Cell Death Differ. 6*, 855–864.
13. Graves, L.M., Guy, H.I., Kozlowski, P., Huang, M., Lazarowski, E., Pope, R.M., Collins, M.A., Dahlstrand, E.N., Earp, H.S., III, and Evans, D.R. (2000) Regulation of Carbamoyl Phosphate Synthetase by MAP Kinase. *Nature 403*, 328–332.
14. Whitmarsh, A.J., and Davis, R.J. (2000) A Central Control for Cell Growth. *Nature 403*, 255–256.
15. Buschmann, T., Adler, V., Matusevich, E., Fuchs, S.Y., and Ronai, Z. (2000) p53 Phosphorylation and Association with Murine Double Minute 2, c-Jun NH2-Terminal Kinase, p14ARF, and p300/CBP During the Cell Cycle and After Exposure to Ultraviolet Irradiation. *Cancer Res. 60*, 896–900.
16. Fuchs, S.Y., Adler, V., Buschmann, T., Yin, Z., Wu, X., Jones, S.N., and Ronai, Z. (1998) JNK Targets p53 Ubiquitination and Degradation in Nonstressed Cells. *Genes Dev. 12*, 2658–2663.
17. Bruls, W.A., Slaper, H., van der Leun, J.C., and Berrens, L. (1984) Transmission of Human Epidermis and Stratum Corneum as a Function of Thickness in the Ultraviolet and Visible Wavelengths. *Photochem. Photobiol. 40*, 485–494.
18. Tyrrell, R.M. (1996) Activation of Mammalian Gene Expression by the UV Component of Sunlight—from Models to Reality. *Bioessays 18*, 139–148.
19. Kvam, E. and Tyrrell, R.M. (1997) Induction of Oxidative DNA Base Damage in Human Skin Cells by UV and near Visible Radiation. *Carcinogenesis 18*, 2379–2384.
20. Basu-Modak, S., Lüscher, P., and Tyrrell, R.M. (1996) Lipid Metabolite Involvement in the Activation of the Human Heme Oxygenase-1 Gene. *Free Radic. Biol. Med. 20*, 887–897.

21. Klotz, L.O., Briviba, K., and Sies, H. (1997) Singlet Oxygen Mediates the Activation of JNK by UVA Radiation in Human Skin Fibroblasts. *FEBS Lett. 408*, 289–291.
22. Klotz, L.O., Pellieux, C., Briviba, K., Pierlot, C., Aubry, J.M., and Sies, H. (1999) Mitogen-Activated Protein Kinase (p38-, JNK-, ERK-) Activation Pattern Induced by Extracellular and Intracellular Singlet Oxygen and UVA. *Eur. J. Biochem. 260*, 917–922.
23. Klotz, L.O., Fritsch, C., Briviba, K., Tsacmacidis, N., Schliess, F., and Sies, H. (1998) Activation of JNK and p38 but Not ERK MAP Kinases in Human Skin Cells by 5-Aminolevulinate Photodynamic Therapy. *Cancer Res. 58*, 4297–4300.
24. Buchczyk, D.P., Klotz, L.O., Lang, K., Fritsch, C., and Sies, H. (2001) High Efficiency of 5-Aminolevulinate-Photodynamic Treatment Using UVA-Irradiaiton, *In Press.*
25. Guyton, K.Z., Liu, Y., Gorospe, M., Xu, Q., and Holbrook, N.J. (1996) Activation of Mitogen-Activated Protein Kinase by H_2O_2. Role in Cell Survival Following Oxidant Injury. *J. Biol. Chem. 271*, 4138–4142.
26. Wang, X., Martindale, J.L., Liu, Y., and Holbrook, N.J. (1998) The Cellular Response to Oxidative Stress: Influences of Mitogen-Activated Protein Kinase Signalling Pathways on Cell Survival. *Biochem. J. 333*, 291–300.
27. Schieke, S.M., Briviba, K., Klotz, L.O., and Sies, H. (1999) Activation Pattern of Mitogen-Activated Protein Kinases Elicited by Peroxynitrite: Attenuation by Selenite Supplementation. *FEBS Lett. 448*, 301–303.
28. Zhang, P., Wang, Y.Z., Kagan, E., and Bonner, J.C. (2000) Peroxynitrite Targets the Epidermal Growth Factor Receptor, Raf-1, and MEK Independently to Activate MAPK. *J. Biol. Chem. 275*, 22479–22486.
29. Knebel, A., Rahmsdorf, H.J., Ullrich, A., and Herrlich, P. (1996) Dephosphorylation of Receptor Tyrosine Kinases as Target of Regulation by Radiation, Oxidants or Alkylating Agents. *EMBO J. 15*, 5314–5325.
30. Cavigelli, M., Li, W.W., Lin, A., Su, B., Yoshioka, K., and Karin, M. (1996) The Tumor Promoter Arsenite Stimulates AP-1 Activity by Inhibiting a JNK Phosphatase. *EMBO J. 15*, 6269–6279.
31. Sullivan, S.G., Chiu, D.T., Errasfa, M., Wang, J.M., Qi, J.S., and Stern, A. (1994) Effects of H_2O_2 on Protein Tyrosine Phosphatase Activity in HER14 Cells. *Free Radic. Biol. Med. 16*, 399–403.
32. Fauman, E.B., and Saper, M.A. (1996) Structure and Function of the Protein Tyrosine Phosphatases. *Trends Biochem. Sci. 21*, 413–417.
33. Zimmermann, S., and Moelling, K. (1999) Phosphorylation and Regulation of Raf by Akt (Protein Kinase B). *Science 286*, 1741–1744.
34. Rommel, C., Clarke, B.A., Zimmermann, S., Nunez, L., Rossman, R., Reid, K., Moelling, K., Yancopoulos, G.D., and Glass, D.J. (1999) Differentiation Stage-Specific Inhibition of the Raf-MEK-ERK Pathway by Akt. *Science 286*, 1738–1741.
35. Datta, S.R., Brunet, A., and Greenberg, M.E. (1999) Cellular Survival: A Play in Three Akts. *Genes Dev. 13*, 2905–2927.
36. Balendran, A., Casamayor, A., Deak, M., Paterson, A., Gaffney, P., Currie, R., Downes, C.P., and Alessi, D.R. (1999) PDK1 Acquires PDK2 Activity in the Presence of a Synthetic Peptide Derived from the Carboxyl Terminus of PRK2. *Curr. Biol. 9*, 393–404.
37. Alessi, D.R., Andjelkovic, M., Caudwell, B., Cron, P., Morrice, N., Cohen, P., and Hemmings, B.A. (1996) Mechanism of Activation of Protein Kinase B by Insulin and IGF-1. *EMBO J. 15*, 6541–6551.

38. Konishi, H., Matsuzaki, H., Tanaka, M., Takemura, Y., Kuroda, S., Ono, Y., and Kikkawa, U. (1997) Activation of Protein Kinase B (Akt/RAC-Protein Kinase) by Cellular Stress and Its Association with Heat Shock Protein hsp27. *FEBS Lett. 410*, 493–498.
39. Shaw, M., Cohen, P., and Alessi, D.R. (1998) The Activation of Protein Kinase B by H_2O_2 or Heat Shock Is Mediated by Phosphoinositide 3-Kinase and Not by Mitogen-Activated Protein Kinase-Activated Protein Kinase-2. *Biochem. J. 336*, 241–246.
40. Sonoda, Y., Watanabe, S., Matsumoto, Y., Aizu-Yokota, E., and Kasahara, T. (1999) FAK Is the Upstream Signal Protein of the Phosphatidylinositol 3-Kinase-Akt Survival Pathway in Hydrogen Peroxide-Induced Apoptosis of a Human Glioblastoma Cell Line. *J. Biol. Chem. 274*, 10566–10570.
41. Wang, X., McCullough, K.D., Franke, T.F., and Holbrook, N.J. (2000) Epidermal Growth Factor Receptor-Dependent Akt Activation by Oxidative Stress Enhances Cell Survival. *J. Biol. Chem. 275*, 14624–14631.
42. Deora, A.A., Win, T., Vanhaesebroeck, B., and Lander, H.M. (1998) A Redox-Triggered ras-Effector Interaction. Recruitment of Phosphatidylinositol 3-Kinase to Ras by Redox Stress. *J. Biol. Chem. 273*, 29923–29928.
43. Klotz, L.O., Schieke, S.M., Sies, H., and Holbrook, N.J. (2000) Peroxynitrite Activates the Phosphoinositide 3-Kinase/Akt Pathway in Human Skin Primary Fibroblasts. *Biochem. J. 352*, 219–225.
44. Cohen, P. (1997) The Search for Physiological Substrates of MAP and SAP Kinases in Mammalian Cells. *Trends Cell Biol. 7*, 353–361.
45. Widmann, C., Gibson, S., Jarpe, M.B., and Johnson, G.L. (1999) Mitogen-Activated Protein Kinase: Conservation of a Three-Kinase Module from Yeast to Human. *Physiol Rev. 79*, 143–180.

Chapter 17

Regulation of the Degradation of Oxidized Proteins

Thomas Reinheckel[a] and Tilman Grune[b]

[a]Institute of Molecular Medicine and Cell Research, Albert-Ludwigs University Freiburg, D-79106 Freiburg, Germany

[b]Neuroscience Research Center, Medical Faculty (Charité), Humboldt University Berlin, D-10098 Berlin, Germany

Introduction

Molecular oxygen is an excellent acceptor of electrons and is therefore employed by nature for a wide variety of highly important biochemical reactions. The chemical reactivity of oxygen, however, also leads to the formation of reactive oxygen species (ROS) as by-products of oxygen metabolism. It was demonstrated in numerous studies that proteins are highly susceptible to ROS attack (1–3). The side chains of amino acids are the primary sites of free radical damage (4). However, oxidative stress represents a complex pattern of radical reactions affecting virtually all cellular constituents. In consequence, secondary protein modifications by glycoxidation or products of lipid peroxidation (e.g., by 4-hydroxynonenal) can occur *in vivo* (5,6). The protein alterations described above give rise to changes in higher-order protein structures. As a consequence, the protein unfolds, surface hydrophobicity increases, and eventually protein function will be impaired (7,8). The increase in surface hydrophobicity may also lead to noncovalent protein aggregation based on hydrophobic interactions. Additionally, covalent intra- or intermolecular protein cross-links as well as protein fragments are generated at high oxidant doses. The accumulation of oxidatively damaged proteins that lack enzymatic activity or other functional properties could lead to a pool of useless cellular debris. More serious complications, such as metabolic disturbances or immunologic problems, are possible. Thus, the removal of oxidized proteins or protein-fragments by proteases and the subsequent reuse of the amino acids produced for energy metabolism or protein synthesis are apparently important for the maintenance of cellular integrity (9).

During the last decade, the proteasomal system was proven to be a sophisticated, highly regulated proteolytic machinery present in the cytosol and nucleus of mammalian cells (10,11). The 700-kDa cylinder-shaped 20S-"core"-proteasome consists of 4 rings, with each ring containing 7 proteins. The outer rings contain 7 homologous α-type subunits, whereas the inner rings are composed of 7 β-type subunits that form the catalytic cavity of the protease. A large number of regulators of proteasomal activity have been described (Fig. 17.1). The association of the 20S-proteasome with the proteasome activator PA 700 is well characterized. This results in the formation of the ATP-stimulated and ubiquitin-dependent 26S-proteasome. Both forms

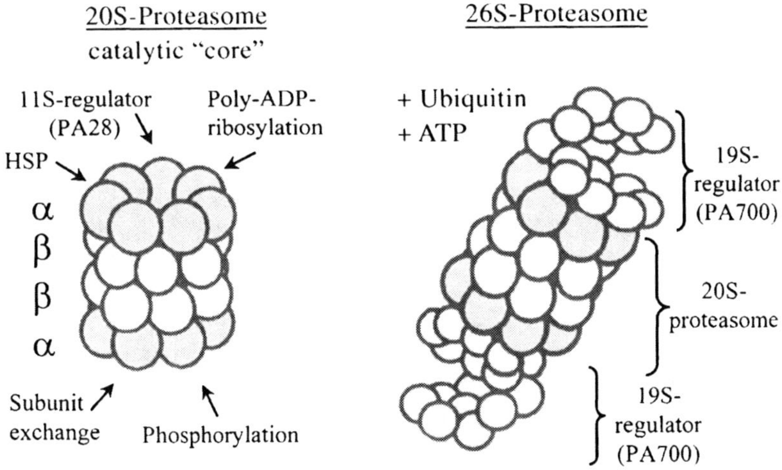

Fig. 17.1. Structure and regulators of the proteasome. The left panel of the figure demonstrates the structure of the 20S-proteasome and indicates the principally known mechanisms of regulation of this complex. In the case of binding of two of the well-known 19S-regulators, a new protease with ATP-stimulable and ubiquitin-recognizing features is formed, i.e., the 26S-proteasome (right panel).

of the proteasomal system, i.e. the 20S-proteasome and the 26S-proteasome, are apparently involved in the degradation of various abnormally folded proteins (11). This paper will discuss the concept of degradation of oxidatively modified proteins with special attention to the influence of oxidative stress toward the 20S- and 26S-components of the proteasomal system.

Discussion

Proteolytic Degradation of Oxidatively Modified Proteins

Over the past years, several investigators have shown that oxidized proteins are preferentially degraded compared with their nonoxidized forms by various proteases *in vitro* (12–16). The picture is, however, more complex. An increased proteolytic susceptibility of a protein requires an optimal ROS dose. Further exposure to oxidizing agents leads to decreased degradation (17–19). This is most likely due to the formation of protein aggregates that limit the access of proteases to their specific cleavage sites (20,21). These *in vitro* findings could be confirmed in viable and dividing cell cultures (18,19,22). Accordingly, increased intracellular proteolysis was found after exposing cell cultures to moderate oxidative stress, whereas an increase of the ROS dose led to diminished proteolysis. Using antisense oligonucleotide techniques and other specific inhibitors, the proteasome could be identified as the protease responsible for the breakdown of cytosolic and nuclear proteins after exposure of cells to ROS (18,19,22).

Activating Effects of Oxidative Stress towards Proteasomes

An explanation for increased intracellular proteolysis after mild oxidative stress could be the activation of proteolytic systems. Importantly, no up-regulation of the cytosolic proteolytic function of the proteasome was found in our work with cell cultures (18,19,23). Therefore, the oxidative stress–induced increase in cellular proteolysis appears to be largely a consequence of enhanced proteolytic susceptibility due to oxidative protein modification. However, mechanisms of 20S-proteasome activation exist under certain oxidative conditions. We have shown that nuclear 20S-proteasome can be transiently activated by poly-ADP ribose polymerase (PARP) during exposure of K562 cells to hydrogen peroxide (24). The activated protease increases the degradation of oxidatively damaged histones in the course of DNA and chromatin repair (25). Strack *et al.* (26) were able to demonstrate enhancement of proteasomal activities by treatment of proteasome preparations with $FeSO_4$-EDTA-ascorbate and hydrogen peroxide. However, there is no *in vivo* evidence to date for proteasome activation mediated by the direct interaction of oxidants with the proteasome molecule.

Comparative Resistance of 20S- and 26S-Proteasomes to Oxidants: In Vitro Studies

The involvement of the 20S-proteasome in the degradation of oxidatively modified proteins was suggested by several authors (9,27–29), but other groups favored a role for the ATP- and ubiquitin-dependent 26S-protease in the degradation of oxidized proteins (10,30–32). One fundamental requirement for the proteolytic removal of oxidized proteins during or after oxidative stress is that the protease involved must be active under these conditions. This raised the question whether the 20S- or the 26S-protease is more susceptible to oxidants *in vitro* and in cell culture. Thus, the effect of various oxidants (hydrogen peroxide, peroxynitrite, hypochlorite/hypochloric acid) toward a chymotrypsin-like peptidase activity (suc-LLVY-MCA) of isolated 20S- and 26S-proteasomes was examined (33,34). It could be demonstrated that the 26S-proteasome was from 4-fold (H_2O_2 and NaOCl) to 16-fold ($ONOO^-$) more susceptible to oxidant treatment than the 20S-protease. Additionally, the 50% inactivation of the 20S-protease was achieved at hydrogen peroxide concentrations of 40 μmol/mg protein which is much higher than the H_2O_2 concentration required for optimal enhanced proteolytic susceptibility of protein substrates after oxidation (i.e. 10 μmol H_2O_2/mg ferritin). The effect of hypochlorite and peroxynitrite on the proteinase activity of the 20S-protease was ~50- to 100-fold (at molar ratio) stronger than the effect of hydrogen peroxide. With the use of a combination of nondenaturing gel electrophoresis and SDS-PAGE, it could be shown that hypochlorite was able to fragment the polypeptide backbones of the proteasome subunits (34). In contrast, with hydrogen peroxide, no fragmentation of the polypeptides could be demonstrated in experiments using up to 40 mol H_2O_2/mg protein. Thus, an inhibition of proteolytic activity due to amino acid residue oxidation is highly likely.

Comparative Resistance of 20S- and 26S-Proteasomes to Oxidants: Findings in Cell Cultures

Because the human hematopoietic cell line K562 was earlier shown to increase its protein turnover after oxidant exposure and to degrade oxidized proteins selectively (19), K562 cells were chosen to evaluate the *in vitro* findings described above (35). Exposure of K562 cells to H_2O_2 concentrations of up to 5 mmol/L for 30 min did not affect the activity of the 20S-proteasome. In contrast, the ATP-stimulated activity of the 26S-proteasome was significantly reduced by 0.4 mmol/L H_2O_2. With as low a concentration as 1 mmol/L H_2O_2, the specific activity of the 26S-proteasome was completely abolished. To give further evidence for the higher oxidant susceptibility of the 26S-proteasome, a nondenaturing gel electrophoresis combined with a protease activity stain was employed. This technique allows the physical separation of the two proteasomal forms and is therefore more accurate in terms of differentiating between the activities of the two protease complexes. In agreement with the proteasome activity assays, a treatment of cells with 1 mmol/L H_2O_2 led to a complete loss of the 26S-proteasome activity in the nondenaturing gel electrophoresis. Western-blot analysis of proteins belonging to the 20S-"core" proteasome and the 19S regulator failed to reveal a decline in staining after treatment of cells with up to 5 mmol/L H_2O_2. Thus, the susceptibility of the 26S-proteasome toward ROS is likely due to the impairment of amino acids essential for the function of the proteasome activator PA 700 or to the binding between particles. On the other hand, heat shock protein 90 has been shown to protect the 20S-proteasome against oxidative inactivation (36,37). This could explain, at least in part, the comparatively high oxidant resistance of this protease during oxidative stress in K562 cells. Consistent with these findings, a differential susceptibility of 26S- and 20S-proteasomes was observed during exposure of vascular cells to oxidized low-density lipoproteins (38). In consideration of the important specific functions of the 26S-proteasome, the reconstitution of its activity after oxidative injury appears to be crucial. In our experiments, the ATP-stimulated 26S activity as well as the specific 26S-band on nondenaturing gels increased again during the 24 h after an incubation of K562 cells with 1 mmol/L H_2O_2. In contrast, treatment with 2 mmol/L H_2O_2 almost completely abolished 26S-proteasome activity for at least 24 h (35).

Summary

In conclusion the proteasomal system appears to play a central role in cellular response to oxidative stress (Fig. 17.2). The 20S-proteasome is able to remove oxidatively modified proteins and short peptides from cells even after a relatively high ROS dose. ROS-induced protein cross-linking with subsequent formation of protein aggregates can limit the accessibility of substrates to the proteasome, thus compromising the 20S-proteasome–mediated proteolysis. Compared with the 20S-protease, the 26S-proteasome is much more susceptible to ROS attack. This raises important questions

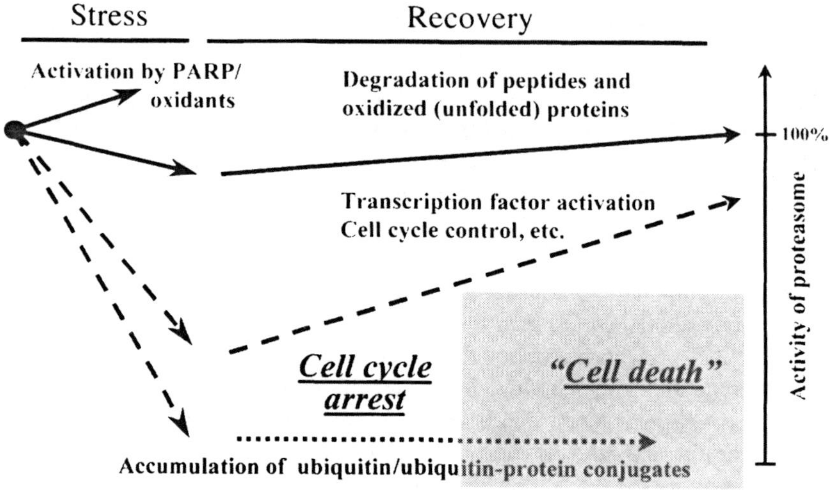

Fig. 17.2. Proteasome function during oxidative stress and recovery. The relationship between proteasome activity and cellular fate after oxidative stress is summarized in this figure. The activity of the 20S-proteasome (continuous line) is largely unimpaired or even increased during oxidative stress (PARP, poly-ADP ribose polymerase). The oxidative stress–related decline of the 26S-proteasome (dashed line) may be dramatic enough to cause a cell cycle arrest. A recovery of the 26S-proteasome activation restores the function of the proteasome in cell cycle control and transcription factor regulation. On the other hand, the failure to reactivate the 26S-proteasome function leads to the accumulation of ubiquitin-conjugates and perhaps to cell death.

concerning the consequences of oxidant-induced 26S-proteasome inactivation for intracellular protein turnover and cell function. For example, proteins that are determined to be degraded by the 26S-proteasome are marked by multiple ubiquitin polypeptides (11). Thus, inactivation of this protease could explain the observed accumulation of ubiquitin and ubiquitinated proteins in stressed and aged tissues (30,39,40). However, the design of the 26S-proteasome is thought to enable controlled proteolysis of specific proteins. In consideration of the involvement of the 26S-proteasome in cell cycle progression, the impairment of this protease could contribute to the transient growth arrest frequently observed in response to oxidative stress (41). Accordingly, the reformation of functional 26S-proteasomes after ROS-mediated inactivation seems to be crucial for the fate of the cell. The ability to reconstitute the 26S-protease complex appears to depend on the degree of oxidative stress (35). Failure to recover the ATP-stimulated and ubiquitin-dependent proteolysis of the 26S-proteasome might ultimately lead to permanent growth arrest or some form of cell death (38).

Acknowledgment

Tilman Grune was supported by DFG (GR1240/10-1 and SFB507/A7).

References

1. Davies, K.J. (1987) Protein Damage and Degradation by Oxygen Radicals. 1. General Aspects. *J. Biol. Chem. 262*, 9895–9901
2. Dean, R.T., Fu, S., Stocker, R., and Davies, M.J. (1997) Biochemistry and Pathology of Radical-Mediated Protein Oxidation. *Biochem. J. 324*, 1–18.
3. Stadtman, E.R. (1993) Oxidation of Free Amino Acids and Amino Acid Residues in Proteins by Radiolysis and by Metal-Catalyzed Reactions. *Annu. Rev. Biochem. 62*, 797–821.
4. Davies, K.J., Delsignore, M.E., and Lin, S. (1987) Protein Damage and Degradation by Oxygen Radicals. II. Modification of Amino Acids. *J. Biol. Chem. 262*, 9902–9907.
5. Uchida, K., and Stadtman, E.R. (1992) Modification of Histidine Residues in Proteins by Reaction with 4-Hydroxynonenal. *Proc. Natl. Acad. Sci. USA 89*, 4544–4548.
6. Lee, Y., and Shacter, E. (1995) Role of Carbohydrates in Oxidative Modification of Fibrinogen and Other Plasma Proteins. *Arch. Biochem. Biophys. 321*, 175–181.
7. Davies, K.J., and Delsignore, M.E. (1987) Protein Damage and Degradation by Oxygen Radicals. III. Modification of Secondary and Tertiary Structure. *J. Biol. Chem. 262*, 9908–9913.
8. Chao, C.C., Ma, Y.S., and Stadtman, E.R. (1997) Modification of Protein Surface Hydrophobicity and Methionine Oxidation by Oxidative Systems. *Proc. Natl. Acad. Sci. USA 94*, 2969–2974.
9. Grune, T., Reinheckel, T., and Davies, K.J. (1997) Degradation of Oxidized Proteins in Mammalian Cells. *FASEB J. 11*, 526–534.
10. Coux, O., Tanaka, K., and Goldberg, A.L. (1996) Structure and Functions of the 20S and 26S Proteasomes. *Annu. Rev. Biochem. 65*, 801–847.
11. Voges, D., Zwickl, P., and Baumeister, W. (1999) The 26S Proteasome: A Molecular Machine Designed for Controlled Proteolysis. *Annu. Rev. Biochem. 68*, 1015–1068.
12. Nakamura, K., and Stadtman, E.R. (1984) Oxidative Inactivation of Glutamine Synthetase Subunits. *Proc. Natl. Acad. Sci. USA 81*, 2011–2015.
13. Rivett, A.J. (1985) The Effect of Mixed-Function Oxidation of Enzymes on Their Susceptibility to Degradation by a Nonlysosomal Cysteine Proteinase. *Arch. Biochem. Biophys. 243*, 624–632.
14. Wolff, S.P., and Dean, R.T. (1986) Fragmentation of Proteins by Free Radicals and Its Effect on Their Susceptibility to Enzymic Hydrolysis. *Biochem. J. 234*, 399–403.
15. Davies, K.J., Lin, S.W., and Pacifici, R.E. (1987) Protein Damage and Degradation by Oxygen Radicals. IV. Degradation of Denatured Protein. *J. Biol. Chem. 262*, 9914–9920.
16. Levine, R.L., Mosoni, L., Berlett, B.S., and Stadtman, E. R. (1996) Methionine Residues as Endogenous Antioxidants in Proteins. *Proc. Natl. Acad. Sci. USA 93*, 15036–15040.
17. Pacifici, R. E., Kono, Y., and Davies, K.J. (1993) Hydrophobicity as the Signal for Selective Degradation of Hydroxyl Radical-Modified Hemoglobin by the Multicatalytic Proteinase Complex, Proteasome. *J. Biol. Chem. 268*, 15405–15411.
18. Grune, T., Reinheckel, T., Joshi, M., and Davies, K.J. (1995) Proteolysis in Cultured Liver Epithelial Cells During Oxidative Stress. Role of the Multicatalytic Proteinase Complex, Proteasome. *J. Biol. Chem. 270*, 2344–2351

19. Grune, T., Reinheckel, T., and Davies, K.J.A. (1996) Degradation of Oxidized Proteins in K562 Human Hematopoietic Cells by Proteasome. *J. Biol. Chem. 271*, 15504–15509.
20. Friguet, B., Stadtman, E.R., and Szweda, L.I. (1994) Modification of Glucose-6- phosphate Dehydrogenase by 4-Hydroxy-2-nonenal. Formation of Cross-Linked Protein That Inhibits the Multicatalytic Protease. *J. Biol. Chem. 269*, 21639–21643.
21. Friguet, B., and Szweda, L.I. (1997) Inhibition of the Multicatalytic Proteinase (Proteasome) by 4-Hydroxy-2-nonenal Cross-Linked Protein. *FEBS Lett. 405*, 21–25.
22. Grune, T., Blasig, I.E., Sitte, N., Roloff, B., Haseloff, R., and Davies, K.J. (1998) Peroxynitrite Increases the Degradation of Aconitase and Other Cellular Proteins by Proteasome. *J. Biol. Chem. 273*, 10857–10862.
23. Grune, T., and Davies, K.J. (1997) Breakdown of Oxidized Proteins as a Part of Secondary Antioxidant Defenses in Mammalian Cells. *Biofactors 6*, 165–172.
24. Ullrich, O., Reinheckel, T., Sitte, N., Haass, R., Grune, T., and Davies, K.J.A. (1999) Poly-ADP Ribose Polymerase Activates Nuclear Proteasome to Degrade Oxidatively Damaged Histones. *Proc. Natl. Acad Sci. USA 96*, 6223–6228.
25. Ullrich, O., Sitte, N., Sommerburg, O., Sandig, V., Davies, K.J., and Grune, T. (1999) Influence of DNA Binding on the Degradation of Oxidized Histones by the 20S Proteasome. *Arch. Biochem. Biophys. 362*, 211–216.
26. Strack, P.R., Waxman, L., and Fagan, J.M. (1996) Activation of the Multicatalytic Endopeptidase by Oxidants. Effects on Enzyme Structure. *Biochemistry 35*, 7142–7149.
27. Rivett, A.J. (1985) Purification of a Liver Alkaline Protease Which Degrades Oxidatively Modified Glutamine Synthetase. Characterization as a High Molecular Weight Cysteine Proteinase. *J. Biol. Chem. 260*, 12600–12606.
28. Stadtman, E.R. (1990) Metal Ion-Catalyzed Oxidation of Proteins: Biochemical Mechanism and Biological Consequences. *Free Radic. Biol. Med. 9*, 315–325.
29. Friguet, B., Bulteau, A.L., Chondrogianni, N., Conconi, M., and Petropoulos, I. (2000) Protein Degradation by the Proteasome and its Implications in Aging. *Ann. N.Y. Acad. Sci. 908*, 143–154.
30. Shang, F., Gong, X., and Taylor, A. (1997) Activity of Ubiquitin Dependent Pathway in Response to Oxidative Stress. *J. Biol. Chem. 272*, 23086–23093.
31. Matthews, W., Driscoll, J., Tanaka, K., Ichihara, A., and Goldberg, A.L. (1989) Involvement of the Proteasome in Various Degradative Processes in Mammalian Cells [published erratum appears in *Proc. Natl. Acad. Sci. USA 86*, 5350]. *Proc. Natl. Acad. Sci. USA 86*, 2597–2601.
32. Iwai, K., Drake, S.K., Wehr, N.B., Weissman, A.M., LaVaute, T., Minato, N., Klausner, R.D., Levine, R.L., and Rouault, T.A. (1998) Iron-Dependent Oxidation, Ubiquitination, and Degradation of Iron Regulatory Protein 2: Implications for Degradation of Oxidized Proteins. *Proc. Natl. Acad. Sci. USA 95*, 4924–4928.
33. Reinheckel, T., Sitte, N., Ullrich, O., Kuckelkorn, U., Davies, K.J., and Grune, T. (1998) Comparative Resistance of the 20S and 26S Proteasome to Oxidative Stress. *Biochem. J. 335*, 637–642.
34. Ullrich, O., Reinheckel, T., Sitte, N., and Grune, T. (1999) Degradation of Hypochlorite- Damaged Glucose-6-phosphate Dehydrogenase by the 20S Proteasome. *Free Radic. Biol. Med. 27*, 487–492.
35. Reinheckel, T., Ullrich, O., Sitte, N., and Grune, T. (2000) Differential Impairment of 20S and 26S Proteasome Activities in Human Hematopoietic K562 Cells During Oxidative Stress. *Arch. Biochem. Biophys. 377*, 65–68.

36. Conconi, M., Szweda, L.I., Levine, R.L., Stadtman, E.R., and Friguet, B. (1996) Age-Related Decline of Rat Liver Multicatalytic Proteinase Activity and Protection from Oxidative Inactivation by Heat-Shock Protein 90. *Arch. Biochem. Biophys. 331*, 232–240.
37. Conconi, M., and Friguet, B. (1997) Proteasome Inactivation upon Aging and on Oxidation-Effect of HSP 90. *Mol. Biol. Rep. 24*, 45–50.
38. Vieira, O., Escargueil-Blanc, I., Jurgens, G., Borner, C., Almeida, L., Salvayre, R., and Negre-Salvayre, A. (2000) Oxidized LDLs Alter the Activity of the Ubiquitin Proteasome Pathway: Potential Role in Oxidized LDL-Induced Apoptosis. *FASEB J. 14*, 532–542.
39. Shang, F., and Taylor, A. (1995) Oxidative Stress and Recovery from Oxidative Stress Are Associated with Altered Ubiquitin Conjugating and Proteolytic Activities in Bovine Lens Epithelial Cells. *Biochem. J. 307*, 297–303.
40. Lowe, J., Blanchard, A., Morrell, K., Lennox, G., Reynolds, L. Billett, M., Landon, M., and Mayer, R.J. (1988) Ubiquitin Is a Common Factor in Intermediate Filament Inclusion Bodies of Diverse Type in Man, Including Those of Parkinson's Disease, Pick's Disease, and Alzheimer's Disease, as Well as Rosenthal Fibres in Cerebellar Astrocytomas, Cytoplasmic Bodies in Muscle, and Mallory Bodies in Alcoholic Liver Disease. *J. Pathol. 155*, 9–15.
41. Janssen, Y.M., Van Houten, B., Bonn, P.J., and Mossman, B.T. (1993) Cell and Tissue Responses to Oxidative Damage. *Lab. Investig. 69*, 261–274.

Chapter 18

Glutathione Depletion Induces Giant DNA Fragmentation Associated with Apoptosis or Necrosis

Yoshihiro Higuchi

Department of Pharmacology, Kanazawa University School of Medicine, Kanazawa 920-8640, Japan

Introduction

The glutathione (GSH) and GSH peroxidase systems play major roles in controlling cellular redox states and in the primary defense against the effects of reactive oxygen species (ROS) damage that may be involved in some neuropathologic disorders (1). Although ROS can activate chemically induced cell death, it is not clear whether ROS are a part of the signal transduction cascade triggered by various inducers for apoptosis or whether they are generated in a parallel pathway that can trigger apoptosis independently. Therefore, it is important to distinguish between ROS molecules involved in such signaling pathways and those that mediate general cellular damage, including giant DNA and high-molecular-weight DNA fragmentation. These DNA fragmentations in chromatin, estimated by the size and the emerging time of fragments, might reveal either apoptosis or necrosis.

Apoptosis and necrosis are two distinct forms of cell death that have profoundly different implications for the surrounding tissues. Apoptosis is characterized by cell shrinkage, chromatin condensation, activation of some caspases, and fragmentation of DNA at internucleosomal linker sites, giving rise to discrete bands of multiples of 180–200 bp (2). In contrast, necrosis is a passive process, typified by cell and organelle swelling, with spillage of the intracellular contents into the extracellular milieu. Necrosis is an uncontrolled event resulting from loss of homeostasis; cell contents are dispersed, which may then have adverse effects on neighboring tissue (3). Excitotoxic and apoptotic cell death of cultured cerebellar granule neurons by glutamate required caspase-3–related cysteine protease activation (4). It has been reported that internucleosomal DNA fragmentation depends on intracellular ATP levels or ATP synthesis (5–7). Furthermore, intracellular ATP level could convert necrosis to apoptosis in oxidant-induced endothelial cell death (8). A decrease in mitochondrial membrane potential in the absence of a functional electron transport system results mainly from the leakage of protons through the membrane and precedes a cell death (9).

We used C6 rat glioma cells as a model of astrocyte glial cells for neuronal cell death (10,11). In this study, we examined 1- to 2-Mbp giant DNA fragmentation during cell death caused by buthionine sulfoximine (BSO) in C6 rat glioma cells. Furthermore, we determined whether BSO-induced cell death is by apoptosis or by necrosis by investigating the effects of polyunsaturated fatty acids (PUFA) on apoptotic or necrotic events such as internucleosomal DNA fragmentation, caspase-3 activity, and change in both ATP levels and mitochondrial membrane potential.

Materials and Methods

Cell Culture. C6 rat glioma cells were grown in Dulbecco's modified Eagle's medium supplemented with 5% fetal calf serum (medium DF-5) containing 25 mmol/L sodium bicarbonate, 100 U/mL penicillin G, and 60 μg/mL kanamycin. C6 cells were generally seeded into 60-mm plastic culture dishes and grown in 5 mL of DF-5 at 37°C in a humidified atmosphere containing 5% CO_2.

Cytotoxic Assay. The ^{51}Cr release assay was carried out according to the method described previously (12). Briefly, C6 cells were labeled with $Na_2{}^{51}CrO_4$ at a final concentration of 370 KBq cells in 500 μL DF-5 for 60 min at 37°C. After being washed several times with chilled Hank's balanced salt solution (pH 7.2), the ^{51}Cr-labeled cells were treated with BSO under various conditions at 37°C in humidified air containing 5% CO_2. Specific ^{51}Cr release, which indicates cytolysis, was calculated by the formula described previously (13).

Determination of Intracellular GSH. Cellular GSH was analyzed by the method described previously, using a high-performance liquid chromatography (HPLC) separating system (10). Briefly, the cell (2×10^6 cells) pellet prepared after the earlier experiments was suspended in 50 μL of 5% trichloroacetic acid (TCA) solution containing 5 mmol/L EDTA and vortexed for 5 min. The suspension was centrifuged at $12{,}000 \times g$ for 10 min; 25 μL of the supernatant was mixed with 100 μL of the solution consisting of 3.5 mmol/L 4-sulfamoyl-7-fluoro-2,1,3-benzoxadiazole, 325 mmol/L sodium borate, pH 9.3, 1 mmol/L EDTA and incubated at 60°C for 5 min. After the mixture was chilled with ice water, the GSH content was determined by HPLC.

Determination of Lipid Peroxides. 2-Thiobarbituric acid reactive substances (TBARS) in cells produced by lipid peroxidation of cell components were measured at 535 nm as malondialdehyde (MDA) formation according to the method described by Buege and Aust (14). Harvested C6 cells (5×10^6 cells) were suspended in 500 μL phosphate-buffered saline (PBS); 1 mL of 2-thiobarbituric acid (TBA) reagent consisting of 0.375% TBA, 15% TCA and 0.25 mol/L HCl was added to the cell suspension. The mixture of cell suspension and TBA reagent was heated in boiling water for 20 min, chilled quickly with ice water to room temperature and centrifuged at $1500 \times g$ for 10 min. The supernatant was measured at 535 nm. The amount of TBARS was calculated according to the molar absorption coefficient of MDA, $\epsilon = 1.56 \times 10^5$ $(mol/L)^{-1} \cdot (cm)^{-1}$ at 535 nm.

Gel Electrophoresis. Pulsed-field gel electrophoresis (PFGE) and agarose gel electrophoresis (AGE) analyses were carried out according to the method described previously (15). Briefly, harvested C6 cells (2×10^6) were suspended in 50 μL PBS and mixed with 50 μL PBS containing 1% low-melting-point agarose. The cell suspension was poured into a template, plugged, and cooled on ice. The hardened agarose gel blocks were incubated with 250 μL of a mixture of proteinase K (1 g/L), *N*-lauroyl sarcosine sodium (1%, wt/vol) and 0.5 mol/L EDTA (pH 9.2) for 48 h at 50°C. After incubation, half of the agarose gel block was loaded into a sample well in a 1% (wt/vol) separating agarose (Sigma type II, St. Louis, MO, USA) gel ($150 \times 150 \times 4.4$ mm) in TBE (89 mmol/L Tris-boric acid, 2 mmol/L EDTA, pH 8.0) for PFGE. PFGE was performed with the Pulsaphor system from LKB and carried out in 0.5X TBE at 14°C for 28 h (constant 150 V, pulse time 90 s for 20 h and 120 s for the next 8 h). The gel was stained with ethidium bromide and photographed under ultraviolet (UV) light. The amount of DNA on the gel was measured densitometrically using the analytical software of the gel documentation system of Epi-Light UV FA1100 from Aishin Cosumosu, Japan.

For AGE, the prepared digest (250 μL) for PFGE was diluted to 500 μL with distilled water and extracted twice with 500 μL of phenol/chloroform (1:1). The DNA in the aqueous phase was precipitated with 70% ethanol, dissolved in 10 μL of TE buffer (10 mmol/L Tris-HCl, 1 mmol/L EDTA, pH 7.4), and treated with 1.6 μg of RNase A for 60 min at 37°C. The sample (5 μL) was electrophoresed on a 1.5% (wt/vol) agarose gel in 0.5X TBE for 90 min at 15 V/cm for AGE. The gel was stained with ethidium bromide.

Caspase-3 Protease Assay. The cell pellet (3×10^6 cells) was treated with 50 μL of the cell lysis buffer, consisting of 10 mmol/L Hepes-KOH, pH 7.4, 2 mmol/L EDTA, 1% Nonident P-40 and 1 mmol/L phenylmethylsulfonyl fluoride (MBL, Japan) for 10 min on ice. The cell suspension was centrifuged at $12{,}000 \times g$ for 2 min. The supernatant was mixed with 50 μL of 2X the reaction buffer consisting of 10 mmol/L dithiothreitol, 20% glycerol, and 50 mmol/L Hepes-KOH, pH 7.4, and then divided into two aliquots. Each aliquot was mixed with (for the sample) or without (for the control) DEVD-pNA (Asp-Glu-Val-Asp-*p*-nitroanilide) substrate. Proteolytic reaction was carried out by mixing the cytosolic extraction with 50 μL of 2X the reaction buffer. The reaction mixture was incubated at 37°C for 2 h, and the formation of *p*-nitroanilide was measured at 405 nm using a spectrometer.

Determination of Intracellular ATP. The harvested cell pellet (2×10^6 cells) was suspended in 25 μL of 0.5 mol/L $HClO_4$ and vortexed vigorously for 5 min. The suspension was centrifuged at $12{,}000 \times g$ for 10 min, and the supernatant was neutralized with 5 μL of 2 mol/L KOH in 0.66 mol/L potassium phosphate buffer, pH 7.5. After precipitates were removed by centrifuging at $12{,}000 \times g$ for 5 min, the supernatant was applied to a HPLC separating system consisting of a TSK-GEL ODS-80T column (4.6×250 mm; Tosoh, Tokyo, Japan) and a UV detector. The gradient protocol for separation of ATP was performed as follows: Eluent A consisting of 0.1 mol/L KH_2PO_4 (pH 5.95) and eluent B consisting of 60% eluent A and 40% methanol. UV absorbance was monitored at 260 nm.

Determination of Mitochondrial Membrane Potentials. Mitochondrial membrane potential was assessed by the retention of [^{3}H]-tetraphenylphosphonium bromide (TPP^+) (16). Briefly, C6 cells were loaded with [^{3}H]-TPP^+ (0.925KBq/mL, Amersham, Tokyo, Japan) for 60 min. After being washed twice with medium, the labeled cells were treated with various drugs for the indicated time. After several washings with PBS, the cells were trapped on a Millipore (Bedford, MA, USA) cellulose membrane (HA). ^{3}H-activity on the membrane was measured. To correct for the nonspecific binding of [^{3}H]-TPP^+, the value from cells treated for 5 min with 0.1% Triton-X100 was subtracted from each value.

Statistical Analysis. Results from experiments were analyzed using Student's *t* test.

Results

PUFA Promoted Cell Death by Enhancing Lipid Peroxidation Without Affecting Intracellular GSH Depletion Induced by BSO in C6 Cells

The intracellular GSH content in C6 cells treated with 10 mmol/L BSO for 18 h was ~0.5 nmol/mg protein and 3% of the control (Fig. 18.1A). The amount of TBARS in the C6 cells treated with BSO increased and was ~0.8 nmol/mg protein after 18 h of incubation. The cytolytic effect of BSO on C6 cells was examined by a ^{51}Cr release assay (Fig. 18.1A). ^{51}Cr release from C6 cells treated with BSO was ~62% at 24 h. α-Tocopherol (α-Toc) strongly inhibited the effect of BSO on TBARS formation and ^{51}Cr release without affecting GSH depletion (Fig. 18.1). The effects of PUFA such as arachidonic acid (Ar.A; $C_{20:4}$), γ-linolenic acid ($C_{18:3}$), linoleic acid ($C_{18:2}$), and oleic acid ($C_{18:1}$) on GSH depletion, lipid peroxidation, and cytolysis induced by BSO were also examined. Ar.A, γ-linolenic acid, and linoleic acid markedly enhanced TBARS formation in C6 cells treated with BSO for 18 h, representing 4.0, 3.5 and 1.7 nmol/mg protein, respectively (Fig. 18.1B), but did not affect the BSO-induced GSH depletion (Fig. 18.1A). Ar.A enhanced ^{51}Cr release from C6 cells treated with BSO, leading to ~98 % ^{51}Cr release, which corresponded to a 1.6-fold increase compared with that by BSO alone at 24 h. Both γ-linolenic acid and linoleic acid also enhanced ^{51}Cr release. The effect of these PUFA on ^{51}Cr release was dose dependent (data not shown). In contrast, oleic acid did not affect GSH depletion; conversely, it suppressed both ^{51}Cr release and TBARS formation induced by BSO. Oleic acid might act as an antioxidant in BSO-caused cell death.

Antioxidants and Iron/Copper Chelators Inhibited Cell Death by Suppressing Lipid Peroxidation Induced by BSO

To evaluate the involvement of ROS in C6 cell death caused by BSO, the effects of antioxidants such as *N*-acetylcysteine (NAC), 5-5′-dimethyl-1-1-pyyroline-*N*-oxide (DMPO), α-Toc, butylated hydroxytoluene (BHT), and *N*-*N*′-diphenyl-1,4-phenylene (DPPD), as well as those of iron/copper chelators such as deferoxamine and

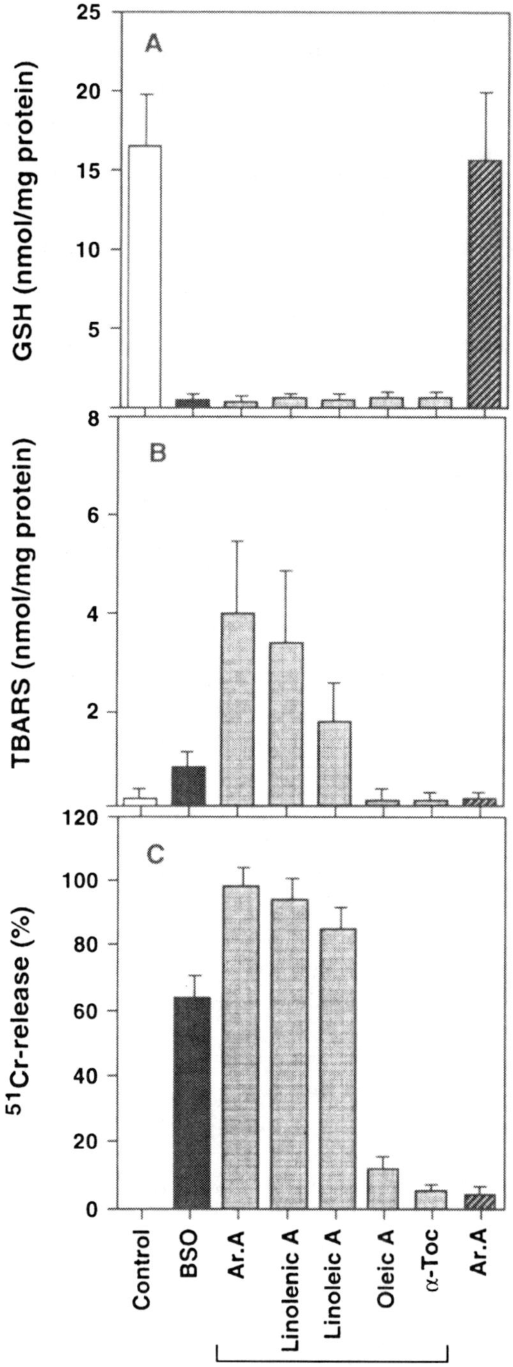

Fig. 18.1. Effect of polyunsaturated fatty acids (PUFA) on depletion of intracellular glutathione (GSH), lipid peroxidation, and cytolysis induced by buthionine sulfoximine (BSO). (A) C6 cells (2×10^6) were treated with 10 mmol/L BSO, with 10 mmol/L BSO plus 100 μmol/L PUFA or 100 μmol/L α-tocopherol (α-Toc), or with 100 μmol/L arachidonic acid (Ar.A). After incubation for (A) 18 h, (B) 18 h, or (C) 24 h, GSH levels in the cells (A), the amount of thiobarbituric acid reactive substances (TBARS) (B), and ^{51}Cr activity released into the medium (C) were determined. Values are the mean ± SD of the three independent experiments.

sodium *N-N*-diethyldithio-carbamate (DDC) on cytotoxicity, GSH depletion, and lipid peroxidation were examined. NAC is deacetylated to cysteine which is a precursor of GSH (17). DMPO can scavenge not only •OH but also $O_2^{\bullet-}$, the lipid radical (L•), and the lipid alkoxyl radical (LO•) (18,19). α-Toc can scavenge L•, LO• and the lipid peroxyl radical (LOO•) and has a chain-breaking antioxidant action within the membrane. DPPD and BHT can scavenge L• and LOO•, respectively (20,21). Deferoxamine can chelate Fe^{3+}/Fe^{2+}. DDC chelates Cu^{+} and has been shown to inhibit Cu/Zn-superoxide dismutase (SOD) activity and other copper proteins (22). NAC, DMPO, α-Toc, BHT, and DPPD did not affect GSH depletion (data not shown), but all inhibited both ^{51}Cr release from C6 cells and TBARS formation. Deferoxamine and DDC also suppressed TBARS formation (Fig. 18.2A), leading to an inhibition of ^{51}Cr release without affecting GSH depletion (Fig. 18.2B) induced by BSO. These iron/copper chelators and antioxidants also inhibited both ^{51}Cr release and TBARS formation, even if Ar.A was present (Fig. 18.2).

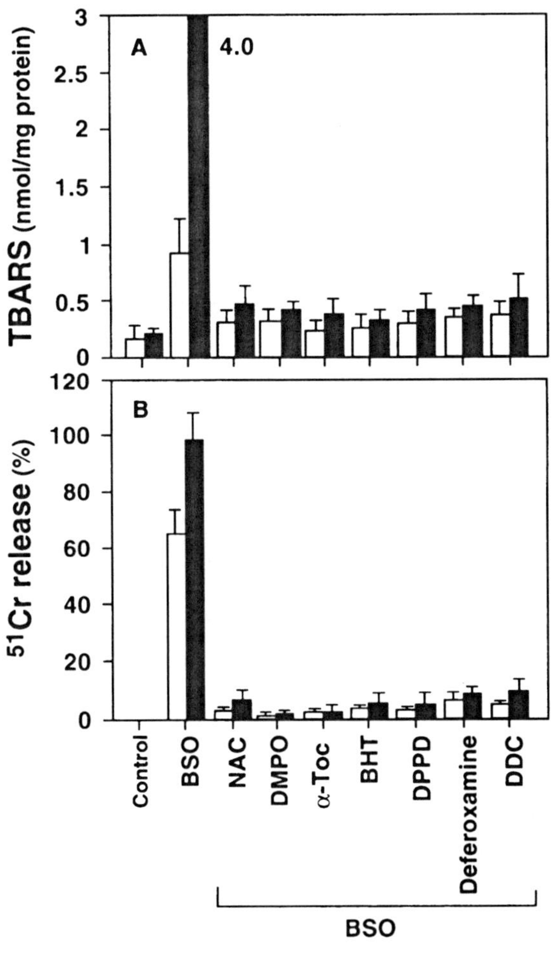

Fig. 18.2. Effect of antioxidants and metal chelators on lipid peroxidation and cytolysis induced by buthionine sulfoximine (BSO) in C6 cells. C6 cells were treated with 10 mmol/L BSO with or without 1 mmol/L *N*-acetylcysteine (NAC), 10 μmol/L sodium *N-N*-diethyldithio-carbamate (DDC), 10 μmol/L deferoxamine, 10 mmol/L 5-5′-dimethyl-1-1-pyyroline-*N*-oxide (DMPO), 100 μmol/L α-tocopherol (α-Toc), 100 μmol/L butylated hydroxytoluene (BHT), or 10 μmol/L *N-N′*-diphenyl-1,4-phenylene (DPPD) in the presence (closed bar) or absence (open bar) of 50 μmol/L Ar.A for (A) 18 h or (B) 24 h. After treatment, (A) thiobarbituric acid reactive substances (TBARS) amounts in the cells and (B) specific ^{51}Cr activity released into medium were determined. Values are the means ± SD of three independent experiments.

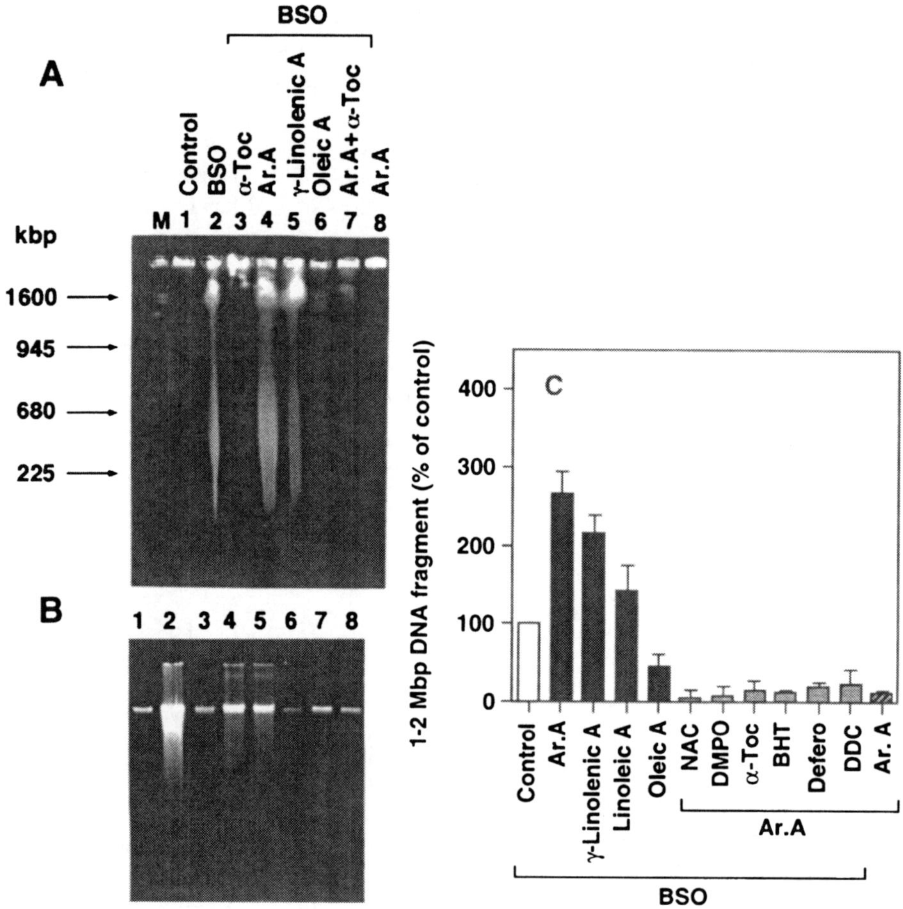

Fig. 18.3. Pulsed-field gel electrophoresis (PFGE) and aragose gel electrophoresis (AGE) analysis of the DNA fragmentation of C6 cells treated with buthionine sulfoximine (BSO). In panel A, each lane indicates the control (lane 1), samples from the cells treated with 10 mmol/L BSO (lane 2) or 50 μmol/L arachidonic acid (Ar.A) alone (lane 8) for 24 h and with 10 mmol/L BSO for 18 h in the presence of 100 mmol/L α-tocopherol (α-Toc) (lane 3), 50 μmol/L Ar.A (lane 4), 50 μmol/L γ-linolenic acid (lane 5), 50 μmol/L oleic acid (lane 6), or 50 μmol/L Ar.A plus 100 μmol/L α-Toc (lane 7). *Saccharomyces cerevisiae* chromosomal DNA (from Bio-Rad, lane M) were used as giant-sized DNA markers. Panel B shows AGE analysis of C6 cells treated with 10 mmol/L BSO. The lane number corresponds to the lane number in panel A. In panel C, the amount of 1- to 2-Mbp giant DNA fragments obtained according to the PFGE analysis as shown in panel A was determined and expressed as a percentage of the control; this indicates the DNA amount in the BSO sample treated for 18 h. The values are the mean ± SD of three independent experiments.

PUFA Promoted Giant DNA Fragmentation but Suppressed Internucleosomal DNA Fragmentation Induced by BSO

The effect of antioxidants and iron/copper chelators on the chromosomal DNA fragmentation during cell death caused by BSO in C6 cells was examined (Fig. 18.3A). DNA fragments 1–2 Mbp in size were observed in C6 cells treated with BSO for 18 h. The giant DNA fragmentation was enhanced by exogenous addition of Ar.A, γ-linolenic acid, or linoleic acid and was dependent on the species of PUFA (Fig. 18.3A). The number of fragments was increased ~2.7-fold by Ar.A, 2.2-fold by γ-linolenic acid, and 1.5-fold by linoleic acid (Fig. 18.3C). In contrast, oleic acid suppressed the giant DNA fragmentation induced by BSO. The giant DNA fragments induced by BSO in the presence of Ar.A were strongly inhibited by NAC, DMPO, α-Toc, BHT, deferoxamine, and DDC (Fig. 18.3C).

The ladder-forming DNA fragments were observed in C6 cells treated with BSO (Fig. 18.3B). Ar.A suppressed the ladder-formed DNA fragmentation in C6 cells induced by BSO in a dose-responsive manner (Fig. 18.3B).

PUFA Inhibited Activation of Caspase-3 Induced by BSO

To determine whether the cell death induced by BSO is based on apoptosis, caspase-3 activity in the cell lysate of C6 cells was first examined. Caspase-3 activity in C6 cells

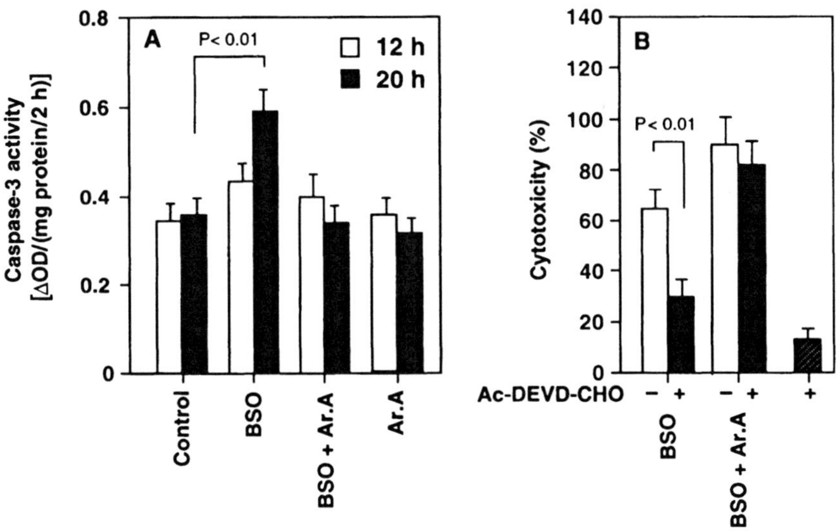

Fig. 18.4. Effect of polyunsaturated fatty acids (PUFA) on caspase-3 activation and the effect of caspase-3 specific inhibitors on the cell death caused by buthionine sulfoximine (BSO). C6 cells were treated with 10 mmol/L BSO with or without 50 µmol/L arachidonic acid (Ar.A) for 12 h (A), 20 h (A), and 24 h (B) in the absence (–) or presence (+) of 20 µmol/L Ac-DEVD- CHO (B). After treatment, caspase 3 activity (A) and ^{51}Cr-release in the cells (B) were determined. Values are the mean ± SD of the four independent experiments.

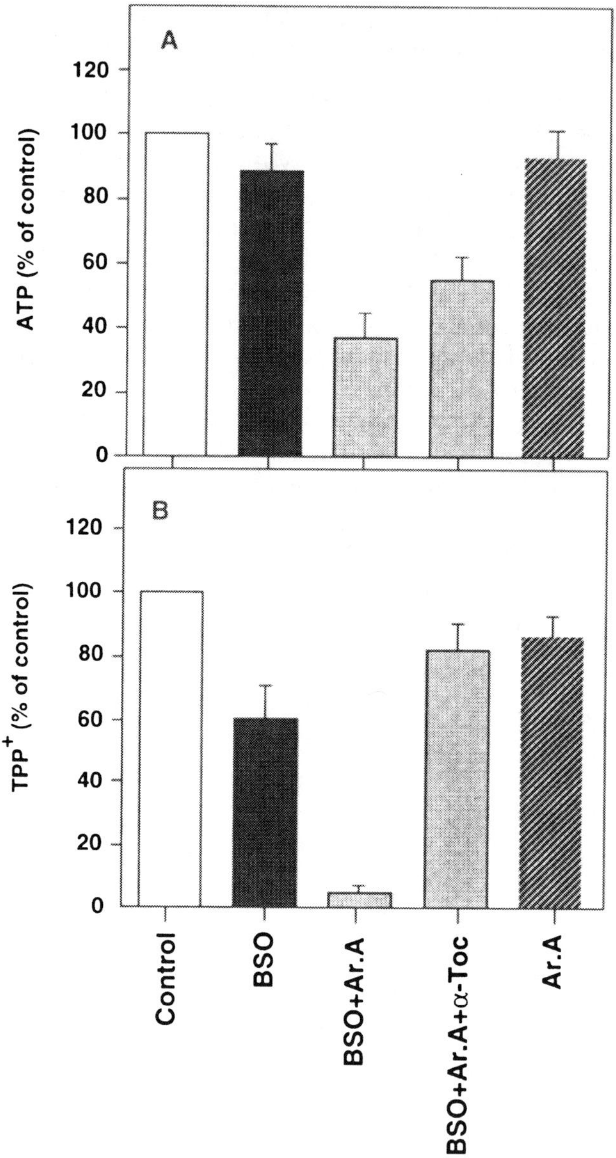

Fig. 18.5. Effect of polyunsaturated fatty acids (PUFA) on reduction of ATP levels and in mitochondrial membrane potential of cells treated with buthionine sulfoximine (BSO). C6 cells were treated with 10 mmol/L BSO, 10 mmol/L BSO plus 50 μmol/L arachidonic acid (Ar.A), 10 mmol/L BSO plus 50 μmol/L Ar.A together with 100 μmol/L α-tocopherol (α-Toc), or 50 μmol/L Ar.A alone. After treatment for 24 h, cellular ATP levels (A) and tetraphenylphosphonium bromide (TPP^+) amount (B) in the C6 cells were determined as described in Materials and Methods. Values are the mean ± SD of the four independent experiments.

treated with BSO for 20 h increased~1.5 fold compared with the control (Fig. 18.4). Caspase-3 activation was suppressed by the addition of not only Ar.A but also α-Toc. Exogenous addition of Ac-DEVD-CHO, a specific inhibitor for caspase-3 significantly suppressed cytolysis of C6 cells caused by BSO for 24 h but did not suppress cytolysis in the presence of Ar.A.

PUFA Reduced Intracellular ATP and TPP^+ Levels During Cell Death Caused by BSO

Intracellular ATP levels and mitochondrial membrane potentials were examined. ATP levels in C6 cells treated with BSO were not significantly reduced. In contrast, Ar.A significantly reduced the ATP level to 38% of the control for 12 h (Fig. 18.5A). The assay using lipophilic TPP^+ indicates membrane potential of permeability as mitochondria damage. Ar.A caused a marked release of TPP^+ in the C6 cells treated with BSO (Fig. 18.5).

Discussion

PUFA such as Ar.A, linolenic acid, and linoleic acid enhanced lipid peroxidation under BSO-induced GSH depletion, leading to C6 cell death without affecting the GSH depletion. Antioxidants and iron or copper chelators inhibited both lipid peroxidation and cell death in C6 cells without affecting GSH depletion, suggesting that not only ROS but also iron and/or copper ions might be involved in lipid peroxidation during cell death caused by BSO in C6 cells. These results support a possible mechanism for lipid peroxidation with a chain reaction initiated by oxygen radicals or by enzyme reaction under GSH depletion as shown in Fig. 18.6A. PUFA are particularly vulnerable to free radical attack because the carbon double bond within PUFA membranes allows easy removal of hydrogen atoms by ROS such as the •OH radical (23). Under aerobic conditions, lipid peroxidation continues because carbon double bonds with doubly allylic hydrogen combine with O_2 to form additional organic LOO•. Auto-oxidizability of PUFA was linearly dependent on the number of doubly allylic positions at 37°C (24,25). LOO• can combine with an abstracted hydrogen atom from adjacent fatty acid acyl chains to form lipid hydroperoxides (LOOH), which are decomposed to LO• by the Fenton reaction in the presence of Fe^{2+} or Cu^+ under the GSH-depleted condition. LOOH produced in this way is ordinarily decayed to lipid hydroxides (LOH) and H_2O by GSH peroxidase using endogenous GSH as a substrate. LOO• can be converted to cycloperoxide hydrolyzing to lipid aldehydes (LCHO), which are detectable as MDA or TBARS by the TBA assay (14). Thus, the action of the •OH molecule initiates a chain reaction that generates numerous toxic reactants, which disrupt membrane integrity, damage membrane proteins, and lead to cell death (26).

In this study, the amount of 1- to 2-Mbp giant DNA fragments in BSO-treated C6 cells was increased by the addition of PUFA. Not only these giant DNA but also 100- to 800-kbp high-molecular-weight DNA fragmentations were suppressed by antioxidants and metal chelators through preventing lipid peroxidation induced by

BSO, even in the presence of Ar.A. It is unclear whether free radicals such as L•, LO•, or LOO• produced during lipid peroxidation directly attack chromosomal DNA or provide certain circumstances favorable for such giant DNA fragmentation by unknown mechanisms. A possible mechanism of giant DNA fragmentation is that lipid peroxidation might proceed not only in the plasma membrane but also in the nuclear membrane close to chromosomes, and lipid radicals might thereafter allow ROS to attack DNA at preferential cleavage sites in the hinge domain of chromatin.

BSO can reduce the GSH level but not the cysteine level. In some types of cells, caspase-3 activation is an early biochemical marker of apoptosis induced by various triggers (27). BSO-induced C6 cell death was associated with caspase-3 activation (Fig. 18.4) (11). Ac-DEVD-CHO inhibited BSO-induced apoptosis but not in the presence of PUFA. Moreover, caspase-3 activity in BSO-treated C6 cells was decreased by the addition of PUFA. Armstrong *et al.* (28) reported activation of caspase-3 in cerebellar granule cells undergoing apoptosis but not necrosis. These findings suggest that caspase-3 activation is involved in the mild cell death induced by BSO but not in the intense cell death in the presence of PUFA under GSH depletion. PUFA might cause necrosis at high concentrations during GSH depletion, promoting 1- to 2-Mbp giant DNA fragmentation of chromatin and suppressing internucleosomal DNA fragmentation (Fig. 18.3). It is likely, therefore, that BSO initiates apoptosis through a caspase activation signaling system in C6 cells, and high concentrations of PUFA turn the

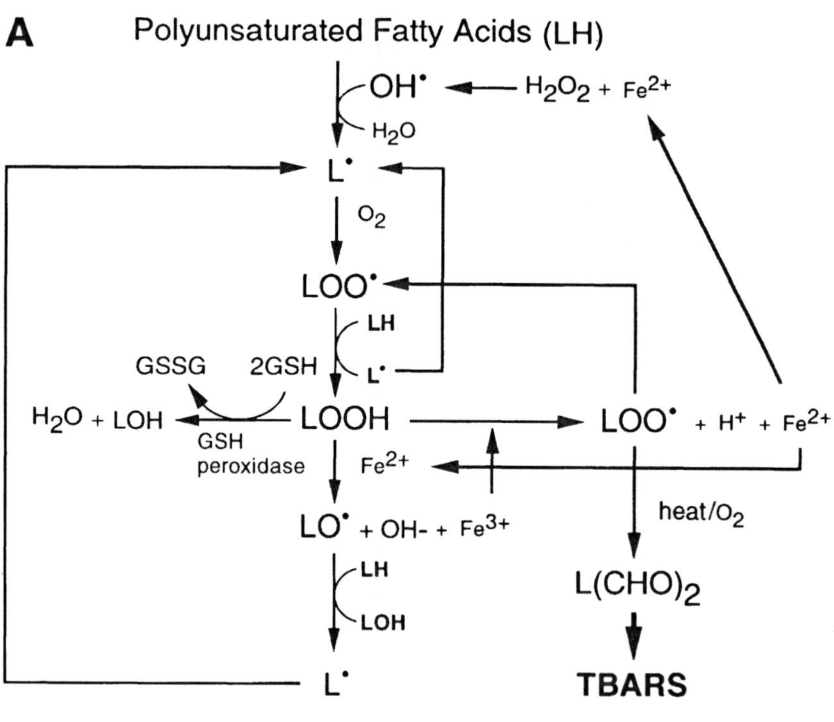

apoptosis into necrosis, as estimated by alterations of not only caspase-3 activation but also internucleosomal DNA fragmentations and cellular ATP levels (2,8). TPP^+ release was observed in BSO-treated cells in both the presence and absence of PUFA. This assay might reflect the cell damage accompanying mitochondrial membrane dysfunction not only in apoptosis but also in necrosis. Alternation of apoptosis and necrosis accompanied by a reduction of internucleosomal DNA fragmentation

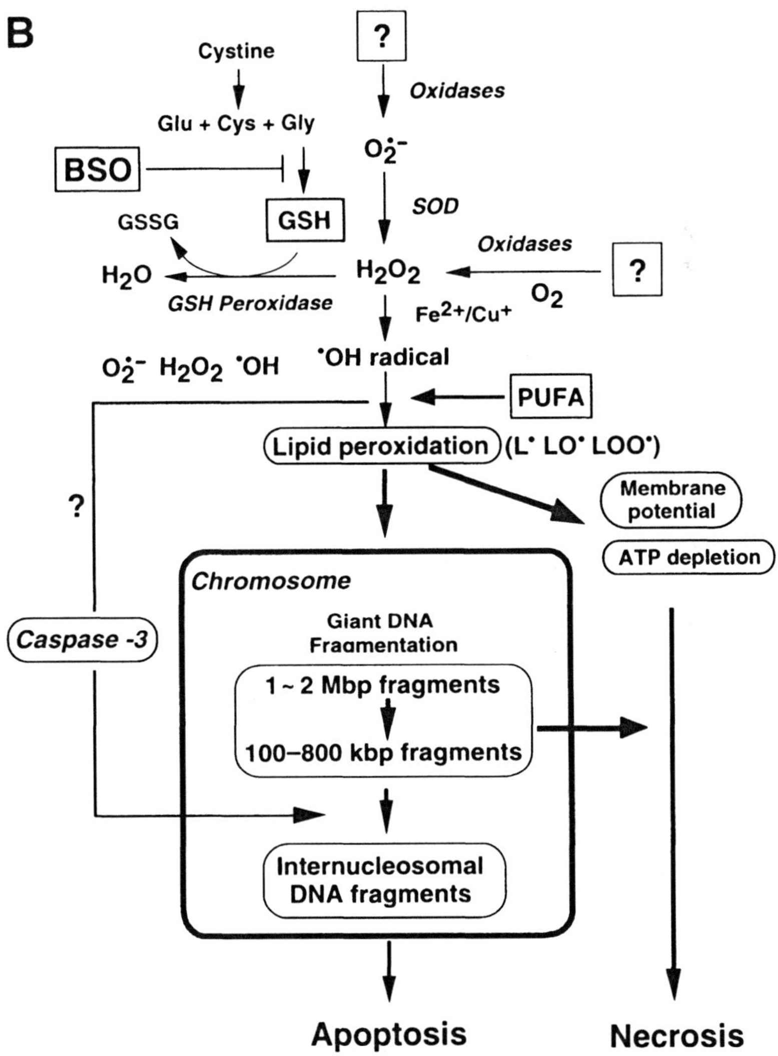

Fig. 18.6. Lipid peroxidation of polyunsaturated fatty acids (PUFA) with (A) lipid chain reaction and (B) a possible mechanism of buthionine sulfoximine (BSO)-induced cell death accompanied by giant DNA fragmentation in C6 rat glioma cells.

in C6 cells might be dependent on the strength of the oxidative stress or lipid peroxidation. Thus, PUFA may promote lipid peroxidation as an oxidant, thereby switching the apoptosis (mild insult) to necrosis (intense insult), which causes rapid cell death. There are a few recent reports of apoptosis and necrosis caused under various conditions, including oxidative stress in neuronal cells. Lysophosphatidic acid induced both apoptosis and necrosis in hippocampal neurons (29). In HT-22 hippocampus-derived cells, the oxidative cell death induced by glutamate demonstrated programmed cell death with characteristics of both apoptosis and necrosis (30).

Hydrogen peroxide, which is continually generated within cells as a result of metabolic pathways, is a major candidate fro ROS. In our previous study, although the source was obscure, release of extracellular accumulation of H_2O_2 without decaying was observed in C6 cells under glutamate-induced GSH depletion (10). In nerve cells, hydrogen peroxide production from the metabolism of catecholamines and indoleamines by monoamine oxidase has been considered (31, 32).

In summary (Fig. 18.6B), hydrogen peroxide is converted to $^{\bullet}OH$ radicals by metals such as iron and copper. The $^{\bullet}OH$ radicals induce lipid peroxidation with a chain reaction in the presence of PUFA. Hydrogen peroxide and lipid hydroperoxide can cause a reduction in intracellular ATP in another step (33), leading to repeated propagation of lipid peroxidation with the $LO^{\bullet}$ radical from PUFA-accelerated 1- to 2-Mbp giant DNA fragmentation associated with necrosis. Excess lipid hydroperoxide accumulation during GSH depletion may be involved in the induction of cell death, with necrosis observed in incidences of neuronal cell death or neuronal decrease.

Acknowledgments

The author thanks Dr. T. Yoshimoto of Kanazawa University School of Medicine for his valuable suggestions. This work was supported in part by a Grant-in-Aid for Scientific Research (C) from the Ministry of Education, Science, Sport and Culture Japan.

References

1. Simonian, N.A., and Coyle, J.T. (1996) Oxidative Stress in Neurodegenerative Diseases. *Annu. Rev. Pharmacol. Toxicol. 36*, 83–106.
2. Carson, D.A., and Ribeiro, J.M. (1993) Apoptosis and Disease. *Lancet 341*, 1251–1254.
3. Swartz, L.M., Smith, S.W., Jone, M.E.E., and Osbone, B.A. (1993) Do All Programmed Cell Deaths Occur via Apoptosis? *Proc. Natl. Acad. Sci. USA 90*, 980–984.
4. Du, Y., Bales, K.R., Dodel, R.C., Hamilton-Byrd, E., Horn, J.W., Czilli, D.L., Simmons, L., Ni, B., and Paul, S.M. (1997) Activation of a Caspase-3 Related Cysteine Protease Is Required for Glutamate-Mediated Apoptosis of Cultured Cerebellar Granule Neurons. *Proc. Natl. Acad. Sci. USA 94*, 11657–11662.
5. Eguchi, Y., Shimizu, S., and Tsujimoto, Y. (1997) Intracellular ATP Levels Determine Cell Death Fate by Apoptosis or Necrosis. *Cancer Res. 57*, 1835–1840.
6. Kass, G.E.N., Eriksson, J.E., Weis, M., Orrenius, S., and Chow, S.C. (1996) Chromatin Condensation During Apoptosis Requires ATP. *Biochem. J. 318*, 749–752.
7. Eguchi, Y., Srinivasan, A., Tomaselli, K.J., Shimizu, S., and Tsujimoto, Y. (1999) ATP-Dependent Steps in Apoptotic Signal Transduction. *Cancer Res. 59*, 2174–2181.

8. Lelli, J.L., Becks, L.L., Dabrowska, M.I., and Hinshaw, D.B. (1998) ATP Converts Necrosis to Apoptosis in Oxidant-Injured Endothelial Cells. *Free Radic. Biol. Med. 25*, 694–702.
9. Ankarcrona, M., Dypbukt, J.M., Bonfoco, E., Zhivotovsky, B., Orrenius, S., Lipton, S.A., and Nicotera, P. (1995) Glutamate-Induced Neuronal Death: A Succession of Necrosis or Apoptosis Depending on Mitochondrial Function. *Neuron 15*, 961–973.
10. Higuchi, Y., and Matsukawa, S. (1998) Active Oxygen-Mediated Chromosomal 1-2 Mbp Giant DNA Fragmentation into Internucleosomal DNA Fragmentation in Apoptosis of Glioma Cells Induced by Glutamate. *Free Radic. Biol. Med. 24*, 418–426.
11. Higuchi, Y., and Matsukawa, S. (1999) Glutathione Depletion Induces Giant DNA and High Molecular Weight DNA Fragmentation Associated with Apoptosis Through Lipid Peroxidation and Protein Kinase C Activation in C6 Glioma Cells. *Arch. Biochem. Biophys. 363*, 33–42.
12. Higuchi, Y. (1996) Antitumor Effect of *Streptococcus pyogenes* by Inducing Hydrogen Peroxide Production. *Jpn. J. Cancer Res. 87*, 1271–1279.
13. Higuchi, Y., and Matsukawa, S. (1997) Appearance of 1-2 Mbp Giant DNA Fragments as an Early Common Response Leading to Cell Death Induced by Various Substances Which Cause Oxidative Stress. *Free Radic. Biol. Med. 23*, 90–99.
14. Buege, J. A., and Aust, S. D. (1978) Microsomal Lipid Peroxidation. *Methods Enzymol. 52*, 302–310.
15. Higuchi, Y. (2001) Measurement of DNA Double-Strand Breaks with Giant DNA and High Molecular Weight DNA Fragments by Pulsed-Field Gel Electrophoresis. *Methods Mol. Biol.*, in press.
16. Shimizu, S., Eguchi, Y., Kamiike, W., Waguri, S., Uchiyama, Y., Matsuda, H., and Tsujimoto, Y. (1996) Bcl-2 Blocks Loss of Mitochondrial Membrane Potential While ICE Inhibitors Act at a Different Step During Inhibition of Death Induced by Respiratory Chain Inhibitors. *Oncogene 13*, 21–29.
17. Meyer, M., Schreck, R., and Baeuerle, P. A. (1993) H_2O_2 and Antioxidants Have Opposite Effects on Activation of NF-κB and AP-1 in Intact Cells: AP-1 as Secondary Antioxidant-Responsive Factor. *EMBO J. 12*, 2005–2015.
18. Rosen, G.M., and Rauckman, E.J. (1984) Spin Trapping of Superoxide and Hydroxyl Radicals. *Methods Enzymol. 105*, 198–208.
19. Kalyanaraman, B., and Sivarajah, K. (1984) in, *Free Radicals in Biology*, (Pryor, W.A., ed.) vol. VI, pp. 149–198, Academic Press, Orlando.
20. Farber, J.L., Kyle, M.E., and Coleman, J.B. (1990) Biology of Disease: Mechanisms of Cell Injury by Activated Oxygen Species. *Lab. Investig. 62*, 670–679.
21. Masaki, N., Kyle, M.E., and Farber, J.L. (1989) *tert*-Butylated Hydroperoxide Kills Cultured Hepatocytes by Peroxidizing Membrane Lipids. *Arch. Biochem. Biophys. 269*, 390–399.
22. Heikkila, R.E., Cabbat, F.S., and Cohen, G. (1976) In Vivo Inhibition of Superoxide Dismutase in Mice by Diethyldithiocarbamate. *J. Biol. Chem. 251*, 2182–2185.
23. Halliwell, B., and Gutteridge, J.M.C. (1989) in, *Free Radicals in Biology and Medicine*, (Halliwell, B. and Gutteridge, J.M.C., eds.) pp. 188–276, Clarendon Press, Oxford.
24. Cosgrove, J.P., Church, D.F., and Pryor, W.A. (1987) The Kinetics of the Autooxidation of Polyunsaturated Fatty Acids. *Lipids 22*, 299–304.
25. Hawkins, R.H., Sangster, K., and Arends, A.M. (1998) Apoptotic Death of Pancreatic Cancer Cells Induced by Polyunsaturated Fatty Acids Varies with Double Bond Number and Involves an Oxidative Mechanism. *J. Pathol. 185*, 61–70.

26. Halliwell, B., and Gutteridge, M.C. (1984) Oxygen Toxicity, Oxygen Radicals, Transition Metals and Disease. *Biochem. J. 219*, 1–14.
27. Ochu, E.E., Rothwell, N.J., and Waters, C.M. (1998) Caspases Mediate 6-Hydroxydopamine-Induced Apoptosis but Not Necrosis in PC12 Cells. *J. Neurochem. 70*, 2637–2640.
28. Armstrong, R.C., Aja, T.J., Hoang, K.D., Gaur, S., Bai, X., Alnemri, E.S., Litwack, G., Karanewsky, D.S., Fritz, C., and Tomaselli, K.J. (1997) Activation of the CED3/ICE-Related Protease CPP32 in Cerebellar Granule Neurons Undergoing Apoptosis but Not Necrosis. *J. Neuroscience 17*, 553–562.
29. Holtsberg, F.W., Steiner, M.R., Keller, J.N., Mark, R.J., Mattson, M P., and Steiner, S.M. (1998) Lysophosphatidic Acid Induces Necrosis and Apoptosis in Hippocampal Neurons. *J. Neurochem. 70*, 66–76.
30. Tan, S., Wood, M., and Maher, P. (1998) Oxidative Stress Induces a Form of Programmed Cell Death with Characteristics of Both Apoptosis and Necrosis in Neuronal Cells. *J. Neurochem. 71*, 95–105.
31. Maher, P., and Davis, J.M. (1996) The Role of Monoamine Metabolism in Oxidative Glutamate Toxicity. *J. Neurosci. 16*, 6394–6401.
32. Cohen, G., Farooqui, R., and Kesler, N. (1997) Parkinson Disease: A New Link Between Monoamine Oxidase and Mitochondrial Electron Flow. *Proc. Natl. Acad. Sci. USA 94*, 4890–4894.
33. Spragg, R.G., Hinshaw, D.B., Hyslop, P.A. Schraufstaller, I.U., and Cochrane, C.G. (1985) Alterations in Adenosine Triphosphate and Energy Change in Cultured Endothelial and P388D1 Cells After Oxidant Injury. *J. Clin. Investig. 76*, 1471–1476.

Chapter 19

Ginkgo biloba Extract and Gene Expression

Kishorchandra Gohil[a] and Lester Packer[b]

[a]Department of Internal Medicine, University of California, Davis, CA
[b]Department of Molecular Pharmacology and Toxicology, School of Pharmacy, University of Southern California, Los Angeles, CA

The real voyage of discovery consists not in seeking new landscapes but in having new eyes.

Marcel Proust

Introduction

A mammalian diploid cell expresses ~2×10^4 mRNAs from the genome of 1.40×10^5 genes. This well-established observation implies complex mechanisms that must selectively transcribe the cell-specific genes within the nucleus and coordinate the transcriptional processes with dynamic events in the extranuclear and extracellular milieu. The analysis of *Ginkgo biloba* extract–sensitive changes in the expression of genes, therefore, is opening a window on the responsiveness of complex transcriptional machinery to a natural extract. *Ginkgo biloba* extract is a flavonoid- and terpenoid-containing extract with antioxidant properties (1). The need for defining the mechanism of action of phytochemical extracts for human consumption has been recognized by clinical and academic researchers. For example, one of the tenets of The Saas Fee Declaration on the significance of antioxidants in preventive medicine (2) stated that "there is a need for further work at the fundamental scientific level ..., which can be expected to lead to more precise information [about antioxidant actions] being made available." Seven years later, the National Institutes for Health's Centers for Dietary Supplements Research recognized that 16 million Americans consume botanical extracts and emphasized four areas of research. One of these research areas was "... identification of active constituents and elucidation of their mechanisms of action." Although the importance of obtaining mechanistic understanding of the effects of plant extracts is accepted, they have not enjoyed the investigative support awarded to purified chemical libraries.

The consumption of botanical extracts for prevention and treatment of human diseases is common in all human cultures. Recent epidemiologic research has given a new impetus to explore the therapeutic potential of botanical extracts. Particularly noteworthy are the results reporting lowered risk of a variety of cancers in human populations consuming diets with more fruits and vegetables (3,4). Also remarkable are the epidemiologic studies that suggest lowered susceptibility to coronary heart disease in populations that consume moderate amounts of wine and alcoholic beverages (5). These observations have fueled the search for the disease-preventive components within a complex mixture of botanical extracts. Because polyphenols are commonly found in plant extracts, they have become primary candidates for investigations.

Flavonoids and terpenoid components of natural extracts such as *Ginkgo biloba* are of particular interest because of their potential activities in regulating cell proliferation and growth. A synthetic flavonoid, flavopiridol, has been shown to inhibit a number of protein kinases including cyclin-dependent kinases and thereby regulate cell cycle and proliferation; it is currently in clinical trials for the treatment of cancers (6). Another bioflavonoid extract, silymarin, has been shown to inhibit activation of nuclear factor (NF)-κB by lipopolysaccharide in a human hepatoma cell line and impair the receptor tyrosine kinase signaling pathway in a human epidermoid cell line (7). Because one of the undisputed activities of *Ginkgo biloba* extract is its antioxidant properties, it is also likely that the flavonoids and terpenoids produce their cellular effects by regulating the status of endogenous reactive oxygen species.

Changes in rates of cell proliferation and death play an important role in initiation and progression of chronic disease and utilize constitutive and inducible metabolic and signaling pathways. In the past decade, the techniques for simultaneous monitoring of changes in the expression of a large number of genes, possibly the entire expressed genome of a cell at mRNA and protein levels, have undergone a revolution. It is now possible to monitor changes in the entire expressed genome of a eukaryotic cell using gene chip technology (10). We recently described the effect of *Ginkgo biloba* extract on the gene expression profile of a human bladder cancer cell line and showed a large transcriptional response (11). In the following pages, we describe the results of applications of different techniques to define changes in the expression of *Ginkgo biloba* extract–sensitive genes in rat neutrophils and in human cancer cells.

Selective Induction of Bcl-2 and Tumor Necrosis Factor (TNF)-α in Rat Neutrophils

Neutrophils are endowed with highly regulated NADPH-oxidase, which generates superoxide radicals and hydrogen peroxide by reduction of molecular oxygen. Superoxide burst is activated in neutrophils as a defense response to the presence of a foreign particle, such as a bacterium or by nanomolar amounts of phorbol 12-myristate 13-acetate (PMA), an activator of protein kinase C. During the production of superoxide, the phagocytic cell is likely to deplete intracellular antioxidants such as glutathione and produce oxidative stress, which in turn may accelerate the intrinsic apoptotic program of neutrophils. Activation of rat neutrophils in the presence of EGb 761 inhibits superoxide production. It has been shown that the apoptotic pathway is regulated by a large number of proteins including Bcl-2, Bcl-xl, and Bax. We therefore examined the effect of EGb 761 on expression of mRNAs for proapoptotic protein Bax and antiapoptotic proteins Bcl-2 and Bcl-xl in rat neutrophils activated by PMA. Figure 19.1 shows that the expression of Bax, Bcl-2 and Bcl-xl was unaffected by PMA. However, EGb 761 doubled the expression of antiapoptotic Bcl-2 without any effect on Bax or Bcl-xl after 18 h following a 15-min stimulation of PMA. EGb

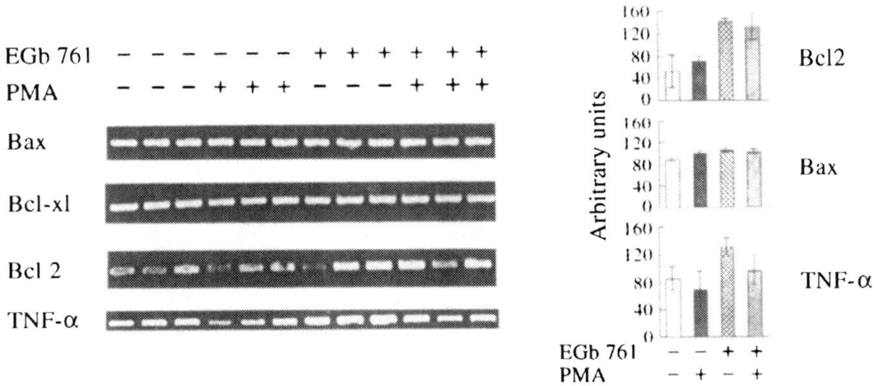

Fig. 19.1. Induction of Bcl 2 and tumor necrosis factor (TNF)-α by EGb 761. Neutrophils from rats were isolated and stimulated with phorbol 12-myristate 13-acetate (PMA) (10 ng/mL) for 15 min and then incubated for a further 18 h *ex vivo* at 37°C under standard conditions. Total RNA was isolated and mRNA for Bcl-2 and TNF-α were estimated by polymerase chain reaction (PCR) with specific primers.

761 also augmented the transcript for TNF-α, an activator of NF-κB, a transcription factor that regulates a large number of cytokine genes and the apoptotic pathways. These observations show that the extract of *Ginkgo biloba* leaves can selectively affect the transcription of mRNAs important in the regulation of the apoptotic process of neutrophils, which play an important role in the defense of the organism and in remodeling of the tissues.

Differential Display of mRNAs

Liang and Pardee (12) described a polymerase chain reaction (PCR)-based method that enabled simultaneous evaluation of upregulated and downregulated expression of mammalian genes in a pair of differently treated cells. The method took advantage of random oligonucleoutide primers, designed to hybridize to all of the cDNAs at sites distal to the oligo-dT tails prepared from mRNAs with four different oligo-dNT primers. mRNA isolated from human bladder cancer cells (T-24 cells) overexpressing the oncogenic G-protein, ras, and exposed to either the vehicle or EGb 761 showed changes in ~40 different transcripts after screening, ~30% of the expressed genome. Figure 19.2 shows a selected region of the differential display autoradiogram. Several amplified products (a,b) showed a decrease in intensity in EGb 761–treated cells. The identities of these transcripts remain to be defined and are likely to be the mRNAs identified by cDNA arrays on nylon filters and oligonucleotide microarrays described below.

cDNA Arrays of Genes or Expressed Sequence Tags (EST)

When EST are dotted on nylon membranes, they offer the advantage of rapid identification of the altered expressions of mRNAs in the presence of the extract. In addition, a good selection of function-specific cDNA arrays are commercially available.

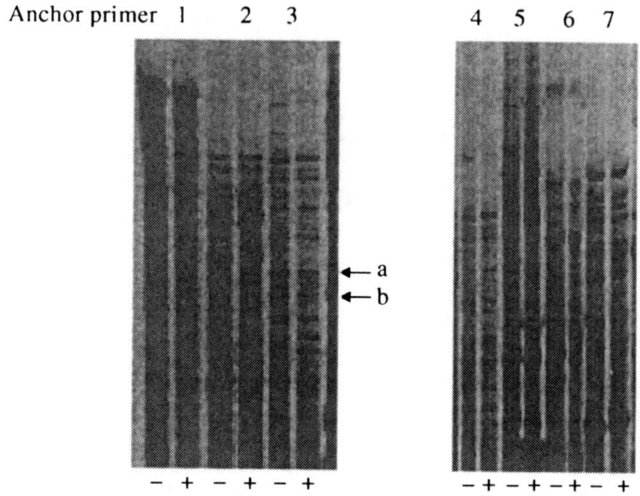

Fig. 19.2. Differential display of mRNAs of human bladder T-24 cells treated with either dimethyl sulfoxide (DMSO) (0.1%) or EGb 761 extract (100 μg/mL) for 72 h at 37°C under standard conditions. Total RNA was isolated and subjected to polymerase chain reaction (PCR) amplication as described by Liang and Pardee (12). The figure shows downregulation of two mRNA fragments, a and b, by incubation with *Ginkgo biloba* extract.

One such cDNA array of human cancer genes was used to screen the changes in the gene expression of human bladder cancer cells in the presence of EGb 761. The array screened for 15 different functional classes of genes, including cell cycle regulators, growth regulators, apoptosis, oncogenes, and genes for DNA damage response and repair. Radiolabeled cDNA prepared from mRNA isolated from T-24 cells hybridized to 131 of the 588 (22% of the genes on the cDNA array) complementary gene fragments on the cDNA array.

An example of differential gene expression in human bladder cancer cells in response to the extract of *Ginkgo biloba*, EGb 761, is shown in Figure 19.3. The figure shows that in the group of apoptosis-related genes, mRNA for EGb 761 downregulated X, whereas the expression of gene Y was upregulated in the same sample. Similarly, in the growth factor and cytokine family of genes, the expression of g1 and g2 was upregulated compared with the two genes in the same area of the blot by the presence of EGb 761 for 72 h in the cell culture medium. These data show that EGb 761 selectively alters the expression of broad functional groups of genes and support the data obtained by differential display of mRNA discussed above.

DNA Microarray Chips

Microarray chips offer a more comprehensive assessment of the transcriptional response of a cell. The technique enables simultaneous screening of changes in the entire expressed genome (up to 20,000 mRNAs) of a cell in response to a variable such

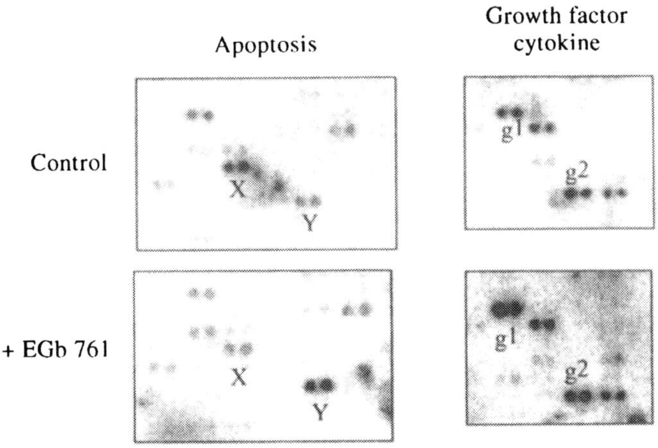

Fig. 19.3. Regulation of growth factor, cytokine and apoptosis mRNAs in human bladder cancer cell line by EGb 761. Total RNA was isolated from the control cells treated with dimethyl sulfoxide (DMSO) (0.1%), or from cells treated with EGb 761 (100 µg/mL) for 72 h. Radiolabeled cDNA was used for hybridization to Human Cancer gene array (Clontech, CA). The figure shows downregulation of apoptosis-related gene X and upregulation of gene Y by the extract. Similarly, genes g1 and g2 from the growth factor and cytokine families of genes were upregulated by the extract.

as a DNA damaging agent, or to serum repletion or to a botanical extract. Currently, there are two distinct techniques available for monitoring changes in gene expression; each technique offers a large amount of data on qualitative and quantitative changes in the gene expression profile of the cell under investigation.

One gene profiling technique, pioneered by Patrick Brown and David Botstein's teams at Stanford University, utilizes PCR-amplified fragments of cloned DNA (cDNA) dotted, robotically, onto a glass microscope slide (1×3 in^2) (8). In a typical DNA microarray slide, up to 6000 different cDNAs can be dotted per slide; each dot is ~200 mm in diameter, containing ~10 ng of DNA. The source of the cDNA determines the comprehensiveness of the data for the transcriptional response of a selected cell to a defined stimulus. If DNAs are randomly selected from the entire human genome data bank of known human genes or expressed sequence tags, then a typical experiment can screen ~10% of the expressed genome in the selected cell type. However, the response of an almost completely (>90%) expressed genome to a selected stimulus can be screened if the cDNAs dotted onto the glass slides are obtained from the cDNA library prepared from the specific cell under investigation. The latter approach, therefore, requires the experimenter to follow an additional step of construction of the cell-specific cDNA library representing every mRNA expressed in that cell. A DNA gene-array generated by the dotting technique is used as microarray probes to define changes in two populations of target cDNAs each of which is specifically tagged with a distinct fluorescently labeled nucleotide. The fluorescent-labeled target cDNAs from control and test cells, immobilized by specific hybridization to their complementary probes on the GeneChip, are visualized by a confocal laser scanner. Mathematical and statistical programs to obtain quantitative information on the number and amount of different mRNAs present in the sample analyze the fluorescent images obtained from the scanner. Such an analysis of data generates a cell-specific gene expression profile that can be compared with similar data from the same cell type under different physiologic and pathologic conditions.

The major difference in the other microarray technique is the manner in which the DNA probes are synthesized on a glass surface (13). The probes are 23-mer oligonucleotides and are synthesized on a glass surface, 1.28 cm × 1.28 cm, by photolithographic techniques. Up to 300,000 oligonucleotides can be present on a single GeneChip to analyze changes in ~7000 different mRNAs (an entire expressed genome of yeast!). The construction of the microarray is such that each target mRNA is probed for specific binding by 20 different oligonucleotides that span from the 5′ end of the message to the 3′ end. Nonspecific binding of the target mRNA is quantitated by hybridization to oligonucleotide probes that are aligned along the specific probes and have a mismatched nucleotide at position 13. Hence each intact target mRNA is simultaneously probed by 20 sense and 20 antisense probes. Target RNA, labeled with a biotinylated nucleotide, is prepared by the following three steps: (i) total or mRNA is isolated from the cells under investigation; (ii) double-stranded DNA is prepared with a specific T7 primer; and (iii) target RNA (cRNA) is amplified in the presence of biotinylated ribose nucleotides by *in vitro* transcription with T7 RNA polymerase. Amplified cRNA is fragmented and mixed into the hybridization solution, which is incubated with the probes on the GeneChips. Bound target cRNAs are detected by incubation with streptavidin phycoerythrin, which binds to biotinylated nucleotides in target cRNAs. Fluorescent-bound target cRNAs are then detected by a chip scanner such as the Hewlett-Packard GeneArray Scanner, and the scanned images are analyzed by the appropriate image-processing software such as GeneChip Expression Analysis.

The transcriptional response of human bladder cancer cells with constitutively active ras was examined *in vitro* by incubation with an extract of *Ginkgo biloba* over a period of 72 h (11). Analysis by GeneChips revealed a net increase in the number of transcripts during the incubation period; after 6 h of incubation, 61 mRNAs were affected more than twofold; at 48 h, a similar number of transcripts were affected, but at 72 h, the total number of mRNAs affected was 114. The abundance of most of the transcripts was increased by the extract, strongly suggesting that the extract either stabilizes mRNAs or increases the transcription of the respective genes. Functional classification of the affected genes showed that the extract altered the expression of genes for intracellular vesicular transport (see Table 19.1), mitochondria, transcription and antioxidants.

In summary, several techniques for the analysis of gene expression at the level of mRNAs have uncovered a complex effect of *Ginkgo biloba* extract that cannot entirely account for its antioxidant properties. Analytical strategies aimed at defining whole-cell responses of gene expression at the level of transcription and translation

TABLE 19.1 Vesicular Transport and the Golgi System

		Fluorescence intensity			
Name	GI #	Control	6 h	48 h	72 h
RAB 1 (ras-related protein)	HG 3521	91	275	228	294
RAB 2 (GTP binding protein)	M28213	125	277	209	300
Krev-1 (ras-related protein)	M22995	333	345	488	900
mp24, transmembrane protein	X92098	214	494	329	250
Synaptobrevin-like novel gene	X92396	169	515	387	408
Synaptophysin-like, hSp1	X68194	161	504	160	132
β-Adaptin	M34175	2059	2449	2772	5457
CDC42	U02570	975	1008	1272	2526
α-Tubulin	X06956	389	332	665	782
Autocrine motility protein	M63175	314	432	538	748
ADP ribosylation factor	M74491	1689	2930	3876	5756
Clathrin light chain B, splice 1	HG 2795	234	4162	2917	2222
Nonmyosin heavy chain	M31013	2086	2630	3645	6791
Kinesin-related protein	D14678	77	103	194	111
Kinesin heavy chain	X65873	88	201	258	229
ELP-1 (Brefeldrin A phenotype–inducing)	X65873	88	201	258	229

(proteomics) will reveal novel molecular targets of complex mixtures of natural extracts. Data from such analysis are essential for more rational and targeted use of natural extracts and their constituents to improve human health.

References

1. Packer, L.C., (1998) *Ginkgo biloba* Extract (EGb 76 1), in *Lessons from Cell Biology*
2. Packer, L., and Fuchs, J. (1996) in *Handbook of Antioxidants*, pp. iii–v, Marcel Dekker, New York.
3. Steinmetz, K.A., and Potter, J.D. (1991) Vegetables, Fruit, and Cancer. I. Epidemiology. *Cancer Causes Control* 2, 325–357.
4. Steinmetz, K.A., and Potter, J.D. (1991) Vegetables, Fruit, and Cancer. II. Mechanisms. *Cancer Causes Control* 2, 427–442.
5. German, J.B., and Walzem, R.L. (2000) The Health Benefits of Wine. *Annu. Rev. Nutr. 20*, 561–593.
6. Drees, M., Dengler, W.A., Roth, T., Labonte, H., Mayo, J., Malspeis, L., Grever, M., Sausville, E.A., and Fiebig, H.H. (1997) Flavopiridol (L86-8275): Selective Antitumor Activity In Vitro and Activity In Vivo for Prostate Carcinoma Cells. *Clin. Cancer Res. 3*, 273–279.
7. Zi, X., Grasso, A.W., Kung, H.J., and Agarwal, R. (1998) A Flavonoid Antioxidant, Silymarin, Inhibits Activation of erbBI Signaling and Induces Cyclin-Dependent Kinase Inhibitors, GI Arrest, and Anticarcinogenic Effects in Human Prostate Carcinoma DU145 Cells. *Cancer Res. 58*, 1920–1929.

8. Schena, M., Shalon, D., Davis, R.W., and Brown, P.O. (1995) Quantitative Monitoring of Gene Expression Patterns with a Complementary DNA Microarray [see comments]. *Science 270,* 467–470.
9. Lockhart, D.J., Dong, H., Byrne, M.C., Follettie, M.T., Gallo, M.V., Chee, M.S., Mittmann, M., Wang, C., Kobayashi, M., Horton, H., and Brown, E.L. (1996) Expression Monitoring by Hybridization to High-Density Oligonucleotide Arrays [see comments]. *Nat. Biotechnol. 14,* 1675–1680.
10. DeRisi, J.L., Iyer, V.R., and Brown, P.O. *(1997)* Exploring the Metabolic and Genetic Control of Gene Expression on a Genomic Scale. *Science 278,* 680–686.
11. Gohil, K., Moy R.K., Farzin S., Rosania G.R., Maguire, J.J., and Packer, L. (2000) *Ginkgo biloba* Extract Alters the mRNA Expression Profile of a Human Cell Line: Induction of Antioxidant Response and the Golgi System. *Free Radic. Res. 33,* 831–849.
12. Liang, P., Zhu, W., Zhang, X., Guo, Z., O'Connell, R P., Averboukh, L., Wang, F., and Pardee, A. B. (1994) Differential Display Using One-Base Anchored Oligo-dT Primers. *Nucleic Acids Res. 22,* 5763–5764.
13. Wodicka, L., Dong, H., Mittmann, M., Ho, M.H., and Lockhart, D.J. (1997) Genome-Wide Expression Monitoring in *Saccharomyces cerevisiae. Nat. Biotechnol. 15,* 1359–1367.

Chapter 20

Conjugated Linoleic Acid: Anticancer Effects

David Kritchevsky

The Wistar Institute, Philadelphia, PA 19104

Introduction

Conjugated linoleic acid (CLA) is an intermediate formed in the course of the conversion of linoleic acid to stearic acid by the rumen bacteria *Butyrivibrio fibrisolvens* (1). The designation CLA covers a mixture of positional and geometric isomers of linoleic acid (18:2, *c*9, *c*12) in which the double bonds are conjugated rather than methylene separated. The predominant isomer of CLA found in foods is the *c*9, *t*11 modification. The level of CLA found in dairy products and meat of ruminant animals is generally in the range of 3–6 mg/g of fat (1).

The CLA used in many of the studies described below is obtained commercially by alkali isomerization of polyunsaturated fats and contains, principally, the *c*9, *t*11 and *t*10, *c*12 modifications.

The antimutagenic effect of CLA was discovered by Pariza *et al.* (2) while studying the formation of carcinogens during the cooking of ground beef. A fraction of the extract of heated beef was found to have antimutagenic properties, and the antimutagenic activity was also found in raw ground beef. The partially purified beef extract was originally designated as a "mutagenesis modulator." The first test in animals of the mutagenesis modulator was as a possible inhibitor of skin papillomas in mice by treatment with 7,12-dimethylbenz[a]anthracene (DMBA). The test compound was found to reduce the incidence of papilloma formation (3). The anticarcinogen in ground beef was identified as a mixture of four isomeric modifications of CLA, namely, the *c*9, *t*11 ; *t*9, *t*11 ; *t*10, *c*12 ; and *t*10, *t*12 modifications (4). CLA was also found to inhibit benzo(a)pyrene (BP)-induced forestomach tumors in mice. The BP was administered orally in olive oil, olive oil plus CLA, or olive oil plus linoleic acid. Linoleic acid reduced tumor incidence by 6% and CLA reduced incidence by 17% (5).

Dietary CLA is also effective in inhibiting experimental carcinogenesis when included in the diet. Ip *et al.* (6) fed varying levels of CLA to rats treated with DMBA. Even when fed at 0.5% of the diet, CLA inhibited tumor incidence (% of rats with tumors) by 17%, tumor multiplicity (tumors/tumor-bearing rat) by 33%, and tumor burden (total weight of all tumors) by 23%. In rats fed 1.5% CLA, tumor incidence, multiplicity, and burden were reduced by 50, 59, and 54%, respectively. A subsequent study (7) showed that, even when fed at a level of 0.05%, CLA inhibited DMBA-induced mammary carcinogenesis by 22%. The level of fat in the diet does not affect CLA inhibition of tumor growth nor does the type of fat (saturated or unsaturated) (8). It has also been shown that the form in which CLA is administered (free acid or triglyceride) does not affect tumor suppression (9). CLA suppresses growth of mammary tumors in rats treated with a direct-acting [methylnitrosourea (MNU)] carcinogen or one requiring metabolic activation (DMBA) (7). Tumor incidence was reduced by 32% ($P < 0.01$) in rats treated with MNU and by 35% ($P < 0.01$) in those given DMBA. It was also found that consumption of CLA for only 5 wk (3 wk postweaning plus 2 wk postcarcinogen administration) was sufficient to inhibit tumor growth (10). CLA has also been reported to inhibit colon carcinogenesis induced by 2-amino-3-methylimidazo [4,5*f*]quinoline (IQ) (10).

When severe combined immunodeficient (SCID) mice are inoculated subcutaneously with human tumor cells, tumors proliferate at the site of injection and eventually metastasize (11). SCID mice were inoculated with 10^7 human breast adenocarcinoma cells (MDA-MB-468) after 2 wk of consuming a diet containing 1% CLA. Twelve weeks later, compared with a control group, tumor weight (g) and volume (mm^3) were significantly reduced and no metastatic spread was observed. The mice were maintained on 1% CLA for the duration of the study (12).

In another study, SCID mice were inoculated with 5×10^6 human prostatic cancer cells. The mice were fed 1% CLA for 2 wk before the inoculation and for 12 wk until the study was terminated. A control group was maintained and a third group was fed 1% linoleic acid (LA). By 6 wk, tumor volume was significantly decreased in the CLA-fed mice. By 12 wk, tumor volume in the linoleic acid-fed mice had increased by ~20% and that in the CLA-fed rats had decreased by ~75% ($P < 0.01$). Tumor mass had increased by ~30% in the LA-fed mice and decreased by 80% in those fed CLA. Metastases to the lungs were observed in 80–100% of the control or LA-fed mice and were seen in only 10% of mice fed CLA (13).

CLA has also been shown to inhibit the growth of a number of human tumor cell lines *in vitro* (14–16). Visonneau *et al.* (17) examined the effects of different dilutions (10^{-4}, 10^{-5}, or 10^{-6}) of CLA and LA on *in vitro* growth of a number of human cell lines. At almost every dilution, CLA inhibited cell growth, whereas LA enhanced it.

The mechanism(s) by which CLA inhibits tumor cell growth are unclear. Ha *et al.* (5) suggested an antioxidant effect. Reduction of carcinogen-DNA adducts has been suggested (10,18,19). Influence on the estrogen response system (20), eicosanoid metabolism (21), and apoptosis (22) have also been suggested as possible factors. CLA treatment of human prostate cells enhances mRNA for glutathione reductase and reduces diacylglycerol content (23). Effects on adhesion molecules such as ICAM have also been observed (13). The specific mode of action of CLA may vary according to tumor cell type. At the moment, it is obvious that CLA is definitely anticarcinogenic, but the mechanism by which it achieves the anticarcinogenic effect is moot.

References

1. Chin, S.F., Liu, W., Storkson, J.M., Ha, Y.L., and Pariza, M.W. (1992) Dietary Sources of Conjugated Dienoic Isomers of Linoleic Acid, a Newly Recognized Class of Anticarcinogens. *J. Food Comp. Anal. 5*, 185–197.
2. Pariza, M.W., Loretz, L.J., Storkson, J.M., and Holland, N.C. (1993) Mutagens and Modulator of Mutagenesis in Fried Ground Beef. *Cancer Res. 43*, 2444S–2446S.

3. Pariza, M.W., and Hargreaves, W.A. (1985) A Beef-Derived Mutagenesis Modulator Inhibits Initiation of Mouse Epidermal Tumors by 7,12-Benz(a)anthracene. *Carcinogenesis 6*, 591–593.
4. Ha, Y.L., Grimm, N.K., and Pariza, M.W. (1987) Anticarcinogens from Fried Ground Beef: Heat-Altered Derivatives of Linoleic Acid. *Carcinogenesis 8*, 1881–1887.
5. Ha, Y.L., Storkson, J., and Pariza, M.W. (1990) Inhibition of Benzo(a)pyrene-Induced Mouse Forestomach Neoplasia by Conjugated Dienoic Derivatives of Linoleic Acid. *Cancer Res. 50*, 1097–1101.
6. Ip, C., Chin, S.F., Scimeca, J.A., and Pariza, M.W. (1991) Mammary Cancer Prevention by Conjugated Dienoic Derivatives of Linoleic Acid. *Cancer Res. 51*, 6118–6124.
7. Ip, C., Singh, M., Thompson, H.J., and Scimeca, J.A. (1994) Conjugated Linoleic Acid Suppresses Mammary Carcinogenesis and Proliferative Activity of the Mammary Gland in the Rat. *Cancer Res. 54*, 1212–1215.
8. Ip, C., and Scimeca, J.A. (1997) Conjugated Linoleic Acid and Linoleic Acid are Distinctive Modulators of Mammary Carcinogenesis. *Nutr. Cancer 27*, 241–247.
9. Ip, C., Scimeca, J.A., and Thompson, H. (1995) Effect of Timing and Duration of Dietary Conjugated Linoleic Acid on Mammary Cancer Prevention. *Nutr. Cancer 24*, 241–247.
10. Liew, C., Schut, H.A.J., Chin, S.F., Pariza, M.W., and Dashwood, R.H. (1995) Protection of Conjugated Linoleic Acids Against 2-Amino-3-methylimidazo (4,5*f*) Quinoline-Induced Colon Carcinogenesis in the F344 Rat: A Study of Inhibitory Mechanisms. *Carcinogenesis 16*, 3037–3043.
11. Cesano, A., Hoxie, J.A., Lange, B., Nowell, P., Bishop, J., and Santoli, D. (1992) The Severe Combined Immunodeficient (SCID) Mouse as a Model for Human Myeloid Leukemia. *Oncogene 7*, 827–836.
12. Visonneau, S., Cesano, A., Tepper, S.A., Scimeca, J.A., Santoli, D., and Kritchevsky, D. (1997) Conjugated Linoleic Acid Suppresses the Growth of Human Breast Cancer Adenoma Cells in SCID Mice. *Anticancer Res. 17*, 969–974.
13. Cesano, A., Visonneau, S., Scimeca, J.A., Kritchevsky, D., and Santoli, D. (1998) Opposite Effects of Linoleic Acid and Conjugated Linoleic Acid on Human Prostate Cancer in SCID Mice. *Anticancer Res. 18*, 833–838.
14. Schultz, T.D., Chew, B.P., and Seaman, W.R. (1992) Differential Stimulatory and Inhibitory Responses of Human MCF-7 Breast Cancer Cells to Linoleic Acid and Conjugated Linoleic Acid in Culture. *Anticancer Res. 12*, 2143–2146.
15. Schonberg, S., and Krokan, H.E. (1995) The Inhibitory Effect of Conjugated Dienoic Derivatives (CLA) of Linoleic Acid on the Growth of Human Tumor Cell Lines Is, in Part, Due to Increased Lipid Peroxidation. *Anticancer Res. 15*, 1241–1246.
16. Cunningham, D.C., Harrison, L.Y., and Schultz, T.D. (1997) Proliferative Responses of Normal Human Mammary and MCF-7 Breast Cancer Cells to Linoleic, Conjugated Linoleic and Eicosanoid Synthesis Inhibitors in Culture. *Anticancer Res. 17*, 197–204.
17. Vissoneau, S., Cesano, A., Tepper, S.A., Scimeca, J.A., Santoli, D., and Kritchevsky, D. (1996) Effect of Different Concentrations of Conjugated Linoleic Acid (CLA) on Tumor Cell Growth *In Vitro*. *FASEB J. 10*, A183 (abstr.).
18. Schut, H.A.J., Cummings, D.A., Smale, H.H.E., Josyula, S., and Friesen, M.D. (1997) DNA Adducts of Heterocyclic Amines: Formation, Removal, and Inhibition by Dietary Components. *Mutat. Res. 376*, 185–194.

19. Josyula, S., and Schut, H.A.J. (1998) Effects of Dietary Conjugated Linoleic Acid on DNA Adduct Formation of PhIP and IQ After Bolus Administration to Female F344 Rats. *Nutr. Cancer 32*, 139–145.
20. Durgam, V.R., and Fernandes, G. (1997) The Growth Inhibitory Effect of Conjugated Linoleic Acid on MCF-7 Cells Is Related to Estrogen Response System. *Cancer Lett. 116*, 121–130.
21. Belury, M.A., and Kempa-Steczko, A. (1997) Conjugated Linoleic Acid Modulates Hepatic Lipid Composition in Mice. *Lipids 32*, 199–204.
22. Schultz, T.D., Chew, B.P., Seaman, W.R., and Luedecke, L.O. (1992) Inhibitory Effect of Conjugated Dienoic Derivatives of Linoleic Acid and β-Carotene on the In Vitro Growth of Human Cancer Cells. *Cancer Lett. 63*, 125–133.
23. Farquharson, A., Wei, H.-C., Grant, J., Graf, B., Choung, J.-J., Eremin, O., Heys, S., and Wahle, K. (1999) Possible Mechanisms for the Putative Antiatherogenic and Antitumorigenic Effects of Conjugated Polyenoic Fatty Acids. *Lipids 34*, S343.

Chapter 21

Molecular Aspects of Age-Related Macular Degeneration in Humans

Marilou G. Nicolas,[a] Keiko Fujiki,[b] Rosie R. Noche,[c] Junie Billones,[a] Marion Abendanio,[c] and Atsushi Kanai[b]

[a]Department of Physical Sciences and Mathematics, College of Arts and Sciences, University of the Philippines Manila, Padre Faura, Ermita, Manila, Philippines
[b]Department of Ophthalmology, Juntendo University School of Medicine, 3-1-3 Hongo Bunkyo-ku Tokyo, Japan
[c]Institute of Ophthalmology, University of the Philippines Manila, Philippine General Hospital Compound, Ermita, Manila, Philippines

Introduction

Macular degeneration is a disease that is normally associated with aging. The disease is characterized by progressive loss of vision, drusen or bright yellow spots that appear in the fovea (macula) (1–3), and lipofuscin (4–6), the age pigment in the retinal pigment epithelium (RPE). The pathogenesis of the disease is unknown but many believe it to be the result of incomplete digestion of the photoreceptors. This subsequently increases the metabolic burden of the RPE, resulting in the formation of drusen and lipofuscin. Incomplete digestion may result from either impaired proteolytic activities (7,8) or modification of the photoreceptors such as that caused, for example, by reactive oxygen species (ROS). The modified or altered structures become unrecognizable and are therefore not degraded by the digestive enzymes.

We found an animal model, three families of cynomolgus monkeys (*Macaca fascicularis*), which manifested familial traits of the disease. The monkeys showed yellow spots that were drusen-like, as well as the aging pigment, lipofuscin. Biochemical studies showed that the concentration of two proteins was altered in the retina of these monkeys (9). These proteins were albumin and glyceraldehyde 3-phosphate dehydrogenase. A decrease in glyceraldehyde 3-phosphate dehydrogenase activity is an indicator of oxidative stress. Additional studies (10) also showed decreases in the activities of two antioxidant enzymes, i.e., catalase and glutathione peroxidase. Thus, oxidative stress could be the result of the decrease in the activity of the antioxidant enzymes.

One of the predisposing factors in macular degeneration is alteration of the zinc concentration. The eye has the highest zinc concentration per gram weight of tissue. This is associated mainly with the melanin pigments. It is thought that changes in zinc concentrations may account for symptoms associated with macular degeneration. Indeed, we detected a fourfold lower zinc concentration in the retina of affected monkeys compared with normal controls. However, there was no significant difference between zinc concentration in plasma of affected monkeys and normal controls.

The eye is also subjected to solar bombardment, which increases free-radical concentration in this tissue. In addition, renewal of photoreceptors involves phagocytosis by the retinal pigment epithelium, which further increases oxidative stress in the retina (11,12). Increased free radical concentrations necessitate increased free radical scavengers. Both oxidative stress and high zinc concentration in the retina are conditions that induce the synthesis of metallothionein, a low-molecular-weight protein that regulates heavy metal concentration in cells and functions as a free radical scavenger.

We detected the presence of metallothionein in the retina of these monkeys. By specifically amplifying metallothionein cDNA, we detected a 300-bp cDNA consistent with metallothionein 2 (MT2) from monkey kidneys (13), which showed 99% cDNA sequence homology and 100% amino acid sequence similarity. Moreover, quantitative polymerase chain reaction (PCR) showed that MT2 synthesis in affected monkey retinas was much lower or suppressed compared with normal controls (10).

The study to determine the pathogenesis of the disease was divided into two parts. The first, described above, used an animal model, cynomolgus monkeys. The second attempts to extrapolate the results in the animal model to studies in humans manifesting age-related macular degeneration (ARMD). Using blood samples from Filipino and Japanese patients, we attempted to validate factors that are thought to predispose humans to macular degeneration.

Materials and Methods

Sample Collection. Blood (10 mL) was taken from each of 35 Filipino patients of the Philippine General Hospital and 37 Japanese patients from Juntendo University School of Medicine and Shinshu University Hospitals. These samples were used for DNA isolation and sequencing studies and plasma zinc as well as glucocorticoid determinations.

Determination of Zinc and Glucocorticoid Concentrations. Plasma was separated by centrifugation using a clinical centrifuge, IEC, and the plasma zinc concentration was determined by Thermo-Jarrel Ash Video 11E Atomic Absorption Spectrophotometer (Fischer Scientific Co., USA) using the graphite furnace detector. This procedure was done at the Natural Science Research Institute, University of the Philippines Diliman, Quezon City, Philippines. Glucocorticoid concentration was determined by radioimmunoassay at a commercial laboratory, New World Laboratory, Manila, Philippines immediately after separation of the red blood cells.

Isolation of DNA from Whole Blood. Whole blood (5 mL) was mixed with lysing solution to separate leukocytes. Total DNA was isolated using the IsoQuick (Orca Research Inc., WA, USA) nucleic acid extraction kit from 100 µL of leukocytes. Isolated DNA was stored at –20°C until use.

Sequencing of Promoter and Exons of MT2. For the specific amplification of the MT2 promoter, the following primers were used: sense, 5′–ATTCCCAGTCC-CGCTTTCAC-3′, and antisense, 5′-ACTCTAGCCGCCTCTTCAGC-3′. PCR used an AMV amplification buffer and enhancer mixture under the following conditions: 95°C denaturation, 55°C annealing and 72°C extension. The PCR product was purified by Qiagen Quick Spin kit (Qiagen, Inc., CA, USA) and the resulting pure DNA was sequenced by dye termination reaction. The three exons were sequenced by the same methodology except that PCR buffer was used in place of the amplification and enhancer mixture. Different primers were also used. The sequencing studies were done at Jutendo University School of Medicine, Tokyo, Japan.

Initial Computer Modeling Studies. Computer models for the MT2 gene and its two clusters, A and B, were obtained from the amino acid sequence determined for metallothionein. A transition state model was also attempted using both molecular mechanics and semiempirical computations with Spartan Pro (Wavefunction, Irvine, CA) software.

Results and Discussion

A total of 72 Filipino and Japanese patients were used in the study, which took place over a period of 2 y. The mean age of the Filipino patients was 63.9 y, whereas the Japanese patients had a mean age of 69.7 y for women and 72.6 y for men. The mean age of the five normal controls was 65.7 y. Indeed, age is a major factor in predisposing individuals to macular degeneration.

The clinical history of the Filipino patients showed histories of hypertension, diabetes, and asthma. Some also had relatives who had eye problems, including blindness as well as macular degeneration. In addition, some were smokers. There were no significant differences in diet among the patients. Almost all of the Filipino patients belonged to the low-income group. However, none were severely malnourished or showed signs of malnutrition. Our studies showed that nutritional factors may not be important in macular degeneration because both low-income Filipino patients and middle-income Japanese patients manifested the disease.

Plasma Zinc and Glucocorticoid Concentrations. The zinc concentration for both normal and ARMD patients showed a broad range of values and a very high SD. The ARMD patients had a plasma zinc concentration range of 121–1750 μg/L compared with normal controls (range, 440–1160 μg/L). Plasma glucocorticoid (cortisone) concentration for ARMD patients was 15.59 ± 3.64 μg/L, whereas normal controls showed a cortisone concentration of 12.79 ± 1.17 μg/L. There was a significant difference between the normal controls and ARMD cortisone concentrations ($P < 0.001$). Both, however, were still within the normal range of values, which is 3–16 μg/L for glucocorticoid (cortisone).

These results showed that plasma zinc concentration in the ARMD patients may not serve as an important marker for macular degeneration as with our monkey model. There was, however, a significant difference in the glucocorticoid concentration of the normal controls and the patients with ARMD, indicating that hormonal changes may also predispose individuals to macular degeneration.

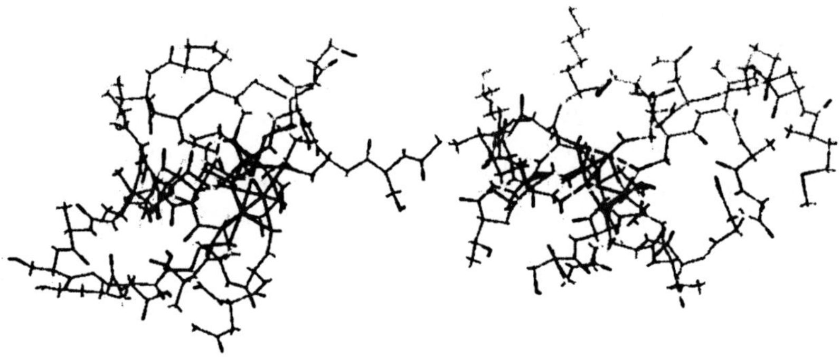

Fig. 21.1. Computer-generated model of metallothionein 2 (MT2) in humans showing clusters A and B and the zinc binding sites (in black). The model was generated from known amino acid sequence using molecular mechanics with Spartan Pro software (Wavefunction, Irvine, CA).

DNA Sequencing Analysis of Promoter Region and Exons of MT2. A 400-bp sequence upstream of the structural gene, which contains the promoter region and other regulatory regions such as the glucocorticoid binding site, was sequenced. We detected an A/A → G/G and A/G → G/G transition near the glucocorticoid binding site in both ARMD and normal controls. The position of this base was 180 upstream of the TATA box. This therefore seemed to be a polymorphism of the promoter gene.

Initial studies determined the sequencing of the three exons of the structural gene for MT2 for both normal controls and ARMD DNA. These initial studies showed an Asp11GlN amino acid change in cluster B of metallothionein in 8 of 37 Japanese patients.

Initial Computer Modeling Studies. The computer model for MT2 is shown in Figure 21.1. This model is consistent with that reported by others and showed two clusters, A and B, formed around a zinc binding site. There were four zinc atoms in cluster A and three in cluster B. All of the zinc atoms were coordinated with the thiol groups of the 20 cysteine molecules found in metallothionein, forming two thiolate clusters. After removal of the apothionein, the zinc binding sites of cluster B showing an Asp11GlN change for normal and altered sequence were compared. The results shown in Figure 21.2 indicate a distortion of the structure of the thiolate cluster for the altered sequence. A comparison of the volume of this site showed that the normal zinc thiolate cluster had a volume of 314.73 (A^3) compared with a volume of 318.79 A^3 for the altered sequence. Equilibrium energy of the normal cluster B was 869.15 vs. 373.99 kcal/mol for the altered sequence. Thus it appears that the altered sequence was more stable than the normal sequence. This was confirmed by initial transition state energy computations, which showed that although zinc was easily

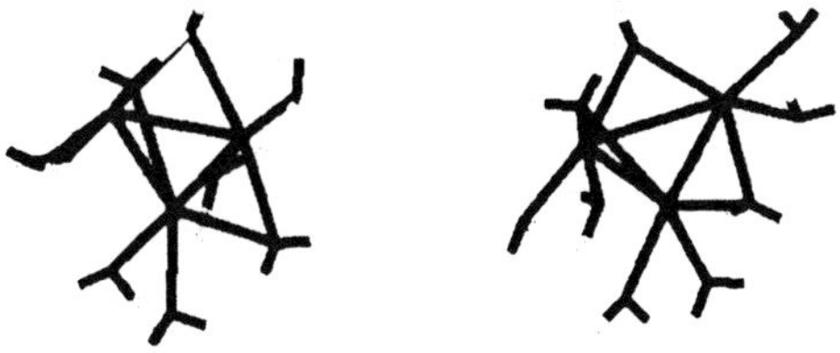

Cluster B (MT2) Zinc site

Cluster BmutB Zinc site (asp 11 gIN)

Fig. 21.2. Zinc binding site in Cluster B of metallothionein 2 (MT2). The site was obtained by cutting the apothionein in computer-generated models using molecular mechanics with Spartan Pro software (Wavefunction, Irvine, CA).

bound to the altered sequence, it was more difficult to remove the bound atoms of zinc. Thus, the altered sequence possessed a lower antioxidant function because the cysteine molecules could not be released from binding with the zinc atoms.

Summary

There are several predisposing factors to macular degeneration, including the following: (i) nutritional deficiencies, notably, zinc deficiency; (ii) age and oxidative stress; (iii) lifestyle or habits such as smoking; (iv) hormonal changes; and (v) genetic factors.

Our studies on macular degeneration showed that age was a major factor predisposing individuals to the disease. However, similar to the monkey model, nutritional deficiency, specifically variations in plasma zinc concentrations, did not necessarily predispose individuals to this disease. Neither did smoking and other factors such as medication and diseases such as hypertension and asthma. These studies also showed that plasma glucocorticoid (cortisone) concentration was significantly higher in the ARMD patients compared with the normal controls although both groups were within the normal range of values. Using our animal model, we extrapolated that oxidative stress could be an important factor in an aging group of individuals who exhibited macular degeneration. Similar to the monkey model, oxidative stress could be brought about by decreased antioxidant activities or free radical–scavenging activities. Other workers reported the induction of metallothionein and catalase gene expression in human RPE as a consequence of phagocytosis and the presence of H_2O_2 (14). In addition, they also reported a decrease in metallothionein concentration in aged human RPE (15). Because glucocorticoid is an inducer of metallothionein synthesis and this was found to be significantly higher in ARMD patients compared with normal controls, it appeared that this was a compensatory mechanism that accounted for increased MT2 synthesis. Consequently, the sequence of regulatory/promoter region and exons of metallothionein was determined. We did not detect any significant difference in the sequence of the MT2 regulatory/promoter region except for an A → G transition that appeared to be a polymorphism of the gene. However, we detected several alterations in the exon region, in particular, an Asp11glN change. Because no linkage analysis could be done, we could not determine whether this was due to a mutation or polymorphism of the structural gene. Molecular mechanics computations using computer software that generated the model of MT2 and its zinc binding site showed that the equilibrium energy for the altered sequence was much lower than that of the normal protein.

Do we now know the mechanism for the pathogenesis of age-related macular degeneration? We still do not, but it would seem that age, hormonal changes, and genetics may play important roles in the etiology of the disease.

Acknowledgments

The authors thank Dr. Vincent Peter Magboo for technical assistance. This work was supported in part by the National Institutes of Health, University of the Philippines, Manila, Department of Ophthalmology. Juntendo University School of Medicine, Tokyo, JASCAA. and the Japan Society for the Promotion of Science (JSPS).

References

1. Farkas, T.G., Sylvester, V., Archer, D., and Altona, M. (1971) The Histochemistry of Drusen. *Am. J. Ophthalmol. 71*, 1206–1215.
2. Ulshafer, R.J., Engel, H.M., Dawson, W.W., Allen, C.B., and Kessler, M.J. (1987) Macular Degeneration in a Community of Rhesus Monkeys: Ultrastructural Observations. *Retina 7*, 198–203.
3. Klein, R., Meuer, S.M., Moss, S.E., and Klein, B.E.K. (1992). Detection of Drusen and Early Signs of Age-Related Maculopathy Using a Nonmydriatic Camera and a Standard Fundus Camera. *Ophthalmology 99*, 1686–1692.
4. Wing, G.L., Blanchard, G.C., and Weiter, J.J. (1978) The Topography and Age Relationship of Lipofuscin Concentration in the Retinal Pigment Epithelium. *Invest. Ophthalmol. Vis. Sci. 17*, 601–607.
5. Feeney-Burns, L., Hilderbrand, E.S., and Eldridge, S. (1984) Aging Human RPE: Morphometric Analysis of Macular, Equatorial and Peripheral Cells. *Investig. Ophthalmol. Vis. Sci. 25*, 195–200.
6. Weiter, J.J., Delori, F.C., Wing, G.L., and Fitch, K.A. (1986) Retinal Pigment Epithelial Lipofuscin and Melanin and Choroidal Melanin in Human Eyes. *Investig. Ophthalmol. Vis. Sci. 27*, 145–152.
7. Ivy, G.O., Kansai, S., Ohta, M., Smith, G., Sato, Y., Kobayashi., M., and Kitani, K. (1990) Lipofuscin-Like Substances Accumulate Rapidly in the Brain, Retina and Internal Organs with Cysteine Protease Inhibition. *Adv. Exp. Med. Biol. 266*, 31–47.
8. Katz, M.L. (1990) Incomplete Proteolysis May Contribute to Lipofuscin Accumulation in the Retinal Pigment Epithelium. *Adv. Exp. Med. Biol. 266*, 109–118.
9. Nicolas, M.G., Fujiki, K., Murayama, K., Suzuki, M.T., Mineki, R., Hayakawa, M., Yoshikawa, Y., Cho, F., and Kanai, A. (1996) Studies on the Mechanisms of Early Onset Macular Degeneration in Cynomolgus Monkeys. I. Abnormal Concentrations of Two Proteins in the Retina. *Exp. Eye Res. 62*, 211–219.
10. Nicolas, M.G., Fujiki, K., Murayama, K., Suzuki, M.T., Shindo, N., Hotta, Y., Iwata, F., Fujimura, T., Yoshikawa, Y., Cho, F., and Kanai, A. (1996) Studies on the Mechanisms of Early Onset Macular Degeneration in Cynomolgus Monkeys. II. Suppression of Metallothionein Synthesis in the Retina in Oxidative Stress. *Exp. Eye Res. 62*, 399–408.

11. Babior, B.M. (1978) Oxygen-Dependent Microbial Killing by Phagocytes. *N. Engl. J. Med. 298*, 659–668.
12. Trenam, C.W., Blake, D.R., and Morris, C.J. (1992) Skin Inflammation: Reactive Oxygen Species and the Role of Iron. *J. Investig. Dermatol. 99*, 675–682.
13. Nicolas, M.G., Fujiki, K., Murayama, K., Iwata, F., Hotta, Y., Suzuki, M.T., Yoshikawa, Y., Cho, F., and Kanai, A. (1995). Synthesis of Metallothionein in the Retina of Cynomolgus Monkeys. *Kimika 11,* 19–24.
14. Tate, D.J., Miceli, M.V., and Newsome, D.A. (1995) Phagocytosis and H_2O_2 Induce Catalase and Metallothionein Gene Expression in Human Retinal Pigment Epithelial Cells. *Investig. Ophthalmol. Vis. Sci. 36*, 1271–1279.
15. Tate, D.J., Newsome, D.A., and Oliver, P.D. (1993) Metallothionein Shows an Age-Related Decrease in Human Macular Retinal Pigment Epithelium. *Investig. Ophthalmol. Vis. Sci. 34*, 2348–2351.

Chapter 22

Antiepileptic Mechanism of Zonisamide Involves Its Antioxidant Effect in the Brain

Akitane Mori,[a] Yasuko Noda,[b] Takao Kaneyuki,[c] and Lester Packer[b]

[a]Okayama University Medical School, Okayama 700-8558, Japan
[b]University of California, Berkeley, CA 94720–3200, U.S.A.
[c]Department of Nutritional Science, Okayama Prefectural University, Soja, Okayama 719-1197, Japan

Introduction

The antiepileptic drug zonisamide (1,2-benzisoxazole-3-methane sulfonamide, ZNS) was first synthesized by Uno and collaborators (1,2) in 1972 (Fig. 22.1). In animal models of epilepsy, ZNS was reported to inhibit experimental seizures, e.g., electroshock- or pentylenetetrazol-induced maximal seizures, or kindled seizures (3–7). ZNS was developed as an antiepileptic drug by Dainippon Pharmaceutical Company (Osaka, Japan); it was launched in Japan in 1989 and in Korea in 1992. The United States Food and Drug Administration approved it as a new antiepileptic drug in 2000. ZNS has excellent clinical efficacy in the treatment of various types of epilepsy, including both partial and generalized seizures (8–15). According to the latest report on 726 newly diagnosed epileptic patients treated with ZNS, seizure control was achieved in ZNS monotherapy in 79% of 99 patients with temporal lobe epilepsy, 84% of 243 with nontemporal lobe epilepsy, and 88% of 17 with unclassified partial epilepsy. ZNS was effective in controlling seizures in 50–100% of 367 patients with generalized epilepsy (16). In spite of its outstanding efficacy, the antiepileptic mechanism of ZNS is not yet fully elucidated. In this chapter, we demonstrate, on the basis of our observations, the antioxidant effect of ZNS to explain in part its antiepileptic mechanism.

Antiepileptic Mechanism of ZNS

ZNS is known to block the voltage-sensitive Na^+ channels. ZNS specifically blocked the sustained repetitive firing of action potentials induced by a depolarizing current pulse in cultured spinal neurons from mouse embryos (17). ZNS caused a hyperpolarizing shift in the steady-state fast inactivation curve and retarded recovery from fast and slow Na^+ inactivation in voltage-clamped Myxicola giant axons (18). In addition, ZNS has been shown to selectively reduce the transient inward current (T-type Ca^{2+} current) in a dose-dependent manner without affecting long-lasting inward current (L-type Ca^{2+} current) in cultured cerebral neurons of rats (19). A reduced voltage-dependent T-type Ca^{2+} current by ZNS was also demonstrated in cultured neuroblastoma cells of human origin (20,21). The effects of ZNS on these ion channels suggest

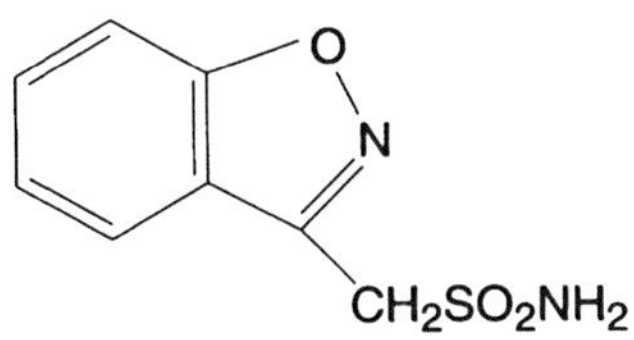

Fig. 22.1. Molecular structure of zonisamide (ZNS).

that ZNS suppresses the epileptiform cellular bursting and limits spread or propagation of seizure activity.

Much evidence has been accumulated to date showing that dopaminergic activity is decreased in epileptic patients. 3,4-Dihydroxyphenylalanine (L-DOPA, a precursor of dopamine), is effective in reducing epileptic seizure frequency, especially in refractory cases (22–24). Reduced dopamine and homovanillic acid levels are observed in cerebrospinal fluid in epileptic patients (25–27). Lower levels of dopamine are demonstrated in epileptic focus tissues compared with surrounding tissues or control tissues, i.e., surgically rejected brain tissue of epileptic patients (28,29). ZNS has been reported to have biphasic effects on dopamine function depending on the dosage level, i.e., therapeutic doses (20–50 mg/kg) enhance dopaminergic function, whereas a supratherapeutic dose (100 mg/kg) inhibits dopaminergic function. This biphasic effect may account for the anticonvulsive effect of therapeutic doses and for the side effects seen with supratherapeutic doses, such as sedation or proconvulsive effects (30).

ZNS is reported to be a weak carbonic anhydrase inhibitor (31). Carbonic anhydrase, such as acetazolamide, blocks the action of brain carbonic anhydrase, resulting in the elevation of interneuronal CO_2, a subsequent decrease in intracellular pH, and depression of neuronal activity (32). However, the inhibitory action of ZNS on carbonic anhydrase may not be a significant component of its anticonvulsant mechanism (15).

ZNS may have specific binding sites in the crude membrane fraction of rat brain, which may relate to benzodiazepine receptors (33). However, ZNS did not alter the postsynaptic response to γ-aminobutyric acid (GABA) in cultured mouse spinal neurons (34). At the same time, ZNS is reported to accelerate GABA release from the hippocampus of epileptic El mice, although it did not accelerate GABA release in control ddY mice (35). The modulation of the GABAergic transmission system may not be the most likely mechanism of action of ZNS.

Antioxidant Activities of ZNS

ZNS is known to have a protective effect on ischemic damage to neonatal rats (36) and gerbils (37). Further, an anticonvulsant dose of ZNS ameliorated brain infarction and the occurrence of neurological deficit after transient focal cerebral ischemia (38). The mechanism of cerebral ischemia involves the generation of oxygen and nitrogen free radicals (39–42). ZNS has been demonstrated to inhibit thiobarbituric acid–reactive substances (TBARS) formation by ferrous chloride and ascorbate in rat cerebral cortex homogenate and in iron-induced epileptic foci of rats (43). We observed the effect

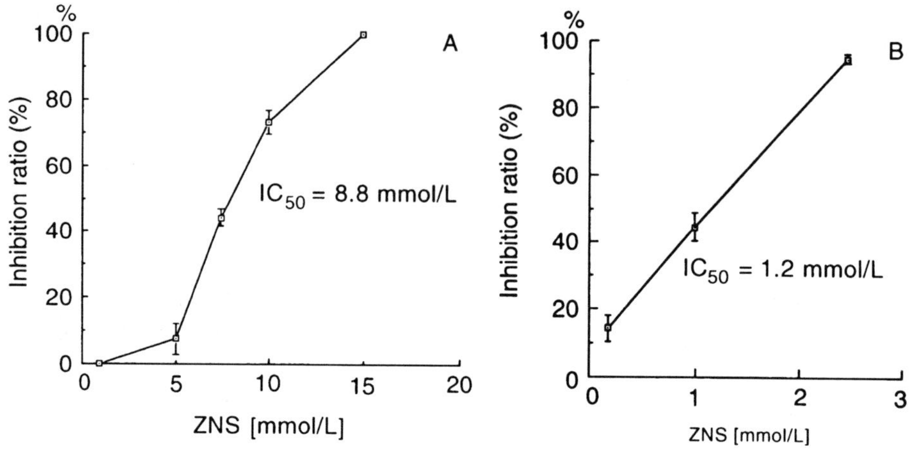

Fig. 22.2. (A) Effect of zonisamide (ZNS) on lipid peroxidation by H_2O_2 in rat brain homogenate. Rat brain homogenate (6% by wt/vol, final) was incubated with H_2O_2 (5 mnmol/L, final) at 37°C for 10 min. (B) Effect of ZNS on lipid peroxidation by $FeCl_2$/ascorbate in rat brain homogenate. Rat brain homogenate (2% by wt/vol, final) was incubated with $FeCl_2$ (0.2 mmol/L, final) and ascorbate (0.02 mmol/L, final) at 37°C for 10 min. *Abbreviation*: IC_{50}, 50% inhibitory concentration.

of ZNS on lipid peroxidation by hydrogen peroxide and by ferrous chloride/ascorbate (44) in the rat brain homogenate. Malondialdehyde plus 4-hydroxyalkenals were measured as an index of lipid peroxidation, using the LPO-586 Kit (OXIS International, Portland, OR). In these experiments, ZNS inhibited lipid peroxidation by both hydrogen peroxide and ferrous chloride/ascorbate in a dose-dependent manner (Fig. 22.2, A and B). On the other hand, ZNS has been shown to reduce the increased levels of 8-hydroxy-2′-deoxyguanosine, a marker for oxidative DNA damage, formed in the brain during iron-induced epileptogenesis in rats (45).

Free Radical–Scavenging Activities of ZNS

The free radical–scavenging activities of ZNS were measured using an electron spin resonance (ESR) spectrometer with spin trap 5,5-dimethyl-1-pyrroline-*N*-oxide (46), and it was observed that ZNS scavenged the hydroxyl radical ($^{\bullet}OH$) in a dose-dependent manner (Fig. 22.3). The 50% inhibitory concentration (IC_{50}) was estimated to be 0.9 mmol/L, and even 0.078 mmol/L of ZNS significantly scavenged $^{\bullet}OH$; this amount could be considered to be in a physiologically relevant range. At the same time, no effect of ZNS on superoxide ($O_2^{\bullet-}$) was observed up to the final concentration of 25 mmol/L (47). Nitric oxide (NO) scavenging activity of ZNS was measured using 1-hydroxy-2-oxo-3-(*N*-methyl-3-aminopropyl)-3-methyl-1-triazene (NOC-7) and 2-(4-carboxyphenyl)-4,4,5,5-tetramethyl-imidazoline-1-oxyl-3-oxide (carboxy-PTIO) according to Akaike *et al* (48). Carboxy-PTIO showed a penta-signal in the ESR recording [Fig. 22.4A (a)]. This signal disappeared and the hepta-signal

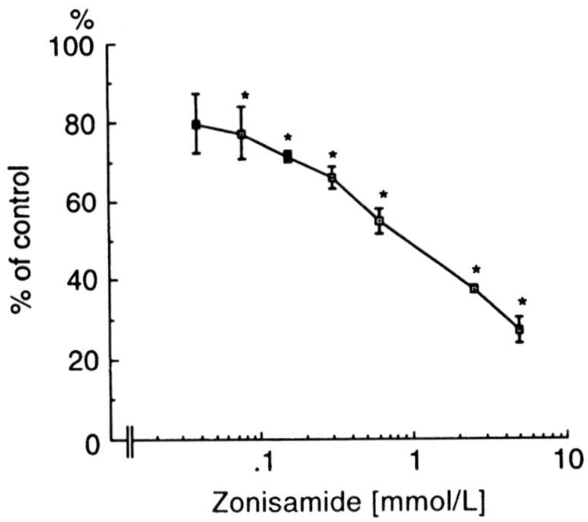

Fig. 22.3. Hydroxyl radical–scavenging activity of zonisamide (ZNS). Hydroxyl radical generation system was as follows: H_2O_2 (0.05 mmol/L, final); $FeSO_4$ (0.005 mmol/L, final); 5-5-dimethylpyrroline-*N*-oxide (DMPO) 0.25 mmol/L (final). Values are expressed as means ± SEM ($n = 4$); *$P < 0.05$, compared with control.

of 2-(4-carboxyphenyl)-4,4,5,5-tetramethylimidazoline-1-oxyl (carboxy-PTI) (theoretically a nine-line signal, but two lines overlapped the other lines) appeared in the ESR recording after addition of a NO generator, NOC-7 [Fig. 22.4A (b)]. The NO scavenging activity of ZNS was dose dependent up to the final concentration of 10 mmol/L (Fig. 22.4B).

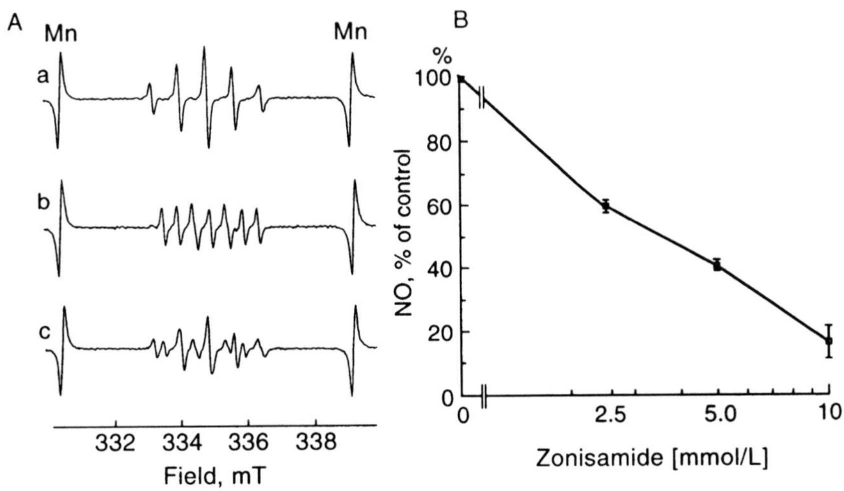

Fig. 22.4. Nitric oxide–scavenging activity of zonisamide (ZNS). (A) Electron spin resonance (ESR) spectra of 2-(4-carboxyphenyl)-4,4,5,5-tetramethyl-imidazoline-1-oxyl-3-oxide (carboxy-PTIO) and 2-(4-carboxyphenyl)-4,4,5,5-tetramethylimidazoline-1-oxyl (carboxy-PTI). (a) Carboxy-PTIO (10 μmol/L) only; (b) Carboxy-PTIO (10 μmol/L) plus nitric oxide [20 min after addition of 1-hydroxy-2-oxo-3-(*N*-methyl-3-aminopropyl)-3-methyl-1-triazene (NOC-7)]; (c) carboxy-PTIO (10 μmol/L) plus nitric oxide with ZNS (10 mmol/L) (20 min after addition of NOC-7). (B) Dose dependence of nitric oxide–scavenging activity by ZNS (2.5–10 mmol/L). Values are expressed as means ± SEM ($n = 3$). *Source*: Ref. 47.

Inhibitory Effect of ZNS on Nitric Oxide Synthase (NOS) Activity by N-Methyl-D-Aspartate (NMDA) and Buthionine Sulfoximine (BSO)

NMDA is a structural analog of the excitatory transmitter, glutamate, and has a potent toxic effect on neurons when applied in an excessive amount in brain tissue either *in vivo* or *in vitro* (49). NMDA receptor activation produces NO and reactive species (50,51). Furthermore, the seizures induced by NMDA administration are accompanied by an enhancement of NO generation and of lipid peroxidation in the brain (52). NO has been implicated as a potent mediator of NMDA neurotoxicity (53,54). That is, overproduction of NO may allow it to react with superoxide to form the potent oxidant peroxynitrite (55), although NO is a putative neurotransmitter in the brain and peripheral nervous system (56) and occurs naturally in the brain without causing overt toxicity.

In the neuronal excitation mechanism, transient glutamate stimulation can lead to sustained opening of NMDA receptor–gated ionic channels; the subsequent rise

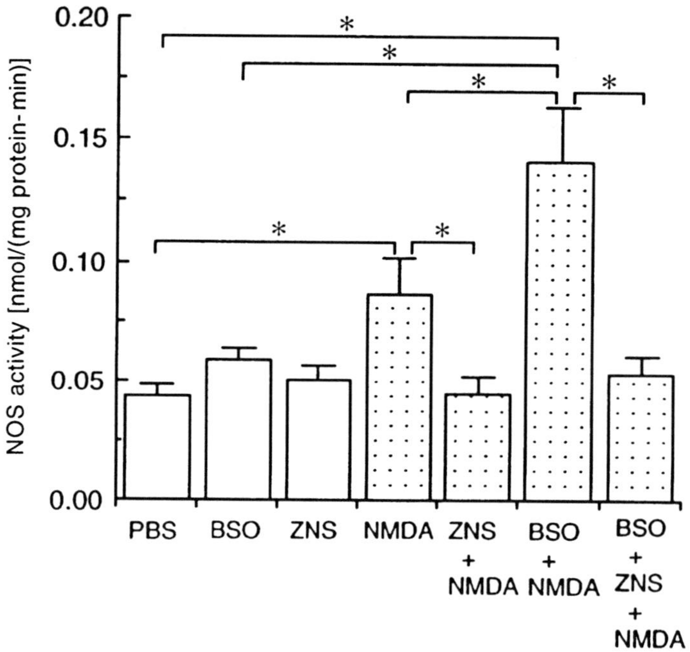

Fig. 22.5. Effect of zonisamide (ZNS) on nitric oxide synthase (NOS) activity in hippocampus of rats. Each group of rats was treated with (1) phosphate-buffered saline (3 h before surgery; control); (2) *N*-methyl-D-aspartate (NMDA) [30 mg/kg, intraperitoneally (i.p.), 3 h]; (3) buthionine sulfoximine (BSO) (150 mg/kg, i.p., 24–27 h); (4) ZNS (50 mg/kg, i.p., 4 h); (5) NMDA (30 mg/kg, i.p., 3 h) for rats pretreated with BSO (150 mg/kg, i.p., 24 h before NMDA injection); (6) ZNS (50 mg/kg, i.p., 1 h before NMDA injection) followed by NMDA (30 mg/kg, i.p., 3 h); or (7) ZNS (50 mg/kg, i.p., 1 h before NMDA injection) and NMDA (30 mg/kg, i.p., 3 h) for rats pretreated with BSO (150 mg/kg, i.p., 24 h before ZNS injection). Data are means ± SEM, (n = 6–10); *significant difference between the two groups ($P < 0.05$). *Source*: Ref. 47.

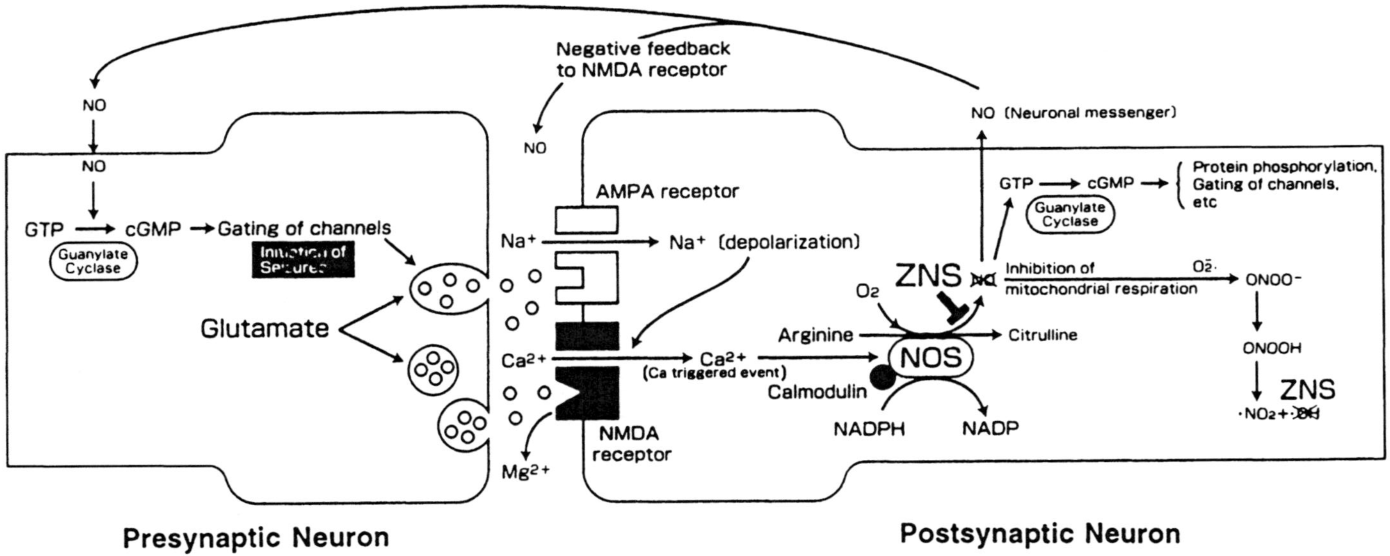

Fig. 22.6. Possible inhibitory effect of zonisamide (ZNS) on excitatory amino acid–induced seizures. ZNS scavenges NO and •OH radicals, and inhibits NO production. To simplify the figure, kainate and metabotropic glutamate receptors were not shown, and NO is illustrated to act on presynaptic neurons, even though NO can actually diffuse as a gas into nearby neuronal cells and act on them. *Abbreviations*: NO, nitric oxide; NOS, nitric oxide synthase; GTP, guanosine 5′-triphosphate; cGMP, cyclic guanosine 3′, 5′-monophosphate; $NADP^+$, nicotinamide adenine dinucleotide phosphate; NADPH, reduced form $NADP^+$; $ONOO^-$, peroxynitrite anion; AMPA, α-amino-3-hydroxy-5-methylisoxazole-4-propionic acid; NMDA, *N*-methyl-D-aspartate. *Source*: Ref. 64.

in cytosolic Ca^{2+} can stimulate NOS (57). Otherwise, NMDA is known to activate Ca^{2+}-independent NOS activity in rat striatum, and this activity is blocked by dexamethasone and aminoguanosine, suggesting the involvement of i-NOS (58).

L-Buthionine-[*S*,*R*]-sulfoximine (BSO), a specific inhibitor of γ–glutamylcysteine synthase, blocks glutathione synthesis and induces endogenous oxidative stress (59–62). Glutathione depletion is known to be accompanied by increased neuronal NOS activity *in vivo* and *in vitro* (63).

We examined the effect of ZNS on NOS activity induced by NMDA and BSO on the rat hippocampus (64). NOS activity was markedly increased by NMDA and BSO treatment. ZNS did not affect the basal level of NOS activity, but inhibited NOS activities, enhanced by NMDA with/without BSO, to the control levels in the hippocampus (Fig. 22.5).

Possible Inhibiting Mechanism of ZNS in NMDA-Induced Seizures

Generally NO is thought to be involved in the seizure mechanism in both initiation and termination of seizures as follows (65): (i) Excitatory neurotransmitter, glutamate release from presynaptic terminal acts on NMDA and α-amino-3-hydroxymethylisoxazole-4-propionic acid (AMPA) receptors. (ii) When the postsynaptic membrane is sufficiently depolarized by Na^+ influx and blocking of NMDA channels by Mg^{2+} is reduced, Ca^{2+} influx is accelerated and activates NOS. (iii) NO production activates guanyl cyclase, and the generated cyclic GMP (cGMP) is related to initiation and propagation of seizures (66). (iv) On the other hand, excess NO generated by accelerated NOS activity inhibits glutamate binding to NMDA receptor in a negative-feedback manner (67,68), i.e., it contributes to the termination of seizures (Fig. 22.6).

In conclusion, ZNS may inhibit initiation and propagation of seizures by inhibiting excess NO production and by controlling cGMP activation; it may also protect neurons from free radical damage by NO and/or •OH (47). ZNS has been known to have a protective effect on ischemic damage (36–38). ZNS may protect neurons from free radical damage, which is a common problem not only in epileptic seizures or ischemic injury but also in other brain disorders such as Parkinson's disease, Alzheimer's disease, and other age-related diseases.

References

1. Uno, H., Kurokawa, M., Masuda, Y., and Nishimura, H. (1979) Studies on 3-Substituted 1,2-Benzisoxazole Derivatives. 6. Synthesis of 3-(Sulfamoylmethyl)-1,2-benzisoxazole Derivatives and Their Anticonvulsant Activities. *J. Med. Chem. 22*, 180–183.
2. Uno, H., Kurokawa, M., Natsuka, K., Yamato, Y., and Nishimura, H. (1976) Studies On 3-Substituted 1,2-Benzisoxazole Derivatives. 1. *Chem. Pharm. Bull. 24*, 632–643.
3. Masuda, Y., Utsui, Y., Shiraishi, Y., Karasawa, T., Yoshida, K., and Shimizu, M. (1979) Relationships Between Plasma Concentrations of Diphenylhydantoin, Phenobarbital, Carbamazepine, and 3-Sulfamoylmethyl-1,2-benzisoxazole (AD-810), a New Anticonvulsant Agent, and Their Anticonvulsant or Neurotoxic Effects in Experimental Animals. *Epilepsia 20*, 23–33.

4. Masuda, Y., Shiraishi, Y., Karasawa, T., Yoshida, K., and Shimizu, M. (1980) Differential Antagonisms of Anticonvulsants to Various Components of Maximal Seizures Induced by Electroshock or Pentylenetetrazol in Mice. *J. Pharmacobio-Dyn. 3*, 526–531.
5. Masuda, Y., Karasawa, T., Shiraishi, Y., Hori, M., Yoshida, K., and Shimizu, M. (1980) 3-Sulfamoylmethyl-1,2-benzisoxazole, a New Type of Anticonvulsant Drug. Pharmacological Profile. *Arzneim.-Forsch. 30*, 477–483.
6. Kamei, C., Oka, M., Masuda, Y., Yoshida, K., and Shimizu, M. (1981) Effects of 3-Sulfamoylmethyl-1,2-benzisoxazole (AD-810) and Some Antiepileptics on the Kindled Seizures in the Neocortex, Hippocampus and Amygdala in Rats. *Arch. Int. Pharmacodyn. Ther. 249*, 164–176.
7. Hamada, K., Ishida, S., Yagi, K., and Seino, M. (1990) Anticonvulsant Effects of Zonisamide on Amygdaloid Kindling in Rats. *Neurosciences 16*, 407–412.
8. Ono, T., Yagi, K., and Seino, M. (1988) Clinical Efficacy and Safety of a New Antiepileptic Drug, Zonisamide. A Multi-Institutional Phase Three Study. *Clin. Psychiatry 30*, 471–482 (in Japanese).
9. Oguni, H., Hayashi, K., Fukuyama, Y., Iimura, K., Seki, T., Seino, M., Watanabe, K., Mimaki, T., Ootahara, S., Kurokawa, T., and Kuriya, N. (1988) Phase III Study of a New Antiepileptic AD-810, Zonisamide in Childhood Epilepsy. *Shohnika Rynsho (Jpn. J. Pediatr.) 41*, 439–450 (in Japanese).
10. Yagi, K., and Seino, M. (1992) Methodological Requirements for Clinical Trials in Refractory Epilepsies—Our Experience with Zonisamide. *Prog. Neuropsycho.-Pharmacol. Biol. Psychiatry 16*, 79–85.
11. Schmidt, D., Jacob, R., Loiseau, P., Deisenhammer, E., Klinger, D., Despland, A., Egli, M., Bauer, G., Stenzel, E., and Blankenhorn, V. (1993) Zonisamide for Add-On Treatment of Refractory Partial Epilepsy: A European Double-Blind Trial. *Epilepsy Res. 15*, 67–73.
12. Leppik, I.E., Willmore, L.J., Homan, R.W., Fromm, G., Oommen, K.J., Penry, J.K., Sackellares, J.C., Smith, D.B., Lesser, R.P., Wallace, J.D., Trudeau, J.L., Lamoreaux, L.K., and Spenser, M. (1993) Efficacy and Safety of Zonisamide: Results of a Multicenter Study. *Epilepsy Res. 14*, 165–173.
13. Seino, M., Naruto, S., Ito, T., and Miyazaki, M. (1995) *Zonisamide in Antiepileptic Drugs*, 4th edn., (Levy, R.H., Rattson, R.M., and Meldrum, B.S., eds.) pp. 1011–1023, Raven Press, New York.
14. Masuda, Y., Ishizaki, M., and Shimizu, M. (1998) Zonisamide: Pharmacology and Clinical Efficacy in Epilepsy. *CNS Drug Rev. 4*, 341–360.
15. Oommen, K.J., and Mathews, S. (1999) Zonisamide: A New Antiepileptic Drug. *Clin. Neuropharmacol. 22*, 192–200.
16. Yagi, K., and Privitera, M.D. (2000) Efficacy of Zonisamide Monotherapy. *Neurology 54 (Suppl. 3)*, A125 (abstr.).
17. Rock, D.M., Macdonald, R.L., and Taylor, C.P. (1989) Blockade of Sustained Repetitive Action Potentials in Cultured Spinal Cord Neurons by Zonisamide (AD-810, CI-912) a Novel Anticonvulsant. *Epilepsy Res. 3*, 138–143.
18. Schauf, C.L. (1987) Zonisamide Enhances Slow Sodium Inactivation in Myxicola. *Brain Res. 413*, 185–188.
19. Suzuki, S., Kawakami, K., Nishimura, S., Watanabe, Y., Yagi, K., Seino, M., and Miyamoto, K. (1992) Zonisamide Blocks T-Type Calcium Channel in Cultured Neurons of Rat Cerebral Cortex. *Epilepsy Res. 12*, 21–27.

20. Kito, M., Maehara, M., and Watanabe, K. (1994) Antiepileptic Drugs—Calcium Current Interaction in Cultured Human Neuroblastoma Cells. *Seizure 3*, 141–149.
21. Kito, M., Maehara, M., and Watanabe, K. (1996) Mechanisms of T-Type Calcium Channel Blockade by Zonisamide. *Seizure 5*, 115–119.
22. Ito, M., Okuno, T., and Mikawa, H. (1982) Brain Monoamine Metabolism and L- DOPA Therapy for Children with Intractable Epilepsy. *Ann. Paediatr. Jpn. 28*, 32–38.
23. Leino, E. (1981) Open Trial with Levodopa-Carbidopa Combination to Patients with Long-Standing Progressive Myoclonus Epilepsy. *Acta Neurol. Scand. 63*, 389–394.
24. Obeso, J.A., Artieda, J., Tuñón, T., Luquin, M.R., and Martinez-Lage, J.M. (1985) Dopamine Agonists Suppress Visual-Cortical Reflux Myoclonus. *J. Neurol. Neurosurg. Psychiatry 48*, 1277–1283.
25. Barolin, G.S., and Hornykiewicz, O. (1967) Zur diagnostischen Wertigkeit der Homovanillinsäure im Liquor cerebrospinalis. *Wien. Med. Wochenschr. 79*, 815–818.
26. Papeschi, R., Molina-Negro, P., Sourkes, T.L. and Erba, G. (1975) The Concentration of Homovanillic Acid and 5-Hydroxyindoleacetic Acid in Ventricular and Lumbar CSF. *Neurology 22*, 1151–1159.
27. Shaywitz, B.A., Cohen, D.J., and Bowers, M.B. (1975) Reduced Cerebrospinal Fluid 5-Hydroxyindoleacetic Acid and Homovanillic Acid in Children with Epilepsy. *Neurology 25*, 72–79.
28. Mori, A., Hiramatsu, M., Namba, S., Nishimoto, A., Ohmoto, T., Mayanagi, Y., and Asakura, T. (1987) Decreased Dopamine Level in Epileptic Focus. *Res. Commun. Chem. Pathol. Pharmacol. 56*, 157–164.
29. Mori, A. (1989) Alterations in Biogenic Amines in Epileptic El Mouse Brain and in Human Epileptic Focus, in *Art and Science of Epilepsy*, (Suzuki, J., Seino, M., Fukuyama, Y., and Komai, S., eds.) pp. 35–38, Elsevier, Amsterdam.
30. Okada, M., Kaneko, S., Hirano, T., Mizuno, K., Kondo, T., Otani, K., and Fukushima, Y. (1995) Effects of Zonisamide on Dopaminergic System. *Epilepsy Res. 13*, 193–205.
31. Masuda, Y., and Karasawa, T. (1993) Inhibitory Effect of Zonisamide on Human Carbonic Anhydrase in Vitro. *Arzneim.-Forsch. 43*, 416–418.
32. Millichap, J.G., Woodbury, D.M., and Goodman, L.S. (1955) Mechanism of the Anticonvulsant Action of Acetazolamide, a Carbonic Anhydrase Inhibitor. *J. Pharmacol. Exp. Ther. 115*, 251–258.
33. Mimaki, T., Suzuki, Y., Tagawa, T., Karasawa, T., and Yabuuchi, H. (1990) Interaction of Zonisamide with Benzodiazepine and GABA Receptors in Rat Brain. *Med. J. Osaka Univ. 39*, 13–17.
34. Taylor, C.P., MacLean, J.R., Bockbrader, N., Buchanan, R.A., Karasawa, T., Miyazaki, M., Rock, D.M., Takemoto, Y., Uno, H., and Walker, R. (1986) Zonisamide (AD-810, CI-912), in *New Anticonvulsant Drugs*, (Meldrum, B.S., and Porter, R.J., eds.) pp. 277–294, John Libbey & Company, London.
35. Endo, A. (1995) Effect of Zonisamide on Neurotransmitter Release from Hippocampal Slice: A Study of Neurotransmitter Release Using an Improved Experimental System. *Okayama Igaku Zasshi 107*, 69–78 (in Japanese).
36. Hayakawa, T., Higuchi, Y., Nigami, H., and Hattori, H. (1994) Zonisamide Reduces Hypoxic-Ischemic Brain Damage in Neonatal Rats Irrespective of Its Anticonvulsive Effect. *Eur. J. Pharmacol. 257*, 131–136.

37. Owen, A., Ijaz, S., Miyashita, H., Wishart, T., Howlett, W., and Shuaib, A. (1997) Zonisamide as a Neuroprotecitve Agent in an Adult Gerbil Model of Global Forebrain Ischemia: A Histological, in Vivo Microdialysis and Behavioral Study. *Brain Res. 770*, 115–122.
38. Minato, H., Kikuta, C., Fujitani, B., and Masuda, Y. (1997) Protective Effect of Zonisamide, an Antiepileptic Drug, Against Transient Focal Cerebral Ischemia with Middle Cerebral Artery Occlusion-Reperfusion in Rats. *Epilepsia 38*, 975–890.
39. Yamaguchi, S., Ogata, H., Hamaguchi, S., and Kitajima, T. (1998) Superoxide Radical Generation and Histopathological Changes in Hippocampal CA1 after Ischemia/Repurfusion in Gerbils. *Can. J. Anaesth. 45*, 226–232.
40. Takamatsu, H., Kondo, K., Ikeda, Y., and Umemura, K. (1998) Hydroxyl Radical Generation After the Third Hour Following Ischemia Contributes to Brain Damage. *Eur. J. Parmacol. 10*, 165–169.
41. Yang, Y., Li. Q., and Shuaib, A. (2000) Neuroprotection by 2-h Postischemia Administration of Two Free Radical Scavengers, α-Phenyl-*N-tert*-butyl-nitrone (PBN) and *N-tert*-Butyl-(2-sulfophenyl)-nitrone (S-PBN), in Rats Subjected to Focal Embolic Cerebral Ischemia. *Exp. Neurol. 163*, 39–45.
42. Love, S. (1999) Oxidative Stress in Brain Ischemia. *Brain Pathol. 9*, 119–131.
43. Komatsu, M., Okamura, Y., and Hiramatsu, M. (1995) Free Radical Scavenging Activity of Zonisamide and Its Inhibitory Effect on Lipid Peroxide Formation in Iron-Induced Epileptogenic Foci of Rats. *Neurosciences 21*, 23–29.
44. Smith, G.J., and Dunkley, W.L. (1962) Initiation of Lipid Peroxidation by a Reduced Metal Ion. *Arch. Biochem. Biophys. 98*, 46–48.
45. Komatsu, M., Hiramatsu, M., and Willmore, L.J. (2000) Zonisamide Reduces The Increase in 8-Hydroxy-2′-deoxyguanosine Levels in the Brain Formed During Iron-Induced Epileptogenesis in Rats. *Epilepsia 41*, 1091–1094.
46. Noda, Y., Anzai, K., Mori, A., Kohno, M., Shimmei, M., and Packer, L. (1997) Hydroxyl and Superoxide Anion Radical Scavenging Activities of Natural Source Antioxidants Using the Computerized JES-FR30 ESR Spectrometer System. *Biochem. Mol. Biol. Int. 42*, 35–44.
47. Mori, A., Noda, Y., and Packer, L. (1998) The Anticonvulsant Zonisamide Scavenges Free Radicals. *Epilepsy Res. 30*, 153–158.
48. Akaike, K., Yoshida, M., Miyamoto, Y., Sato, K., Kohno, M., Sakamoto, K., Miyazaki, K., Ueda, S., and Maeda, M. (1993) Antagonistic Action of Imidazolineoxyl *N*-Oxidase Against Endothelium-Derived Relaxing Factor/•NO Through a Radical Reaction. *Biochemistry 32*, 827–832.
49. Meldrum, B., and Garthwaite, J. (1990) Excitatory Amino Acid Neurotoxicity and Neurodegenerative Disease. *Trends Pharmacol. Sci. 11*, 379–387.
50. Gunasekar, P.G., Kanthasamy, A.G., Borowitz, J.L., and Isom, G.E. (1995) NMDA Receptor Activation Produces Concurrent Generation of Nitric Oxide and Reactive Oxygen Species: Implication for Cell Death. *J. Neurochem. 65*, 2016–2021.
51. Gunasekar, P.G., Sun, P.W., Kanthasamy, A.G., Borowitz, J.L., and Isom, G.E. (1996) Cyanide-Induced Neurotoxicity Involves Nitric Oxide and Reactive Oxygen Species Generation after *N*-Methyl-D-aspartate Receptor Activation. *J. Pharmacol. Exp. Ther. 277*, 150–155.

52. Raevskii, K.S., Bashkatova, V.G., Vitskova, G.I.U., Narkevich, V.B., Mikoian, V.D., and Vanin, A.F. (1998) The Seizures Induced by *N*-Methyl-D, L-aspartate Administration Are Accompanied with an Enhancement of Nitric Oxide Generation and of Lipid Peroxidation Process in the Rat Brain. *Eksp. Klin. Farmakol. 61*, 13–16 (in Russian).
53. Dawson, T.M., Dawson, V.L., and Snyder, S.H. (1992) A Novel Neuronal Messenger Molecule in Brain: The Free Radical, Nitric Oxide. *Ann. Neurol. 32*, 297–311.
54. Zhang, J., Dawson, V.L., Dawson, T.M., and Snyder, S.H. (1994) Nitric Oxide Activation of Poly (ADP-ribose) Synthetase in Neurotoxicity. *Science 263*, 687–689.
55. Beckman, J.S., Beckman, T.W., Chen, J., Marshall, P.A., and Freeman, B.A. (1990) Apparent Hydroxyl Radical Production by Peroxynitrite: Implications for Endothelial Injury from Nitric Oxide and Superoxide. *Proc. Natl. Acad. Sci. USA 87*, 1620–1624.
56. Holscher, C. (1997) Nitric Oxide, the Enigmatic Neuronal Messenger: Its Role in Synaptic Plasticity. *Trends Neurosci. 20*, 298–303.
57. Akira, T., Henry, D., and Wasterlain, C.G. (1994) Nitric Oxide Mediates the Sustained Opening of NMDA Receptor-Gated Ionic Channels Which Follows Transient Excitotoxic Exposure in Hippocampal Slices. *Brain Res. 652*, 190–194.
58. Lecanu, L., Verrecchia, C., Margaill, I., Boulu, R.G., and Plotkine, M. (1998) iNOS Contribution to the NMDA-Induced Excitotoxic Lesion in the Rat Striatum. *Br. J. Pharmacol. 125*, 584–590.
59. Jain, A., Martensson, J., Stole, E., Auld, P.A., and Meister, A. (1991) Glutathione Deficiency Leads to Mitochondrial Damage in Brain. *Proc. Natl. Acad. Sci. USA 88*, 1913–1917.
60. Martensson, J., Jain, A., Stole, E., Frayer, W., Auld, P.A., and Meister, A. (1991) Inhibition of Glutathione Synthesis in the Newborn Rat: A Model for Endogenously Produced Oxidative Stress. *Proc. Natl. Acad. Sci. USA 88*, 9360–9364.
61. Meister, A. (1991) Glutathione Deficiency Produced by Inhibition of Its Synthesis, and Its Reversal; Applications in Research and Therapy. *Pharmacol. Ther. 51*, 155–194.
62. Mizui, T., Kinouchi, H., and Chan, P.H. (1992) Depletion of Brain Glutathione by Buthionine Sulfoximine Enhances Cerebral Ischemic Injury in Rats. *Am. J. Physiol. 262*, H313–H317.
63. Heales, S.J.R., Bolaños, J.P., and Clark, J.B. (1996) Glutathione Depletion Is Accompanied by Increased Neuronal Nitric Oxide Synthase Activity. *Neurochem. Res. 21*, 35–39.
64. Noda, Y., Mori, A., and Packer, L. (1999) Zonisamide Inhibits Nitric Oxide Synthase Activity Induced by *N*-Methyl-D-aspartate and Buthionine Sulfoximine in the Rat Hippocampus. *Res. Commun. Mol. Pathol. Pharmacol. 105*, 23–33.
65. Mori, A. (1996) Reactive Oxygen Species and Mechanism of Induction of Seizures by Guanidino Compounds, in *Free Radicals in Brain Physiology and Disorders*, (Packer, L., Hiramatsu, M., and Yoshikawa, T., eds.) pp. 3–15, Academic Press, San Diego.
66. Ferrendelli, J.A., Blank, A.C., and Gross, R.A. (1980) Relationships Between Seizure Activity and Cyclic Nucleotide Levels in Brain. *Brain Res. 200*, 93–103.
67. Manzoni, O., Prezeau, L., Martin, P., Deshager, S., Bockaert, L., and Fagni, L. (1992) Nitric Oxide-Induced Blockade of NMDA Receptors. *Neuron 8*, 653–662.
68. Lipton, S.A. (1996) Distinctive Chemistries of NO-Related Species. *Neurochem. Int. 29*, 111–114.

Chapter 23

Determination of Antioxidant Effects by ESR-CT Imaging of Rat Brain Tissue Damage Formed During Iron-Induced Epileptogenesis in Rats

Midori Hiramatsu,[a] Makiko Komatsu,[a] Katsuki Imao,[b] and Hitoshi Kamada[a]

[a]Institute for Life Support Technology, Yamagata Technopolis Foundation, 2-2-1 Matsuei, Yamagata 990-2473

[b]Saido Company, Imaizumi, Chuoh-ku, Fukuoka 810-0021, Japan.

Introduction

When we digest food, fight infections, and detoxify pollutants, the metabolic processes generate free radicals. Most are neutralized by antioxidants, but some injure proteins and lipids in membranes, and DNA in our cells, leading to aging and most of the chronic and degenerative diseases. In the case of diseases involving brain degeneration, e.g., Alzheimer's disease, Parkinson's disease, and stroke, neuronal cell death is markedly progressed; this cell death is thought to be associated with reactive oxygen and nitrogen species. Antioxidants of free radical scavengers quench these free radicals, reduce the accumulation of oxidative damage, and prolong life span.

Recently we were able to detect brain tissue damage induced by injection of ferric chloride solution into rat hippocampus using L-band electron spin resonance–computed tomography (ESR-CT). Here we describe the effects of free radical scavengers on brain tissue damage, using an L-band ESR-CT system in rats.

Brain Imaging

Because the ESR-CT system cannot detect endogenous free radicals in rats and mice, spin labels have been used to detect free radicals such as the nitroxide radical in brain (1–3) and liver (4) of rats and mice after their injection. Because spin labels are reduced by endogenous antioxidants, a redox state can be found in concentrations of nitroxide radicals. Although carbamoyl-PROXYL does not cross the blood-brain barrier, accumulated nitroxide radicals could be detected in brain tissue, which would lead to membrane damage. We found accumulated nitroxide radicals in the ipsilateral striatum 60 min after injection of 30 μL of 0.1 mol/L $FeCl_3$ into the left striatum of rats (3), which suggests the appearance of tissue damage in the striatum induced by $FeCl_3$. Recently, we detected the accumulation of nitroxide radicals in the ipsilateral hippocampus 3 h after injection of 10 μL of 0.1 mol/L $FeCl_3$ into the left hippocampus of rats (Fig. 23.1A).

The mechanism of brain tissue damage induced by $FeCl_3$ is suggested to result from the generation of free radicals in the neuronal membranes after injection of

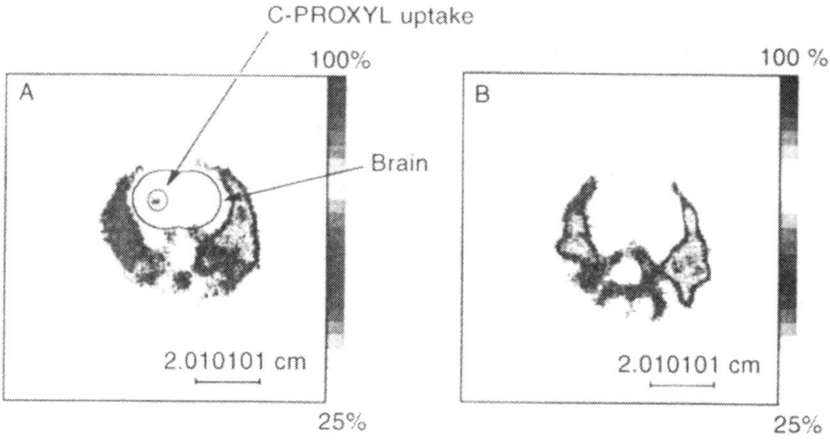

Fig. 23.1. (A) The images of nitroxide radicals in the ipsilateral hippocampus 3 h after injection of 10 μL of 0.1 mol/L ferric chloride into the left hippocampus and intraperitoneal injection of carbamoyl-PROXYL using the L-band ESR-CT system. (B) Preventive effect of zonisamide on the brain tissue damage. Images of the nitroxide radical were not found in the brain area.

$FeCl_3$, which leads to lipid peroxidation after damage in neuronal membranes. Therefore, we examined the effects of free radical scavengers on the tissue damage in the hippocampus of rats using the ESR-CT technique.

Free Radical Scavengers

Zonisamide. Zonisamide, 1,2-benzisoxazole-3-methanesulfonamide, was developed as an antiepileptic by Dainippon Pharmaceutical Company (Osaka, Japan). Its efficacies were reported in the amygdaloid kindling in rats (5,6), photosensitive kindled cats (7), and in epilepsy (8). Zonisamide has free radical–scavenging activity against 1,1-diphenyl-2-picrylhydrazy radical (9), hydroxyl and nitric oxide radicals (10). It diminished lipid peroxidation measured as thiobarbituric acid–reactive substances (TBARS) formation in rat brain homogenate induced by $FeCl_2$ and ascorbic acid, and in the ipsilateral cortex after injection of $FeCl_3$ solution into the left cortex of rats (9). Recently we found that the Fenton reaction accelerates the formation of 8-hydroxy-2′-deoxyguanosine (8-OHdG) in the thymus of calves (Fig. 23.2). Zonisamide inhibited the elevation of 8-OHdG levels in the ipsilateral cortex 30 min after injection of 5 μL of 0.1 mol/L $FeCl_3$ into the left cortex of rats (11).

Fermented Papaya Preparation. The fermented papaya preparation (PS-501) is a sweet, white, granular substance that is sold as a natural functional health food in Japan. It is made by yeast fermentation of *Carica papaya* L., which is popular as a medicinal fruit in the Philippines. We found that PS-501 has free radical–scavenging activity against hydroxyl and DPPH radicals (12) and reduced TBARS formation in

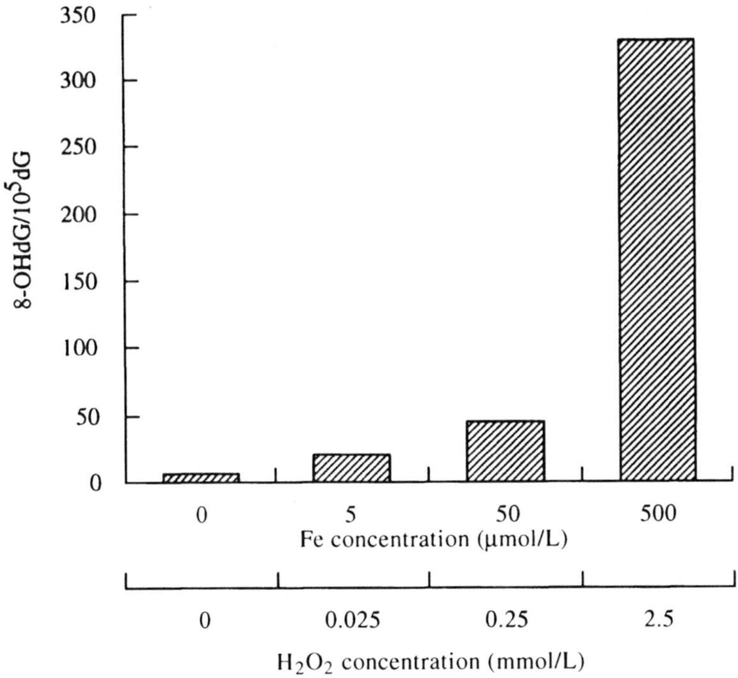

Fig. 23.2. The formation of 8-hydroxy-2′-deoxyguanosine (8-OHdG) in the thymus of calves by Fenton's reaction.

the plasma, hippocampus, and striatum of rats 4 wk after oral administration in drinking water (13). It also reduced the increase in TBARS formation and 8-OHdG level in the ipsilateral cortex 30 min after injection of 5 μL of 0.1 mol/L $FeCl_3$ solution into the left cortex of rats (12,14). These effects are thought to be due to its free radical–scavenging activities.

Petal Extract of Safflower. Dried petals of safflower (*Carthamus tinctorius* L.) have been used in dyes and as herbs from ancient times in countries including Egypt, Ethiopia, Italy, India, China, and Japan. The safflower petal is yellow and red, and its components include safflower yellow and its derivatives, as well as carthamin (Fig. 23.3).

Water and methanol extracts of safflower petals have free radical–scavenging activities against superoxide, hydroxyl, and DPPH radicals. Pigments of yellow and red safflower also scavenge these radicals; a comparison of scavenging activity between yellow and red for DPPH is shown in Table 23.1. The state of scavenging activity in carthamin is almost the same as that of vitamin C, epicatechin gallate, and epigallocatechin gallate (15).

The methanol extract of safflower petals inhibited the elevation of TBARS formation and 8-OHdG level in the ipsilateral cortex of rats 30 min after injection of

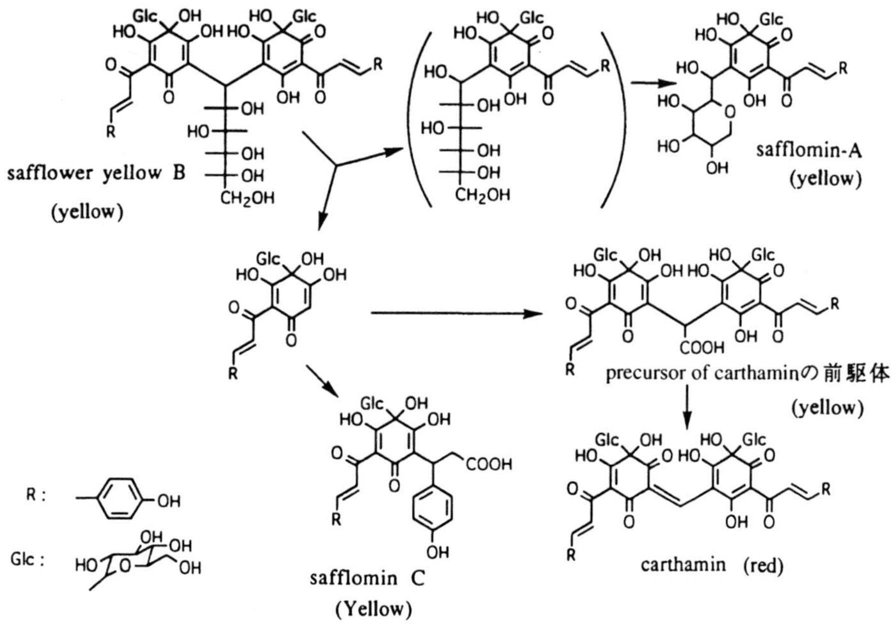

Fig. 23.3. Possible pathway for formation of carthamin from safflower yellow B in petals of safflower. *Source*: Ref. 23.

$FeCl_3$ solution into the left cortex. Carthamin also reduced the increase in 8-OHdG levels in the same model. These effects were thought to be due to the free radical–scavenging activity.

Efficacy of Free Radical Scavengers on Brain Tissue Damage Induced by Iron Injection into the Hippocampus of Rats Using ESR-CT

Injection of microliter volumes of ferric chloride into rodent isocortex induces acute and chronic epileptiform discharges and behavioral seizures. These effects are thought to reflect the neurochemical changes that are initiated in head trauma, with subsequent hemorrhage and the development of post-traumatic epilepsy (16). We injected 10 μL of 0.1 mol/L ferric chloride solution into the hippocampus of rats and observed the appearance of epileptiform discharges. In addition, using the L-band ESR-CT system, we detected the presence of nitroxide radicals in the ipsilateral hippocampus of rats 3 h after injection of 10 μL of 0.1 mol/L ferric chloride solution into the left hippocampus, indicating the induction of tissue damage in the left hippocampus. Pretreatment with three kinds of free radical scavengers, i.e., zonisamide, fermented papaya preparation, and methanol extract of petal safflower, inhibited the brain tissue damage resulting from the injection of the iron solution. That is, no nitroxide radicals were detected in the brain area (Fig. 23.1B).

TABLE 23.1 Comparison of Radical-Scavenging Activity Against 1,1-Diphenyl-2-picrylhydrazy (DPPH) Radical

	Concentration for 50% inhibition	
	(μg/mL)	(μmol/L)
Vitamin C (H_2O)	1.0	5.0
Vitamin E (C_2H_5OH)	30.0	700.0
Safflower yellow (H_2O)	15.0	
Carthamin (DMSO)[a]	1.5	3.3
(-)-Epicatechin 3-O-gallate	1.4	3.2
(-)-Epigallocatechin 3-O-gallate	1.4	3.1
Dried petals of *Carthamus tinctorius* L.	300.0	

[a]DMSO, dimethyl sulfoxide.

Discussion

Memory lapses associated with aging and degenerative neurological disorders, including dementia, stroke, and Parkinson's disease, are the result of neuronal cell death. Neuronal cell death is suggested to be related to peroxynitrite through glutamate.

We found previously that free radical–scavenger activity of the Japanese herb, Sho-saiko-to- go-keishi-ka-shakuyaku-to, inhibited TBARS formation in the aged rat brain (17) and iron-injected rat cortex (18). The herb also led to an increase in life span of senescence accelerated mice (SAMP8) (19). Although choline acetyltransferase activity was decreased in aged rat brain compared with the adult brain, the herb increased choline acetyltransferase activity in aged rat brain (20). The Japanese herb, Toki-shakuyaku-san, also has free radical–scavenging activity against superoxide, hydroxyl and DPPH radicals (21), and it decreased TBARS formation in the cortex, hippocampus and striatum of aged rats. It enhanced the function of cholinergic neurons in aged rats compared with adult rats (22). These data suggest that herbs with free radical–scavenger activity may help maintain neuronal functions during aging, and may be prophylactic against degenerative neurological diseases associated with free radicals.

In consideration of the efficacies of free radical scavengers on lipid peroxidation, proteins, and DNA induced by oxidative stress in brain tissue and our direct and clear data using L-band ESR-CT system, daily intake of free radical scavengers may be essential to maintain a healthy anti-aging state.

Summary

In this study, we found that an intraperitoneal injection of zonisamide and oral administration of the safflower petal extract into the stomach once a day for 7 d inhibited the brain tissue damage 3 h after injection of iron solution into the left hippocampus of rats using L-band ESR-CT system. In addition, oral administration of the fermented papaya preparation in the drinking water for 1 mo also inhibited brain tissue damage. These *in vivo* results revealed that the presence of a free radical scavenger against even one kind of free radical could inhibit tissue damage in addition to lipid peroxide formation and DNA damage in rat brain induced by oxygen stress. Daily intake of free radical scavengers may protect against age-related degenerative neurological disorders and even the memory lapses associated with aging.

References

1. Hiramatsu, M., Oikawa, K., Noda, H., Mori, A., Ogata, T., and Kamada, H. (1996) Free Radical Imaging by Electron Spin Resonance Computed Tomography in Rat Brain. *Brain Res. 697*, 44–47.
2. Hiramatsu, M., Komatsu, M., Oikawa, H., Noda, R., Niwa, R., Konaka, R., Mori, A., and Kamada, H. (1995) in *Bioradicals Detected by ESR Spectroscopy*, (Ohya-Nishiguchi, H., and Packer, L., eds.) pp. 193–202, Birkhauser Verlag, Basel.
3. Hiramatsu, M., Nakajima, M., Komatsu, M., Oikawa, K., Ueda, Y., Nakai, O., and Willmore, L.J. (1996) in *Free Radicals in Brain Physiology and Disorders*, (Packer, L., Hiramatsu, M., and Yoshikawa, T., eds.) pp.185–195, Academic Press, San Diego.
4. Yoshimura, T., Yokoyama, H., Fujii, S., Takayama, F., Oikawa, K., and Kamada, H. (1996) *In Vivo* EPR Detection and Imaging of Endogenous Nitric Oxide in Lipopolysaccharide-Treated Mice. *Nat. Biotechnol. 14*, 992–994.
5. Kamei, C., Oka, M., Masuda, Y., Yoshida, K., and Shimizu, M. (1981) Effects of 3-Sulfamoylmethyl-1,2-benzisoxazole (AD-810) and Some Antiepileptics on the Kindled Seizures in the Neocortex, Hippocampus and Amygdala in Rats. *Arch. Int. Pharmacol. Ther. 249*, 164–176.
6. Hamada, K., Ishida, S., Yagi, K., and Seino, M. (1990) Anticonvulsant Effects of Zonisamide on Amygdaloid Kindling in Rats. *Neurosciences 16*, 407–412.
7. Wada, Y., Hasegawa, H., and Yamaguchi, N. (1990) Effect of a Novel Anticonvulsant, Zonisamide (AD-810, CI-912), in an Experimental Model of Photosensitive Epilepsy. *Epilepsy Res. 7*, 117–120.
8. Masuda, Y., Ishizaki, M., and Shimizu, M. (1998) Zonisamide: Pharmacology and Clinical Efficacy in Epilepsy. *CNS Drug Rev. 4*, 341–360.
9. Komatsu, M., Okamura, Y., and Hiramatsu, M. (1995) Free Radical Scavenging Activity of Zonisamide and Its Inhibitory Effect on Lipid Peroxide Formation in Iron-Induced Epileptogenic Foci of Rats. *Neurosciences 21*, 23–29.
10. Mori, A., Noda, Y., and Packer, L. (1998) The Anticonvulsant Zonisamide Scavenges Free Radicals. *Epilepsy Res. 30*, 153–158.
11. Komatsu, M., Hiramatsu, M., and Willmore, L.J. (2000) Zonisamide Reduces the Increase in 8-Hydroxy-2′-deoxyguanosine Levels Formed During Iron-Induced Epileptogenesis in the Brains of Rats. *Epilepsia 41*, 1091–1094.
12. Imao, K., Wang, H., Komatsu, M., and Hiramatsu, M. (1998) Free Radical Scavenging Activity of Fermented Papaya Preparation and Its Effect on Lipid Peroxide Levels and Superoxide Dismutase Activity in Iron-Induced Epileptic Foci of Rats. *Biochem. Mol. Biol. Int. 45*, 11–23.
13. Wang, H., Komatsu, M., and Hiramatsu, M. (2000) Antioxidant Property of Fermented Papaya Preparation. *Res. Commun. Biochem. Cell Mol. Biol. 4*, 141–147.

14. Imao, K., Komatsu, M., Wang, H., and Hiramatsu, M. (1999) Inhibitory Effect of Fermented Papaya Preparation on Oxidative DNA Damage and Tissue Injury in the Brain Formed During Iron-Induced Epileptogenesis in Rats. *J. Brain Sci. 25*, 71–77.
15. Uchida, S., Edamatsu, R., Hiramatsu, M., Mori, A., Nonaka G., Nishioka, I., Niwa, M., and Ozaki, M. (1987) Condensed Tannins Scavenge Active Oxygen Free Radicals. *Med. Sci. Res. 15*, 831–832.
16. Willmore, L.J., Sypert, G.W., and Munson, J.B. (1978) Chronic Focal Epileptiform Discharges Induced by Injection of Iron into Rat and Cat Cortex. *Science 200*, 1501–1503.
17. Hiramatsu, M., Edamatsu, R., Kabuto, H., and Mori, A. (1987) Inhibitory Effect of Tsumura Sho-saiko-to-go-keishi-ka-shakuyaku-to (TJ-960) on Iron-Induced Epileptic Discharges in Rats. *Clin. Rep. 21*, 59–65.
18. Hiramatsu, M., Edamatsu, R., Ohyama, H., and Mori, A. (1992) in *Lipid Soluble Antioxidants: Biochemistry and Clinical Applications*, (Ong, A.S.H., and Packer, L., eds.) pp. 535–552, Birkhauser Verlag, Basel.
19. Hiramatsu, M., Komatsu, M., and Ueda, Y. (1996) in *Proceedings of the International Symposium on Natural Antioxidants Molecular Mechanisms and Health Effects*, (Packer, L., Traber, M.G., and Xin, W., eds.) pp. 54–63, AOCS Press, Champaign, IL.
20. Hiramatsu, M., Haba, K., Edamatsu, R. Hamada, H., and Mori, A. (1989) Increased Choline Acetyltransferase Activity by Chinese Herbal Medicine Sho-saiko-to-go-keishi-ka-shakuyaku-to in Aged Rat Brain. *Neurochem. Res. 14*, 249–251.
21. Ueda, Y., Komatsu, M., and Hiramatsu, M. (1996) Free Radical Scavenging Activity of the Japanese Herbal Medicine, Toki-shakuyaku-san (TJ-23), and Its Effect on Superoxide Dismutase Activity, Lipid Peroxides, Glutamate and Monoamine Metabolites in Aged Rat Brain. *Neurochem. Res. 21*, 909–914.
22. Hiramatsu, M., Komatsu, M., Yuzurihara T., Ishige, A., and Komatsu, M. (1999) Herbal Medicine, Toki-shakuyaku-san Enhanced Cholinergic Neuronal Functions in the Striatum of Aged Rats. *J. Anti-Aging Med. 2*, 51–57.
23. Kawamoto, K. (1996) Abstract of the 39th Meeting of the Society of Natural Organic Compounds, p. 421.

Chapter 24

Extreme Longevity: The Role of Antioxidant Enzymes, Vitamins, and Micronutrients

Maria Cristina Polidori,[a,b] Antonio Cherubini,[a] Wilhelm Stahl,[b] Leonarda Troiano,[c] Claudio Franceschi,[d] Umberto Senin,[a] Helmut Sies,[b] and Patrizia Mecocci[a]

[a]Institute of Gerontology and Geriatrics, Perugia University Hospital, Perugia, Italy
[b]Institute of Physiological Chemistry I, Heinrich-Heine University, Duesseldorf, Germany
[c]Department of Biomedical Sciences, Section of General Pathology, University of Modena and Reggio Emilia, Italy
[d]Department of Experimental Pathology, University of Bologna, Bologna, Italy

Introduction

Among several theories that have been postulated over the years to explain changes associated with aging, the "free radical" theory remains popular (1) and has been examined for 50 years. It is indeed in these last decades that developed countries have faced an impressive demographic phenomenon, i.e., the remarkable growth of the elderly population as a consequence of the lengthening of life expectancy. That span has grown from ~50 y for a person born in the year 1900 to ~80 years for an individual born in the year 2000 (2–4). Although this has an important effect on the research examining the economic implications and social needs of the growing elderly population, and despite the large number of studies on the biology and pathophysiology of senescence and age-related diseases, the selected population of subjects who reach ≥85 y has not been characterized biologically.

Very old subjects for whom advanced age has come either with disease ("usual aging") or without ("successful aging") (5), are to be considered unique sources of new information on the mechanisms underlying aging and longevity. In contrast to a few decades ago, when individuals with Down's syndrome or progeria were studied to explain age-associated changes, it is possible now to evaluate the type and occurrence of factors influencing these modifications in nonagenarians and centenarians (6). Therefore, in the near future, it will be not only useful, but also mandatory to study critical aspects of biological senescence in these subjects, as follows: (i) whether the age-related increased production of free radicals in the organisms is responsible for the occurrence of age-associated changes (1,7); (ii) whether these changes can be substantially influenced by endogenous antioxidants or by antioxidant supplementation (8); and (iii) whether oxidative stress (9) acts independently of, synergistically, or additively with genetics and defense network systems of the senescent individual.

This paper describes recent advances in the field of oxidative stress and extreme longevity, highlighting the role of the antioxidant defense system of the organism in reaching the most advanced years of life.

Antioxidant Enzymes, Vitamins, and Susceptibility to Oxidative Stress in Centenarians

A large body of experimental research supports the association between oxidative stress and aging; until few years ago, however, data on physiologic human aging were scarce and inconsistent, mainly because research in this field was hindered by a shorter lifespan in humans. Even despite the considerable growth in the number of centenarians in Italy in the last decades (from 49 in 1921 to 1660 in 1990), however, available data on centenarians have been purely epidemiological and clinical (10–12). Nevertheless, in the early 1990s, Franceschi and colleagues (6) published the results of elegant experiments performed on peripheral blood lymphocytes from Down's syndrome and centenarian donors. In these experiments, they exposed cells for 1 h to oxidants produced extracellularly by the xanthine oxidase/hypoxanthine system, and then washed and stimulated them with phytohemagglutinin. The authors observed that the sensitivity of lymphocytes (as assessed by the percentage of ^{3}H-thymidine incorporation into cultures) to oxidant exposure was significantly higher in older patients with Down's syndrome compared with children with Down's syndrome (6), and that this age-related trend of the response to free radicals was present also in healthy subjects, although several years later (13). As opposed to Down's syndrome and usual aging, however, the ability to proliferate after phytohemagglutinin stimulation was found to be preserved in lymphocytes from 17 centenarians, which, unlike cells from younger subjects, also showed a resistance to oxidative stress before the occurrence of irreversible cell damage (6).

In a more recent study performed on 21 healthy centenarians, Pinzani and colleagues (14) assessed serum antioxidant capacity compared with that of 37 healthy subjects aged 18-91 y. Serum antioxidant capacity was 306 ± 108 μmol/L Trolox equivalents in centenarians, which was significantly lower than that in younger subjects (493 ± 183 μmol/L Trolox equivalents) (14). The authors, recognizing the lack of specificity of the assay (15), measured serum levels of urate and bilirubin as well. They found similar serum urate levels in centenarians and younger subjects, whereas total bilirubin was significantly lower in centenarians (14).

Subsequently, Paolisso and colleagues (16) published the results of a study performed to assess plasma levels of vitamin C and E and the reduced/oxidized glutathione ratio (GSH/GSSG), as well as indices of lipid peroxidation [malondialdehyde (MDA)/thiobarbituric acid–reactive substances (TBARS) and lipid hydroperoxides (LPO)] in 30 young adults (<50 y old), in 30 aged subjects (70–99 y old) and in 22 centenarians. Plasma lipid peroxidation, as assessed by TBARS and LPO levels, was found to be significantly more pronounced in centenarians than in young adults, but lower than in aged subjects. In contrast, plasma GSH/GSSG, vitamin C and E were significantly higher in centenarians than in aged subjects, and the authors concluded that healthy centenarians show a low degree of oxidative stress compared with younger subjects (16).

These two studies (14,16) did not use the same measures of oxidative stress and are therefore not directly comparable. We recently evaluated plasma levels of MDA [by high-performance liquid chromatography (HPLC) with fluorescence detection]

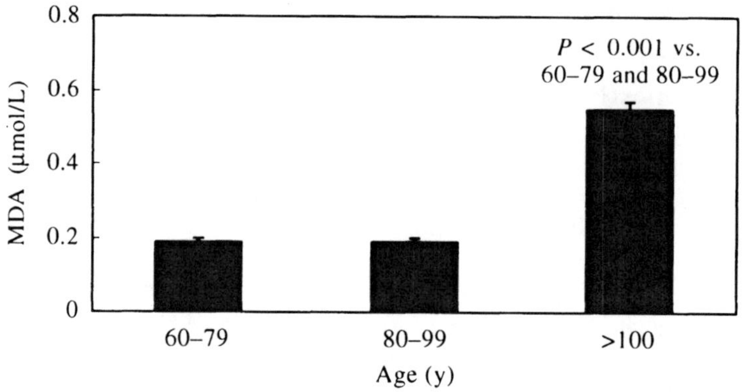

Fig. 24.1. Plasma malondialdehyde (MDA) concentrations in 16 healthy subjects aged 60–79 y, in 12 healthy subjects aged 80–99 y, and in 17 centenarians. Values are means ± SEM.

and of vitamin C (by HPLC with electrochemical detection) in 16 healthy subjects aged 60–79 y, in 12 healthy subjects aged 80–99 y and in 17 centenarians (4 men, 13 women, 101.5 ± 0.4 y) (17).

As shown in Figures 24.1 and 24.2, we found significantly higher levels of plasma MDA and significantly lower levels of plasma vitamin C in centenarians compared with younger subjects. Vitamin C was also significantly lower in subjects aged 80–99 y compared with subjects aged 60–79 y (Fig. 24.2). Subjects from the two studies were similarly selected in terms of vitamin intake and health status (16,17). In this preliminary report, we expected lower MDA and higher vitamin C plasma levels in centenarians than in younger subjects, thus confirming a strong defense status of healthy centenarians. Surprisingly, our data were not consistent with those published by Paolisso and colleagues, although some variation could be due to geographical/nutritional and laboratory/methodological differences (16, 17). We also hypothesized that a depleted

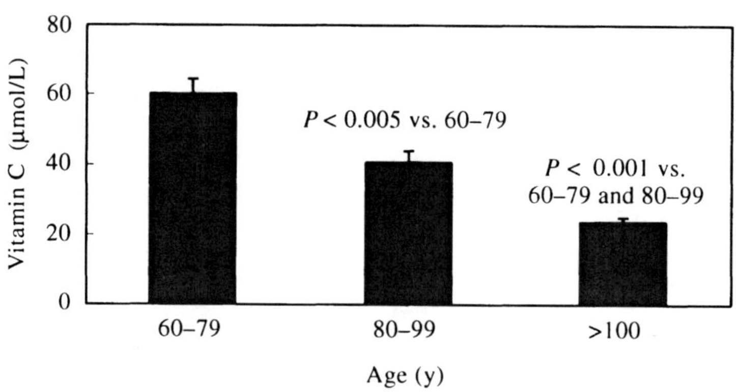

Fig. 24.2. Plasma vitamin C concentrations in 16 healthy subjects aged 60–79 y, in 12 healthy subjects aged 80–99 y, and in 17 centenarians. Values are means ± SEM.

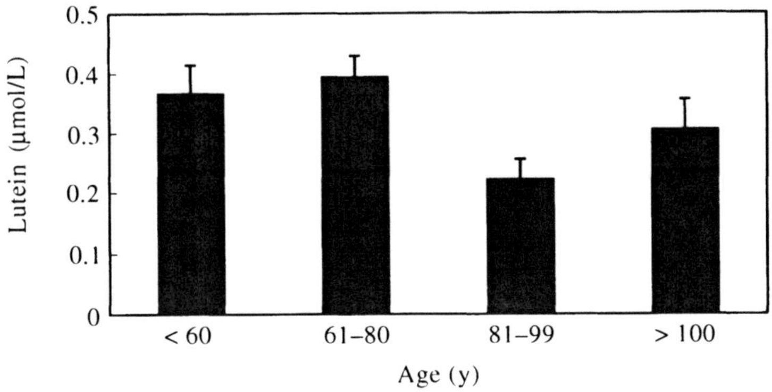

Fig. 24.3. Plasma lutein concentrations in 24 healthy subjects aged <60 y, 34 healthy subjects aged 61–80 y, 17 healthy subjects aged 81–99 y, and 32 centenarians. Values are means ± SEM.

reservoir of vitamin C, the only antioxidant able to completely prevent lipid peroxidation even in the presence of free iron (18), along with increased lipid peroxidation in centenarians, could reflect the progressive impairment of the ability of the aged organism to combat stressing insults (17).

To test this hypothesis, and to verify the antioxidant status of centenarians through the evaluation of a much broader spectrum of antioxidant vitamins and enzyme activities, we recently performed a biological study on 24 young adults aged <60 y, 34 young-old subjects aged 61–80 y, 17 old-old subjects aged 81–99 y and 32 centenarians (19). All subjects were healthy, nonsmokers, and community-dwellers; they were not taking antioxidant supplements and had normal serum levels of albumin, cholesterol, and triglycerides. We obtained blood from all subjects and measured plasma levels of water-soluble antioxidants including vitamin C and uric acid by

TABLE 24.1 Plasma Carotenoid Concentrations and Antioxidant Enzyme Activities in Healthy Subjects < 60 y, Aged 61–80 y, Aged 81–99 y, and in Healthy Centenarians[a,b]

	<60 y	61–80 y	81–99 y	>100 y
Zeaxanthin (μmol/L)	0.133 ± 0.02	0.136 ± 0.014[c]	0.092 ± 0.019	0.078 ± 0.01
β-Cryptoxanthin (μmol/L)	0.344 ± 0.096	0.452 ± 0.072	0.153 ± 0.047	0.142 ± 0.031
Lycopene (μmol/L)	0.9 ± 0.092[d,e]	0.577 ± 0.06[e]	0.396 ± 0.086	0.239 ± 0.033
α-Carotene (μmol/L)	0.141 ± 0.048[f,g]	0.082 ± 0.015	0.042 ± 0.009	0.04 ± 0.009
β-Carotene (μmol/L)	0.772 ± 0.22	0.796 ± 0.173[g]	0.251 ± 0.057	0.214 ± 0.036
Plasma SOD (U/mL)	28.1 ± 1.9[f]	30.3 ± 1.7	34.3 ± 1.1	27.2 ± 0.9[f]
RBC SOD (U/g Hb)	2582 ± 97[f]	2803 ± 116.4[f]	3239 ± 109	2782 ± 89[f]
Plasma GPX [nmol NADPH/(min•mL)]	0.112 ± 0.005	0.126 ± 0.007	0.139 ± 0.009	0.141 ± 0.026

[a]Values are means ± SEM.
[b]Abbreviations: SOD, superoxide dismutase; RBC, red blood cell; Hb, hemoglobin; GPX, glutathione peroxidase.
[c]$P < 0.01$ vs. > 100 y; [d]$P < 0.0001$ vs. 81–99 y; [e]$P < 0.0001$ vs. >100 y; [f]$P < 0.01$ vs. 81–99 y;
[g]$P < 0.001$ vs. >100 y.

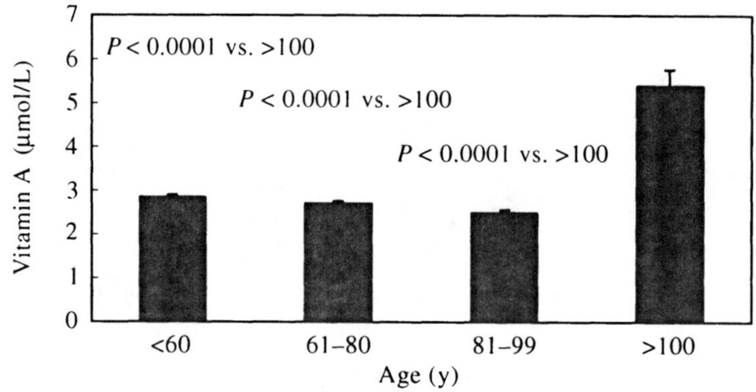

Fig. 24.4. Plasma vitamin A concentrations in 24 healthy subjects aged <60 y, 34 healthy subjects aged 61–80 y, 17 healthy subjects aged 81–99 y, and 32 centenarians. Values are means ± SEM.

HPLC with electrochemical detection and total thiols by spectrophotometry; plasma levels of lipophilic antioxidants including vitamin A, vitamin E and carotenoids (lutein, zeaxanthin, β-cryptoxanthin, lycopene, α-carotene and β-carotene) by HPLC with UV/vis detection; and plasma superoxide dismutase (SOD), glutathione peroxidase (GPX) and red blood cell (RBC) SOD activities by spectrophotometry (19).

Plasma carotenoid levels, with the exception of lutein (Fig. 24.3), showed a trend towards an age-dependent decrease (Table 24.1) (19). We found that both vitamin A and vitamin E plasma levels were significantly higher in centenarians compared to younger subjects (Figs. 24.4 and 24.5). Plasma vitamin A concentrations, in fact, were roughly doubled in centenarians compared with all three groups of younger subjects ($P < 0.0001$) (Fig. 24.4), and vitamin E concentrations were higher in centenarians by ~10% than in subjects <60 y old ($P < 0.01$), by ~17% vs. subjects 61–80 y old ($P < 0.0001$),

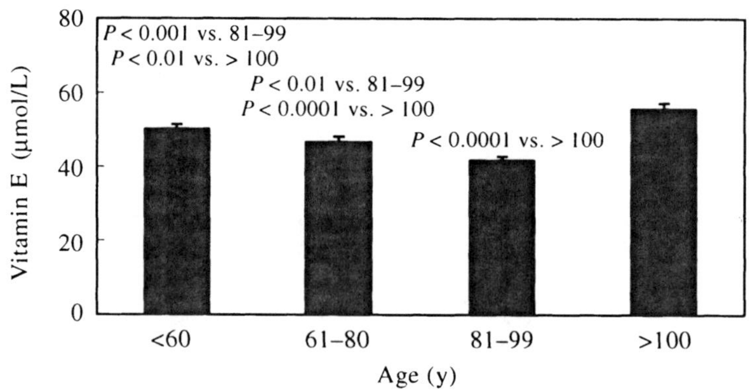

Fig. 24.5. Plasma vitamin E concentrations in 24 healthy subjects aged <60 y, 34 healthy subjects aged 61–80 y, 17 healthy subjects aged 81–99 y, and 32 centenarians. Values are means ± SEM.

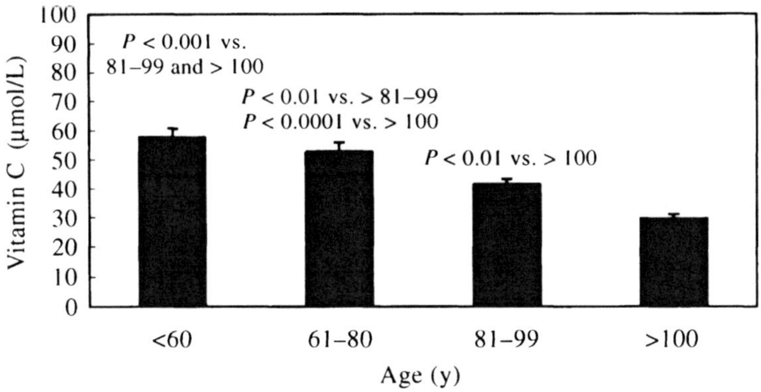

Fig. 24.6. Plasma vitamin C concentrations in 24 healthy subjects aged <60 y, 34 healthy subjects aged 61–80 y, 17 healthy subjects aged 81–99 y, and 32 centenarians. Values are means ± SEM.

and by ~24% vs. subjects 81–99 y old ($P < 0.0001$) (Fig. 24.5) (19). Thus, vitamins A and E show an age-dependent decrease until the tenth decade of age, whereas a marked increase appears to occur after the threshold of 100 y of age. Our findings on vitamin E plasma levels in centenarians are in agreement with data from Paolisso and co-workers (16) as well as with those from a recent study conducted on 16 centenarians from Poland (20), suggesting that this vitamin, along with vitamin A (21), is of particular importance for longevity, perhaps not only in their role as antioxidants, but also due to their broad spectrum of biological activities. It is indeed known that vitamin E deficiency leads to impaired immune function (22–24), neurological disorders, cardiovascular diseases, and cancer (25–27), all conditions from which our centenarians were completely free (19).

On the other hand, plasma levels of water-soluble antioxidants including vitamin C (Fig. 24.6), uric acid (Fig. 24.7) and thiols (Fig. 24.8) were found to be significantly

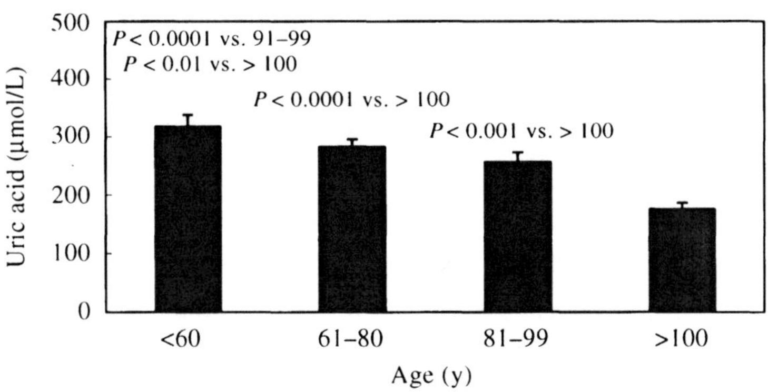

Fig. 24.7. Plasma uric acid concentrations in 24 healthy subjects aged <60 y, 34 healthy subjects aged 61–80 y, 17 healthy subjects aged 81–99 y, and 32 centenarians. Values are means ± SEM.

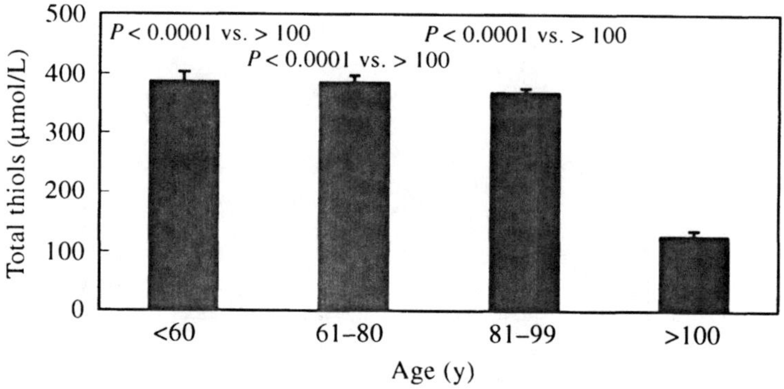

Fig. 24.8. Plasma thiol concentrations in 24 healthy subjects aged <60 y, 34 healthy subjects aged 61–80 y, 17 healthy subjects aged 81–99 y, and 32 centenarians. Values are means ± SEM.

lower in centenarians compared with younger subjects, and to be inversely correlated with age when all subjects, including centenarians, were considered ($r = -0.6$ for vitamin C and uric acid, $P < 0.0001$; $r = -0.7$ for thiols, $P < 0.0001$).These data, along with the findings of higher vitamin A and E levels in centenarians than in younger individuals, could also allow us to hypothesize that age-related oxidative stress consumes water-soluble antioxidants before the lipophilic ones, and that the latter are indeed preserved and maintained at higher levels in individuals who have aged successfully (19).

Finally, we observed an overall age-dependent increase of plasma SOD, RBC SOD, and plasma GPX activities (Table 24.1) (19). Plasma SOD activity was found to be significantly lower in centenarians and subjects <60 y old compared with the 81- to 99-y-old group ($P < 0.01$), which showed the highest enzyme activity level before the ninth decade of age (Table 24.1). Similarly, RBC SOD activity was highest in subjects 81–99 y old compared with the other age groups ($P < 0.01$) (Table 24.1). Finally, an age-dependent increase in GPX activity was shown until the very last decade of age, although this was not significant (Table 24.1). With respect to changes of antioxidant enzyme activities with aging, the literature is rather inconsistent, mainly because antioxidant enzymes in various stressing conditions may be induced and increased or consumed and decreased (26). A recent study of 16 healthy Polish centenarians showed significantly higher RBC glutathione reductase and catalase activities in centenarians compared with younger subjects (20).

Summary

Healthy centenarians represent a fascinating, highly selected group of individuals, not simply from the human and clinical point of view. They are, in fact, impressive in that their ability to remember, perform activities of daily living, keep interested, and make a variety of useful things during the day is in all ways comparable to that of persons five decades younger. They did not have much to eat during their lives; they cultivated fields, and their diet was made up of fruits and vegetables. They often presented a deficit of antioxidants (14,17,19) and micronutrients (19,28), but their routine blood analyses were perfectly normal. The results of our studies on healthy centenarians suggest that although longevity is not associated with an overall strong antioxidant status of blood plasma, the activities of vitamins A and E and preserving the ability to combat stressing events may play critical roles in allowing humans to reach the most advanced decades of age free of disease and therefore able to enjoy a good quality of life. These aspects, along with the study of the effect of energy intake in aging organisms (29,30), will constitute an important research field for scientists in the near future.

Acknowledgments

The authors thank Mrs. Roberta Cecchetti, Mrs. Heide Krahl, and Mrs. Annette Reimann for technical assistance. Dr. Polidori would like to thank Dr. Emilio Foá for helping in visiting centenarians at home. Dr. Helmut Sies is a NFCR Fellow.

References

1. Harman, D. (1956) Aging: A Theory Based on Free Radical and Radiation Chemistry. *J. Gerontol. 11*, 298–300.
2. United Nations (1991) *World Population Prospects 1990*, United Nations, New York.
3. U.S. Senate Committee on Aging (1992) *Aging America: Trends and Projections*, p. 144, U.S. Government Printing Office, Washington, DC.
4. Wilmoth, J.R. (1998) The Future of Human Longevity: A Demographer's Perspective. *Science 280*, 395–397.
5. Rowe, J., and Kahn, R.L. (1987) Human Aging: Usual and Successful. *Science 237*, 143–149.
6. Franceschi, C., Monti, D., Cossarizza, A., Fagnoni, F., Passeri, G., and Sansoni, P. (1991) Aging, Longevity, and Cancer: Studies in Down's Syndrome and Centenarians. *Ann. N.Y. Acad. Sci. 621*, 428–440.
7. Harman, D. (1993) Free Radicals Involvement in Aging. Pathophysiology and Therapeutic Implications. *Drugs Aging 3*, 60–80.
8. Schlienger, J.L., Pradignac, A., and Grunenberger, F. (1995) Nutrition of the Elderly: A Challenge Between Facts and Needs. *Horm. Res. 43*, 46–51.
9. Sies, H. (2000) in *Oxidative Stress and Vascular Disease*, (Keaney J.F., Jr., ed.) pp. 1–8, Kluwer Academic Publishers, Boston.
10. The Italian Multicentric Study on Centenarians (1997) Epidemiological and Socioeconomical Aspects of Italian Centenarians. *Arch. Gerontol. Geriatr. 25*, 149–157.
11. The Italian Multicentric Study on Centenarians (1998) Assessment of Sense of Taste in Italian Centenarians. *Arch. Gerontol. Geriatr. 26*, 177–183.
12. The Italian Multicentric Study on Centenarians (1998) Laboratory Parameters of Italian Centenarians. *Arch. Gerontol. Geriatr. 27*, 67–74.
13. Monti, D., Cossarizza, A., Troiano, L., Tomasi, A., Sartor, G., Comaschi, V., Farruggia, G., Masotti, L., and Franceschi, C. (1990) in *Protein Metabolism in Aging*, pp. 381–386, A.R. Liss, New York.
14. Pinzani, P., Petruzzi, E., Orlando, C. Stefanescu, A.M., Antonini, M.F., Serio, M., and Pazzagli, M. (1997) Reduced Serum Antioxidant Capacity in Healthy Centenarians. *Clin. Chem. 43*, 855–856.

15. Stocker, R., and Frei B. (1991) in *Oxidative Stress: Oxidants and Antioxidants*, (Sies H., ed.) pp. 213–243, Academic Press, London.
16. Paolisso, G., Tagliamonte, M.R., Rizzo, M.R., Manzella, D., Gambardella, A., and Varricchio, M. (1998) Oxidative Stress and Advancing Age: Results in Healthy Centenarians. *J. Am. Geriatr. Soc. 46*, 833–838.
17. Polidori, M.C., Mecocci, P., Reimann, A., Cherubini, A., Cecchetti, R., Briviba, K., Stahl, W., Sies, H., and Senin, U. (1999) Plasma Lipid Peroxidation and Vitamin C Status in Healthy Centenarians. *J. Am. Geriatr. Soc. 47*, 1038–1039.
18. Berger, T., Polidori, M.C., Morrow, J., Evans, P., Halliwell, B., and Frei, B. (1997) Antioxidant Properties of Vitamin C in Presence of Bleomicyn-Detectable Free Iron in Cord Plasma of Preterm Infants. *J. Biol. Chem. 272*, 15656–15660.
19. Mecocci, P., Polidori, M.C., Troiano, L., Cherubini, A., Cecchetti, R., Pini, G., Straatman, M., Monti, D., Stahl, W., Sies, H., Franceschi, C., and Senin, U. (2000) Plasma Antioxidants and Longevity: A Study on Healthy Centenarians. *Free Radic. Biol. Med. 28*, 1243–1248.
20. Kapcinska, B., Derejczyk, J., Wieczorowska-Tobis, K., Sobczak, A., Sadowska-Krepa, E., and Danch, A. (2000) Antioxidant Defense in Centenarians (A Preliminary Study). *Acta Biochim. Pol. 47*, 281–292.
21. Livrea, M.A., and Packer, L. (1994) in *Retinoids: From Basic Science to Clinical Applications*, (Livrea, M.A., and Vidali, G., eds.) pp. 293–303, Birkhäuser-Verlag, Basel.
22. Mariotti, S., Sansoni, P., Barbesino, G., Caturegli, P., Monti, D., Cossarizza, A., Giacomelli, T., Passeri, G., Fagiolo, U., Pinchera, A., and Franceschi, C. (1992) Thyroid and Other Organ-Specific Autoantibodies in Healthy Centenarians. *Lancet 339*, 1506–1508.
23. Sansoni, P., Cossarizza, A., Brianti, V., Fagnoni, F., Snelli, G., Monti, D., Marcato, A., Passeri, G., Ortolani, C., Forti, E., Fagiolo, U., Passeri, M., and Franceschi, C. (1993) Lymphocyte Subsets and Natural Killer Cell Activity in Healthy Old People and Centenarians. *Blood 9*, 1–7.
24. Meydani, S.N., Meydani, M., Blumberg, J.B., Leka, L.S., Siber, G., Loszewski, R., Thompson, C., Pedrosa, M.C., Diamond, R.D., and Stollar, B.D. (1997) Vitamin E Supplementation and In Vivo Immune Response in Healthy Elderly Subjects: A Randomized Trial. *J. Am. Med. Assoc. 277*, 1380–1386.
25. Diplock, A.T. (1997) Will the "Good Fairies" Please Prove to Us That Vitamin E Lessens Human Degenerative Disease? *Free Radic. Res. 27*, 511–532.
26. Beckman, K., and Ames, B.N. (1998) The Free Radical Theory of Aging Matures. *Physiol. Rev. 78*, 547–581.
27. Ashok, B.T., and Ali, R. (1999) The Aging Paradox: Free Radical Theory of Aging. *Exp. Gerontol. 34*, 293–303.
28. Ravaglia, G., Forti, P., Maioli, F., Bastagli, L., Facchini, A., Mariani, E., Savarino, L., Sassi, S., Cucinotta, D., and Lenaz, G. (2000) Effect of Micrinutrient Status on Natural Killer Cell Immune Function in Healthy Free-Living Subjects Aged ≥ 90 y. *Am. J. Clin. Nutr. 71*, 590–598.
29. Jacques P.F., Halpner A.D., and Blumberg, J.B. (1995) Influence of Combined Antioxidant Nutrient Intakes on Their Plasma Concentrations in an Elderly Population. *Am. J. Clin. Nutr. 62*, 1228–1233.
30. Weindruch, R., and Sohal, R.S. (1997) Caloric Intake and Aging. *New Engl. J. Med. 337*, 986–994.

Chapter 25

Mechanisms of Cholesterol- or Homocysteine-Induced Atherosclerosis: Role of Vitamin E

Nesrin K. Özer

Department of Biochemistry, Faculty of Medicine, Marmara University, 81326 Haydarpasa, Istanbul, Turkey

Introduction

Atherosclerosis is a life-threatening disease, which affects critical organs including heart and brain. Therefore, it is the major cause of age-related disease and death in the world. One of the major risks for atherosclerosis is the presence of hypercholesterolemia with elevated levels of cholesterol-rich low density lipoprotein (LDL). In combination with other factors, high plasma concentrations of LDL promote the development of atherosclerosis. Smooth muscle cell (SMC) migration and proliferation, and the accumulation of oxidized LDL in macrophages and SMC result in foam cell formation, an initial step in atherosclerosis (1–3). Some epidemiologic studies have shown an association between high dietary intake and high serum concentrations of vitamin E and lower rates of ischemic heart disease (4–8). In cell culture studies, it has been shown that α-tocopherol inhibits vascular SMC proliferation. This event takes place *via* inhibition of protein kinase C (PKC) activity. α-Tocopherol also inhibits low density lipoprotein–stimulated SMC proliferation and PKC activity (9–12). Because β-tocopherol and other potent antioxidants are not inhibitory, the effect of α-tocopherol likely occurs through a nonoxidant mechanism (13)

Epidemiologic studies in the general population have suggested associations between elevated circulating homocysteine levels and premature coronary, cerebral, and peripheral atherosclerosis (14–19). In baboons, it was demonstrated that blood infusion of homocysteine resulted in human atheroma-like myointimal lesions (20). In another study, homocysteine was shown to induce atherosclerosis-like alterations of the aorta in normotensive and hypertensive rats (21). Because SMC migration and proliferation are hallmarks of atherosclerosis, it was suggested that homocysteine may contribute to the clinical presentation of this vascular disease through such a process. In smooth muscle culture studies, it was reported that homocysteine stimulates aortic cyclin-dependent kinase; as a consequence, aortic cells would proliferate (22). On the other hand, it has been shown to act as an inducer of c-fos and c-myc (23). However, the mechanisms by which homocysteine promotes atherosclerosis formation are not clearly defined.

Because hypercholesterolemia and hyperhomocysteinemia are important risk factors for atherosclerosis, these animal and cell culture studies were conducted to investigate the mechanism of cholesterol- or homocysteine-induced atherosclerosis and the effect of vitamin E in protecting against the disease.

Materials and Methods

Materials. Culture media and serum for cell culture were obtained from Gibco Laboratories (Grand Island, NY, USA). A7r5 rat aortic SMC were obtained from the American Type Culture Collection (Rockville, MD). Methyl-^{3}H thymidine (925GBq/mmol) was purchased from Amersham International (UK). *RRR*-α-tocopherol was a generous gift from Henkel Corporation (La Grange, IL). Vitamin E–free rabbit diet and vitamin E (Ephynal) were kindly donated by Hoffman La Roche (Basel, Switzerland and Istanbul, Turkey). The kit for measurement of PKC activity was obtained from Upstate Biotechnology, Lake Placid, NY. DL-Homocysteine and catalase were from Sigma Chemical (St. Louis, MO). All other chemicals used were of the purest grade commercially available.

Animal Experiments. Male New Zealand albino rabbits (n = 30), 2–4 mo old, were used in this study. They were fed 100 g/d of a diet poor in vitamin E. Cholesterol was added to the diet as a diethyl ether solution. The control diet was treated with the same amount of pure solvent. All diets were dried of the solvent before use. The concentrations of cholesterol and vitamin E used were based on previous literature reports (24–28).

The rabbits were randomly assigned to one of the following four groups. One group of rabbits was fed only the diet, without additions or treatments. The second group was fed the same diet and received daily injections of 50 mg/kg of vitamin E intramuscularly on alternate rear legs. The diet of the third group contained 2% cholesterol. The diet of the fourth group also contained 2% cholesterol, and the rabbits received daily injections of 50 mg/kg of vitamin E. After 4 wk, plasma samples were taken and thoracic aortas were removed. Samples were taken from the media of thoracic aortas to measure SMC PKC activity by using a nonradioactive kit (Upstate Biotechnology). Plasma cholesterol levels were determined using an automated enzymatic technique. Vitamin E levels were measured by reverse-phase high-pressure liquid chromatography (29).

Cell Culture. A7r5 cells were maintained in Dulbecco's modified Eagle's medium (DMEM) supplemented with 10% (vol/vol) fetal calf serum (FCS). Cells in a subconfluent state were made quiescent by incubation in DMEM containing 0.2% FCS for 48 h. Cells were then washed with phosphate-buffered saline (PBS) and treated as indicated in the figure legends. Viability was determined by the trypan blue dye method.

Determination of Cell Number and [^{3}H]Thymidine Incorporation. Quiescent A7r5 cells were restimulated to grow by the addition of 10% FCS. Homocysteine (different concentrations) and/or catalase (2600 U/mL) was added to cells. Cell number was determined 48 h later by using a hemocytometer.

To measure DNA synthesis, the cells that had been made quiescent in 12-well plates were restimulated to grow by the addition of 10% FCS, homocysteine, and catalase for 20 h. Plates were pulsed with [^{3}H]thymidine (1 μCi/well) during the last

2 h of incubation. After labeling, cells were washed twice with PBS, fixed for 20 min with ice-cold 5% trichloroacetic acid, and solubilized in 0.1 mol/L NaOH/2% Na_2CO_3/1% SDS. The radioactivity incorporated into the acid-insoluble material was determined with a liquid scintillation analyzer. [^{3}H]Thymidine incorporation was expressed as cpm/mg protein. Protein concentration was measured by the method of Lowry *et al.* (30).

Statistics. Values are expressed as means ± SD. The significance of the difference between mean values was analyzed by Student's *t*-test.

Results

The animal experiments addressed the question whether vitamin E can prevent development of cholesterol-induced atherosclerosis *in vivo*. Cholesterol and vitamin E plasma concentrations of the 4 rabbit groups are shown in Table 25.1. Supplementation of the diet with 2% cholesterol for 4 wk resulted in an ~20-fold increase in plasma cholesterol. After additional supplementation with vitamin E, plasma cholesterol increased 12- and 13-fold respectively, relative to control. Plasma vitamin E concentrations were higher in the cholesterol-fed rabbits, consistent with the data in the literature (31–35); however, the values corrected for the plasma cholesterol concentrations were of a similar order of magnitude.

Previous results have shown that PKC activity and expression were up-regulated by cholesterol, whereas vitamin E antagonism, although visible as a tendency, was not significant (36). In this study (Table 25.2), in the total absence of vitamin E in the diet, the activity of SMC PKC was 8.4 Δ Absorbance units/(min·mg protein). After vitamin E treatment, an ~50% reduction of PKC activity was seen. With cholesterol supplementation, the activity of PKC increased to 10.2 Δ Absorbance units/(min·mg protein). Vitamin E treatment was able in this case to reduce values for PKC activity to those measured in the absence of cholesterol [4.5 Δ Absorbance units/(min·mg protein)].

TABLE 25.1 Effect of Cholesterol and Vitamin E Treatment on Their Respective Plasma Levels in Rabbits[a]

Group	Cholesterol (mmol/L)	Vitamin E (mmol/L)	Vitamin E/Cholesterol ratio
Control	1.0 ± 0.5	5.2 ± 2.4	5.2
Vitamin E	0.9 ± 0.1	50.7 ± 10.2[b]	56.3
Cholesterol	21.1 ± 10.7[b]	14.6 ± 6.5[c]	0.7
Cholesterol + Vitamin E	12.4 ± 6.1[b]	216.2 ± 70.2[b]	17.4

[a]The plasma levels of cholesterol and vitamin E were measured in the four diet groups (n = 5 rabbits/group). Values are means ± SD and represent the plasma values measured after 1 mo of consuming the diet.
[b]$P < 0.01$.
[c]Not significant.

TABLE 25.2 Protein Kinase C (PKC) Activity from Smooth Muscle Cell Homogenates Obtained from Rabbits Receiving Different Treatments[a]

Group	Total PKC activity [Δ Absorbance/(min•mg protein)]	
Control	8.4 ± 1.1	
Vitamin E	4.5 ± 2.5	$P < 0.01$[b]
Cholesterol	10.2 ± 2.4	
Cholesterol + Vitamin E	4.5 ± 1.0	$P < 0.02$[c]

[a]Aortic medias were minced, homogenized, and nuclei sedimented by centrifugation. Supernatants were centrifuged again at 100,000 × *g* to obtain cytosolic fractions. Pellets were used for preparation of membrane fractions. PKC activity was measured in both fractions. Because differences in membrane/cytosol distribution were not significant, only the values of total PKC activity are reported. Results are means ± SD ($n = 5$).
[b]Referred to control group.
[c]Referred to cholesterol group

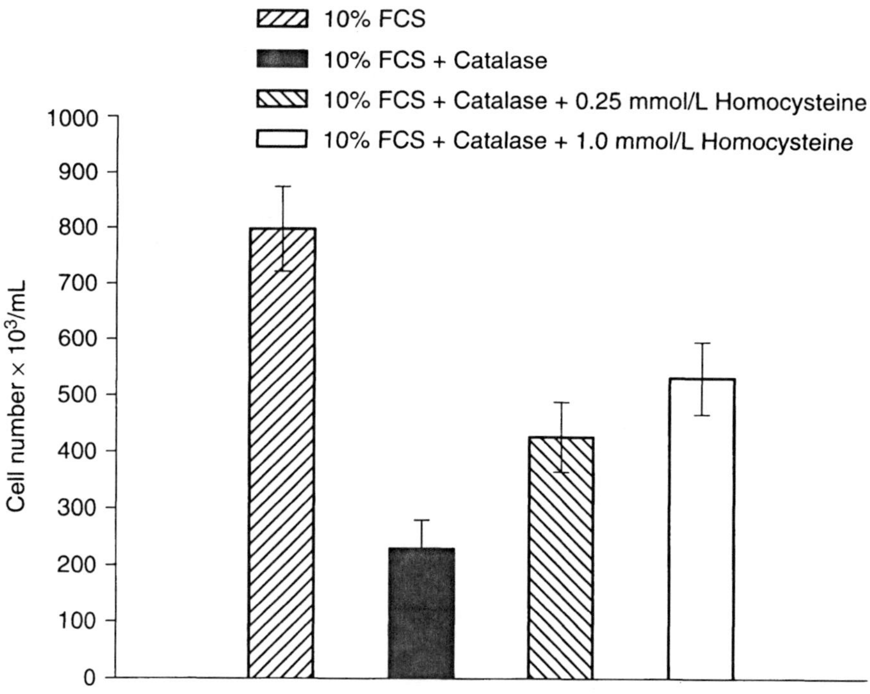

Fig 25.1. Effect of homocysteine on vascular smooth muscle cell proliferation. Serum-deprived quiescent cells were stimulated to grow by fetal calf serum (FCS) in the presence of 2600 U/mL catalase and different concentrations of homocysteine. After 48 h, the cell number was measured as described in Materials and Methods. Viability was >95%. Results are expressed as the mean ± SD of 10 independent experiments.

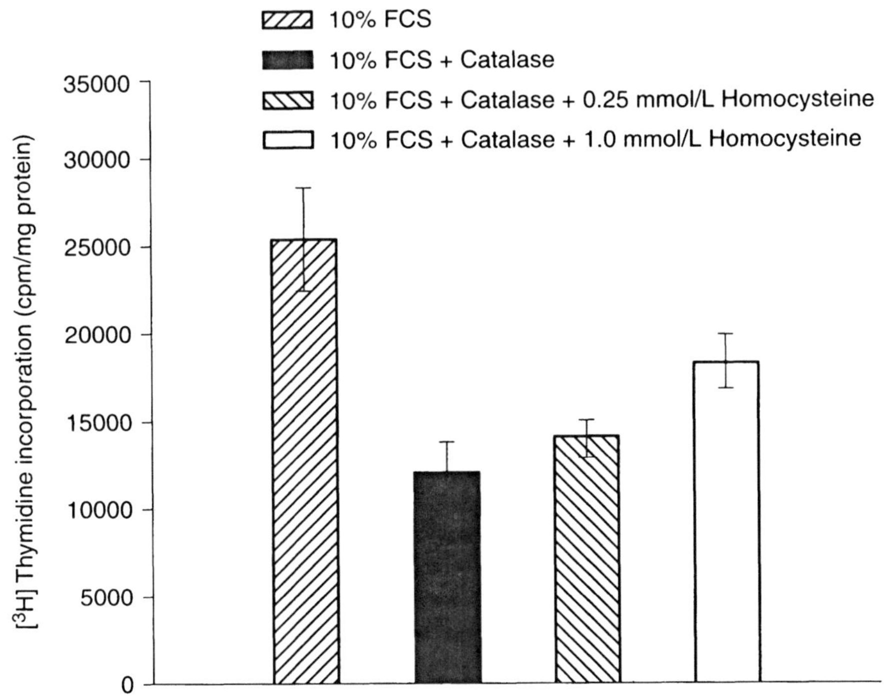

Fig 25.2. Effect of homocysteine on DNA synthesis in vascular smooth muscle cells. Quiescent cells were stimulated to grow by calf serum (FCS) in the presence of 2600 U/mL catalase and different concentrations of homocysteine for 20 h. The cells were pulsed with [^{3}H]thymidine during the last 2 h of incubation. [^{3}H]Thymidine incorporation was determined as described in Materials and Methods. Results are expressed as the mean ± SD of 10 independent experiments.

To determine whether homocysteine can induce vascular SMC proliferation, the cells were starved of serum for 48 h and restimulated to grow with 10% FCS in the presence of increasing homocysteine concentrations. To establish whether H_2O_2 has a role in homocysteine-initiated signal transduction, vascular SMC were treated with FCS and homocysteine in the presence of 2600 U/mL catalase. Under these conditions, no other effects of catalase could be seen on vascular SMC, particularly on the viability as assessed by trypan blue exclusion. As shown in Figure 25.1, homocysteine increased proliferation of the cells in the presence of catalase.

[^{3}H]Thymidine incorporation was studied as a measure of DNA synthesis. It was evaluated after 20 h of incubation with FCS, a time that represents a peak in [^{3}H]thymidine incorporation (data not shown). [^{3}H]Thymidine incorporation was increased in the presence of homocysteine and catalase (Fig 25.2). At 1.0 mmol/L homocysteine concentration, the response was maximal in terms of both increased cell proliferation and [^{3}H]thymidine incorporation (Figs. 25.1 and 25.2).

Discussion

An early event in the development of atherosclerosis is the intimal deposition of lipids, including cholesterol. This deposition arises from a combination of extra- and intracellular processes and has been shown, in some animal models, to be inhibited by antioxidants (37). We observed a specific inhibition of proliferation *in vitro* of SMC by α-tocopherol at physiologic concentrations. Of particular relevance was the finding of an antiproliferative effect of α-tocopherol on rat and human SMC. Proliferation of these cells is fundamental in the onset of accelerated atherosclerosis, after cardiac transplantation, and restenosis. Multiple pathways are involved in the proliferative response of SMC to an extracellular stimulus, which has rendered difficult the identification of precise targets of antiproliferative agents. One of the important elements in signal transduction cascades is PKC, and its inhibition appears to be sufficient to cause inhibition of SMC proliferation *in vitro*.

Several groups have reported that antioxidant vitamins and especially vitamin E have an important antiatherogenic role (3–6,38). The questions posed in this study include the following: (i) Does hypercholesterolemia affect smooth muscle cells at the level of PKC, a key enzyme in the control of proliferation? (ii) Is vitamin E capable of protecting against the molecular modifications induced by hypercholesterolemia at the level of SMC? The present *in vivo* data of cholesterol stimulation and vitamin E inhibition of PKC activity agree with previous results obtained both *in vitro* (9,11,13,39,40) and *in vivo* (36). It appears also that among the molecular events that may be responsible for the protection by vitamin E against atherosclerotic plaque formation, the inhibition of smooth muscle PKC may play a crucial role. These studies provide a molecular interpretation of the epidemiologic information linking a decrease in plasma α-tocopherol with an increased risk of ischemic heart disease.

The mechanism by which homocysteine induces coronary atherosclerotic lesions is unknown. The development of a complicated atherosclerotic plaque in humans involves proliferation of SMC. It is unclear, however, whether the effects on DNA synthesis and cell proliferation are produced by homocysteine itself or by some of its metabolites. How these effects are mediated also remains obscure. Possible explanations include the role of free radicals and H_2O_2 produced through the oxidation of homocysteine to the thiolactone (41). Furthermore, it has been demonstrated that the signal transduction induced by platelet-derived growth factor (PDGF) requires the generation of H_2O_2, which may act as a signaling molecule for SMC growth (42).

Studies have shown that the action of homocysteine on SMC is associated with the induction of genes important for cell proliferation (c-fos and c-myc) (23). Tsai *et al.* (43) showed that mRNA levels of cyclins D_1 and A are elevated by homocysteine. It was demonstrated recently that homocysteine activates the ERK2 signal transduction pathway and originates growth-promoting signals in SMC (44). To understand whether H_2O_2 is an early signal for proliferation in vascular SMC, we decreased its concentration by adding the peroxide-scavenging enzyme catalase. This enzyme rapidly degrades H_2O_2 to water and molecular oxygen. In the conditions of this study, the increase in catalase prevented the stimulation of cell proliferation and DNA synthesis. These results are very similar to results reported by Sundearesan *et al.* (42). In this study, we showed that homocysteine produces a twofold stimulation of cell growth and a 1.5-fold increase of DNA synthesis in catalase-treated vascular SMC, i.e., through an H_2O_2-independent pathway. Experiments relating the role of vitamin E in homocysteine-induced SMC proliferation are in progress.

In conclusion, the data shown in this study with animal and cell culture strongly suggest that the mitogenic signals of cholesterol or homocysteine in vascular SMC cause proliferation of SMC. By promoting the proliferation of vascular SMC via a pathway, the effects of cholesterol or homocysteine may act synergistically; the known initiating events are produced by an oxidative stress, and the result is an acceleration of the progression of atherosclerosis. It is at this level that the protective effect of vitamin E against atherosclerosis is exerted.

References

1. Raines, E.W., and Ross, R. (1993) Smooth Muscle Cells and the Pathogenesis of the Lesions of Atherosclerosis. *Br. Heart J. 69*, S30–S37.
2. Ross, R. (1993) The Pathogenesis of Atherosclerosis: A Perspective for the 1990s. *Nature 362*, 801–809.
3. Steinberg, D. (1995) Clinical Trials of Antioxidants in Atherosclerosis: Are We Doing the Right Thing? *Lancet 346*, 36–38.
4. Rimm, E.B., Stampfer, M.J., Ascherio, A., Giovannucci, E., Colditz, G.A., and Willett, W.C. (1993) Vitamin E Consumption and the Risk of Coronary Heart Disease in Men. *N. Engl. J. Med. 328*, 1450–1456.
5. Stampfer, M.J., Hennekens, C.H., Manson, J.E., Colditz, G.A., Rosner, B., and Willett, W.C. (1993) Vitamin E Consumption and the Risk of Coronary Disease in Women. *N. Engl. J. Med. 328*, 1444–1449.
6. Gey, K.F., Moser, U.K., Jordan, P., Stahelin, H.B., Eichholzer, M., and Ludin, E. (1993) Increased Risk of Cardiovascular Disease at Suboptimal Plasma Concentrations of Essential Antioxidants: An Epidemiological Update with Special Attention to Carotene and Vitamin C. *Am. J. Clin. Nutr. 57*, 787S–797S.
7. Gey, K.F. (1990) The Antioxidant Hypothesis of Cardiovascular Disease: Epidemiology and Mechanisms. *Biochem. Soc. Trans. 18*, 1041–1045.
8. Stephens, N.G., Parsons, A., Schofield, P.M., Kelly, F., Cheeseman, K., Mitchinson, M.J., and Brown, M.J. (1996) Randomised Controlled Trial of Vitamin E in Patients with Coronary Disease: Cambridge Heart Antioxidant Study (CHAOS). *Lancet 347*, 781–786.
9. Boscoboinik, D., Szewczyk, A., Hensey, C., and Azzi, A. (1991) Inhibition of Cell Proliferation by Alpha-Tocopherol. Role of Protein Kinase C. *J. Biol. Chem. 266*, 6188–6194.
10. Azzi, A., Boscoboinik, D., Chatelain, E., Özer, N.K., and Stäuble, B. (1993) *d*-α-Tocopherol Control of Cell Proliferation. *Mol. Asp. Med. 14*, 265–271.
11. Boscoboinik, D., Özer, N.K., Moser, U., and Azzi, A. (1995) Tocopherols and 6-Hydroxy-chroman-2-carbonitrile Derivatives Inhibit Vascular Smooth Muscle Cell Proliferation by a Nonantioxidant Mechanism. *Arch. Biochem. Biophys. 318*, 241–246.

12. Azzi, A., Boscoboinik, D., Marilley, D., Özer, N.K., Stäuble, B., and Tasinato, A. (1995) Vitamin E: A Sensor and an Information Transducer of the Cell Oxidation State. *Am. J. Clin. Nutr. (Suppl.) 62,* 1337S–1346S.
13. Özer, N.K., Palozza, P., Boscoboinik, D., and Azzi, A. (1993) *d*-α-Tocopherol Inhibits Low Density Lipoprotein Induced Proliferation and Protein Kinase C Activity in Vascular Smooth Muscle Cells. *FEBS Lett. 322*, 307–310.
14. Clarke, R., Daly, L., Robinson, K., Naugten, E., Cahalane, S., and Fowler, B.G. (1991) Hyperhomocysteinemia: An Independent Risk Factor for Vascular Disease. *N. Engl. J. Med. 324*, 1149–1155.
15. Taylor, LM., De Frang, R.D., Harris, E.J., and Porter, J.M. (1991) The Association of Elevated Plasma Homocysteine with Progression of Symptomatic Peripheral Arterial Disease. *J. Vasc. Surg. 13*, 128–136.
16. Nygard, O., Vollset, S.E., and Refsum, H. (1995) Total Plasma Homocysteine and Cardiovascular Risk Profile. *J. Am. Med. Assoc. 274*, 1526–1533.
17. Miner, S., Evrovski, E., and Cole, D. (1997) Clinical Chemistry and Molecular Biology of Homocysteine Metabolism: An Update. *Clin. Biochem. 30*, 189–201.
18. Stehouver, C.D.A., Weijenberg, M.P., Van den Berg, M., Jakobs, C., Feskens, E.J.M., and Kromhout, D. (1998) Serum Homocysteine and Risk of Coronary Heart Disease and Cerebrovascular Disease in Elderly Men—A 10 Year Follow-Up. *Arterioscler. Thromb. Vasc. Biol. 18*, 1895–1901.
19. Welch, G.N., Upchurch, G., and Loscalzo, J, (1997) in *Annals of the New York Academy of Sciences, Atherosclerosis IV: Recent Advances in Atherosclerosis Research*, (Numano, F., and Russ, R., eds.) vol. 811, pp. 48–59, The New York Academy of Sciences, New York.
20. Harker, L.A., Harlau, JM., and Ross, R. (1983) Effect of Sulfinpyraizone on Homocyst(e)ine-Induced Endothelial Injury and Arteriosclerosis in Baboons. *Circ. Res. 53*, 731–739.
21. Matthias, D., Becker, C.H., Riezler, R., and Kindling, P.H. (1996) Homocysteine Induced Arteriosclerosis-Like Alterations of the Aorta in Normotensive and Hypertensive Rats Following Application of High Doses of Methionine. *Atherosclerosis 122*, 201–216.
22. Tsai, J., Wang, H., Perrella, M.A., Yoshizumi, M., Sibinga, N.E.S., Tan, L.C., Haber, E., Chang, T.H., Schlegel, R., and Lee, M. (1996) Induction of Cyclin A Gene Expression by Homocysteine in Vascular Smooth Muscle Cells. *J. Clin. Investig. 97*, 146–153.
23. Dalton, M.L., Gadson, P.F., Wrenn, R.W., and Rosenquist, T.H. (1997) Homocysteine Signal Cascade: Production of Phospholipids, Activation of Protein Kinase C, and the Induction of c-fos and c-myc in Smooth Muscle Cells. *FASEB J. 11*, 703–711.
24. Stein, Y., Stein, O., Delplanque, B., Fesmire, J.D., Lee, D.M., and Alaupovic, P. (1989) Lack of Effect of Probucol on Atheroma Formation in Cholesterol-Fed Rabbits Kept at Comparable Plasma Cholesterol Levels. *Atherosclerosis 75*, 145–155.
25. Ferns, G.A., Forster, L., Stewart Lee, A., Konneh, M., Nourooz Zadeh, J., and Anggard, E.E. (1992) Probucol Inhibits Neointimal Thickening and Macrophage Accumulation After Balloon Injury in the Cholesterol-Fed Rabbit. *Proc. Natl. Acad. Sci. USA 89*, 11312–11316.
26. Bocan, T.M., Mueller, S.B., Mazur, M.J., Uhlendorf, P.D., Brown, E.Q., and Kieft, K.A. (1993) The Relationship Between the Degree of Dietary-Induced Hypercholesterolemia in the Rabbit and Atherosclerotic Lesion Formation. *Atherosclerosis 102*, 9–22.

27. Mantha, S.V., Prasad, M., Kalra, J., and Prasad, K. (1993) Antioxidant Enzymes in Hypercholesterolemia and Effects of Vitamin E in Rabbits. *Atherosclerosis 101*, 135–144.
28. Konneh, M.K., Rutherford, C., Li, S.-R., Änggård, E.E., and Ferns, G.A.A. (1995) Vitamin E Inhibits the Intimal Response to Balloon Catheter Injury in the Carotid Artery of the Cholesterol-Fed Rat. *Atherosclerosis 113*, 29–39.
29. Nierenberg, D.W., and Nann, S.L. (1992) A Method for Determining Concentrations of Retinol, Tocopherol, and Five Carotenoids in Human Plasma and Tissue Samples. *Am. J. Clin. Nutr. 56*, 417–426.
30. Lowry, O.H., Rosenbrough, N.J., Farr, A.L., and Randall, R.J. (1951) Protein Measurements with the Folin Phenol Reagent. *J. Biol. Chem. 193*, 265–271.
31. Godfried, S.L., Combs, G.F., Jr., Saroka, J.M., and Dillingham, L.A. (1989) Potentiation of Atherosclerotic Lesions in Rabbits by a High Dietary Level of Vitamin E. *Br. J. Nutr. 61*, 607–617.
32. Wilson, R.B., Middleton, C.C., and Sun, G.Y. (1978) Vitamin E, Antioxidants and Lipid Peroxidation in Experimental Atherosclerosis of Rabbits. *J. Nutr. 108*, 1858–1867.
33. Bitman, J., Weyant, J., Wood, D.L., and Wrenn, T.R. (1976) Vitamin E, Cholesterol, and Lipids During Atherogenesis in Rabbits. *Lipids 11*, 449–461.
34. Bjorkhem, I., Henriksson-Freyschuss, A., Breuer, O., Diczfalusy, U., Berglund, L., and Henriksson, P. (1991) The Antioxidant Butylated Hydroxytoluene Protects Against Atherosclerosis. *Arterioscler. Thromb. 11*, 15–22.
35. Morel, D.W., De la Llera-Moya, M., and Friday, K.E. (1994) Treatment of Cholesterol-Fed Rabbits with Dietary Vitamins E and C Inhibits Lipoprotein Oxidation but Not Development of Atherosclerosis. *J. Nutr. 124*, 2123–2130.
36. Sirikci, Ö., Özer, N.K., and Azzi, A. (1996) Dietary Cholesterol-Induced Changes of Protein Kinase C and the Effect of Vitamin E in Rabbit Aortic Smooth Muscle Cells. *Atherosclerosis 126*, 253–263.
37. Esterbauer, H., Waeg, G., Puhl, H., Dieber Rotheneder, M., and Tatzber, F. (1992) Inhibition of LDL Oxidation by Antioxidants. *EXS 62*, 145–157.
38. Stahelin, H.B., Eichholzer, M., and Gey, K.F. (1992) Nutritional Factors Correlating with Cardiovascular Disease: Results of the Basel Study. *Bibl. Nutr. Dieta 49*, 24–35.
39. Özer, N.K., Boscoboinik, D., and Azzi, A. (1995) New Roles of Low Density Lipoproteins and Vitamin E in the Pathogenesis of Atherosclerosis. *Biochem. Mol. Biol. Int. 35*, 117–124.
40. Boscoboinik, D., Szewczyk, A., and Azzi, A.(1991) Alpha-Tocopherol (Vitamin E) Regulates Vascular Smooth Muscle Cell Proliferation and Protein Kinase C Activity. *Arch. Biochem. Biophys. 286*, 264–269.
41. Starkebaum, G., and Harlan, J.M. (1986) Endothelial Cell Injury Due to Copper-Catalyzed Hydrogen Peroxide Generation from Homocyst(e)ine. *J. Clin. Investig. 77*, 1370–1376.
42. Sundearesan, M., Yu, Z., Ferrans, V., Irani, K., and Finkel, T. (1995) Requirement for Generation of H_2O_2 for Platelet-Derived Growth Factor Signal Transduction. *Science 270*, 296–299.
43. Tsai, J., Perrella, M.A., Yoshizumi, M, Hsieh, C., Haber, E., Schlegel, R, and Lee, M. (1994) Promotion of Vascular Smooth Muscle Cell Growth by Homocysteine: A Link to Atherosclerosis. *Proc. Natl. Acad. Sci. USA 91*, 6369–6373.
44. Brown, J.C., Rosenquist, T.H., and Monaghan, D.T. (1998) ERK2 Activation by Homocysteine in Vascular Smooth Muscle Cells. *Biochem. Biophys. Res. Commun. 251*, 669–676.

Chapter 26

Biomarkers of Oxidative Stress and of Antioxidative Defense: Relationship to Intervention with Antioxidant-Rich Foods

Lars O. Dragsted,[a] Jette F. Young,[b] Steffen Loft,[c] and Brittmarie Sandström[b]

[a]Danish Food Administration, Søborg, Denmark
[b]Research Institute of Human Nutrition, The Royal Veterinary and Agricultural University, Frederiksberg, Denmark
[c]Institute of Public Health, University of Copenhagen, Denmark

Introduction

Dietary fruits and vegetables are known to reduce the risk of cancer (1,2) and cardiovascular disease (3–5). These actions have been ascribed to their high content of antioxidants, which are supposed to protect vital cellular structures against damage from free radicals (6–8). However, the outcome of most clinical trials has been disappointing; to date, the antioxidant vitamins, ascorbate, and β-carotene, have not been shown unequivocally to be protective against chronic diseases in humans (9), whereas vitamin E (*RRR*-α-tocopherol), which is not derived mainly from fruits or vegetables in our diets, has been observed to have a possible protective effect against prostate cancer only (10). We hypothesize that other antioxidants in fruits and vegetables such as the nonnutritive flavonoids and other polyphenols might therefore be the true human health protectants in foods of plant origin. The polyphenols seem particularly interesting because they are good antioxidants and they are highly prevalent in the normal diet in most of the world at levels at least as high as those of ascorbate. The flavonoids have been recognized as particularly efficient *in vitro* antioxidants among the polyphenols. If the flavonoids protect against oxidation in humans, intervention with an increased intake of foods and extracts rich in these compounds should affect either markers of oxidative damage or antioxidant defense homeostasis. To test this, we performed a series of controlled short-term human trials evaluating the antioxidant actions of single food items or extracts rich in flavonoids, e.g., apple and black currant juice, grape skin extract, tea extract, and the herb, parsley. All of these trials were performed as crossover studies in which the volunteers were kept on a strictly controlled diet, otherwise free from all flavonoid-containing dietary items, including juices, wines, teas, fruits, vegetables, and chocolate. The flavonoid-free root vegetables, potatoes and carrots, were allowed in the basic diet, however. The biomarker analyses included some or all of the following: oxidative damage to plasma protein and lipids, excretion of 8-oxo-deoxyguanosine (8-oxo-dG), red blood cell antioxidant enzyme activities, and plasma ascorbate. The analyses were performed in a completely blinded manner, and when possible, the nature of the extract was not known by the volunteers.

Discussion

The results of the four crossover intervention studies performed (11–14) can be divided into effects due to the intervention and effects related to the basic diet used throughout. These effects are summarized in Tables 26.1 and 26.2.

Apples and black currants are rich in flavonols, mainly quercetin and myricetin, and black currants are additionally rich in anthocyanins. The apple and black currant crossover intervention study was performed with three doses of a 1:1 mixture of apple and black currant juices, 750, 1000, and 1500 mL/d. The juices had a known content of flavonoids and were given to five volunteers in a randomized fashion during three 1-wk intervention periods divided by 14-d wash-out intervals (13). Quercetin excretion was used to monitor exposure (15), and we observed a dose- and time-dependent increase in this marker. The black currant juice was rich in vitamin C, which was also observed to increase in a time-dependent manner in plasma of the volunteers during intervention. The juice intakes corresponding to ~150, 200, or 300 mg vitamin C/d had a dose- and time-dependent prooxidant action on plasma proteins, and a weak antioxidant action on plasma lipids at the highest dose level. During juice intervention, oxidative DNA damage assessed by urinary excretion of 8-oxo-dG tended to increase (17%, on average), although this possible effect was not significant and lacked any apparent relationship with dose (unpublished data). Otherwise the flavonoid-containing juice resulted in only a minor increase in the erythrocyte antioxidant enzyme, glutathione peroxidase (Gpx), whereas there was no effect on the other three enzymes monitored, catalase (CAT), superoxide dismutase (SOD), and glutathione reductase (GR) (see Table 26.1). No effects were observed on markers of plasma antioxidant capacity.

The parsley intervention study was performed because parsley is rich in the flavone, apigenin, which is otherwise uncommon in the diet. Parsley is also rich in lutein. The study was a blinded 2 × 1 wk double crossover study with 16 volunteers divided into two groups (12). Parsley (20 g/10 MJ) was mixed into the dishes during the intervention week. Apigenin excretion was monitored as a marker of exposure (16). No effects of parsley intervention were observed on markers of protein or lipid oxidative damage but the antioxidant enzymes, GR and SOD, increased.

Grape skin extract is rich in catechins and anthocyanins. We performed the intervention study with this extract with the same design used in the parsley study, except that grape skin extract was used for intervention (14). No exposure marker was used. The grape skin extract had a sparing effect on vitamin C as determined by a less pronounced decrease in this vitamin during the periods in which the extract was added to the basic diet. This was accompanied by a weak prooxidant effect on plasma proteins.

The green tea extract study had a slightly different design compared with the former two in that the intervention was performed with green tea extract mixed into two different dietary matrices, i.e., dissolved in a drink or mixed into meat patties (11). However, the two groups in this crossover study were further subdivided into low-dose (100 mg/d) and high-dose (400 mg/d) groups. No food matrix effects were

TABLE 26.1 Summary of Findings in Four Human Crossover Intervention Studies: Effects of Intervention on Biomarkers of Oxidative Damage and Antioxidant Defense[a,b]

Biomarker:	PPO	8-oxo	P-MDA	LDL-MDA	Gpx	GR	SOD	CAT	Vit C-PL
Apple and black currant juices (I)	↑	—	[↓]	ND	↑	—	—	—	↑
Parsley (II)	—	ND	ND	ND	—	↑	↑	—	ND
Grape skin extract (III)	—	ND	—	—	↑	↑	—	—	—
Green tea extract (IV)	—	ND	ND	ND	ND	ND	ND	ND	—

[a]Abbreviations: PPO, plasma protein oxidation; 8-oxo, urinary 8-oxo-deguanosine; P-MDA, plasma malondialdehyde; LDL-MDA, low density lipoprotein malondialdehyde; Gpx, glutathione peroxidase; GR, glutathione reductase; SOD, superoxide dismutase; CAT, catalase; Vit C-PL, plasma vitamin C.
[b]Symbols: ↑, increase; —, no effect observed; ↓, decrease; ND, not determined. Brackets indicate an effect in

TABLE 26.2 Effect of Flavonoid-Free Basic Diet in Three Human Crossover Intervention Studies[a,b]

Biomarker:	PPO	P-MDA	LDL-MDA	Gpx	GR	SOD	CAT	Vit C-PL
Parsley study (II)	—	ND	ND	↓	↓	↓	↓	ND
Grape skin extract study (III)	↓	↑	—	—	↓	—	↓	↓
Green tea extract study (IV)	↓	ND	ND	ND	ND	ND	ND	↓

[a]Abbreviations: PPO, plasma protein oxidation; P-MDA, plasma malondialdehyde; LDL-MDA, low density lipoprotein malondialdehyde; Gpx, glutathione peroxidase; GR, glutathione reductase; SOD, superoxide dismutase; CAT, catalase; Vit C-PL, plasma vitamin C.
[b]Symbols: ↑, increase; —, no effect observed; ↓, decrease; ND, not determined.

observed. The uptake of catechins was determined in a separate study (Young *et al.*, unpublished). The green tea extract had a transient protective action against oxidation in plasma proteins at the highest dose level but no other effects were observed.

Taken together, these studies provide only weak evidence for a direct antioxidant effect of flavonoid-rich food items at ordinary dietary levels in humans (see Table 26.1). Only a few other studies have been reported with which to compare these results. A study using spinach intervention was published by a cooperating group (17). The study had a parallel design with a control group and groups receiving spinach or carotenoids (β-carotene and a lutein-rich extract). There was evidence for a spinach-dependent increase in glutathione reductase in that study, which correlated with plasma lutein. This might explain the effect on this enzyme reported above in the parsley intervention study because parsley is also rich in this carotenoid; however, it cannot explain our findings in the grape skin extract study. In a study on red grape juice intervention among seven individuals consuming an uncontrolled diet, a favorable effect was observed on plasma antioxidant capacity and on low density lipoprotein oxidation (18). This is in agreement with other studies using citrus juice intervention in which lipoprotein oxidation also decreased (19,20). A decrease in lipid peroxidation was also observed after tomato juice intervention. We observed a weak similar effect after intervention with another noncitrus fruit juice, indicating that lipid oxidation may be favorably affected by fruit juices. In a fruit and vegetable intervention study in which the number of servings increased by four to five in the intervention group but only by one in the control group, a slight relative decrease in plasma malondialdehyde was similarly reported after 3 and 6 mo (21); however, the difference was small and not significant. In most of these studies, as in ours, the effects of flavonoids and other nonnutritive antioxidants cannot be distinguished from potential effects of vitamin C. A pro-oxidant effect of fruit juices rich in polyphenols and vitamin C toward plasma proteins and possibly toward DNA was observed in our juice intervention study. In a previous intervention study with pure vitamin C in smokers, a nonsignificant increase in 8-oxo-dG excretion of ~26% was apparent from the data (22), implicating vitamin C as a possible prooxidant factor in the juice.

In most published short-term intervention studies, total or specific fruit and vegetable intake is increased. In our four intervention studies, we used a basic diet essentially devoid of fruits and vegetables. In the juice study, we could not distinguish the effects of intervention and the effects of the basic diet because there were no periods with basic diet only. Effect of the basic diet could be monitored in the parsley and grape skin extract studies because in these studies, there were 1-wk controlled interventions with the basic diet. In the grape skin extract study, no effects of the extract were found; thus, this study serves essentially as a short-term fruit and vegetable depletion study. The basic diet was essentially free from flavonoids, but also had a low content of vitamin C and a relatively high content of β-carotene (Young et al., unpublished). This resulted in decreased plasma ascorbate levels in the studies using grape skin or green tea extracts (see Table 26.2). Plasma lipid oxidation was determined only in the former in which it was weakly increased by the basic diet within the trial periods. This supports the observations by others mentioned above.

In the grape skin and green tea extract studies, the flavonoid-free basic diet also had a profound decreasing effect on plasma protein oxidation. This is in agreement with the effects seen in our juice study in which increases in urinary quercetin and in plasma vitamin C were accompanied by increased plasma protein oxidation. In the parsley study, we observed increased excretion of the flavone, apigenin, but we did not monitor plasma vitamin C. In that study, there was no significant effect of the intervention or of the basic diet on protein oxidation. In the spinach study, a significant positive correlation was observed between plasma vitamin C and plasma protein oxidation (17). The overall picture is that a strong and specific pro-oxidant effect toward plasma proteins exists, which is caused by vitamin C or compounds with a closely similar dietary distribution, possibly flavonols or some polyphenols more bioavailable than the flavonols. The vitamin C mimetic effects observed from the grape skin extract support the latter possibility. We speculate that one of the lysine residues in plasma albumin serves as a molecular biosensor for plasma Fenton-type oxidation potential, and that our specific protein oxidation marker is monitoring this sensor. The possible signal pathway and molecular consequences are currently under investigation.

The flavonoid-free diet also tended to decrease the activities of erythrocyte antioxidant enzymes. In the parsley study, all four activities (CAT, SOD, Gpx and GR) decreased significantly with time while the basic diet was consumed. In the grape skin extract study, only weak decreases in GR and CAT were observed. In the green tea extract study, antioxidant enzymes were not determined. As already discussed, decreased GR might be related to decreases in plasma levels of the carotenoid, lutein, which was unfortunately not determined in these studies. In the case of both GR and the other antioxidant enzyme activities, the molecular mechanism behind this effect seems obscure at present because erythrocytes have no nuclei and, hence, cannot regulate DNA transcription. We speculate therefore that a post-translational mechanism must be in effect.

In conclusion, in our short-term intervention studies, we observed an overall weak trend toward decreased lipid oxidation with increased polyphenol intake, which parallels most of the results in the literature. In contrast, we observed an increased oxidative stress response toward plasma proteins from food items rich in polyphenols and vitamin C and a decreased response when fruits and vegetables were omitted using a controlled diet. The data available could even be compatible with increased oxidation of DNA by high vitamin C intake. We also observed a similar trend toward increased antioxidant enzymes in red blood cells, particularly GR and Gpx, with increased polyphenols or vitamin C. This is in contrast to expectations and does not seem to be in agreement with the hypothesis that general relief of oxidative stress is a major protective mechanism by which dietary fruits and vegetables ameliorate chronic diseases. We find it likely that redox homeostasis is highly compartmentalized, even within the blood compartments, and that several mechanisms, both antioxidant and prooxidant, exist to keep the right redox balance within each of these compartments. Basic molecular studies are warranted to elucidate the regulatory mechanisms of the redox homeostasis in the various biological compartments and the effects of polyphenols and other redox-active compounds on these basic regulatory systems.

Acknowledgments

This work was supported in part by the Danish FØTEK3 Food Technology Programme funded by the Danish Research Councils as part of the project "Antioxidative Defense—Interactions Between Nutritive and Non-Nutritive Antioxidants."

References

1. Steinmetz, K.A., and Potter, J.D. (1996) Vegetables, Fruit, and Cancer Prevention: A Review. *J. Am. Diet. Assoc. 96*, 1027–1039.
2. World Cancer Research Fund (1997) *Food, Nutrition and the Prevention of Cancer: A Global Perspective*. Cannon, G. (ed.) American Institute for Cancer Research, Washington, DC.
3. Kushi, L.H., Lew, R.A., Stare, F.J., Ellison, C.R., el Lozy, M., Bourke, G., Daly, L., Graham, I., Hickey, N., and Mulcahy, R. (1985) Diet and 20-year Mortality from Coronary Heart Disease. The Ireland-Boston Diet-Heart Study. *N. Engl. J. Med. 312*, 811–818.
4. Gaziano, J.M., Manson, J.E., Branch, L.G., Colditz, G.A., Willett, W.C., and Buring, J.E. (1995) A Prospective Study of Consumption of Carotenoids in Fruits and Vegetables and Decreased Cardiovascular Mortality in the Elderly. *Ann. Epidemiol. 5*, 255–260.
5. Law, M.R., and Morris, J.K. (1998) By How Much Does Fruit and Vegetable Consumption Reduce the Risk of Ischaemic Heart Disease? *Eur. J. Clin. Nutr. 52*, 549–556.
6. Block, G. (1991) Epidemiologic Evidence Regarding Vitamin C and Cancer. *Am. J. Clin. Nutr. 54*, 1310S–1314S.
7. Peto, R., Doll, R., Buckley, J.D., and Sporn, M.B. (1981) Can Dietary β-Carotene Materially Reduce Human Cancer Rates? *Nature 290*, 201–208.
8. Weisburger, J.H. (1991) Nutrional Approach to Cancer Prevention with Emphasis on Vitamins, Antioxidants, and Carotenoids. *Am. J. Clin. Nutr. 53*, 226S–237S.
9. van Poppel, G., and van den Berg, H. (1997) Vitamins and Cancer. *Cancer Lett. 114*, 195–202.
10. Alpha Tocopherol Beta Carotene Cancer Prevention Study Group (1994) The Effect of Vitamin E and Beta Carotene on the Incidence of Lung Cancer and Other Cancers in Male Smokers. *N. Engl. J. Med. 330*, 1029–1035.
11. Dragsted, L.O., Nilsson, L., Háraldsdottir, J., Daneshvar, B., Kall, M., Young, J.F., and Sandstrom, B. (2000) Green Tea Extract Influences Plasma Protein Oxidation in a Short-Term Human Intervention Study, in *Polyphenols Commun. 2000* (Martens, S., Treutter, D., and Forkmann, G., eds.), pp. 489–490, Technical University of München, München.
12. Nielsen, S.E., Young, J.F., Daneshvar, B., Lauridsen, S.T., Knuthsen, P., Sandstrom, B., and Dragsted, L.O. (1999) Effect of Parsley (*Petroselinum crispum*) Intake on Urinary Apigenin Excretion, Blood Antioxidant Enzymes and Biomarkers for Oxidative Stress in Human Subjects [see comments]. *Br. J. Nutr. 81*, 447–455.

13. Young, J.F., Nielsen, S.E., Haraldsdóttir, J., Daneshvar, B., Lauridsen, S.T., Knuthsen, P., Crozier, A., Sandström, B., and Dragsted, L.O. Effect of Fruit Juice Intake on Urinary Quercetin Excretion and Biomarkers of Antioxidative Status. *Am. J. Clin. Nutr. 69*, 87–94. 1999.
14. Young, J.F., Dragsted, L.O., Daneshvar, B., Lauridsen, S.T., Hansen, M., and Sandström, B. (2000) The Effect of Grape Skin Extract on Oxidative Status. *Br. J. Nutr. 84,* 505–513.
15. Nielsen, S.E., and Dragsted, L.O. (1998) Column-Switching High-Performance Liquid Chromatographic Assay for Determination of Apigenin and Acacetin in Human Urine with Ultraviolet Absorbance Detection. *J. Chromatogr. B 713*, 379–386.
16. Nielsen, S.E., and Dragsted, L.O. (1998) Column-Switching High-Performance Liquid Chromatographic Assay for the Determination of Quercetin in Human Urine with Ultraviolet Absorbance Detection. *J. Chromatogr. B 707*, 81–89.
17. Castenmiller, J.J.M., Lauridsen, S.T., Dragsted, L.O., van het Hof, K.H., Linssen, J.P.H., and West, C.E. (1999) β-Carotene Does Not Change Markers of Enzymatic and Nonenzymatic Antioxidant Activity in Human Blood. *J. Nutr. 129*, 2162–2169.
18. Day, A.P., Kemp, H.J., Bolton, C., Hartog, M., and Stansbie, D. (1997) Effect of Concentrated Red Grape Juice Consumption on Serum Antioxidant Capacity and Low-Density Lipoprotein Oxidation. *Ann. Nutr. Metab. 41*, 353–357.
19. Abbey, M., Noakes, M., and Nestel, P.J. (1995) Dietary Supplementation with Orange and Carrot Juice in Cigarette Smokers Lowers Oxidation Products in Copper-Oxidized Low-Density Lipoproteins. *J. Am. Diet. Assoc. 95*, 671–675.
20. Harats, D., Chevion, S., Nahir, M., Norman, Y., Sagee, O., and Berry, E.M. (1998) Citrus Fruit Supplementation Reduces Lipoprotein Oxidation in Young Men Ingesting a Diet High in Saturated Fat: Presumptive Evidence for an Interaction Between Vitamins C and E *In Vivo. Am. J. Clin. Nutr. 67*, 240–245.
21. Maskarinec, G., Chan, C.L., Meng, L., Franke, A.A., and Cooney, R.V. (1999) Exploring the Feasibility and Effects of a High-Fruit and -Vegetable Diet in Healthy Women. *Cancer Epidemiol. Biomark. Prev. 8*, 919–924.
22. Prieme, H., Loft, S., Nyyssonen, K., Salonen, J.T., and Poulsen, H.E. (1997) No Effect of Supplementation with Vitamin E, Ascorbic Acid, or Coenzyme Q10 on Oxidative DNA Damage Estimated by 8-Oxo-7,8-dihydro-2′-deoxyguanosine Excretion in Smokers. *Am. J. Clin. Nutr. 65*, 503–507.
23. Daneshvar, B., Frandsen, H., Autrup, H., and Dragsted, L.O. (1997) γ-Glutamyl Semialdehyde and 2-Amino-adipic Semialdehyde: Biomarkers of Oxidative Damage to Proteins. *Biomarkers 2*, 117–123.

Chapter 27

Redox Regulation of Antioxidant Protection of the Heart

Dipak K. Das and Nilanjana Maulik

Cardiovascular Research Center, University of Connecticut School of Medicine, Farmington, CT 06030

Introduction

A large number of degenerative diseases, including coronary heart disease, have been linked with the overproduction of oxygen-derived free radicals. The results of many studies, including our own, have demonstrated that excessive production of reactive oxygen species (ROS), in concert with drastic reduction of antioxidant reserve, plays a crucial role in the pathophysiology of ischemic heart disease (1–4). Myocardial ischemia and reperfusion cause the cardiomyocytes to face conditions that shift their redox status and to undergo a drastic change that subjects them to oxidative stress (5). Interventions with oxygen free radical scavengers or antioxidant therapy have been found to be cardioprotective against ischemic reperfusion injury (6–8).

Recent studies have documented that coronary heart diseases cause cardiomyocyte death not only by necrosis but also by apoptosis (9–11). Reperfusion of the ischemic myocardium results in apoptotic cell death and DNA fragmentation (12). In concert, ischemia/reperfusion is associated with the induction of a number of both pro- and antiapoptotic genes and transcription factors (13,14). Ebselen, a glutathione peroxidase (GSHPx) mimic and a functional antioxidant, was found to reduce cardiomyocyte apoptosis (15). The hearts from the transgenic mice overexpressing the GSHPx-1 gene were resistant to ischemia/reperfusion injury, whereas those from the GSHPx-1 knockout mice, devoid of any copy of GSHPx-1, were extremely vulnerable to cellular injury compared with wild-type controls (16).

Three Lines of Antioxidant Defense

ROS are continuously generated in the heart during incomplete reduction of the oxygen molecule. The ROS include superoxide anions and hydroxyl radicals as well as oxidants such as hydrogen peroxide. These ROS lead to the production of a number of secondary free radicals, including peroxyl and hydroperoxyl radicals. Nitric oxide generated in the tissue can produce extremely cytotoxic peroxynitrites. Virtually every biomolecule, including lipids, proteins, and DNA molecules, are potential targets of free radical attack. The mammalian heart is equipped with its own antioxidant defense to fight any free radical attack (17). Constitutive cellular protection against acute stress can be provided by various intracellular antioxidants such as glutathione, α-tocopherol, ascorbic acid, β-carotene, and antioxidant enzymes that include superoxide dismutase (SOD), catalase, and GSHPx. These cellular compounds reduce/eliminate oxidative stress by directly quenching the ROS before they damage vital cellular components; therefore, they can be considered as part of the *first line of defense* against the external stress (Fig. 27.1). Often, because of the inadequacy of the intracellular antioxidants or due to the presence of increased amount of oxidative stress in pathophysiologic conditions such as ischemia and heart failure, the ROS may reach their targets, which include nucleic acid, protein, and lipids. This results in injury to the cellular components, causing DNA strand breaks, protein degradation, and lipid peroxidation. Mammalian hearts are also protected by a *second line of defense* system consisting of several lipolytic and proteolytic enzymes, proteases and phospholipases that are involved in the systematic recognition and removal of injured components.

In view of the increasing evidence for the involvement of cellular oxidation and oxidative stress in various pathophysiologic conditions of heart disease, it is of considerable interest to examine whether myocardial cells possess an inducible pathway for antioxidant defense. The signal transduction pathways by which various stress signals are translated into oxidative stress leading to the modulation of antioxidants/antioxidant enzymes, are likely to be different, but the induction of the expression of their mRNAs and/or the increased translation of mRNA accumulation as a result of

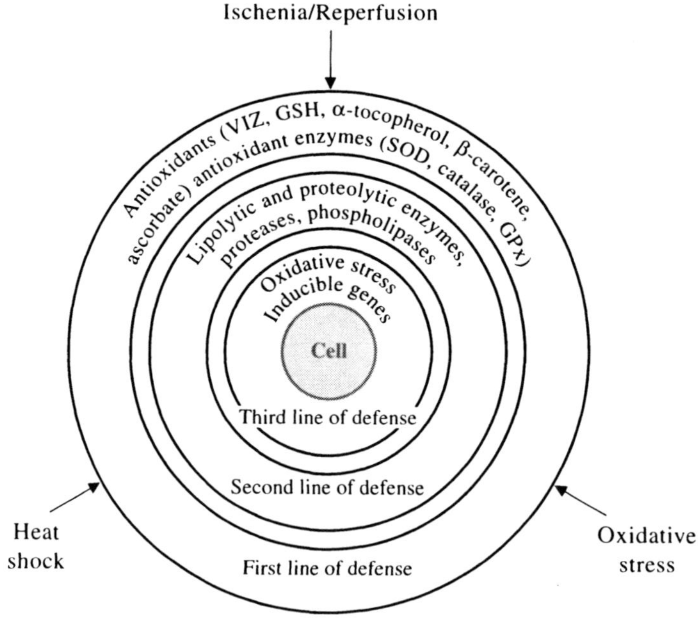

Fig. 27.1. Antioxidant defense system against ischemic heart disease.

changes at the level of RNA transcription or stability seem to be the most plausible mechanisms. This could lead to the synthesis of proteins involved in cellular protection or repair of injury. These phenomena related to specific gene expression could be viewed as a *third line of defense* and may reflect the ultimate adaptive responses.

Antioxidant Protection of the Heart

It should be clear from the above discussion that despite the presence of adequate antioxidant defense, hearts becomes helpless in pathologic conditions because of the reduction of antioxidants in conjunction with the massive production of ROS. There is general agreement that the amounts of several antioxidants and antioxidant enzymes are significantly reduced after ischemia and reperfusion. For example, reduced amounts of SOD, catalase, and GSHPx enzymes as well as α-tocopherol and ascorbic acid have been found in the ischemic reperfused myocardium (18). The loss of the key antioxidant enzymes and antioxidants thus reduces the overall antioxidant reserve of the heart, making it susceptible to ischemia/reperfusion injury. One of the major functions of antioxidants is to block free radical formation. Thus, reduced antioxidant reserve in conjunction with increased free radical generation leads to the cellular injury associated with ischemia/reperfusion.

It is believed that antioxidants such as SOD, catalase, and GSHPx enzymes as well as α-tocopherol comprise the first line of defense against many degenerative diseases, including myocardial ischemic reperfusion injury (19). Additionally, induction of the expression of the oxidative stress inducible genes can be viewed as a stress survival signal for the heart and suggests another line of defense for the ischemic myocardium (19).

Antioxidant supplementation to the heart in the face of ischemia has been found to be cardioprotective. Treatment of hyperthyroid rats with α-tocopherol protected the heart from ischemic reperfusion injury (20). Antioxidant therapy with SOD plus catalase prevented apoptotic cardiomyocyte death induced by ischemia and reperfusion (21). Selenium deficiency led to an increase in myocardial ischemic injury to rats (22). IRFI 042, a novel vitamin E-like antioxidant, inhibited activation of nuclear factor (NF)-κB and reduced the inflammatory response in myocardial ischemia/reperfusion injury (23). Grape seed proanthocyanidins protected rat hearts from ischemic injury by scavenging hydroxyl and peroxyl radicals generated during ischemia and reperfusion (24). In another related study, the red wine antioxidant resveratrol protected isolated rat hearts from ischemia reperfusion injury (25). Ischemia/reperfusion-induced oxidative stress was reduced by vitamin E treatment (26). Recombinant adenovirus-mediated cardiac gene transfer of SOD and catalase attenuated postischemic contractile dysfunction (27). Another study showed that overexpression of MnSOD protected against myocardial ischemia/reperfusion injury in transgenic mice (28). Pretreatment of the heart with SOD plus catalase also ameliorated ischemic reperfusion injury (29).

Thus, it is clear that exogenous antioxidants can reduce myocardial ischemia reperfusion injury by improving postischemic contractile dysfunction and decreasing tissue injury by reducing both necrotic and apoptotic cell death. The potential for antioxidant therapy to combat ischemic heart disease appears to be enormous.

Micronutrients, Antioxidants, and Heart

Micronutrients are essential for survival because they play a key role in metabolism. A growing body of evidence indicates a crucial role of several micronutrients in cardioprotection. Of particular importance are vitamins A, C, and E, folate, β-carotene, coenzyme Q_{10}, zinc and selenium because the absence of one or more of these micronutrients constitutes an important risk factor for cardiac diseases.

Clinical use of antioxidant vitamin supplementation may help prevent coronary heart disease. Beneficial effects of vitamin E treatment in acute myocardial infarction are well recognized (30). Vitamin A is another essential micronutrients throughout the development of heart. Its active form, retinoic acid, is involved in intracellular signaling, regulating development. Vitamin A has recently been found to play an antioxidant role in cardioprotection against ischemic heart disease (31). Low serum carotene has been linked with the increased risk of ischemic heart disease (32).

Folic acid (vitamin B-9), a member of the B-complex family of vitamins, functions by *S*-methylation of homocysteine to generate methionine (33). Homocysteine, which is an intermediate formed during the metabolism of methionine, has recently been found to be an important risk factor for vascular disease, including coronary atherosclerosis (34). Recently, folic acid was found to possess an antioxidant-like function. Folic acid may be used to reduce increased homocysteine concentration in patients with coronary artery disease.

Several metal ions, especially divalent cations, are important members of the essential micronutrient group. Copper is a catalytic cofactor for Cu/Zn-SOD and ceruloplasmin, both of which have been implicated in cardioprotection (35). Manganese is also a cofactor for Mn-SOD, which plays an important role in cardioprotection. Targeted MnSOD gene delivery was found to ameliorate ischemia/reperfusion injury. MnSOD can also be induced in the heart during myocardial adaptation to ischemic stress (36). GSHPx, which detoxifies hydrogen peroxide, is an important member of the first line of antioxidant defense. Hearts of transgenic mice overexpressing extra copies of GSHPx-1 gene are resistant, whereas knockout mice devoid of any copies of GSHPx-1 are susceptible to ischemia reperfusion injury (37). Selenium is a cofactor for GSHPx. The activity of GSHPx is decreased by selenium deficiency, which renders the myocardium susceptible to ischemic reperfusion injury (38). Selenium is also essential for humans because it protects the heart against cardiomyopathy (39). Two other metal ions, zinc and magnesium, also play an important role in cardioprotection. Recently, the antioxidant effect of magnesium was found to play a role in its cardioprotective ability against ischemic reperfusion injury (40).

Lycopene, the pigment responsible for the characteristic deep-red color of ripe tomatoes, has recently been added to the ever-growing essential micronutrient list because this pigment can quench singlet oxygen twice as efficiently as β-carotene (41). Dietary supplementation of lycopene significantly increased serum lycopene levels and lowered lipid peroxidation and low density lipoprotein (LDL) oxidation, two important risk factors in coronary heart disease (42). Coenzyme Q_{10} is another important factor; it can provide cardioprotection against ischemia reperfusion injury (43). A recent study showed that supplementation of CoQ_{10} in the diet leads to the induction of ubiquitin gene expression, simultaneously ameliorating ischemic injury to the heart (44).

Antioxidants and Redox Signaling

Despite the overwhelming evidence indicating that ROS are detrimental factors, it is becoming increasingly clear that these free radicals can also function as signaling molecules, and hence, may be essential for the biological and physiologic function of the cells. Biological cells including cardiomyocytes contain enzymes that can simultaneously generate ROS and intracellular redox buffer in response to a specific stress. Depending on the amounts of antioxidant reserve and oxygen free radicals, the ROS are either destroyed or persist. Thus, the oxygen free radicals fulfill the definition of a second messenger; they are either upregulated or downregulated after physiologic stimuli such as ischemia. A number of growth factors and cytokines have been found to induce oxidative stress and overproduce specific antioxidant enzymes (45). Environmental stresses, including heat stress, oxidative stress, and ischemia/reperfusion also produce oxidative stress, which is then translated into the induction of antioxidant enzymes (46).

Perhaps the finding that the production of ROS during the agonist-induced activation of the nuclear transcription factor, NF-κB, provided the first concrete evidence for the role of ROS as a second messenger. NF-κB regulates the inducible expression of a number of genes involved in cell survival and execution. For example, NF-κB has been found to control the antiapoptotic gene, bcl-2, and the proapoptotic factors, bax and p53, in the ischemic/reperfused myocardium (47). Diverse extracellular signals from interleukin (IL)-1, tumor necrosis factor (TNF)-α, H_2O_2, and others converge into development of oxidative stress, which leads to activation of NF-κB (48). Such activation of NF-κB can be blocked by antioxidants such as vitamin E (49) or α-lipoic acid (50). Antioxidants such as *N*-acetyl cystein can prevent NF-κB activation by diverse stimuli, including H_2O_2, by suppressing the generation of ROS (51).

Although ischemia/reperfusion has been found to manipulate cardiomyocyte life and death through redox signaling, the precise physiologic role of the signaling process is not clear. Ischemia/reperfusion, especially intermittent ischemia, commonly known as ischemic preconditioning or adaptation, leads to the activation of both G-proteins and receptor tyrosine kinases, potentiating a signaling cascade that results in the activation of multiple kinases (52–55). These sequential events lead to the induction of the activation of several redox-sensing transcription factors and genes (56,57). Such intracellular events ultimately dictate whether the cells survive or die. The changes in gene expression are likely to influence the physiologic function of the cardiomyocyte during postischemic survival.

A number of recent studies clearly demonstrated that redox signaling plays a physiologic role in myocardial survival during the postischemic period. As mentioned earlier, oxygen free radicals are generated during ischemia/reperfusion. When the heart is adapted to ischemic stress by repeated short-term ischemia and reperfusion, the generation of ROS increases rapidly, but does not increase at the same rate during subsequent ischemia and reperfusion. The same pattern of development of oxidative stress is observed when hearts are treated with endotoxin, IL-1, or TNFα. Interestingly, these interventions lead to the development of oxidative stress within a very short period, but reduce/inhibit subsequent oxidative stress development when hearts are subjected to ischemia/reperfusion. Additionally, such an adaptive response is associated with the induction of the expression of a number of stress proteins, including HSP 27, HSP 70, and heme oxygenase, and antioxidant enzymes, including Mn-SOD and GSHPx (58). Such adaptive response is also associated with the increased binding activity of NF-κB. Increased activity of NF-κB and induction of the protective proteins can be blocked by pretreating the hearts with an oxygen free radical scavenger such as DMTU (59). More interestingly, an endotoxin-derived compound, monophosphoryl lipid A (MLA), was found to induce iNOS mRNA through a tyrosine kinase–dependent mechanism and protect the heart from ischemic reperfusion injury (60).

Thus, it seems likely that one of the major functions of redox signaling in the ischemic myocardium is to synthesize stress-inducible proteins, comprising the *third line of defense* through the activation of transcription factors such as NF-κB or by potentiating induction of other inducible proteins such as iNOS. However, more study is required to unveil completely the physiologic function of redox cycling.

Summary and Conclusion

It should be clear from the above discussion that the potential for antioxidant therapy in cardiovascular diseases is enormous. The fact that the primary defense of heart against cellular injury comprises antioxidants and that these antioxidants are lowered in the pathophysiologic conditions in concert with massive production of ROS warrants administration of exogenous antioxidants as potential therapy. Such antioxidant therapy may be manifested by nutritional supplement of the antioxidants or by direct administration into the blood circulation. Many of these antioxidants are found as polyphenolic compounds in fruits and vegetables. Regular consumption of fresh fruits and vegetables is expected to upregulate the body's defense system against cardiovascular diseases. Antioxidant gene therapy has also great potential and is gaining popularity.

It is also important to remember that the same detrimental and cytotoxic ROS can function as second messengers and become responsible for redox signaling leading to the induction of the expression of many cardioprotective genes. These genes, which include the antideath gene Bcl-2, transmit survival signals and tend to protect the ischemic myocardium from cellular injury, especially from apoptotic cell death. Antioxidants, by eliminating the oxidative stress, may simply block this important survival signal (Fig. 27.2).

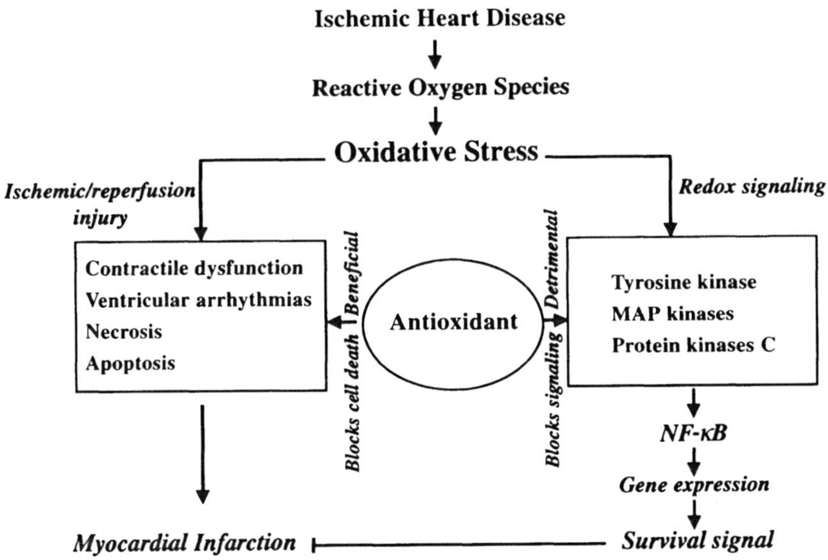

Fig. 27.2. Beneficial and detrimental components of antioxidants.

Acknowledgments

This study was supported by National Institutes of Health grants HL 33889, HL 56421, HL 22559 and HL 56803.

References

1. Otani, H., Engelman, R.M., Rousou, J.A., Breyer, R.H., and Das, D.K. (1986) Enhanced Prostaglandin Synthesis Due to Phospholipase Breakdown in Ischemic-Reperfused Myocardium. Control of Its Production by a Phospholipase Inhibitor or Free Radical Scavengers. *J. Mol. Cell. Cardiol. 18*, 953–961.
2. Simpson, P.J., and Lucchesi, B.R. (1987) Free Radicals and Myocardial Ischemia and Reperfusion Injury. *J. Lab. Clin. Med. 110*, 13–18.
3. Baker, J.E., Felix, C.C., Olinger, G.N., and Kalyanaraman, B. (1988) Myocardial Ischemia and Reperfusion: Direct Evidence for Free Radical Generation by Electron Spin Resonance Spectroscopy. *Proc. Natl. Acad. Sci. USA 85*, 2786–2788.
4. Zweier, J.L. (1988) Measurement of Superoxide-Derived Free Radicals in the Reperfused Heart: Evidence for a Free Radical Mechanism in Reperfusion Injury. *J. Biol. Chem. 263*, 1353–1356.
5. Tosaki, A., Bagchi, D., Hellegouarch, A., Pali, T., Cordis,G.A., and Das, D.K. (1993), Comparisons of ESR and HPLC Methods for the Detection of Hydroxyl Radicals in Ischemic/Reperfused Hearts. A Relationship Between the Genesis of Oxygen-Free Radicals and Reperfusion-Induced Arrhythmias. *Biochem. Pharmacol. 45*, 961–969.
6. Ambrosio, G., Jacobus, W.E., Weisfeldt, M.L., and Flaherty, J.T. (1987) Evidence for a Reversible Oxygen Radical-Mediated Component of Reperfusion Injury: Reduction by Human Recombinant Superoxide Dismutase Administered at the Time of Reflow. *Circulation 75*, 282–287.

7. Bolli, R., Zhi, W.X., and Hartley, C.J. (1987) Attenuation of Dysfunction in the Post- Ischemic Stunned Myocardium by Dimethylthiourea. *Circulation 76*, 458–462.
8. Myers, C.L., Weiss, S.J., Kirsh, M.M., Shepard, B.M., and Shlafer, M. (1986) Effects of Supplementing Hypothermic Crystalloid Cardioplegic Solution with Catalase, Superoxide Dismutase, Allopurinol, on Ischemic and Reperfused Hearts. *J. Thorac. Cardiovasc. Surg. 91*, 281–285.
9. Maulik, N., Yoshida, T., and Das, D.K. (1998) Oxidative Stress Developed During the Reperfusion of Ischemic Myocardium Induces Apoptosis. *Free Radic. Biol. Med. 24*, 869–875.
10. Maulik, N., Kagan, V., and Das, D.K. (1998) Redistribution of Phosphatidylserine and Phosphatidylethanolamine Precedes Reperfusion-Induced Apoptosis. *Am. J. Physiol. 274*, H242–H248.
11. Maulik, N., and Das, D.K. (1999) Apoptosis, Heart Failure, Ischemic Heart Disease. *Heart Failure Rev. 4*, 165–173.
12. Maulik, N., Yoshida, T., Engelman, R.M., Deaton, D., Flack, J.E., Rousou, J.A., and Das, D.K. (1998) Ischemic Preconditioning Attenuates Apoptotic Cell Death Associated with Ischemia/Reperfusion. *Mol. Cell. Biochem. 186*, 139–145.
13. Maulik, N., Goswami, S., Galang, N., and Das, D.K. (1999) Differential Regulation of Bcl-2, AP-1 and NFκB on Cardiomyocyte Apoptosis During Myocardial Ischemic Stress Adaptation. *FEBS Lett. 443*, 331–336.
14. Maulik, N., Sasaki, H., Addya, S., and Das, D.K. (2000) Regulation of Cardiomyocyte Apoptosis by Redox-Sensitive Transcription Factors. *FEBS Lett. 485*, 7–12.
15. Maulik, N., and Yoshida, T. (2000) Oxidative Stress Development During Open Heart Surgery Induces Apoptosis: Reduction of Apoptolic Cell Death—by Ebselem, a Glutathione Peroxidase Mimic. *J. Cardiovasc. Pharmacol. 36*, 601–608.
16. Yoshida, T., Watanabe, M., Engelman, D.T., Engelman, R.M., Schley, J., Maulik, N., Ho, Y.-S., Oberly, T.D., and Das, D.K. (1996) Transgenic Mice Overexpressing Glutathione Peroxidase Are Resistant to Myocardial Ischemia Reperfusion Injury. *J. Mol. Cell. Cardiol. 28*, 1759–1767.
17. Engelman, D., Watanabe, M., Engelman, R.M., Rousou, J.A., Kisin, E., Kagan, V.E., Maulik, N., and Das, D.K. (1995) Hypoxic Preconditioning Preserves Antioxidant Reserve in the Working Rat Heart. *Cardiovasc. Res. 29*, 133–140.
18. Das, D.K., Engelman, R.M., Rousou, J.A., Breyer, R.H., Otani, H., and Lemeshow, S. (1986) Pathophysiology of Superoxide Radical as Potential Mediator of Ischemic and Reperfusion Injury in Pig Heart. *Basic Res. Cardiol. 81*, 155–166.
19. Das, D.K., Maulik, N., and Moraru, I.I. (1995) Gene Expression in Acute Myocardial Stress. Induction by Hypoxia, Ischemia, Reperfusion, Hyperthermia and Oxidative Stress. *J. Mol. Cell. Cardiol. 27*, 181–193
20. Venditti, P., Masullo, P., Agnisola, C., and Di Meo, S. (2000) Effect of Vitamin E on the Response to Ischemia-Reperfusion of Langendorff Heart Preparations from Hyperthyroid Rats. *Life Sci. 66*, 697–708.
21. Galang, N., Sasaki, H., and Maulik, N. (2000) Apoptotic Cell Death During Ischemia/Reperfusion and Its Attenuation by Antioxidant Therapy. *Toxicology 148*, 111–118.
22. Toufektsian, M.C., Boucher, F., Pucheu S., Tanguy, S., Ribuot, C., Sanou, D., Tresallet, N., and de Leiris, J. (2000) Effects of Selenium Deficiency on the Response of Cardiac Tissue to Ischemia and Reperfusion. *Toxicology 148*, 125–132.

23. Altavilla, D., Deodate, B., Campo, G.M., Arlotta, M., Miano, M., Squadrito, G., Saitta, A., Cucinotta, D., Ceccarelli, S., Ferlito, M., Tringali, M., Minutoli, L., Caputi, A.P., and Squadrito, F. (2000) IRF1 042, a Novel Dual Vitamin E-Like Antioxidant, Inhibits Activation of Nuclear Factor Kappa B and Reduces the Inflammatory Response in Myocardial Ischemia-Reperfusion Injury. *Cardiovasc. Res. 47*, 515–528.
24. Sato, M., Maulik, G., Ray, P.S., Bagchi, D., and Das, D.K. (1999) Cardioprotective Effects of Grape Seed Proanthocyanidin Against Ischemic Reperfusion Injury. *J. Mol. Cell. Cardiol. 31*, 1289–1297.
25. Ray, P.S., Maulik, G., Cordis, G.A, Bertelli, A.A., Bertelli, A., and Das, D.K. (1999) The Red Wine Antioxidant Resveratrol Protects Isolated Rat Hearts from Ischemia Reperfusion Injury. *Free Radic. Biol. Med. 27*, 160–169.
26. Venditti, P., Masullo, P., Di Meo, S., and Agnisola, C. (1999) Protection Against Ischemia-Reperfusion Induced Oxidative Stress by Vitamin E Treatment. *Arch. Physiol. Biochem. 107*, 27–34.
27. Woo, Y.J., Zhang, J.C., Vijayasarathy, C., Zwacka, R.M., Englehardt, J.F., Gardner, T.J., and Sweeney, H.L. (1998) Recombinant Adenovirus-Mediated Cardiac Gene Transfer of Superoxide Dismutase and Catalase Attenuates Postischemic Contractile Dysfunction. *Circulation 98*, II255–260.
28. Chen, Z., Siu, B., Ho, Y.S., Vincent, R., Chua, C.C., Hamdy, R.C., and Shua, B.H. (1998) Overexpression of MnSOD Protects Against Myocardial Ischemia/Reperfusion Injury in Transgenic Mice. *J. Mol. Cell. Cardiol. 30*, 2281–2289.
29. Otani, H., Engelman, R.M., Rousou, J.A., Breyer, R.H., Lemeshow, S., and Das, D.K. (1986) Cardiac Performance During Reperfusion Improved by Pretreatment with Oxygen-Free Radical Scavengers. *J. Thorac. Cardiovasc. Surg. 91*, 290–295.
30. Sethi, R., Takeda, N., Nagano, M., and Dhalla, N.S. (2000) Beneficial Effects of Vitamin E Treatment in Acute Myocardial Infarction. *J. Cardiovasc. Pharmacol. Ther. 5*, 51–58.
31. Todd, S., Tunstall-Pedoe, H., Woodward M., and Bolton-Smith, C. (1999) Dietary Antioxidant Vitamins and Fiber in the Etiology of Cardiovascular Disease and All-Causes Mortality, Results from the Scottish Heart Health Study. *Am. J. Epidemiol. 150*, 1073–1080.
32. Hsueh, Y.M, Wu, W.L., Huang, Y.L., Chiou, H.Y., Tseng, C.H., and Chen, C.J. (1998) Low Serum Carotene Level and Increased Risk of Ischemic Heart Disease Related to Long-Term Arsenic Exposure. *Atherosclerosis 141*, 249–257.
33. Brattstrom, L., and Wilcken, D.E. (2000) Homocysteine and Cardiovascular Disease: Cause or Effect? *Am. J. Clin. Nutr. 72*, 315–323.
34. Title, L.M., Cummings, P.M., Giddens, K., Genest, J.J., and Nassar, B.A. (2000) Effect of Folic Acid and Antioxidant Vitamins on Endothelial Dysfunction in Patients with Coronary Artery Disease. *J. Am. Coll. Cardiol. 36*, 758–765.
35. Yoshida, T., Maulik, N., Engelman, R.M., Ho, Y.S., and Das, D.K. (2000) Targeted Disruption of the Mouse SOD1 Gene Makes the Heart Vulnerable to Ischemic Reperfusion Injury. *Circ. Res. 86*, 264–269.
36. Ibrahim, W., Lee, U.S., Yen, H.C., St Clair, D.K., and Chow, C.K. (2000) Antioxidant and Oxidative Status in Tissues of Manganese Superoxide Dismutase Transgenic Mice. *Free Radic. Biol. Med. 28*, 397–402.
37. Maulik, N., Yoshida, T., and Das, D.K. (1999) Regulation of Cardiomyocyte Apoptosis in Ischemic Reperfused Mouse Heart by Glutathione Peroxidase. *Mol. Cell. Biochem. 196*, 13–21.

38. Toufektsian, M.C., Boucher, F., Pucheu, S., Tanguy, S., Ribuot, C., Sanou, D., Tresallet, N., and de Lairis, J. (2000) Effects of Selenium Deficiency on the Response of Cardiac Tissue to Ischemia and Reperfusion. *Toxicology 148*, 125–132.
39. Dhindsa, H.S., Bermingham, M.A., Mierzwa, J., and Sullivan, D. (1998) Plasma Selenium Concentrations in a Sikh Population in Sydney, Australia. *Analyst 123*, 885–887.
40. Maulik, M., Maulik, S.K., and Kumari, R. (1999) Importance of Timing of Magnesium Administration: A Study on the Isolated Ischemic-Reperfused Rat Heart. *Magnes. Res. 12*, 37–42.
41. Shi, J., and Le Maguer, M. (2000) Lycopene in Tomatoes: Chemical and Physical Properties Affected by Food Processing. *Crit. Res. Food Sci. Nutr. 40*, 1–42.
42. Agarwal, S., and Rao, A.V. (1998) Tomato Lycopene and Low Density Lipoprotein Oxidation: A Human Dietary Intervention Study. *Lipids 33*, 981–984.
43. Otani, H., and Das, D.K. (2000) Role of Coenzyme Q10 in Myocardial Tolerance to Ischemia and Reperfusion, in *Coenzyme Q: Molecular Mechanisms in Health and Disease* (Kagan, V.E. and Quinn, P.J., eds.) pp. 277–284, CRC Press, Boca Raton.
44. Maulik, N., Yoshida, T., Engelman, R.M., Bagchi, D., Otani, H., and Das, D.K. (2000) Dietary Coenzyme Q_{10} Supplementation Renders Swine Hearts Resistant to Ischemia Reperfusion Injury. *Am. J. Physiol. 278,* H1084–H1090.
45. Maulik, N., Watanabe, M., Engelman, D., Engelman, R.M., Kagan, V.E., Kisin, E., Tyurin, V., Cordis, G.A., and Das, D.K. (1995) Myocardial Adaptation to Ischemia by Oxidative Stress Induced by Endotoxin. *Am. J. Physiol. 269*, C907–C916.
46. Maulik, N., Watanabe, M., Engelman, D., Engelman, R.M., and Das, D.K. (1995) Oxidative Stress Adaptation Improves Postischemic Ventricular Recovery. *Mol. Cell. Biochem. 144*, 67–74.
47. Bromme, H.J., and Holz, J. (1996) Apoptosis in the Heart; When and Why. *Mol. Cell. Biochem. 163/164*, 261–275.
48. Beg, A.A., and Baltimore, D. (1996) An Essential Role for NFB in Preventing TNF-Alpha-Induced Cell Death. *Science 274*, 787–789.
49. Suzuki, Y.J, and Packer, L. (1993) Inhibition of NFB DNA Binding Activity by α-Tocopheryl Succinate. *Biochem. Mol. Biol. Int. 31*, 693–700.
50. Suzuki, Y.J., Aggarwal, B.B., and Packer, L. (1992) α-Lipoic Acid Is a Potent Inhibitor of NFκB Activation in Human T Cells. *Biochem. Biophys. Res. Commun. 189*, 1709–1715.
51. Screck, R., Rieber, P., and Baeuerle, P.A. (1991) Reactive Oxygen Intermediates as Apparently Widely Used Messengers in the Activation of the NFκB Transcription Factor and HIV-1. *EMBO J. 10*, 2247–2258.
52. Maulik, N.,Yoshida, T., Zu, Y.L., Sato, M., Banerjee, A., and Das, D.K. (1998) Ischemic Preconditioning Triggers Tyrosine Kinase Signaling: Potential Role for MAPKAP Kinase 2. *Am. J. Physiol. 275*, H1857–H1864.
53. Tosaki, A., Cordis, G.A., Szerdahelyi, P., Engelman, R.M., and Das, D.K. (1996) Role of Protein Kinase C in Ischemic Preconditioning of Rat Hearts. *J. Cardiovasc. Pharmacol. 28*, 723–731.
54. Maulik, N., and Das, D.K. (1996) Ischemic Preconditioning Triggers the Activation of MAP Kinases and MAPKAP Kinase 2 in Rat Hearts. *FEBS Lett. 396*, 233–237.
55. Sato, M., Cordis, G.A., Maulik, N., and Das, D.K. (2000) SAPKs Regulation of Ischemic Preconditioning. *Am. J. Physiol. 279*, H901–H907.

56. Das, D.K., Maulik, N., and Moraru, I.I. (1995) Gene Expression in Acute Myocardial Stress. *J. Mol. Cell. Cardiol. 27*, 181–193.
57. Das, D.K., Maulik, N., Engelman, R.M., Rousou, J.A., Deaton, D., and Flack, J.E. (1998) Signal Transduction Pathway for HSP 27 and HSP 70 Gene Expression During Myocardial Adaptation to Stress. *Ann. N.Y. Acad. Sci. 851*, 129–138.
58. Das, D.K., Engelman, R.M., and Kimura, Y. (1993) Molecular Adaptation to Cellular Defences Following Preconditioning of the Heart by Repeated Ischemia. *Cardiovasc. Res. 27*, 578–584.
59. Das, D.K., Maulik, N., Sato, M., and Ray, P. (1999) Reactive Oxygen Species Function as Second Messenger During Ischemic Preconditioning of Heart. *Mol. Cell. Biol. 196*, 59–67.
60. Yoshida, T., Engelman, R.M., Engelman, D.T., Rousou, J.A., Maulik. N., Sato, M., Elliott, G.T., and Das, D.K. (2000) Preconditioning of Swine Heart with Monophosphoryl Lipid A Improves Myocardial Preservation. *Ann. Thorac. Surg. 70*, 895–900.

Chapter 28

Imbalanced Antioxidant Status in Transfusion-Dependent Thalassemia Patients in Jakarta, Indonesia

S. Handayani,[d] C. Adhiyanto,[d] I.R. Fani,[d] J. Hidayat,[d] D.R. Laksmitawati,[d] V. Kurniati,[d] R.R. Soegianto,[d] D.H.S. Dillon,[c] R. Pudiantari,[a] B.G. Munthe,[a] R. Wirawan,[b] S. Kusnandar,[b] S.K.U. Freisleben,[d] W. Ramelan,[d] and H.-J. Freisleben[d]

[a]Thalassemia Center and [b]Clinical Pathology, Cipto Mangunkusumo General Hospital, [c]SEAMEO-TROPMED Nutrition and [d]Study Program Biomedical Science, Faculty of Medicine, University of Indonesia, Salemba Raya No. 4, Jakarta, Indonesia.

Introduction

Thalassemias are inborn disorders of globin chain synthesis and the most frequent single gene-derived group of inherited diseases in the world. Of the worlds population, >3% carry thalassemia genes, with the highest incidence (up to 40%) in South East Asia (α-thalassemia, 30 million; β-thalassemia, 60 million; hemoglobin [Hb]E/β-thalassemia, 84 million [1]rsqb). Various mutations and deletions on α- and the β-globin gene clusters (>100 in the α- and ~200 in the β-gene are known) diminish globin chain synthesis to varying extents and result in the thalassemia trait or clinical presentation of thalassemia. In the Indonesian population, a frequency of β-globin genes of ~6–10% is estimated (2). The β-thalassemic phenotype shows wide variations among transfusion-dependent thalassemia major, different severities of thalassemia intermedia and thalassemia minor (trait) and is determined by the combination of two different alleles and coinheritance of different kinds of thalassemia/Hb anomalies. The influence of the globin haplotype on the clinical expression of thalassemias has been discussed (3).

The clinical picture of thalassemias is dominated by chronic anemia caused by ineffective erythropoesis, intra- and extramedullary hemolysis, and by iron overload after increased intestinal iron absorption and blood supply to transfusion-dependent patients. Imbalanced excessive globin chains tend to precipitate near the red blood cell (RBC) membrane, causing either intramedullary cell death or increased clearance of the erythrocyte from the peripheral circulation. Hemochromes, heme (protoporphyrin), and released iron contribute to the damage conferred by the precipitated globin chains (inclusion bodies) (4,5).

Transition metals such as iron and some iron-containing low-molecular-weight compounds play an important role in the generation of reactive oxygen species (ROS) and free radicals, which damage cellular and subcellular structures and cause metabolic dysfunction (6–8). Due to the disturbed iron metabolism, intense production of oxygen-derived free radicals occurs in thalassemias. This condition, together with impaired natural factors and mechanisms involved in detoxication of ROS and free radicals, results in extensive oxidative stress (9).

To clarify the iron-related changes in thalassemia patients in Jakarta, transfusion-dependent and insufficiently chelated patients (n = 5) were compared with healthy controls (n = 5) in this preliminary study.

Subjects and Methods

Subjects. Transfusion-dependent and not regularly chelated α-thalassemia major patients (n = 5) from Cipto Mangunkusumo General Hospital, in an age range of 19–30 y were investigated (group T). These patients had been transfused regularly for 12–25 y, and deferoxamine chelation was applied only once with each transfusion. The controls (n = 5; group C) were student volunteers without diagnosis or clinical signs of thalassemia in the same age range (20–30 y); each group consisted of 3 women and 2 men. All participants were nonsmokers, did not have other metabolic diseases or acute infections, and indicated that they had not taken specific vitamin supplementation.

The study was approved by the Ethical Clearance Board of the Faculty of Medicine, University of Indonesia, and all blood samples from controls and patients were obtained with fully informed consent. Citrate (20 mL) and EDTA (5 mL) blood were collected from each participant (for transfusion-dependent patients, just before transfusion). Transfusion intervals and amounts of transfused blood and clinical status were taken from the patients' hospital records.

Hemoglobin analysis. Hb-screening was done in the laboratory of the thalassemia ward with a Variant Hemoglobin Testing System using cation-exchange high-performance liquid chromatography (HPLC) connected with a dual wavelength filter photometer. EDTA blood was processed and analyzed according to the Variant β-Thalassemia Short Program with retention time for HbA_2 and HbE of 3.83 min. Differentiation between the two hemoglobins was done by the area percentage calculation on the sample record; HbE was considered to be present if the HbA_2 band exceeded 30%.

Lipid-Soluble Antioxidants. β-Carotene and vitamins A and E were measured in the SEAMEO-TROPMED Nutrition laboratory by means of HPLC especially set up for determination of lipid-soluble antioxidants. For determination of α-tocopherol (vitamin E), retinol (vitamin A), and β-carotene, 40 μL of plasma was mixed vigorously in a 0.5-mL cup for 10 s with 100 μL ethanol/water (2:1, vol/vol), then for 5 min with 120 μL of hexane containing 42 μg butyl hydroxytoluene. This mixture was centrifuged at 12,000 × g for 3 min, and 40 μL of the supernatant was transferred to a new tube and evaporated with nitrogen. The residue was dissolved in 50 mL dioxane/ethanol/acetonitrile (20:20:60, by vol) and 20 μL was applied for HPLC analysis using a Nova-Pack C-18 60 A 4-μm column, 3.9 × 150 mm, eluted with acetonitrile/tetrahydrofurane/methanol/ammonium acetate 1% (684:220:68:28, by vol) at a flow rate of 1.0 mL/min. For detection with an ultraviolet visible (UV-VIS) spectrophotometer, wavelengths were changed from 325 nm for retinol (0–3 min) to 292 nm for α-tocopherol (3–6 min), and finally to 450 nm for β-carotene (6–10 min). For quantification, international certified NIST standards were used.

Clinical Pathology. All other hematological parameters and investigations were performed from 10 mL of citrate blood in the Laboratory of Clinical Pathology according to standard methods.

Statistical Evaluation. Mean values, standard deviations, and probability were calculated. Using Student's *t*-test, $P < 0.05$ was considered significant for differences between the two groups. Because of the low number of observations for covariants ($n = 5$), regression and correlations are mentioned only if $r^2 > 0.5$.

Results

All subjects (patients and healthy volunteers) were in the same age range (between 19 and 30 y). One patient (Table 28.1, no. 1) died at the age of 27.

Blood Analysis. RBC and hematocrit (HCT) were significantly lower in patients than in controls: 3.32×10^6 vs. $4.57 \times 10^6/\mu L$ and 25.5 vs. 39.6%, respectively. Leukocytes (white blood cells, WBC) were increased fourfold in patients (Table 1). WBC differentiation was different between patients and controls: 61 vs. 33% of lymphocytes and 34 vs. 61% segmented neutrophils, whereas monocytes did not differ significantly. Platelets were $401 \times 10^3/\mu L$ in patients and $244 \times 10^3/\mu L$ in healthy control subjects.

Hemoglobin Analysis and Bilirubin. Total Hb was 8.5 g/dL (5.3 mmol/L) in patients and 13.5 g/dL (8.4 mmol/L) in controls. Fetal Hb (HbF) was detected in all patients in a range between 1.4 and 5.6%. Two patients had HbA_2 <10%, and one >20%; the remaining two were >30%. HbA_2 bands with >30% in Hb analysis should contain HbE by definition, and the sample with >20% HbA_2 should contain HbE as well. Total bilirubin was 1.37 mg/dL in patients vs. 0.64 mg/dL in controls, and direct bilirubin was 0.34 vs. 0.16 mg/dL, respectively.

Serum Proteins. Serum protein, in general, did not differ greatly between the control group and patients: total serum protein, 7.7 vs. 8.2 g/dL; albumin, 5.0 vs. 4.5 g/dL; globulin, 2.8 vs. 3.8 g/dL. However, serum activities of glutamate-oxaloacetate transaminase (SGOT), glutamate pyruvate transaminase (SGPT), and γ-glutamyltransferase (γ-GT) were significantly increased in patients: C vs. T: SGOT 42.4 vs. 116.6 IU/L; SGPT 34.2 vs. 98.8 IU/L; γ-GT 17.0 vs. 61.2 IU/L.

Serum Lipids. Relative to controls, triglycerides were doubled in thalassemic patients (group C vs. group T; 72 vs. 141 mg/dL) whereas total cholesterol was lower

(188 vs. 142 mg/dL) mainly due to strongly decreased high density lipoprotein (HDL) values in patients (71 vs. 20 mg/dL); low density lipoprotein (LDL) did not vary greatly (103 vs. 90 mg/dL). Thus, the LDL/HDL ratio differed significantly between controls (1.45) and patients (4.5).

Iron Status. Serum iron (SI) was almost doubled in patients relative to controls, 194 vs. 103 mg/dL, and ferritin ~100 times that of controls, 7573.4 vs. 78.9 ng/mL. Total iron-binding capacity (TIBC) was decreased in patients, 244 vs. 339 mg/dL in controls, and transferrin saturation was 30% in controls vs. 80% in patients.

Lipid-Soluble Antioxidants. α-Tocopherol (vitamin E) was 21.68 μmol/L in controls and 5.86 μmol/L in patients. Retinol (vitamin A) was 1.51 μmol/L (C) vs. 0.91 μmol/L (T) and β-carotene (pro-vitamin A) 0.34 μmol/L (C) vs. 0.07 μmol/L (T).

Correlations. Positive correlations with the years of transfusion (i.e., how many years a patient had already regularly obtained blood transfusions) were calculated for serum transferases SGOT (r = 0.92), SGPT (r = 0.96), and γ-GT (r = 0.83). Similar correlations were also found with the age of patients, SGOT (r = 0.88); SGPT (r = 0.82); γ-GT (r = 0.81). Further correlations were calculated with years of transfusions for TIBC (r = 0.79), ferritin (r = 0.73), total cholesterol (r = 0.89), and LDL (r = 0.91). Increase in serum iron was correlated with both years of transfusion and age of the patients, whereas HCT (r = 0.96) was correlated only with age.

Discussion

A study of thalassemia patients in Jakarta was initiated to obtain a comprehensive picture of metabolic dysfunction, iron overload, oxidative stress, and cell damage. Although thalassemia is a genetic disease characterized by the imbalanced expression of globin genes, an excess of impaired globin chains, as well as iron overload due to increased intestinal iron absorption and regular blood transfusions, causes a sequence of secondary events leading to severe oxidative stress in thalassemia patients.

Imbalanced globin gene expression generates HbH and Hb Bart's in the case of α-thalassemia, and increased levels of HbF, HbA_2/HbE, and α-globin precipitation in β-thalassemic RBC. These globin chains, which are associated with the cytoskeleton and the membrane of erythrocytes, are unstable, oxidizable, and easily release their heme moiety (protoporphyrin) and iron ions into the environment of the erythrocyte membrane (10–13).

Increased intestinal iron absorption due to the anemic situation in thalassemia and regular blood transfusions to thalassemia major patients lead to iron overload and hemochromatosis. Improvement can be achieved by iron chelation therapy to transfusion-dependent patients even though they continue to exhibit symptoms of severe oxidative stress (9).

TABLE 28.1 Hematological Parameters

Patient	1	2	3
Age	27 (†)	19	30
Transfusion therapy (y)	25	18	18
Red blood cells ($10^6/\mu L$)	2.93	3.8	3.54
Hematocrit (%)	24	30	27
Hemoglobin (Hb; g/dL)	7.8	10.6	8.8
HbF (%)	4.8	1.4	5.6
HbE/A_2 (%)			33.3
HbA_2 (%)	4.2	9.7	
Leukocytes (10^9/L; white blood cells, WBC)	48	5.8	44
Lymphocytes (%)	69	59	73
Monocytes (%)	6	5	3
Segmented neutrophils (%)	25	35	24
Platelets (10^9/L)	280	168	491
Protein (g/dL)	8.9	7.4	8.4
Albumin (g/dL)	4.2	4.5	4.6
Globulin (g/dL)	4.7	2.9	3.8
Serum glutamate-oxaloacetate transanimase (SGOT; IU/L)	206	84	87
Serum glutamate-pyruvate transanimase (SGPT; IU/L)	155	93	113
Serum γ-glutamyltransferase (γ-GT; IU/L)	104	30	68
Total bilirubin (mg/dL)	1.09	1.56	1.21
Direct bilirubin (mg/dL)	0.4	0.4	0.2
Triglycerides (mg/dL)	134	139	144
Total cholesterol (mg/dL)	179	121	140
Low density lipoprotein (mg/dL)	124	81	80
High density lipoprotein (mg/dL)	19	19	28
Serum iron (SI; µg/dL)	241	186	179
Total iron-binding capacity (µg Fe/dL)	287	268	222
Unsaturated iron-binding capacity (TIBC-SI; µg Fe/dL)	46	82	43
Transferrin saturation (SI/TIBC × 100; %)	84	69	84
Ferritin (ng/mL)	15219	14286	4614.4
β-Carotene (µmol/L)	0.062	0.12	0.041
Vitamin A (µmol/L)	0.873	0.978	0.83
Vitamin E (µmol/L)	12.375	2.075	10.354

[a]ND, not determined.

The five patients in our preliminary study obtained iron chelation with desferoxamine only once with each blood transfusion, which is (due mainly to high costs) the generally applied therapy in Indonesia, although it is considered to be insufficient. In other countries, chelation with desferoxamine is regularly applied 5 times per week; unwanted (side) effects of that therapy will not to be discussed here.

In this preliminary study, we investigated five patients who had been transfused for >10 y. Hemoglobin analysis excluded other hemoglobinopathies, e.g. HbE/F or hereditary persistence of fetal Hb (HPHF), which are also very common in South East Asia and often associated with thalassemia. However, it must be clearly stated that Hb

4	5	Mean ± SD	Control mean ± SD	*P* (*t* test)
24	21	24.2 ± 4.4	27.8 ±2.8	ND[a]
13	19	ND		
3.1	3.25	3.324 ± 0.311	4.574 ± 0.58	0.002
21	26	25.5 ± 3.007	39.6 ± 5.0	0.0004
7	8.2	8.48 ± 1.211	13.46 ±1.93	0.0004
3	3.2			ND
40.3	23.5			ND
				ND
4.0	38.7	27.7 ± 19.66	6.22 ± 0.71	0.05
34	67	61 ± 14.0	33 ± 5.0	0.01
5	5	5 ± 0.98	6 ± 1.79	0.15
60	28	34 ± 14.9	61 ± 7.03	0.02
509	559	401.4 ±150.8	243.8 ± 14.43	0.06
7.6	8.9	8.24 ± 0.63	7.74 ± 0.27	0.14
4.6	4.4	5.22 ± 1.60	4.96 ± 0.22	0.37
3	4.5	3.78 ± 0.74	2.78 ± 0.17	0.15
67	139	116.6 ± 51.0	42.4 ± 3.26	0.025
33	100	98.8 ± 39.3	34.2 ± 10.8	0.018
40	64	61.2 ± 25.7	17.0 ± 7.13	0.012
1.38	1.62	1.372 ± 0.201	0.63 ± 0.18	0.0017
0.2	0.5	0.34 ± 0.12	0.16 ± 0.05	0.027
130	157	140.8 ± 9.4	71.6 ± 13.48	0.001
123	148	142.2 ± 21.03	188.2 ± 20.21	0.0014
77	88	90 ± 17.4	103.0 ± 18.4	0.21
7	28	20.2 ± 7.7	71.0 ± 18.29	0.004
174	189	193.8 ± 24.18	102.8 ± 35.15	0.006
215	226	243.8 ± 28.54	338.6 ± 54.92	0.013
41	37	49.8 ± 18.3	235.8 ± 50.87	ND
81	81	80 ± 6	30 ± 10	ND
719.2	3028.6	7573.4 ± 5998	78.9 ± 41.3	0.033
0.067	0.058	0.07 ± 0.027	0.34 ± 0.1	0.005
1.171	0.717	0.91 ± 0.153	1.51 ± 0.26	0.014
3.597	0.919	5.86 ± 4.761	21.68 ± 5.24	0.02

analysis of patients who have been regularly transfused for years is often not consistent with the clinical picture of thalassemia major because the blood of these patients contains mixtures of endogenous and exogenous (= transfused) erythrocytes and Hb.

Although all patients were regularly transfused, their RBC counts, HCT, and total Hb were only 65–70% of controls. On the one hand, this is due to decreased erythropoiesis and, on the other hand, to rapid degradation of both endogenous and transfused erythrocytes and Hb. The latter event results in bilirubin as a degradation product, a further increase in serum iron levels, and a decrease in iron-binding capacity. This is consistent with the doubled serum iron levels in our patients relative to controls, their decreased total iron–binding capacity (TIBC), and their extremely low unsaturated iron–binding capacity (UIBC) of only 21% compared with controls.

Our data can be compared with results of a study of thalassemia major patients in Sicily; in that study, serum iron was even higher in patients (254 μg/dL) than in our patients (194 μg/dL), although the Sicilian patients obtained regular chelation therapy. TIBC was only slightly increased (4%) in these patients, whereas it was decreased by 28% in our patients. Transferrin saturation increased from 30% in controls to 80% in our patients, which was ~10% higher than in the Sicilian patients; the ferritin level was 7573 ng/mL, almost 100 times that of controls, whereas in the Sicilian study, the level rose in patients by a factor of 23 to 1866 ng/mL. Generally accepted threshold blood values of pathology are ferritin levels of 700 ng/mL and transferrin saturation of 55%.

Leukocytes were ~4 times higher in our patients and WBC differentiation was different between the two groups, i.e., lymphocyte counts were almost doubled, whereas segmented neutrophils amounted to only half the control value. Platelets were also higher in patients. Although this picture clearly indicates a pathologic condition, these results should not be overinterpreted because our automated blood cell counts did not correct for increased amounts of circulating immature erythroblasts, which still contain residual nuclei and may falsify WBC counts.

Serum lipids and lipid-soluble antioxidants were imbalanced in patients, i.e., triglycerides were twofold higher and total cholesterol lower than in controls, whereas LDL was not altered significantly; HDL decreased to 28% of controls, leading to significantly different LDL/HDL ratios between controls (1.45) and patients (4.5). Abnormal serum lipid and lipoprotein patterns have been reported in thalassemia patients (14,15).

In patients, vitamin E (α-tocopherol) was 36%, vitamin A (retinol) 62%, and β-carotene 20% of control values. A similar tendency was reported in the above-mentioned study in Sicily, although the β-carotene level in their patients was still 71%. However, another carotenoid, lycopene, which was not measured in our study, was only 33% in Sicilian patients compared with their controls.

Iron overload and oxidant-antioxidant imbalance arising from blood circulation progressively affect tissues and organs in thalassemia major patients, leading to a sequence of metabolic disorders. In the beginning, liver (16) and spleen are affected; later, other tissues and glands are affected, with symptoms such as growth retardation or diabetes mellitus. Finally, the effects on the heart (17) and myocardial insufficiency are often the ultimate reason for the patients' death.

Transferase activities were greatly increased in patients' serum vs. controls: SGOT 116.6 vs. 42.4 IU/L, SGPT 98.8 vs. 34.2 IU/L, and γ-GT 61.2 vs. 17.0 IU/L. Glutamate-oxaloacetate transaminase (GOT) = γ aspartate aminotransferase (EC 2.6.1.1) and glutamate pyruvate transaminase (GPT) = alanine aminotransferase (EC 2.6.1.2) are both present in liver, with GOT also in heart muscle cells. If these enzymes (SGOT, SGPT) occur in serum, their activity indicates tissue damage, such as inflammation, acute or chronic liver disease, or, in the case of SGOT, myocardial injury. γ-Glutamyltransferase (γ-GT) = γ-glutamyltranspeptidase (GTP) is normally present in kidneys, liver, spleen, and pancreas. Increased enzyme activity in serum indicates liver injury. It must be considered that many regularly transfused patients suffer from hepatitis and from hemochromatosis and inflammation in various tissues, with release of acute phase proteins, all of which may contribute to increased globulins and enzymatic activities in serum.

Increase of bilirubin in serum is a pathological parameter, indicating increased Hb degradation, impaired liver cell function, and/or cholestatic complications. In our study, direct or conjugated bilirubin, although doubled in patients, was still in the normal range, whereas total bilirubin, doubled as well in patients, already exceeded the normal range. With the imbalanced antioxidant status in thalassemic patients and loss of physiologic antioxidants, serum bilirubin can serve as an antioxidant metabolite and may contribute in part to the total antioxidant capacity in the blood. This would explain why in the Sicilian study this parameter, measured as Trolox equivalent antioxidant capacity (TEAC), decreased by only 14% in thalassemia major patients (9). Total bilirubin in that study showed the same mean value in patients (1.36 mg/dL) as in our study (1.37 mg/dL).

A correlation of several parameters of oxidative stress and metabolic dysfunction with the years of transfusion therapy and also with the age of patients was observed in our study. Although we are very careful in our interpretation because of the small number of patients ($n = 5$), it can be stated that serum transferases, TIBC, ferritin, and cholesterol appear more closely correlated with the years of transfusions than with the age of the patients.

Summary

In this preliminary study, iron overload, antioxidant imbalance in the blood, inflammation, and severe liver dysfunction were detected in thalassemia major patients. Regular blood transfusions and the lack of adequate chelating therapy supposedly contribute to their metabolic disorders, although serum iron levels were even lower in our patients than those in a Sicilian study with chelated patients (9). A further set of measurements must be carried out for ascorbate, urate, thiols, lipid peroxidation, and other membrane parameters. Furthermore, thalassemia intermedia patients who have not yet been transfused should be included, and the entire study requires extended numbers of subjects. The results will be reported in the future.

Acknowledgment

This study was supported by the URGE Project of the Indonesian Government.

References

1. WHO (1983), *Bull. WHO 61*, 63–80.
2. Sofro, A.S.M. (1995) Molecular Pathology of β-Thalassemia in Indonesia. *Southeast Asian J. Trop. Med. Public Health 26 (Suppl.1)*, 221–224.

3. Lie-Injo, L.E., Cai, S.P., Wahidiyat, I., Moeslichan, S., Lim, M.L., Evangelista, L., Doherty, M., and Khan, Y.W. (1989) Beta-Thalssemia Mutations in Indonesia and Their Linkage to Different Haplotypes. *Am. J. Hum. Genet. 45*, 971–975.
4. Shinar, E., and Rachmilewitz, E.A. (1990) Oxidative Denaturation of Red Blood Cells in Thalassemia. *Semin. Hematol. 27*, 70–82.
5. Williamson, D. (1993) The Unstable Hemoglobins. *Blood Rev. 7*, 146–163.
6. Hershko, C., Graham, G., Bates, G.W., and Rachmilewitz, E.A. (1978) Non-Specific Serum Iron in Thalassemia: An Abnormal Serum Iron Fraction of Potential Toxicity. *Br. J. Haematol. 40*, 255–263.
7. Graham, G., Bates, G.W., Rachmilewitz, E.A., and Hershko, C. (1979) Non-Specific Serum Iron in Thalassemia: Quantitation and Chemical Reactivity. *Am. J. Hematol. 6*, 207–217.
8. Halliwell, B., and Gutteridge, J.M.C. (1988) *Free Radicals in Biology and Medicine* (Halliwell, B., and Gutteridge, J.M.C., eds.) 2nd ed., Oxford University Press, Oxford, UK.
9. Livrea, M.A., Tesoriere, L., Pintaudi, A.M., Calabrese, A., Maggio, A., Freisleben, H.-J., D'Arpa, A., D'Anna, R., and Bongiorno, A. (1996) Oxidative Stress and Antioxidant Status in β-Thalassemia Major: Iron Overload and Depletion of Lipid-Soluble Antioxidants. *Blood 88*, 3608–3614.
10. Wilairat, P., Kittikalayawong, A., and Chaicharoen, S. (1992) The Thalassemic Red Cell Membrane, *Southeast Asian J. Trop. Med. Public Health 23*, 74–78.
11. Repka, T., Shalev, O., Reddy, R., Yuan, J., Abrahamov, A., Rachmilewitz, E.A., Low, P.S., and Hebbel, R.P. (1993) Nonrandom Association of Free Iron with the Membranes of Sickle and Beta-Thalassemic Erythrocytes. *Blood 82*, 3204–3210.
12. Scott, M.D., van den Berg, J.J., Repka, T., Rouver-Fessaerd, P., Hebbel, R.P., Beuzard, Y., and Lubin, B. (1993) Effect of Excess Alpha-Globin Chain on Cellular and Membrane Oxidation in Model Beta-Thalassemic Erythrocytes. *J. Clin. Investig. 91*, 1706–1712.
13. Chiu, D.T.-J., Van den Berg, J., Kuypers, F.A., Hung, I.-J., Wie, J.-S., and Liu, T.-Z. (1996) Correlation of Membrane Lipid Peroxidation with Oxidation of Hemoglobin Variants: Possibly Related to the Rates of Hemin Release. *Free Radic. Biol. Med. 21*, 89–95.
14. Giardini, O., Murgia, F., Martino, F., Mannarino, O., Corrado, G., and Maggiono, G. (1978) Serum Lipid Pattern in β-Thalassaemia. *Acta Haematol. 60*, 100–107.
15. Maioli, M., Cuccuru, G.B., Pranzetti, P., Pacifico, A., and Cherchi, G.M. (1984) Plasma Lipids and Lipoprotein Pattern in Beta-Thalassemia Major. *Acta Haematol. 71*, 106.
16. Britton, R.S. (1996) Metal-Induced Hepatotoxicity. *Semin. Liver Dis. 16*, 3–12.
17. Brili, S.V., Tzonou, A.I., Castelanos, S.S., Aggeli, C.J., Tentolouris, C.A., Pitsavos, C.E., and Toutouzas, P.K. (1997) The Effect of Iron Overload in the Hearts of Patients with Beta-Thalassemia. *Clin. Cardiol. 20*, 541–546.

Chapter 29

Red Palm Oil, Vitamin A, and the Antioxidant Enzymes

H.T. Khor and R. Raajeswari

Department of Biochemistry, Faculty of Medicine, University of Malaya, Kuala Lumpur, Malaysia

Introduction

Crude palm oil has the highest content of natural carotenes, ranging from 600 to 1000 parts per million (ppm), and a high content of vitamin E, tocopherols, and tocotrienols (500–800 ppm). Conventional refining processes, which produce refined, bleached, and deodorized palm olein (RBDPO), remove practically all of the carotenes, but retain substantial amounts of the vitamin E present in crude palm oil. Red palm oil (RPO) is a refined palm oil produced by a nonconventional process that retains >80% of the carotenes in addition to the vitamin E present in crude palm oil (1). Therefore, the major difference between RPO and RBDPO is their carotene content, which gives RPO a strong reddish color compared with the straw-yellow color of RBDPO. The carotene content of red palm oil is composed mainly of α- and β-carotene as the major components (~85% of its total carotenes), and the vitamin E content of RPO is slightly higher than that of RBDPO (1).

Carotenes have been shown to possess provitamin A and natural antioxidant activities. As provitamin A, carotenes are converted to vitamin A in the intestinal mucosa of mammals and humans, and stored in the liver as vitamin A esters. Different carotene isomers have different vitamin A potency. Previous studies have shown that supplementation of red palm oil to rural school children greatly enhanced vitamin A status in the blood (2–4). In addition to its provitamin A activity, carotenes may have other biological functions such as antioxidant (5) and anticancer activities (6). As natural antioxidants, carotenes act to prevent lipid peroxidation and scavenge free radicals generated by oxidative processes. A number of antioxidant enzymes exist in the body to convert harmful oxidative products into safe metabolites or wastes. The effect of natural carotenes on the activity of these antioxidant enzymes has not been widely explored. In this study, the provitamin A potency and the effect of palm oil carotenes on the activity of the antioxidant enzymes, i.e., glutathione-*S*-transferase (GST), glutathione peroxidase (GSH-Px), superoxide dismutase (SOD), and catalase, were investigated by using red palm oil as a source of palm oil natural carotenes.

Materials and Methods

Treatment of Animals. Golden Syrian hamsters were purchased from the Animal Research Center, University Malaya. They were separated into four groups of approximately equal mean body weight; each hamster was kept individually in a cage with dimensions of 44.0 cm × 28.0 cm × 12.0 cm. The hamsters were housed in the experimental room with a controlled 12-h light:dark cycle. Room temperature was set at 25 ± 2°C. The hamsters were allowed to adapt to the new environment for ~2 wk before they were fed the experimental diets for a period of 45 d. The basic compositions of the experimental diets are shown in Table 29.1 and the preparation of these diets was described previously (7). The fat for group I was palm olein (PO); for group II it was 25% red palm oil in palm olein (PO-RPO); for group III it was corn oil (CO); and for group IV it was 25% red palm oil in corn oil (CO-RPO).

At the end of the experimental period, the hamsters were killed after overnight food deprivation. Blood was taken by cardiac puncture while the hamsters were under ether anesthesia. The liver was quickly excised, wiped clean, weighed, and kept in the freezer at –80°C. Sera were prepared by centrifugation at 2000 × *g* for 20 min after the blood was allowed to stand at room temperature for 45 min (8).

Extraction of Serum Vitamin E and A. Serum vitamin E and A were extracted by a micromethod as described by Khor and Chieng (7) with some modifications. Clear serum (200 µL) was pipetted into a microfuge tube and 200 µL methanol [high-performance liquid chromatography (HPLC) grade] was added. The tubes were then vortexed vigorously at maximum speed for ~1 min to precipitate the proteins. Then, 800 µL hexane (HPLC grade) was added and the tubes were again vortexed intermittently for 2 min. The tubes were then centrifuged at 10,000 × *g* for 5 min, and 700 µL of the upper hexane layer was transferred to another microfuge tube. The solvent was evaporated under a stream of nitrogen at room temperature. The dried extract was dissolved in 20 µL hexane for vitamin E analysis, or 5% isopropanol (IPA) in hexane for vitamin A analysis. An aliquot of the final extract was used for HPLC analysis.

Extraction of Hepatic Vitamin E and A. Frozen liver was thawed and a 100-mg portion was minced in 400 µL IPA in a microfuge tube using a pair of scissors. The tip of the scissors and the inner sides of the microfuge tube were rinsed with another 600 µL IPA. The tubes were capped tightly and vortexed intermittently at maximum

TABLE 29.1 Composition of the Semisynthetic Diets

Ingredient	(g/100 g diet)	Ingredient	(g/100 g diet)
Corn flour	29.0	Choline bitartrate	0.2
Dextrose	23.0	Cholesterol	0
Cellulose	5.0	Mineral mix (AIN 76)	4.5
Casein	27.0	Vitamin mix (AIN 76)	1.0
DL-Methionine	0.3		
Fats[a]	10.0		

[a]Consisting of palm olein, 25% red palm oil (RPO) in palm olein, corn oil, or 25% RPO in corn oil.

speed for 2 min. The suspension obtained was then microfuged for 10 min at 5000 × *g*. The deproteinized supernatant was decanted into another microfuge tube and dried under a flow of nitrogen gas at low temperature. The dried extract was dissolved in a suitable volume of hexane or 5% IPA in hexane for HPLC analysis of vitamin E or A.

HPLC Analysis of Vitamin E. Serum and hepatic vitamin E levels were analyzed by normal phase HPLC with silica column (250 mm × 4.6 mm, 5-μm film) and a fluorescent detector. A binary solvent mixture of 0.5% IPA in hexane was used as the eluting solvent for the system, which was run in isocratic mode. The detector was set for excitation wavelength at 295 nm and for emission wavelength at 325 nm (7). Pure α-, β-, γ-, and δ-tocopherol were used to construct the calibration curves for the quantification of serum and hepatic vitamin E levels.

HPLC Analysis of Vitamin A. Serum and hepatic vitamin A were analyzed by normal phase HPLC with a silica column (250 mm × 4 mm; 5-μm film) and a fluorescent detector (Shimadzu RF-535). A binary solvent mixture of 5% IPA in hexane was used as the eluting solvent for the system, which was run in isocratic mode. The fluorescent detector was set for excitation wavelength at 325 nm and for emission wavelength at 470 nm. Pure retinol and retinyl palmitate were used to construct the calibration curves for the quantification of serum and hepatic vitamin A levels.

Assay of the Activity of the Antioxidant Enzymes

Preparation of Liver Subcellular Fractions. Liver was thawed and a 1-g portion was rinsed with ice-cold 0.88% KCl solution and homogenized in 4 volumes of homogenization buffer, pH 7.2, consisting of 0.32 mol/L sucrose, 0.01 mol/L Tris-HCl and 1 mmol/L EDTA. Homogenization was carried out using a Potter-Elvehjem glass homogenizer. All of these steps were carried out on ice. Subcellular fractions were isolated by differential centrifugation. Initial pelleting was done to remove nuclei, red blood cells, and debris at 1000 × *g* for 10 min at 4°C. This was followed by centrifugation at 10,000 × *g* for 20 min at 4°C to pellet mitochondria and peroxisomes. The supernatant that was obtained was subjected to further ultracentrifugation at 100,000 × *g* for 60 min at 4°C to obtain the microsomal pellets and the final 100,000 × *g* supernatant. These subcellular fractions were used for the estimation of the activities of the antioxidant enzymes. Protein determination of the subcellular fractions was done according to the method of Bradford (9).

Assay of Glutathione-S-Transferase Activity. GST activity was assayed using the 100,000 × *g* supernatant as the source of enzyme because preliminary results indicated that this fraction has the highest enzyme activity in the liver. The principle of the assay was based on the conjugation of 1-chloro-2, 4-dinitrobenzene (CDNB) to glutathione (GSH) by GST and the changes in absorbance at 344 nm (10). The incubation mixture consisted of 200 μL of 0.5 mol/L phosphate buffer, pH 8.0, and 20 μL of 0.05 mol/L CDNB in 95% ethanol. A sufficient volume of distilled water was also added to obtain a final volume of 1 mL. The incubation mixture was preincubated at 37°C for 10 min before 50 μL of 20 mmol/L GSH and 5 μL of the enzyme were added to initiate the reaction. Changes in absorbance at 344 nm were followed for 5 min. A reagent blank without the enzyme was also carried out for every test sample. One unit of enzyme activity is defined as the amount of enzyme catalyzing the formation of 1 nmol product/(min/mg protein) under the conditions of the assay.

Assay of Glutathione Peroxidase Activity. GSH-Px activity was determined by coupling the reactions catalyzed by GSH-Px to that catalyzed by NADPH-dependent glutathione reductase and by measuring the changes in absorbance at 340 nm due to the formation of $NADP^+$ (11). GSH-Px activity was determined using the 10,000 × *g* supernatant as the source of enzyme because preliminary results indicated that this fraction has the highest enzyme activity. *t*-Butyl hydroperoxide was used as the substrate, and the incubation mixture consisted of 100 μL of 1 mol/L Tris-HCl, pH 8.0, containing 5 mmol/L EDTA. 20 μL of 0.1 mol/L GSH, 100 μL of glutathione reductase, 10 U/mL, 100 μL of 2 mmol/L NADPH and an aliquot, 10 μL, of the enzyme plus a sufficient volume of distilled water to obtain a total volume of 1 mL. The above incubation mixture was preincubated at 37°C for 10 min. Finally 10 μL of 7 mmol/L *t*-butyl hydroperoxide was added to the incubation mixture to initiate the reaction, and the changes in absorbance at 340 nm were followed for 5 min in a 1-cm cuvette. A complete incubation mixture without the enzyme served as the blank for the assay.

Superoxide Dismutase Assay. SOD activity was determined spectrophotometrically according to the method of Marklund and Marklund (12) and Roth and Gilbert (13) by measuring the autoxidation of pyrogallol at 420 nm. Pyrogallol autoxidizes rapidly in aqueous solution to produce a yellow color that can be read at 420 nm. This process is dependent on the presence of superoxide anions. The enzyme SOD inhibits the autoxidation of pyrogallol by catalyzing the breakdown of superoxide. The amount of enzyme producing 50% inhibition is defined as 1 unit of enzyme activity.

Liver SOD was assayed using the 10,000 × *g* supernatant as the source of the enzyme because preliminary results indicated that this fraction has the highest enzyme activity. The incubation mixture, consisting of 100 μL of 1 mol/L Tris-HCl, pH 8.0, containing 5 mmol/L EDTA and 20 μL of enzyme plus a sufficient volume of distilled water to obtain a final volume of 1 mL, was preincubated at 37°C for 10 min. Then, 27 μL of 10 mmol/L pyrogallol in 10 mmol/L HCl was added to initiate the reaction, and the increases in absorbance at 420 nm were monitored for 5 min. A complete incubation mixture without the enzyme served as the blank for the assay.

Assay of Catalase Activity. Catalase activity was estimated by measuring the disappearance of H_2O_2 as catalyzed by catalase spectrophotometrically at 240 nm (14). Catalase activity was assayed using the 10,000 × *g* supernatant as the source of enzyme because preliminary results indicated that this fraction has the highest activity. The incubation mixture consisted of 50 μL of 1 mol/L phosphate buffer, pH 7.0, 900 μL of 59 mmol/L hydrogen peroxide (H_2O_2) and a sufficient volume of distilled water to obtain a final volume of 1 mL. The incubation mixture was preincubated at 37°C for 10 min before 20 μL of the enzyme was added to initiate the reaction. The changes/decreases in absorbance at 240 nm were monitored for 5 min in a 1-cm cuvette. A complete incubation mixture without the H_2O_2 served as the blank.

Statistical Analaysis. Student's t test was used to compare the differences of means, and $P < 0.05$ was considered significant.

Results

The fatty acid composition of the PO, RPO, and CO is shown in Table 29.2. PO and RPO have very similar fatty acid compositions, which differ significantly from that of CO. PO and RPO contain ~33% $C_{16:0}$, 42% $C_{18:1}$, and 18% $C_{18:2}$, whereas CO contains 12% $C_{16:0}$, 34% $C_{18:1}$, and 48% $C_{18:2}$. In addition to the differences in fatty acid composition, PO, RPO, and CO also differ in their content and composition of carotenes and vitamin E. PO and CO have no detectable carotenes, but RPO has ~560 ppm of carotenes.

The vitamin E content and composition of PO, RPO, and CO are shown in Table 29.3. RPO has a somewhat higher total vitamin E content (842 ppm) than do PO (664 ppm) and CO (653 ppm). The vitamin E of PO and RPO consists of both tocopherols and tocotrienols, whereas the vitamin E of CO consists of tocopherols only. The com-

TABLE 29.2 Fatty Acid Profiles of Red Palm Oil (RPO), Palm Olein (PO), and Corn Oil (CO)[a]

	Composition (wt %)		
Fatty acid	RPO	PO	CO
12:0	0.2	0.3	ND
14:0	1.2	1.1	0.1
16:0	33.5	32.9	12.5
16:1(n-7)	0.2	0.5	0.2
18:0	2.4	2.6	2.7
18:1(n-9)	42.4	41.3	34.2
18:2(n-6)	18.1	17.9	48.3
18:3(n-6)	tr	tr	0.6
18:3(n-3)	0.7	1.5	0.7
20:0	0.3	0.7	0.3
20:1(n-9)	0.4	0.3	0.1
20:1(n-11)	tr	tr	0.2
22:0	0.1	0.5	0.1
22:1(n-9)	0.5	0.4	tr

[a]Abbreviations: ND, not detected; tr, trace, <0.1%.

TABLE 29.3 Vitamin E Profiles of Red Palm Oil (RPO), Palm Olein (PO), and Corn Oil (CO)[a]

Vitamin E isomers	Vitamin E content (ppm)		
Tocopherol	Red palm oil	Palm olein	Corn oil
α	180.5	157.1	223.8
β	ND	ND	36.5
γ	40.3	21.3	354.1
δ	ND	ND	39.2
Tocotrienol			
α	216.8	148.0	ND
β	ND	ND	ND
γ	328.6	275.5	ND
δ	76.2	62.4	ND
Total vitamin E	842.4	664.3	653.6

[a]Abbreviations: ppm, parts per million; ND, not detected.

position of vitamin E in PO is as follows: α-tocopherol (α-T; 157 ppm), γ-tocopherol (γ-T; 21 ppm), α-tocotrienol (α-T3; 148 ppm), γ-tocotrienol (γ-T3; 275 ppm), and δ-tocotrienol (δ-T3; 62 ppm). The composition of vitamin E in RPO is as follows: α-T (180 ppm), γ-T (40 ppm), α-T3 (216.8 ppm), γ-T3 (328.6 ppm), and δ-T3 (76.2 ppm). The vitamin E of CO, on the other hand, is made up of α-T (223.8 ppm), β-tocopherol (β-T; 36.5 ppm) γ-T (354.1 ppm) and δ-tocopherol (δ-T; 39.2 ppm). Therefore PO and RPO have a similar vitamin E profile but differ significantly from CO both qualitatively and quantitatively.

The body, heart, and liver weights of hamsters fed the semisynthetic diets are shown in Table 29.4. These results indicate that there were no significant differences in body, heart, and liver weights after consumption of semisynthetic diets supplemented with 25% RPO for 45 d.

TABLE 29.4 Body, Liver, and Heart Weights of Hamsters Fed Semisynthetic Diets[a,b]

		Body weight		Liver weight	Heart weight
		(g)			
Diet	*n*	Initial	Final		
PO	5	160.4 ± 0.7	171.6 ± 3.2	5.02 ± 0.62	0.59 ± 0.02
PO-RPO	6	163.2 ± 3.2	169.1 ± 4.3	5.69 ± 0.24	0.60 ± 0.05
CO	5	163.2 ± 3.2	172.0 ± 2.1	4.47 ± 0.34	0.55 ± 0.05
CO-RPO	6	161.9 ± 1.2	170.6 ± 4.1	4.80 ± 0.60	0.54 ± 0.05

[a]Values are means ± SEM; *n* = number of hamsters.
[b]Abbreviations: PO, palm olein; PO-RPO, 25% red palm oil in palm olein; CO, corn oil; CO- RPO, 25% red palm oil in corn oil.

The serum and liver vitamin A levels of hamsters fed the semisynthetic diets containing PO, PO-RPO, CO, and CO-RPO are shown in Table 29.5. Only retinol, the free form of vitamin A, was detected in serum. The serum retinol levels of hamsters fed the semisynthetic diets containing PO and CO were comparable because neither oils contains carotenes. However, in hamsters fed the semisynthetic diet containing RPO in PO (PO-RPO), the serum retinol level was significantly higher ($P < 0.05$) than that of hamsters fed the diet containing PO. Similarly, hamsters fed the semisynthetic diet containing RPO with CO (CO-RPO) had serum retinol levels higher than those of hamsters fed the diet containing CO; however, in this case, the elevation in serum vitamin A level was not significant ($P > 0.05$).

Analyses of the liver vitamin A content revealed that both retinol and retinol esters were present (Table 29.5). These results show that hamsters fed semisynthetic diets containing PO and CO had comparable liver vitamin A content. However, hamsters fed semisynthetic diets containing RPO with PO (PO-RPO) and RPO with CO (CO-RPO) showed significant increases in the hepatic content of retinol and retinol esters ($P < 0.05$). There was a fourfold increase in the concentration of retinol esters and an approximately two- to threefold increase in that of retinol in hamsters fed RPO-supplemented diets compared with those fed the PO or CO diet. It appears that RPO supplementation effectively elevated liver concentrations of vitamin A, retinol, and retinol esters, irrespective of the nature of the oil to which RPO was blended.

Because RPO is rich in tocopherols and tocotrienols, the effect of RPO supplementation to PO and CO on serum and hepatic vitamin E level was assessed. Supplementation of RPO to the PO diet (PO-RPO group) resulted in a significant ($P < 0.05$) increase in serum α-T level compared with hamsters fed the PO diet. In spite of increased intake of α-T3 in the diet, no α-T3 was detected in the serum of hamsters fed the PO-RPO diet. On the other hand, the effect of RPO supplementation

TABLE 29.5 Serum and Liver Vitamin A Levels of Hamsters Fed Red Palm Oil (RPO)-Supplemented Semisynthetic Diets[a,b]

Dietary group	Serum level Retinol (ng/dL)	Liver content Retinol (mg/g)	Liver content Retinol esters (mg/g)
PO	40.16 ± 2.07[c]	4.85 ± 1.22[c]	109.99 ± 8.92[c]
PO-RPO	47.45 ± 2.81[d]	10.57 ± 1.49[d]	472.53 ± 6.50[d,e]
CO	37.56 ± 2.12[c]	3.03 ± 2.62[c]	97.45 ± 4.31[c]
CO-RPO	42.72 ± 1.83[c]	9.15 ± 1.73[d]	440.12 ± 7.23[d,f]

[a]Values are means ± SEM; values in a column with different superscripts are significantly different, $P < 0.05$.
[b]Abbreviations: PO, palm oil; PO-RPO, 25% red palm oil in palm olein; CO, corn oil; CO-RPO, 25% red palm oil in corn oil.

TABLE 29.6 Serum Vitamin E Levels of Hamsters Fed Red Palm Oil (RPO)-Supplemented Semisynthetic Diets[a,b]

Dietary group	Serum α-tocopherol level (mg/dL)
PO	1.57 ± 0.06[c]
PO-RPO	1.79 ± 0.04[d]
CO	1.62 ± 0.08[c]
CO-RPO	1.71 ± 0.10[c]

[a]Values are means ± SEM; values in a column with different superscripts are significantly different, $P < 0.05$.
[b]Abbreviations: PO, palm oil; PO-RPO, 25% red palm oil in palm olein; CO, corn oil; CO-RPO, 25% red palm oil in corn oil.

to the CO diet on serum vitamin E level was not as clear-cut because the increase in serum vitamin E was not significant compared with the CO group (Table 29.6).

The vitamin E content in the liver of hamsters fed semisynthetic diets containing PO, PO-RPO, CO and CO-RPO is shown in Table 29.7. Because of the basic differences in the vitamin E composition in PO and CO, hamsters fed the PO diet had hepatic vitamin E profiles completely different from those of hamsters fed the CO diet. Both tocopherols and tocotrienols, i.e., α-T, γ-T, α-T3, γ-T3, and δ-T3 were detected in the liver of hamsters fed the PO diet, whereas only the tocopherols, α-T and γ-T, were detected in the liver of hamsters fed the CO diet. These results indicate that the liver vitamin E profiles reflected the dietary vitamin E intake of the hamsters. Moreover, RPO supplementation to the PO diet resulted in a significant increase in α-T, γ-T, α-T3, γ-T3, and δ-T3 content in the liver compared with those fed the PO

TABLE 29.7 Hepatic Vitamin E Level of Hamsters Fed Red Palm Oil (RPO)-Supplemented Semisynthetic Diets[a,b]

	Hepatic vitamin E levels (μg/g)				
	Tocopherols		Tocotrienols		
Dietary group	α	γ	α	γ	δ
PO	38.24 ± 1.21[c]	0.12 ± 0.03[c]	0.37 ± 0.04[c]	0.32 ± 0.10	0.22 ± 0.06
PO-RPO	68.51 ± 0.96[d,e]	0.34 ± 0.04[d]	0.51 ± 0.10[d]	0.59 ± 0.24	0.26 ± 0.07
CO	41.73 ± 1.30[c]	0.28 ± .06[d]	ND	ND	ND
CO-RPO	72.16 ± 0.43[e]	0.48 ± 0.10[e]	0.30 ± 0.08[c]	0.23 ± 0.06	0.21 ± 0.05

[a]Values are means ± SEM; values in a column with different superscripts are significantly different, $P < 0.05$.
[b]Abbreviations: PO, palm oil; PO-RPO, 25% red palm oil in palm olein; CO, corn oil; CO-RPO, 25% red palm oil in corn oil; ND, not detected.

TABLE 29.8 Hepatic Glutathione-*S*-Transferase (GST) and Glutathione Peroxidase (GSH-Px) Activities in Hamsters Fed Red Palm Oil (RPO)-Supplemented Semisynthetic Diets[a,b]

Dietary group	GST [nmol/(min•mg protein)]	GSH-Px [mol/(min•mg protein)]
PO	520.85 ± 10.30[c]	80.88 ± 9.15[c]
PO-RPO	730. 73 ± 10.23[d]	175.03 ± 9.20[d]
CO	498.98 ± 12.29[c]	62.77 ± 9.29[c]
CO-RPO	566.31 ± 16.52[e]	117.46 ± 8.31[e]

[a]Values are means ± SEM; values in a column with different superscripts are significantly different, $P < 0.05$.
[b]Abbreviations: PO, palm oil; PO-RPO, 25% red palm oil in palm olein; CO, corn oil; CO-RPO, 25% red palm oil in corn oil.

diet. RPO supplementation to the CO diet also resulted in significant increases in α-T and γ-T and the appearance of α-T3, γ-T3, and δ-T3 in the liver, which was not seen in the CO group. β-T, δ-T, and β-T3 were not detected in any of the dietary groups.

Four antioxidant enzymes, i.e., GST, GSH-Px, SOD, and catalase, in the liver were assayed. The effect of RPO supplementation on the activity of GST and GSH-Px is shown in Table 29.8. Despite the basic differences in the chemical composition of PO and CO, cytosolic GST activity was not affected because both groups had comparable enzyme activity. However, RPO supplementation to the PO and CO diets resulted in a significant increase in hepatic GST activity (Table 29.8). The margin of increase in activity of GST appeared to be greater in the PO-RPO group than in the CO-RPO group, indicating that GST activity may be affected by factors common to both PO and RPO. Therefore, there was an additive effect of these factors on GST in the PO-RPO group.

The effect of PO, CO, PO-RPO, and CO-RPO on hepatic GSH-Px activity in hamsters is shown in Table 29.8. Although hamsters fed the PO diet had somewhat higher GSH-Px activity than those fed the CO diet, the difference was not significant ($P > 0.05$). RPO supplementation to the PO and CO diets effectively enhanced the

TABLE 29.9 Hepatic Catalase and Superoxide Dismutase (SOD) Activities in Hamsters Fed Red Palm Oil (RPO)-Supplemented Semisynthetic Diets[a,b]

Dietary group	Catalase [μmol/(min•mg protein)]	SOD [mol/(min•mg protein)]
PO	64.60 ± 9.97	10.00 ± 1.59
PO-RPO	90.82 ± 4.52	10.68 ± 2.10
CO	67.04 ± 5.94	12.66 ± 1.17
CO-RPO	80.14 ± 7.29	10.00 ± 1.18

[a]Values are means ± SEM.
[b]Abbreviations: PO, palm oil; PO-RPO, 25% red palm oil in palm olein; CO, corn oil; CO-RPO, 25% red palm oil in corn oil.

TABLE 29.10 Serum Lipid Levels of Hamsters Fed Red Palm Oil (RPO)-Supplemented Semisynthetic Diets[a,b]

	Serum lipid levels (mg/dL)			
Dietary group	Total cholesterol	HDL-C	LDL-C	Triacylglycerol
PO	96.21 ± 3.51[c,d]	62.33 ± 1.70[c]	26.58 ± 1.40[c]	144.07 ± 3.64
PO-RPO	105.64 ± 5.07[c]	73.12 ± 2.56[d]	22.02 ± 3.21[d]	133.70 ± 5.07
CO	82.13 ± 4.42[c,d]	49.76 ± 2.13[e]	25.17 ± 3.08[c]	145.16 ± 4.31
CO-RPO	88.92 ± 3.32[c,d]	56.71± 2.68[f]	24.85 ± 1.42[c]	137.83 ± 3.22

[a]Values are means ± SEM; values in a column with different superscripts are significantly different, $P < 0.05$.
[b]Abbreviations: HDL-C, high density lipoprotein cholesterol; LDL-C, low density lipoprotein cholesterol; PO, palm oil; PO-RPO, 25% red palm oil in palm olein; CO, corn oil; CO-RPO, 25% red palm oil in corn oil.

activity of GSH-Px in liver. The magnitude of increase in activity was comparable (twofold) in the PO-RPO and CO-RPO groups compared with the PO and CO groups, respectively.

The nature of dietary fats appeared to have no effect on the activity of hepatic catalase and SOD (Table 29.9). RPO supplementation to the PO and CO diets also did not result in any significant change in the activity of hepatic catalase and SOD.

The effect of PO, CO, and RPO-supplemented PO and CO on the serum lipids of hamsters is shown in Table 10. Hamsters fed the CO diet had significantly lower serum total cholesterol (TC) and high density lipoprotein cholesterol (HDL-C) levels than those fed the PO diet. No significant differences were observed in low density lipoprotein cholesterol (LDL-C) and serum triacylglycerol (TAG) levels between the PO and CO groups. RPO supplementation to the PO diet (PO-RPO group) resulted in increases in serum TC and HDL-C levels and reductions in LDL-C and TAG levels. The increase in TC level was not significant ($P > 0.05$), but the increase in HDL-C level was significant ($P < 0.05$). The reduction in LDL-C level was significant, but the reduction in serum TAG level was not significant between the PO and PO-RPO groups. Similarly, RPO supplementation to CO resulted in increases in serum TC and HDL-C levels and in reduction in LDL-C and serum TAG levels compared with the CO group. However, the changes in serum TC, HDL-C, LDL-C, and TAG levels were not significant ($P > 0.05$).

Discussion

Carotenoids are natural yellow, orange and red pigments that are widely distributed in the plant kingdom (15). They may be divided into the following two main groups: (i) carotenes or hydrocarotenoids and (ii) xanthophylls or oxycarotenoids, and their oxygenated derivatives (16). Carotenes are a group of C-40 polyunsaturated hydrocarbons that impart an orange-red color to the red palm oil. Different carotene isomers are found in red palm oil with α- and β-carotene as the two major isomers (1,17). Different carotene isomers exhibit different provitamin A activity and β-carotene has the highest vitamin A potency (18). Provitamin A carotenes are converted enzymatically to retinol or vitamin A in the intestinal mucosa and stored as retinol esters in the liver (18). Vitamin A has a wide spectrum of physiologic and biochemical functions in humans, and its role in vision and night blindness is well established.

Vitamin A deficiency is a prevailing problem in many developing countries, especially among children. Various attempts have been made to improve the vitamin A status in children of the developing countries by dietary supplementation with synthetic vitamin A and provitamin A carotenes. Synthetic vitamin A is readily available and has been used with some degree of success; however, overdoses of synthetic vitamin A have given rise to the problem of hypervitaminosis or vitamin A toxicity, which can have serious consequences. An alternative means is dietary supplementation with natural provitamin A carotenes. Crude palm oil (CPO) and red palm oil (RPO) are rich sources of natural provitamin A carotenes. Dietary or oral supplementation of CPO and RPO to schoolchildren has been attempted. Lian *et al.* (2) treated preschool children in two selected villages in Indonesia with RPO and observed significant improvement in vitamin A status and a decrease in xerophthalmia in the treated groups. Similar trials were conducted by Manorama *et al.* (3) in school children in India, and they observed improved serum vitamin A status in these children. Solomons (4), reviewing studies in India and elsewhere, concluded that RPO is an excellent source of provitamin A β-carotene and is as effective as synthetic retinol palmitate in restoring and preserving vitamin A nutriture in school children. Our results in hamsters (Table 29.5) provide further evidence to strengthen the clinical findings that RPO could serve as an excellent source of provitamin A β-carotene because RPO supplementation in the diet improved both serum vitamin A level and vitamin A stores in the liver. In addition to the improved vitamin A status, the serum vitamin E level and liver vitamin E content in RPO-supplemented groups were also significantly increased (Tables 29.6 and 29.7). Thus, our results show that RPO supplementation improved both vitamin A and E status in the treated groups compared with the untreated groups, and that RPO could serve as an excellent source of natural carotenes.

β-Carotene and other carotenoids serve not only as provitamin A but also as natural antioxidants. Serbinova *et al.* (19) studied the antioxidant activity of a palm oil carotene concentrate and observed an inverse correlation between tissue carotenoid level and the accumulation of lipid peroxidation products. The antioxidant functions of the carotenoids could be mediated through the action of the antioxidant enzymes, i.e., GST, GSH-Px, SOD, and catalase. These antioxidant enzymes catalyze the conversion of harmful oxidative products into nonharmful metabolites for excretion or scavenge reactive free radicals that are generated during oxidative metabolic processes, thus preventing the spread of oxidative damage in cells.

GST is both a detoxification enzyme and an antioxidant enzyme. It catalyzes the conjugation of GSH to foreign compounds and makes these foreign compounds more water soluble and readily excreted (10). GSH protects cells against a number of potential cytotoxic agents, including reactive oxygen species (ROS), hydroperoxides, drugs, and steroids (20). Manorama *et al.* (21) reported that RPO caused an induction of GST production in rats. Our results (Table 29.8) show that there was a significant increase in liver GST activity in hamsters fed the diet supplemented with RPO.

GSH-Px is a selenium-dependent enzyme (22). Its function is to catalyze the reduction of H_2O_2 and lipid hydroperoxides by oxidation of the reduced GSH so that the proliferation of oxygen-derived radical species is prevented. It protects against free radical damage by catalyzing their inactivation, thereby consuming GSH (23). Our results (Table 29.8) show that RPO supplementation in the diet greatly enhanced GSH-Px activity in the liver.

SOD catalyzes the destruction of the superoxide ($O_2^{-\bullet}$) free radical. The superoxide anion can be scavenged by SOD, which catalyzes the conversion of two of these radicals into hydrogen peroxide (H_2O_2) and molecular oxygen (24). The H_2O_2 is then converted to water, H_2O, and molecular oxygen, O_2. Thus, the SOD and catalase act in concert to protect oxygen-metabolizing cells against harmful effects of superoxide free radicals (25–27). The $O_2^{-\bullet}$ ion, is formed by the univalent reduction of oxygen during various enzymatic reactions or by ionizing radiation (28,29). Protonation of $O_2^{-\bullet}$ yields a hydroperoxyl radical, which can react spontaneously with another $O_2^{-\bullet}$ to form H_2O_2. Our results (Table 29.9) indicate that RPO supplementation had no significant effect on the activity of these two antioxidant enzymes.

The effect of β-carotene supplementation on serum lipids in humans has been investigated previously. Carughi and Hooper (30) observed that β-carotene supplementation for 4 wk did not produce any significant change in serum TC, TAG, HDL-C, or LDL-C levels in men and women. Similarly Allard *et al.* (31) reported that β-carotene supplementation did not result in any significant change in serum TC, TG, HDL-C, or LDL-C levels in smokers and nonsmokers. Our results (Table 29.10) showed that there was no significant change in serum TC level between the RPO-supplemented groups and the groups that were not supplemented. However, our results (Table 29.10) indicated that there may be a redistribution of cholesterol between HDL and LDL, resulting in higher HDL-C levels and lower LDL-C levels in the PO-RPO group compared with the PO group. A similar redistribution of cholesterol between HDL and LDL was also observed in the CO-RPO and CO groups, but the results were less obvious.

Acknowledgements

This work was supported by research funds from the University of Malaya and Palm Oil Research Institute of Malaysia.

References

1. Choo, Y.M. (1996) Antioxidants in Red Palm Oil. *MOST 5*, 15–16.
2. Lian, O.K., Liem, T.T., Rose, C.S., Prawiranegra, D.D., and Gyorgy, P. (1967) Red Palm Oil in the Prevention of Vitamin A Deficiency. A Trial on Preschool Children in Indonesia. *Am. J. Clin. Nutr. 20*, 11267–1274.

3. Manorama, R., Brahman, G.N., and Rukmini, C. (1996) Red Palm Oil as a Source of β-Carotene for Combating Vitamin A Deficiency. *Plant Foods Hum. Nutr. 49*, 75–81.
4. Solomons, N.W. (1998) Plant Sources of Vitamin A and Human Nutrition: Red Palm Oil Does the Job. *Nutr. Rev. 56*, 309–311.
5. Paiva, S.A., and Russell, R.M. (1999) β-Carotene and Carotenoids as Antioxidants. *J. Am. Coll. Nutr. 18*, 426–433.
6. Wang, X.D., and. Russell, R.M. (1999) Procarcinogenic and Anticarcinogenic Effects of β-Carotene. *Nutr. Rev. 57*, 263–72.
7. Khor, H.T., and Chieng, D.Y. (1996) Effect of Dietary Supplementation of Tocotrienols and Tocopherols on Serum Lipids in the Hamster. *Nutr Res. 16*, 1393–1401.
8. Tan, D.T.S., Khor, H.T., Low, W.H., Ali, A., and Gapor, A. (1991) Effect of a Palm Oil Vitamin E Concentrate on the Serum and Lipoprotein Lipids of Humans. *Am. J. Clin. Nutr. 53*, 1027s–1030s.
9. Bradford, M.M. (1967) A Rapid and Sensitive Method for the Quantitation of Microgram Quantities of Protein Utilizing the Principle of Protein Dye Binding. *Anal. Biochem. 72*, 248–254.
10. Habig, W.H., Pabst, M.J., and Jakoby, W.B. (1974) Glutathione-*S*-Transferase. The First Enzymatic Step in Mercapturic Acid Formation. *J. Biol. Chem. 249*, 7130–7136.
11. Lawrence, R., and Burk, R. (1976) Glutathione Peroxidase Activity in Selenium-Deficient Rat Liver. *Biochem. Biophys. Res. Commun. 55*, 350–353.
12. Marklund, S., and Marklund, G. (1974) Involvement of the Superoxide Anion Radical in the Autoxidation of Pyrogallol and a Convenient Assay for Peroxide Dismutase. *Eur. J. Biochem. 47*, 469–474.
13. Roth, E.F., Jr., and Gilbert, H.S. (1984) The Pyrogallol Assay for Superoxide Dismutase: Absence of a Glutathione Artifact. *Anal. Biochem. 137*, 50–53.
14. Bears, R.F., and Sizers, J.W. (1952) A Spectrophotometric Method of Measuring The Breakdown of Hydrogen Peroxide by Catalase. *J. Biol. Chem. 195*, 133–140.
15. Mangels, A.R., Holden, J.M., Beecher, G.R., Forman, M.R., and Lanza, E. (1993) Carotenoid Content of Fruits and Vegetables: An Evaluation of Analytical Data. *J Am Diet. Assoc. 93*, 284–296.
16. Thane, C., and Reddy, S. (1997) Processing of Fruits and Vegetables: Effect on Carotenoids. *Nutr. Food Sci. 2*, 58–65.
17. Hamid, H.A., Choo, Y.M., Khor, H.T., and Goh, S.H. (1995) Ubiquinone of Palm Oil, in *Nutrition, Lipids, Health and Diseases*, (Ong A.S.H., Niki, E., and Packer, L., eds) pp. 122–128, AOCS Press, Champaign, IL.
18. Mayne, S.T. (1996) β-Carotene, Carotenoids and Disease Prevention in Humans. *FASEB J. 10*, 690–701.
19. Serbinova, E., Choo, Y.M., and Packer, L. (1992) Distribution and Antioxidant Activity of a Palm Oil Carotene Fraction in Rats. *Biochem. Int. 28*, 881–886.
20. McIntosh, M.K, Goldfarb, A.H., Curtis, L.N., and Cote, P.S. (1993) Vitamin E Alters Antioxidant Enzymes in Rats Treated with Dehydroepiandrosterone (DHEA). *J. Nutr. 123*, 216–224.
21. Manorama, R., Chinnasamy, N., and Rukmini, C. (1993) Effect of Red Palm Oil on Some Hepatic Drug Metabolizing Enzymes in Rats. *Food Chem. Toxicol. 31*, 583–588.
22. Mehiert, A., and Diplock, A.T. (1985) The Glutathione-*S*-Transferases in Selenium and Vitamin E Deficiency. *Biochem. J. 227*, 823–831.

23. Van Lieshout, E.M., Ekkel, M.B., Bedaf, M.M., Nijhoff, W.A., and Peters, W.H. (1998) Effects of Dietary Anticarcinogens on Rat Gastrointestinal Glutathione Peroxidase Activity. *Oncol. Rep. 5*, 959–963.
24. Stryer L. (1988) Biosynthesis of Membrane Lipids and Steroid Hormones, in *Biochemistry*, (Kudlacik, A., ed.) pp. 547–574, W.H. Freeman and Company, New York.
25. Petkau, A., Chelack, W., Pleskach, S., Meeker, B., and Brady, C. (1975) Radioprotection of Mice by Superoxide Dismutase. *Biochem. Biophys. Res. Commun. 65*, 886–888.
26. Paschen, W., and Wesser, U. (1973) Singlet Oxygen Decontaminating Activity of Erythrocuprein (Superoxide Dismutase). *Biochem. Biophys. Acta 327*, 217–219.
27. Lavelle, F., Michelson, A., and Dimitrijevic, L. (1973) Biological Protection by Superoxide Dismutase. *Biochem. Biophys. Res. Commun. 55*, 350–353.
28. Fee, J., and Tettelbaum, H. (1972) Evidence That Superoxide Dismutase Plays a Role in Protecting Red Blood Cells Against Peroxidative Hemolysis. *Biochem. Biophys. Res. commun. 49*, 150–152.
29. Fee, J., Bergamini, R., and Briggs, R. (1975) Observations on the Mechanism of the Oxygen Dialuric Acid Induced Hemolysis of Vitamin E Deficient Red Blood Cells and the Protective Roles of Catalase and Superoxide Dismutase. *Arch. Biochem. Biophys. 169*, 160–163.
30. Carughi A., and Hooper, F.G. (1994). Plasma Carotenoid Concentrations Before and After Supplementation with a Carotenoid Mixture. *Am. J. Clin. Nutr. 59* 896–899.
31. Allard J.P., Royall, D., Kurian R., Mugghi, R., and Jeejeebhoy, K. (1994) Effects of β-Carotene Supplementation on Lipid Peroxidation in Humans. *Am. J. Clin. Nutr. 59*, 884–890.

Chapter 30

Effect of Flavonoids and Trace Elements on Murine Immune Response

U.R. Kuppusamy,[a] M. Kasthuri Bai,[a] and M.S. Kanthimathi[b]

[a]Department of Allied Health Sciences, Faculty of Medicine, University of Malaya, Kuala Lumpur
[b]Department of Biochemistry, Faculty of Medicine, University of Malaya, Kuala Lumpur

Introduction

The immune system involves interaction of two major responses, i.e., humoral and cell-mediated immunity (1). T lymphocytes play myriad roles in the defense against certain viruses, fungi, tumor cells, and facultative intracellular bacterial pathogens. T lymphocytes may accomplish these functions *via* fundamental effector cell activation, inhibition of cell migration, activation of macrophages, and cooperation with B lymphocytes for antibody production (1). Thus, patients whose immune responses are suppressed, such as in cancer and acquired immunodeficiency syndrome (AIDS), would be susceptible to other infections/complications that may even lead to death.

Oxygen free radicals, which are generated by xanthine oxidase (XO; EC 1.1.3.22) *in vivo*, have been implicated in the etiology of cancer and numerous other diseases (2). In a normal healthy individual, the antioxidant enzymes such as superoxide dismutase (SOD; EC 1.15.1.1), catalase (CAT; EC 1.11.1.6), and glutathione peroxidase (GPX; EC 1.11.1.9) are able to eliminate the damaging oxygen radicals (3). These enzyme activities may be compromised in individuals who lack essential nutrients that are required for the optimal enzyme activities due to poor dietary habit or the disease condition. Several trace elements and flavonoids have been reported to have the ability to scavenge/destroy free radicals, and some of the trace elements have also been reported to stimulate T lymphocyte proliferation (4–8).

In the present study, the trace elements, zinc, selenium, iron, and copper as well as the flavonoids, quercetin (3,3′,4′,5,7-pentahydroxyflavone), fisetin (3,3′,4′,7-tetrahydroxyflavone), naringenin (4′,5,7-trihydroxyflavanonone), and genistein (4′,5,7-trihydroxyisoflavone), were tested for their proliferative response on murine thymocytes. The activities of xanthine oxidase and catalase in thymocyte cultures incubated with iron or selenium were also estimated.

Materials and Methods

Materials. Copper(II)chloride anhydrous, iron(II)sulfate heptahydrate, selenium dioxide sublimed, zinc(II)chloride anhydrous, sodium hydroxide, potassium dihydrogen orthophosphate, dipotassium hydrogen phosphate anhydrous, and perchloric acid were obtained from Merck, Darmstadt, Germany; quercetin, naringenin, fisetin, genistein, dimethyl sulfoxide (DMSO), hypoxanthine (6-hydroxypurine), uricase (urate oxidase; EC 1.7.3.3.), and peroxidase (hydrogen-peroxide oxidoreductase; EC 1.11.1.7) were obtained from Sigma Chemical, St.Louis, MO; tritiated thymidine (thymidine-5'-3H) was obtained from Amersham Life Sciences, UK; scintillation fluid was obtained from ICN Biomedicals, Amsterdam, The Netherlands; RPMI 1640 with penicillin and glutamine and FBS (fetal bovine serum) were obtained from Biosciences, Australia; ABTS (2,2′-azino-bis(3-ethylbenzthiozoline-6-sulfonic acid) diammonium salt was obtained from Boehringer Mannheim, Germany; hydrogen peroxide and hypochloride were obtained from Fischer Chemicals, St. Louis, MO, and mice (BALB/cj strain) were obtained from the Animal House, Faculty of Medicine, University of Malaya, Kuala Lumpur, Malaysia.

Thymocyte Culture. A BALB/cj strain mouse (6–8 wk old) was killed by cervical dislocation and the thymus removed and placed in cold phosphate-buffered saline (PBS). The thymocytes were released by teasing with forceps. The cell suspension was then centrifuged at 2000 rpm for 5 min. The washed pellet was resuspended in RPMI containing 10% FBS and diluted to yield 10^6 cells/mL.

The thymocyte proliferation response was quantitated by the incorporation of ^{3}H-thymidine into newly formed DNA. The trace elements and flavonoids were dissolved in double-distilled water and DMSO, respectively. Each culture well contained 100 µL cell suspension, 20 µL test compound, and 80 µL of complete media (RPMI with 10% FBS). In the control culture, 20 µL water or DMSO was added instead of the test compound. The cultures were incubated at 37°C in humidified air containing 5% CO_2 for 48 h, after which 1 µL of tritiated thymidine was added to each well. The cells were harvested after a further incubation of 18–24 h and the radioactivity counted in a liquid scintillation counter.

Enzyme Assays. Thymocytes were grown in the presence of various concentrations of selenium or iron for 60 h. The cell suspension was then removed from the well and sonicated (two 10-s pulses with a 10-s interval). The sonicate was centrifuged at 13000 rpm for 10 min at 4°C. The supernatant was then used in the xanthine oxidase and catalase assays.

Xanthine Oxidase Assay. This assay was carried out according to the method of Singh *et.al.* (9). In this assay, the chromogen ABTS is stoichiometrically oxidized in the following coupled reactions:

$$\text{Hypoxanthine} + 2H_2O + 2O_2 \xrightarrow{XO} \text{Uric acid} + 2H_2O_2$$

$$\text{Uric acid} + O_2 \xrightarrow{Uricase} \text{allantoin} + H_2O_2 + CO_2$$

$$H_2O_2 + \text{ABTS}_{(red)} \xrightarrow{Peroxidase} \text{ABTS}_{(ox)} + 2H_2O$$

The absorbance of oxidized ABTS, measured at 410 nm, is directly proportional to XO activity.

The incubation mixture contained 10 µmol hypoxanthine in 1 mL of 66.7 mmol/L KH_2PO_4 solution (pH 7.9), 5 µL of 100 g/L uricase and 50 µL of sonicate. The mixture was incubated at 37°C for 10 min, after which 1 mL of phosphate buffer (66.7 mmol/L, pH7.9) containing 2 µmol ABTS and 250 U peroxidase was added and vortex-mixed. The reaction was terminated by the addition of 1 mL perchloric acid (2 mol/L). The absorbance of the clear supernatant obtained after centrifugation at 3500 rpm (5 min) was read at 410 nm against a sample blank that did not contain hypoxanthine. The activity was calculated as $A_{410nm} \times 79.9$ on the basis of $ABTS_{ox}$ molar lineic absorbance, which is 2550 m^2/mol.

Catalase Assay. Catalase activity was measured according to the method proposed by Flescher (10). The supernatant obtained from the sonicated cells (50 µL) was mixed with 600 µL H_2O_2 (15 mmol/L) in a cuvette, and the decrease in the absorbance at 240 nm over a period of 3 min was monitored spectrophotometrically.

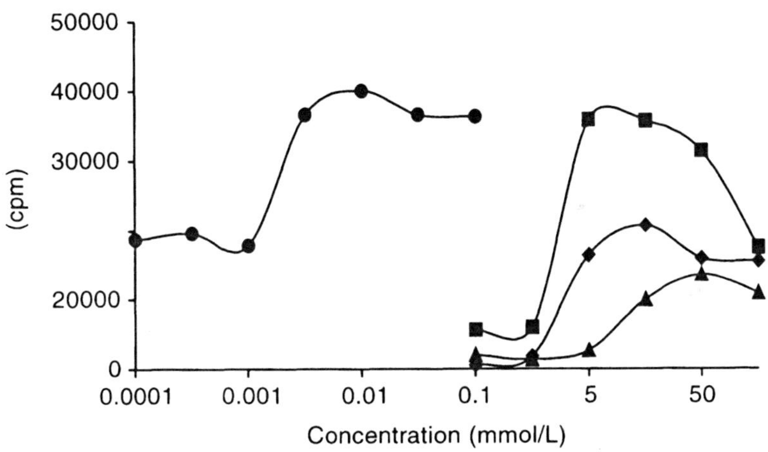

Fig. 30.1. Effect of trace elements on the proliferation of murine thymocytes. The graph presents the effect of the trace elements tested on mouse thymocyte proliferation. Mouse thymocytes (1 × 10^6 cells/100 µL) in RPMI containing 10% fetal calf serum were incubated at 37°C in humidified air containing 5% CO_2 with different concentrations of trace elements, ranging from 0.1 µmol/L to 100 mmol/L. ^{3}H-thymidine (1 µL/well) was added after a 48-h incubation. After a further 18–24 h of incubation, cells were harvested onto glass fiber filters and the radioactivity counted. The *x*-axis represents the concentration of trace element used; the *y*- axis represents the counts per minute (cpm) measured above that of control values (controls contained cells without trace element). The symbols are as follows: ●, selenium; ■, copper; ▲, iron; and ◆, zinc. Selenium stimulated thymocyte proliferation at 0.1–100 µmol/L; other trace elements were stimulatory at 0.1–100 mmol/L.

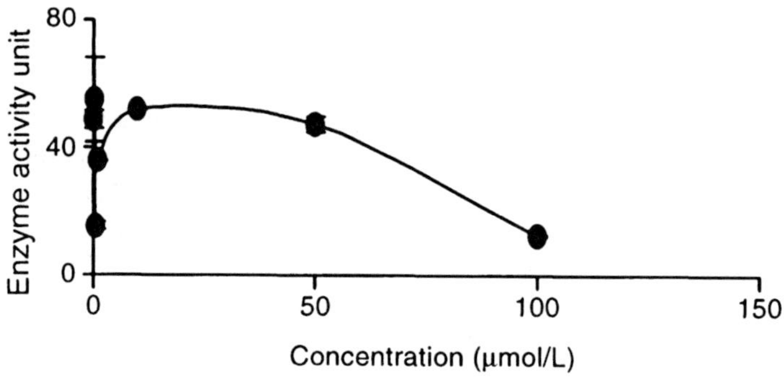

Fig. 30.2. Effect of selenium on catalase activity in murine thymocytes. The graph presents the mean + SEM for triplicate assays of catalase activity in selenium-induced T lymphocytes in an *in vitro* study. Catalase activity was estimated by the method of Flescher (10). Enzyme activity (*y*- axis) is expressed as the rate constant of a first-order-reaction (*k*) divided by the protein concentration for each concentration of iron. The enzyme activity is expressed per minute per milligram protein. The *x*-axis represents the concentration of selenium used in mmol/L. Selenium inhibited catalase activity in a dose-dependent manner at a concentration range of 10–100 mol/L. The decrease at this concentration range is significant (Student's *t* test; $P < 0.05$). The initial increase shown is not significantly different from the control (thymocytes without selenium).

The activity was expressed as the rate constant of a first-order reaction per mg protein as follows: $k = (2.3/t)(\log A1/A2)/(\text{min}\cdot\text{mg protein})$.

Results and Discussion

Selenium exerted a stimulatory effect even at the low dose range of 1–100 μmol/L (final concentration), whereas zinc, iron, and copper were able to stimulate thymocyte proliferation only at a dose range of 5-100 mmol/L (final concentration, Fig. 30.1). The order of potency of the trace elements in stimulating thymocyte proliferation was selenium >> zinc > copper > iron.

The effects of selenium and iron on thymocytes were further evaluated by estimating key enzyme activities. Thymocytes that were incubated with selenium did not show any xanthine oxidase activity (result not shown), whereas catalase activity was not significantly different from that of the control (Fig. 30.2). Selenium has been reported to be a potent inhibitor of xanthine oxidase (11). Thus, it is possible that selenium could enhance cell proliferation by maintaining an oxygen radical–free environment. The insignificant catalase activity was probably due to the lack of endogenous generation of its substrate, hydrogen peroxide. The efficient inhibition of xanthine oxidase by selenium could possibly prevent or minimize the subsequent generation of hydrogen peroxide; as a result, catalase activity might not be induced. Further investigations would have to be conducted to verify this hypothesis. Selenium has also been reported to be a component of DNA repair en-

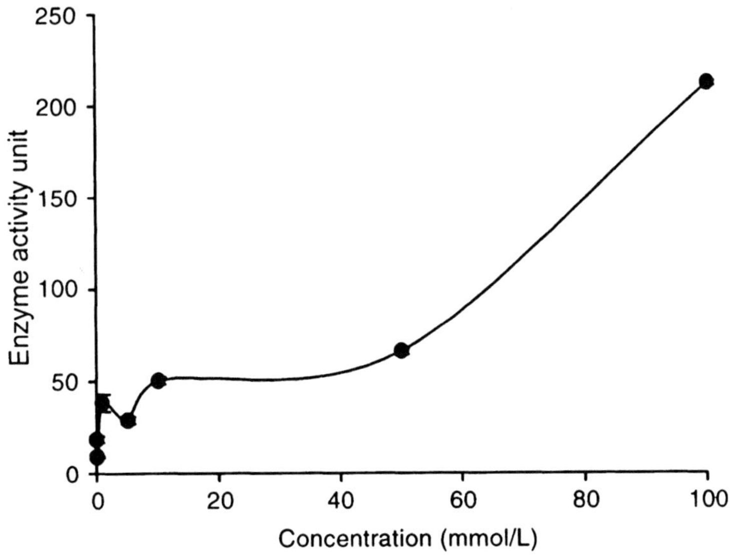

Fig. 30.3. Effect of iron on catalase activity in murine thymocytes. The graph presents the mean + SEM for triplicate assays on catalase activity in iron-induced thymocytes in an *in vitro* study. Catalase activity was estimated by the method of Flescher (10). Enzyme activity (*y*-axis) is expressed as the rate constant of a first-order reaction (*k*) divided by the protein concentration for each concentration of iron. The enzyme activity is expressed per minute per milligram protein. The *x*-axis represents the concentration of iron used in mmol/L. There was a dose-dependent increase in catalase activity above 5 mmol/L. The increase in enzyme activity between 5 and 100 mmol/L was significantly different (Student's *t* test; $P < 0.05$).

zymes, thus preventing or minimizing errors in protein synthesis that may lead to the destruction of cells (5).

The xanthine oxidase activity in thymocytes incubated with iron was detectable only at a high concentration of 100 mmol/L (result not shown), whereas catalase activity increased in a dose-dependent manner within a range of 0–100 mmol/L (Fig. 30.3). These results indicate that catalase activity might be induced only when there are free radicals produced by xanthine oxidase. The hydrogen peroxide–scavenging enzyme, catalase, decreases the generation of $^{\bullet}OH$ produced by xanthine oxidase in the Fenton reaction (12). The cell proliferation curve in the presence of iron showed a slight decrease at 100 mmol/L (Fig. 30.1) despite having high catalase activity (Fig. 30.3). It could be due to the toxicity of iron, which might have overwhelmed the protective effect of catalase, leading to the inevitable cellular damage.

The stimulatory effects of zinc were consistent with other reports (13,14). Zinc may be involved in the cell cycle during mid- to G_1 phase in promotion of thymidine kinase expression. It is well known that zinc deficiency may impair the M phase of the cell cycle and that numerous enzymes at the basic level of replication and transcription require zinc for their activity. Zinc has been reported to be able to activate protein kinase C, which mediates the phosphorylation of intracellular proteins that regulate activation and cell regulation (4).

Copper has been shown to be an essential element for the production of interleukin–2 (IL- 2) (15). IL-2 promotes ^{3}H-thymidine incorporation in the *in vitro* system. IL-2 has also been reported as a characteristic marker of early T-cell activation.

Of the four flavonoids tested, only fisetin significantly stimulated murine thymocyte proliferation at a dose range of 100–500 µmol/L (final concentration) (Fig. 30.4). Naringenin, genistein, and quercetin significantly inhibited thymocyte proliferation (Fig. 30.4). Genistein, naringenin, quercetin, and fisetin have been reported to exert inhibitory effects on breast tumors and various cancer cell lines. Herrera (16) reported that naringenin has the ability to inhibit protein kinase C, which in turn could result in the inhibition of T-lymphocyte proliferation. Genistein, an isoflavone that has the same hydroxylation pattern as naringenin, a flavonone, has been shown to inhibit prostate cancer and MCF-T human breast cancer cells (17). Genistein has also been shown to cause tumor cell cycle derangements that lead to cell death by apoptosis (18). However, the mode of action for the inhibitory effect of genistein on thymocyte proliferation is not yet known.

It is interesting to note that quercetin (3,3′,4′,5,7-pentahydroxyflavone) and fisetin (3,3′,4′,7-tetrahydroxyflavone), which differ structurally by only one hydroxyl

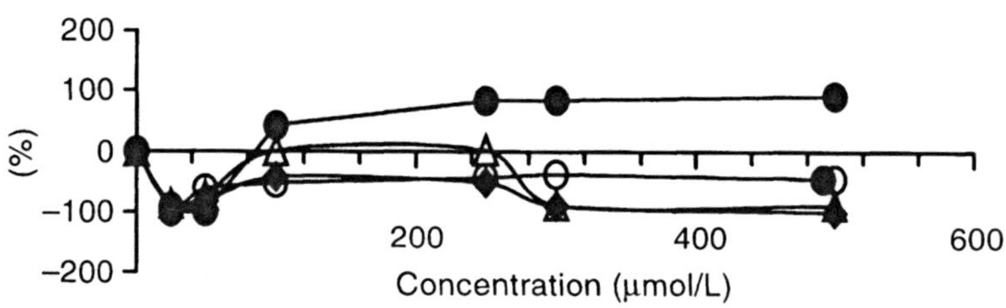

Fig. 30.4. Effect of flavonoids on murine thymocytes. The graph presents the effect of flavonoids on mouse thymocyte proliferation. Mouse thymocytes (1 × 10^6 cells/100 µL) in RPMI containing 10% fetal calf serum, were incubated at 37°C in humidified air containing 5% CO_2, with different concentrations of flavonoid, ranging from 0 to 500 mmol/L. ^{3}H-thymidine (1 µL/well) was added after a 48-h incubation. After a further 18–24 h of incubation, cells were harvested onto glass fiber filters and the radioactivity counted. The *x*-axis represents the concentration of flavonoid used; the *y*-axis represents the counts per minute as a percentage (%) of values for controls, which contained cells without flavonoid. The (+) sign along the *y*-axis indicates a stimulatory response and the (–) sign indicates an inhibitory response of the flavonoid compounds on thymocyte proliferation. The basal level is 0, shown by the control. Flavonoids used were fisetin (●), quercetin (θ), genistein (Δ), and naringenin (◆). Fisetin shows a stimulatory response, whereas all other flavonoids tested showed inhibition. The slight stimulatory response shown by genistein between a dose range of 100 and 250 µmol/L is not significant (Student's *t* test; $P < 0.05$).

group, are able to exert contrasting effects on the cell proliferation. Preliminary *in vitro* work carried out in our laboratory has shown that fisetin is a more potent inhibitor of catalase than quercetin (result not shown), whereas quercetin has been reported to be a more potent xanthine oxidase inhibitor (19). The mode of action of fisetin on thymocyte proliferation probably does not involve the prevention of xanthine oxidase–mediated oxygen radical formation in the culture system. Further investigations would have to be carried out to confirm the mechanism of action of fisetin on thymocyte proliferation. Fisetin may be a better candidate as an antitumorigenic agent because it has the ability to stimulate thymocyte proliferation.

This preliminary study on murine thymocyte immune response has shown some interesting results; further investigations using human T cells must be conducted before these compounds could be exploited as therapeutic agents or boosters.

References

1. Sheffy, B.E., and Schultz, R.D. (1979) Influence of Vitamin E and Selenium on Immune Response Mechanisms. *Fed. Proc. 38*, 2139–2142.
2. Bolann, B.J., and Rune, J.U. (1990) The Limited Ability of Superoxide to Release Iron From Ferritin. *Eur. J. Biochem.*, 899–904.
3. Kuppusamy, P., and Zweier, J.L.(1988) Characterization of Free Radical Generation by Xanthine Oxidase. *J. Biol. Chem. 264*, 9880–9884.
4. Moulder, K., and Steward, M.W. (1989) Experimental Zinc Deficiency: Effects on Cellular Responses and the Affinity of Humoral Antibody. *Clin. Exp. Immunol. 77*, 269–274.
5. Dutta, S.K., Miller, P.A., Greenberg, L.B., and Levander, O.A. (1983) Selenium and Acute Alcoholism. *Am. J. Clin. Nutr. 38*, 713–718.
6. Kelly, D.S., Daudu, P.A., Taylor, P.C., Mackey, B.E., and Turnlund, J.R. (1995) Effects of Low Copper Diets on Human Immune Response. *Am. J. Clin. Nutr. 62*, 412–416.
7. Middleton, E.J.R., and Kandaswami, C. (1992) Effects of Flavonoids on Immune and Inflammatory Cell Functions. *J. Immunol. 43*, 1167–1179.
8. Kuppusamy, U.R., and Das, N.P. (1992) Effects of Flavonoids on Cyclic AMP Phosphodiesterase and Lipid Mobilization in Rat Adipocytes. *Biochem. Pharmacol. 44*, 1307–1315.
9. Singh, N.M., Bogavac, L., Kalimanovska, V., Jelic, Z., and Spasic, S. (1987) Spectrophotometric Assay of Xanthine Oxidase with ABTS as Chromogen. *Clin. Chim. Acta 162*, 29–36.
10. Flescher, E. (1998) Oxidative Stress Suppresses Transcription Factor Activities in Stimulated Lymphocytes. *Clin. Exp. Immunol. 112*, 242–247.
11. Kuppusamy, U.R., Law, C.H., and Ong, G. (1998) Studies on the Effects of Glucose, Iron and Selenium on Blood Lipid Peroxidation and Xanthine Oxidase Activity. *Abstracts of the 8th FAOBMB Congress*, p. 64, Kuala Lumpur, Malaysia.
12. Brigitan, B.E., Sovitaj, P., Rosen, G.M., Lilleg, D.M., and Buettner, G.R. (1990) Hydroxyl Radical Is Not a Product of the Reaction of Xanthine Oxidase and Xanthine. *J. Biol. Chem. 265*, 17533–17538.
13. Csermely, P., Szamel, M., Resch, K., and Somogyi, J. (1988) Zinc Can Increase the Activity of Protein Kinase C and Contribute to Its Binding to Plasma Membranes in T-Lymphocytes. *J. Biol. Chem. 263*, 6487–6490.

14. Shankar, A.H., and Prasad, A. (1998) Zinc and Immune Function: The Biological Basis of Altered Resistance to Infection. *Am. J. Clin. Nutr.*, 447S–463S.
15. Failla, M.L., and Hopkins, R.G. (1981) Is Low Copper Status Immunosuppressive? *Nutr. Rev. 56*, S59–S64.
16. Herrera, M.D. (1996) Effects of Flavonoids on Rat Aortic Smooth Muscle Contractility; Structure-Activity Relationship. *Gen. Pharmacol. 27*, 273–277.
17. Pagliacci, M.C., Smacchia, M., Migliorati, G., Grignani, F., Riccardi, C., and Nicoletti, I. (1994) Growth Inhibitory Effects of the Natural Phytooestrogen Genistein in MCF-7 Human Breast Cancer Cells. *Eur. J. Cancer 30A*, 1675–1682.
18. Markovitz, J., Linassier, C., Fosse, P., Couprie, J., Pierre, J., Jacquemin-Sablon, A., Saucier, J., Le Pecq, J.B., and Larsen, A.K. (1989) Inhibitory Effects of the Thyrosine Kinase Inhibitor Genistein on Mammalian DNA Topoisomerase II. *Cancer Res. 49*, 5111–5117.
19. Kuppusamy, U.R., and Law, C.S. (2000) Effects of Trace Elements and Flavonoids on Bovine and Human Milk Xanthine Oxidase Activity. *Abstracts of the 15th Scientific Meeting of the Malaysian Society of Pharmacology and Physiology,* Poster 8, Kelantan, Malaysia.

Chapter 31

Antibodies of All Isotypes to Oxysterols in Normal Human Sera: A Parameter for *In Vivo* Oxidative Status?

S.L. Tung,[a] H.M. Cheng,[a] C.K. Sam,[a] and K. Sundram[b]

[a]Institute of Postgraduate Studies, University of Malaya, Kuala Lumpur, Malaysia
[b]Division of Nutrition, Malaysian Palm Oil Board, Malaysia

Introduction

Oxysterols are the oxidation products of cholesterols. Oxidation can occur at different carbon atoms of the cholesterol molecule. For example, 7-β-hydroxycholesterol and 7-ketocholesterol are the oxysterols oxidized at carbon number seven. Oxysterols are generated by enzymatic reactions during cholesterol catabolism, through the peroxidation of lipoproteins in vivo or as contaminants of cholesterol-rich processed foods.

Oxysterols are associated with lipoproteins or albumin in the blood circulation. Unlike cholesterol, oxysterols are distributed almost equally between lipoprotein-containing and lipoprotein-deficient serum. Esterification of oxysterols may enhance their incorporation into high density lipoproteins (HDL) and low density lipoproteins (LDL) but decrease their distribution in serum (1).

Data from Patel *et al.* (2) showed that oxidized LDL (oxLDL) are produced by secondary oxidation events involving the fatty acid peroxyl/alkoxyl radicals at the 7-position of cholesterol in LDL. Furthermore, peroxynitrite, copper, and myoglobin are capable of generating oxLDL.

Oxysterols have been shown to be proatherogenic compared with cholesterol. The enrichment of native human HDL (especially HDL_3) with oxysterols caused a reduced capacity to simulate the cholesterol efflux from peripheral tissues to liver (3). The decreased cholesterol efflux is due to an unregulated uptake by macrophage scavenger receptors belonging to class A type I and II (4). A high level of lipid deposition within the macrophages endowed them with a foamy appearance, which is a characteristic feature of the atherosclerotic lesion (5).

Oxysterols are found in human atherosclerotic plaque (6,7). Zieden *et al.* (8) indicated a relationship between the plasma levels of oxysterols and atherosclerosis. They found that high plasma levels of 7-β-hydroxycholesterol were associated with a high risk of cardiovascular diseases in a Lithuanian population. Oxysterols, especially 7-ketocholesterols, are the major component of oxLDL (9). Serum antibodies to oxLDL (anti-oxLDL) are elevated in atherosclerosis (10) and may participate in the vascular pathology. In this case, the anti-oxLDL are proatherogenic. In contrast, in a study with experimental animals that were immunized with oxLDL, the induced anti-oxLDL appeared to suppress the progression of atherosclerosis (11). In this study, an immunoassay was used to detect the serum natural antibodies to oxysterols (antioxysterols). The presence of antioxysterols in this *in vitro* system was presumed to reflect a raised level of anti-oxLDL.

Materials and Methods

Enzyme-Linked Immunosorbent Assay (ELISA). The solid-phase indirect ELISA system was used for antioxysterol detection. The oxysterols, dissolved in absolute ethanol, were allowed to evaporate off in 96-well microtiter plates (50 μL/well; Nunc, Denmark) at 4°C overnight. Diluent buffer [100 μL; phosphate buffered saline (PBS)/1% bovine serum albumin] was dispensed into each well. The plate was covered by parafilm and incubated for 2 h at room temperature. Then the plate was washed twice (200 μL/well). Diluted serum (50 μL; 1:100) was dispensed into each well. The plate was covered by parafilm and incubated for 2 h at room temperature, then washed three times. Horseradish peroxidase-conjugated rabbit anti-human immunoglobulin (Ig; Dako) was prepared at 1:1000 dilution. Then 50 μL/well of this second antibody was added and incubated for 2 h at room temperature, then washed four times. Substrate buffer was prepared with 1 g/L *o*-phenylenediamine (OPD) in citrate-phosphate buffer (pH 5.6) and 1 μL/mL of 30% hydrogen peroxide. Substrate buffer (50 μL/well) was dispensed. The plate was incubated at room temperature for 10 min, and the colorimetric reaction stopped with 50 μL/well of 4 mol/L sulfuric acid. The optical absorbance at 490 nm was measured in an automated MRX Microplate Reader (Dynex Technologies) The reaction was considered to be positive when the value of mean optical density (dOD) was ≥0.3.

TABLE 31.1 The Binding of Naturally Occurring IgG, IgM, and IgA to Cholesterol and Four Different Oxysterols[a,b]

Antibody in NHS	Cholesterol	Cholesterol epoxide	19-OH	7-Keto	7-β-OH
IgG	12/22 (54.5%)	11/11 (100%)	0/11 (0%)	22/22 (100%)	7/11 (63.6%)
IgM	17/22 (77.3%)	10/11 (90.0%)	9/11 (81.8%)	22/22 (100%)	7/11 (63.6%)
IgA	4/22 (18.2%)	11/11 (100%)	0/11 (0%)	21/22 (95.5%)	0/11 (0%)

[a]The reaction is considered to be positive when the value of the mean optical density (dOD) is ≥0.3.
[b]Abbreviations: Ig, immunoglobulin; NHS, normal human sera; 19-OH, 19-hydroxycholesterol; 7-keto, 7-ketocholesterol; 7-β-OH, 7-β-hydroxycholesterol.

Results

Natural Antibodies to Cholesterol and Oxysterols. The oxysterols tested in this study were cholesterol epoxide (CE), 7-ketocholesterol (7-keto), 7-β-hydroxycholesterol (7-β-OH) and 19-hydroxycholesterol (19-OH). Detection of natural antibodies was done for IgG, IgM, and IgA.

Natural IgG to Cholesterol and Oxysterols. IgG in normal human sera (NHS) bound to cholesterol (Cho), CE, 7-keto, and 7-β-OH (Table 31.1 and Fig. 31.1). All eleven NHS did not show binding of IgG to 19-OH. The relative binding capacity of IgG to these molecules in decreasing order was as follows: CE = 7-keto > 7-β-OH > Cho > 19-OH.

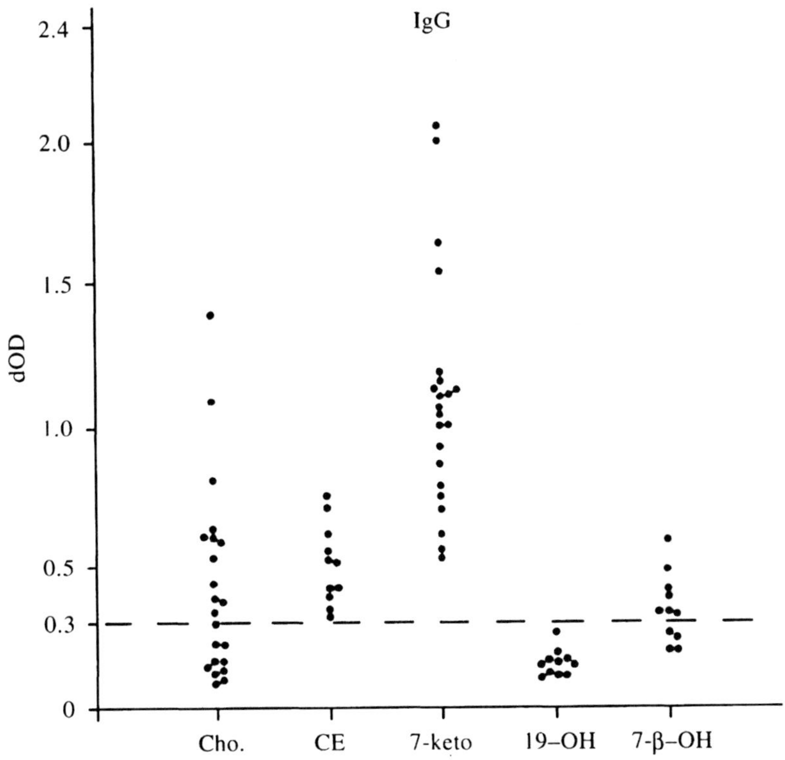

Fig. 31.1. Normal serum immunoglobulin (Ig)G binding to cholesterol (Cho), cholesterol epoxide (CE), 7-ketocholesterol (7-keto), 19-hydroxycholesterol (19-OH), and 7-β-hydroxycholesterol (7-β-OH). The vertical scale shows the mean optical density (dOD) readings between the test sample and antigen-negative wells. The reaction is considered to be positive when the dOD value is ≥0.3.

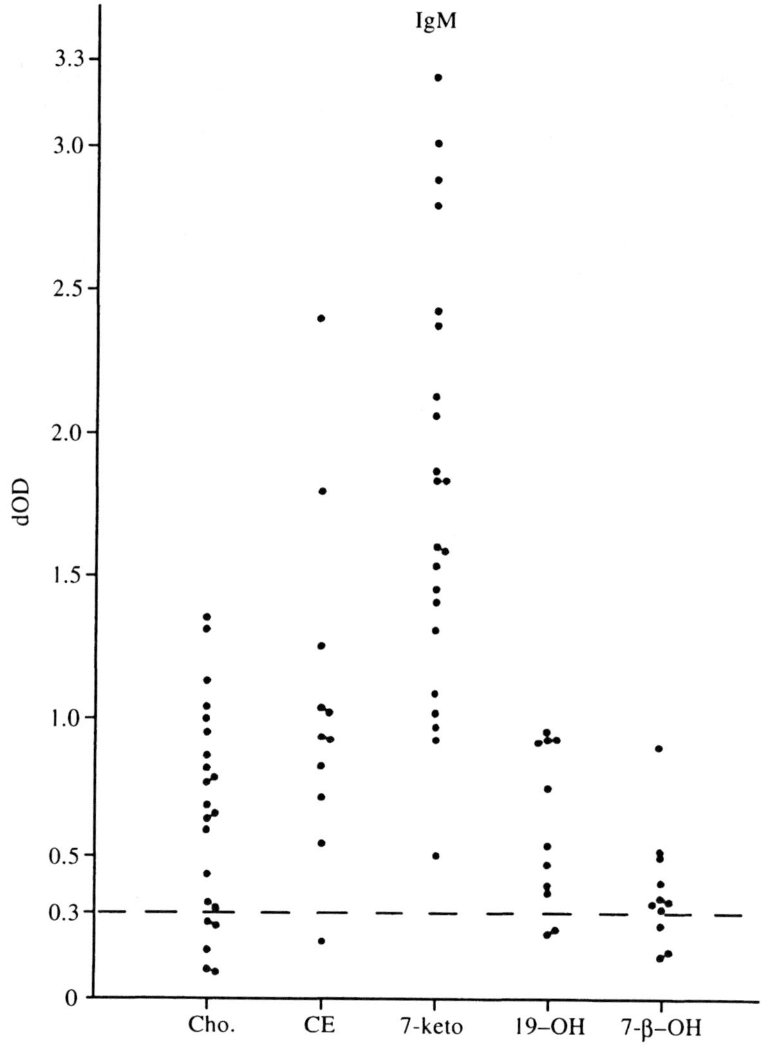

Fig. 31.2. Normal serum immunoglobulin (Ig)M binding to cholesterol (Cho), cholesterol epoxide (CE), 7-ketocholesterol (7-keto), 19-hydroxycholesterol (19-OH) and 7-β-hydroxycholesterol (7-β-OH). The vertical scale shows the mean optical density (dOD) readings between the test sample and antigen-negative wells. The reaction is considered to be positive when the dOD value is ≥0.3.

Natural IgM to Cholesterol and Oxysterols. Natural IgM to oxysterols were detected also. From the ELISA result, all 22 NHS had IgM binding to 7-keto (Table 31.1 and Fig. 31.2). CE is another target for IgM binding. Ten of eleven NHS had IgM binding to CE. Natural IgM has a higher binding frequency to 19-OH (9/11) than Cho (17/22). Natural IgM bound less to 7-β-OH compared with the other oxysterols.

Only 7/11 NHS contained IgM against 7-β-OH although this represents >50% binding. The relative binding capacity of IgM antioxysterol was as follows: 7-keto > CE > 19-OH > Cho > 7-β-OH.

Natural IgA to Cholesterol and Oxysterols. Natural IgA against Cho, CE, 7-keto, 7-β-OH, and 19-OH were also determined (Table 31.1 and Fig. 31.3). IgA bound only to Cho, CE, and 7-keto. IgA reacted mainly with CE (10/11) followed by 7-keto (21/22) and Cho (4/22). No natural IgA binding was observed for IgA against 19-OH and 7-β-OH. The relative binding capacity of IgA was as follows: CE > 7-keto > Cho > 19-OH = 7-β-OH.

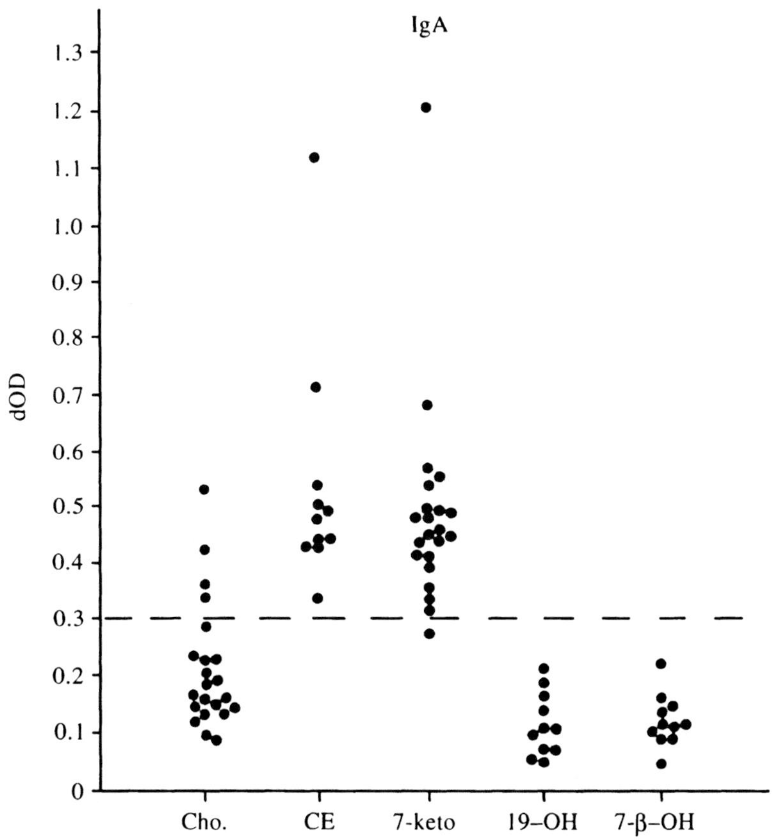

Fig. 31.3. Normal serum immunoglobulin (Ig)A binding to cholesterol (Cho), cholesterol epoxide (CE), 7-ketocholesterol (7-keto), 19-hydroxycholesterol (19-OH) and 7-β-hydroxycholesterol (7-β-OH). The vertical scale shows the mean optical density (dOD) readings between the test sample and antigen-negative wells. The reaction is considered to be positive when the dOD value is ≥0.3.

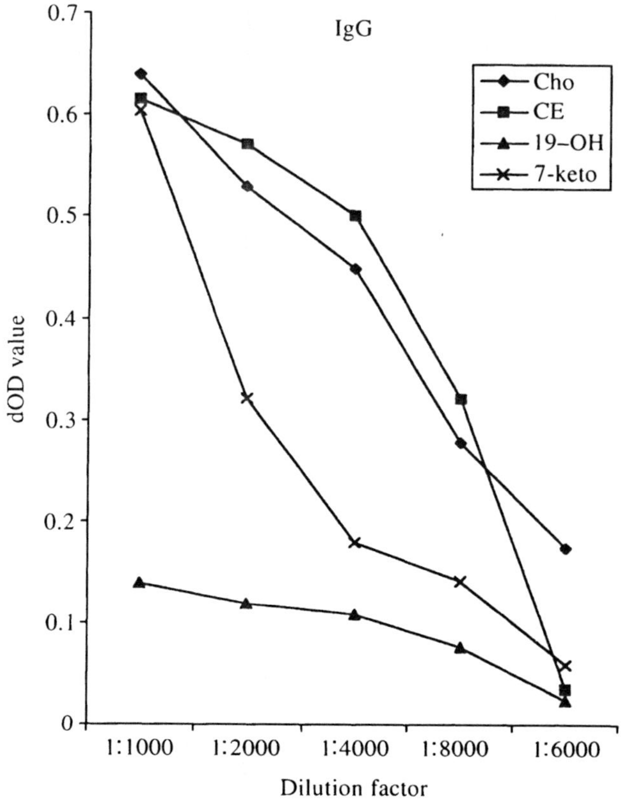

Fig. 31.4. Dilution curve of natural immunoglobulin (Ig)G to cholesterol and three different oxysterols. A dilution of 1:100 was equivalent to 50 µg/mL antigen. Abbreviations: dOD, mean optical density; Cho, cholesterol; CE, cholesterol epoxide; 19-OH, 19-hydroxycholesterol; 7-keto, 7-ketocholesterol; dOD, mean optical density.

Comparison Between IgG, IgM and IgA Antibody to Oxysterols. Results for IgG, IgM, and IgA binding patterns were compared. The results in Table 31.1 demonstrate that IgM is the predominant immunoglobulin in NHS that reacted with cholesterol and other oxysterols. The binding of IgM for cholesterol and other oxysterols was high (>63.6%). Natural IgG is the second major isotype that binds to these oxidized cholesterol antigens. The frequency of binding ranged from 54.5 to 100%. The binding of IgA was quite different. IgA showed different reactivity to the various oxysterols. Natural IgA bound more to CE (100%) and 7-keto (95.5%), but bound less to cholesterol (18.2%), and showed no binding to 19-OH and 7-β-OH.

Comparison Between Cholesterol and Oxysterols Bound by Natural Antibodies. 7-Keto was the dominant antigen among the oxysterols. All three antibody isotypes of anti-7-keto were present at a high frequency, especially IgG and

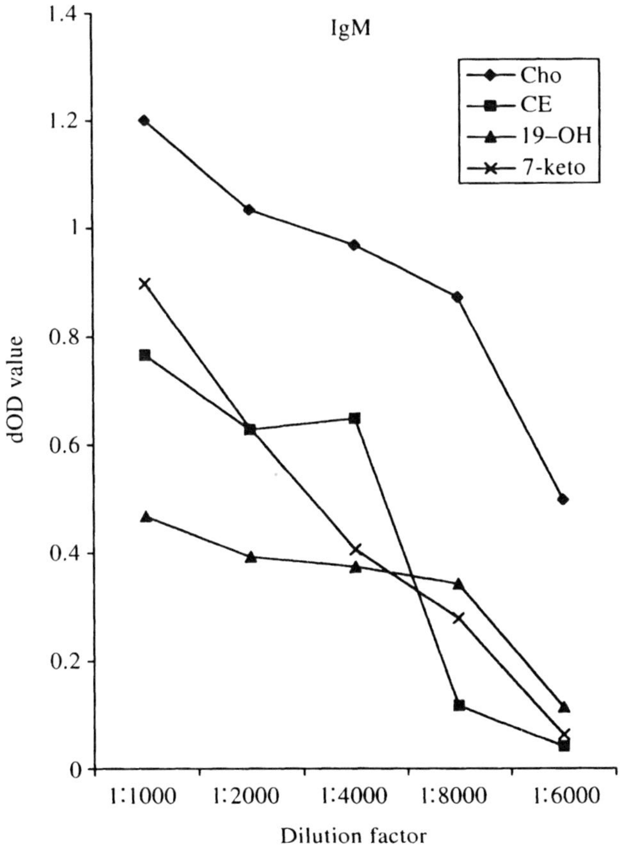

Fig. 31.5. Dilution curve of natural immunoglobulin (Ig)M to cholesterol and three different oxysterols. A dilution of 1:100 was equivalent to 50 μg/mL of antigen. Abbreviations: dOD, mean optical density; Cho, cholesterol; CE, cholesterol epoxide; 19-OH, 19-hydroxycholesterol; 7-keto, 7-ketocholesterol; dOD, mean optical density.

IgM (100%). CE were also bound by IgG, IgA, and IgM at high frequency (>90%). The binding of IgM to CE was slightly less than that of IgG and IgA. Cholesterol was bound mainly by natural IgM, followed by IgG and IgA.

Natural IgM and IgG have the same binding reactivity to 7-β-OH. IgA had no reaction to this molecule. 19-OH was a weak antigen for natural antibody binding except for IgM (72%), whereas natural IgG and IgA showed no binding.

In summary, the relative antigenicity of cholesterol-derived antigen as measured by ELISA for natural antibodies is as follows: 7-keto > CE > Cho > 7-β-OH > 19-OH. The dilution curves for IgG, IgM and IgA natural antibodies to oxysterols are shown in Figures 31.4–6.

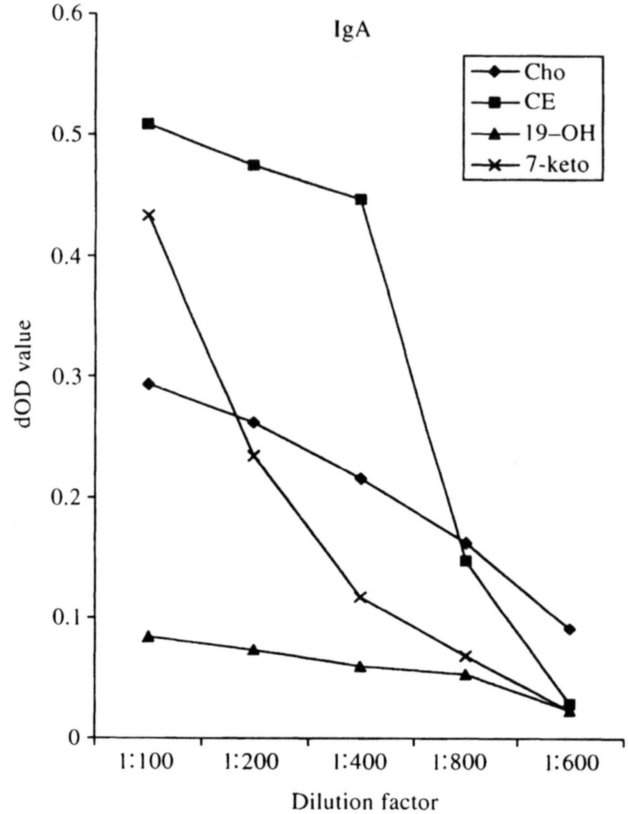

Fig. 31.6. Dilution curve of natural immunoglobulin (Ig)A to cholesterol and three different oxysterols. A dilution of 1:100 was equivalent to 50 μg/mL of antigen. Abbreviations: dOD, mean optical density; Cho, cholesterol; CE, cholesterol epoxide; 19-OH, 19-hydroxycholesterol; 7-keto, 7-ketocholesterol; dOD, mean optical density.

Discussion

Natural Antibodies Against Oxysterols. In this study, natural autoantibodies (NAA) were found to bind to cholesterol and four different oxysterols including cholesterol epoxide (CE), 7-ketocholesterol (7-keto), 7-β-hydroxycholesterol (7-β-OH) and 19-hydroxycholesterol (19-OH). Results showed that 7-keto and CE are the main oxysterol antigens for natural antibody binding. This may suggest that the oxygen atom at the side chain of 7-keto and CE may play an important role for antibody recognition rather than the hydroxyl group (-OH) at the side chain of 19-OH and 7-β-OH. All three antibody isotypes (IgG, IgA, and IgM) were detected. IgM was the predominant immunoglobulin that bound cholesterol and oxysterols. Cheng and Sundram (12) found that IgG bound to oxysterols as follows: 7-keto >CE = 19-OH >

7-OH. In this study, natural IgG, IgM, and IgA also reacted strongly with both 7-keto and CE as follows: CE = 7-keto > 7-β-OH > cholesterol > 19-OH.

According to Zieden *et al.* (8), CE are easily formed in sample handling. This may indicate, therefore, that the source of CE can come from the diet in addition to *in vivo* oxidation. By binding to oxysterols, natural antibodies may regulate their free plasma concentration. When the level of NAA is decreased, this presumably can cause an increased plasma level of these oxysterols. The binding of NAA to oxysterols indicated that they may be involved in some aspects of immunophysiologic homeostasis. The functions of NAA in this case may include the immunoclearance of aged and modified HDL, LDL, and cell membranes that contain a substantial amount of cholesterol (12). Thus natural antibodies could serve a "housekeeping" function.

An earlier study showed that IgM and IgA were the major plasma proteins in normal human blood responsible for LDL binding (13). Usually oxysterols are found at a low level in plasma. They are the main components of oxidized lipoproteins, especially oxLDL. Thus, natural antibodies could bind to these modified lipoproteins to attenuate their pathophysiologic activities. In 130 healthy Japanese subjects, Shoji *et al.* (14) found an inverse association between natural anti-oxLDL levels and plasma oxLDL concentration. They proposed that anti-oxLDL could clear oxLDL from the circulation. The oxysterols in oxLDL might also be bound by cross-reactive natural anticholesterol antibodies, and this would also attenuate the pathobiologic activity of oxLDL (15).

Because oxysterols are involved in the development of atherosclerosis, natural antioxysterol antibodies might reduce their potential in inducing the pathogenesis of atherosclerosis. The data from this study suggested that antioxysterol and, by implication, anti-oxLDL may be antiatherogenic. Natural antibodies to oxysterols and oxLDL may serve to modulate pathobiologic effects of oxLDL on the endothelium, platelets, and macrophages. Thus, the natural activities of antibodies can supplement antioxidants in regulating the amount and activity of circulating oxLDL (16). The role of anti-oxLDL in atherosclerosis warrants further evaluation; it is possible that a temporal difference exists between the effects of antioxysterol in health and disease progression in atherogenesis.

7-β-Hydroxycholesterol and 7-ketocholesterol are the potent inducers of apoptosis (17). Thus, when bound by natural autoantibodies, the process of apoptosis may be reduced or blocked. Inhibition of apoptosis by antioxidant therapies (which may reduce cholesterol oxidation) can reduce vascular dysfunctions in hypercholesterolemic patients. Thus, it is conceivable that by binding to cholesterol, natural antibodies might also reduce its oxidation. In this way, natural antibodies would function indirectly as antioxidants.

Oxysterols are found in cholesterol-rich processed foods. These dietary oxysterols increase the atherogenicity of LDL in animal models (18,19). The effects of oxysterols in foods might be modulated by natural antibodies. By complexing with dietary oxysterols, the natural antibodies may help to prevent an unfavorable rise in the concentration of these oxysterols in blood circulation.

In this study, naturally occurring IgM and IgG were found to bind to unmodified cholesterol. Anticholesterol antibodies might contribute to normal homeostasis of LDL metabolism. These antibodies do not have any apparent deleterious effect on normal cells and tissues. On the basis of their accumulated data, Alving and Wassef (20) recently proposed that in addition to LDL receptor mechanisms, immunoregulation of LDL by natural antibodies to cholesterol can mediate LDL cholesterol turnover in healthy individuals.

Whether the different isotypes, IgG, IgA, and IgM antioxysterols, serve unique immunophysiologic functions remains to be determined. If oxysterols in oxLDL are among the primary immunogens, then the levels of such natural autoantibodies may be used as a serological indicator of *in vivo* oxidative status. It also follows that in antioxidant intervention studies, the measurement of antioxysterols in volunteers could be exploited as an additional parameter with which to assess the efficacy of the inhibition of circulating LDL oxidation.

Acknowledgments

This work was initiated and partially supported during a sabbatical of Dr. H.M. Cheng with the Malaysian Palm Oil Board (MPOB). We also thank MPOB for a travel grant to present this data at the Micronutrient and Health Workshop, July 2000, Langkawi Island, Malaysia.

References

1. Lin, C.Y., and Morel, D.W. (1996) Esterification of Oxysterols in Human Serum: Effects on Distribution and Cellular Uptake. *J. Lipid Res. 37*, 168–178.
2. Patel, R.P., Diczfalusy, U., Dzeletovic, S., Wilson, M.T., and Darley-Usmar, V.M. (1996) Formation of Oxysterols During Oxidation of Low Density Lipoprotein by Peroxynitrite, Myoglobin, and Copper. *J. Lipid Res. 37*, 2361–2371.
3. Gesquiere, L., Loreau, N., and Blache, N. (1997) Impaired Cellular Cholesterol Efflux by Oxysterol-Enriched High Density Lipoprotein. *Free Radic. Biol. Med. 23*, 541–547.
4. Kodama, T., Freeman, M., Rohrer, L., Zabrecky, J., Matsudaira, P., and Krieger, M. (1990) Type I Macrophage Scavenger Receptor Contains A-Helical and Collagen-Like Coiled Coils. *Nature 343*, 531–535.
5. Goldstein, E.M., and Brown, M.S. (1977) The Low-Density Lipoprotein Pathway and Its Relation to Atherosclerosis. *Annu. Rev. Biochem. 46*, 108–115.
6. Schroepfer, G.J. (2000) Oxysterols—Modulation of Cholesterol Metabolism and Other Processes. *Physiol. Rev. 80*, 361–381.
7. Brown, A.J., and Jessup, W. (1999) Oxysterols and Atherosclerosis. *Atherosclerosis 142*, 1–28.
8. Zieden, B., Kaminskas, A., Kristenson, M., Kucinskiene, Z., Vessby, B., Olsson, A.G., and Diczfalusy, U. (1999) Increased Plasma 7β- Hydroxycholesterol Concentrations in a Population with a High Risk for Cardiovascular Disease. *Arterioscler. Thromb. Vasc. Biol. 19*, 967–971.
9. Brown, A.J., Mander, E.L., Gelissen, I.C., Kritharides, L., Dean, R.T., and Jessup, W. (2000) Cholesterol and Oxysterol Metabolism and Subcellular Distribution in Macrophage Foam Cells. Accumulation of Oxidized Esters in Lysosomes. *J. Lipid Res. 41*, 226–237.

10. Salonen, J.T., Yla-Herttula, S., Yamamoto, R., Butler, S., Korpela, H., Salonen, R., Nyyssonen, K., Palinski, W., and Witstum, J.L. (1992) Autoantibody Against Oxidized LDL and Progression of Carotid Atherosclerosis. *Lancet 339*, 883–887.
11. Ameli, S., Hultgardh-Nilsson, A., Regnstrom, J., Calara, F., Yano, J., Cercek, B., Shah, P.K., and Nilsson, J. (1996) Effect of Immunization with Homologous LDL and Oxidized LDL on Early Atherosclerosis in Hypercholesterolemic Rabbits. *Arterioscler. Thromb. Vasc. Biol. 16*, 1074–1079.
12. Cheng, H.M., and Sundram, K. (1998) Cholesterol Oxides and Natural Autoantibodies. *Atherosclerosis 141*, 347–348.
13. Bauer, B.J., Blashfield, K., Norris, R., Buthala, D.A., and Ginsberg, L.C. (1982) Immunoglobulin as the Major Low Density Lipoprotein Binding Protein in Plasma. *Atherosclerosis 44*, 153–160.
14. Shoji, T., Nishizawa, Y., Fukumoto, M., Shimamura, K., Kimura, J., Kanda, H., Emoto, M., Kawagishi, T., and Morii, H. (2000) Inverse Relationship Between Circulating Oxidized Low Density Lipoprotein (oxLDL) and Anti-oxLDL Antibody Levels in Healthy Subjects. *Atherosclerosis* 148, 171–177.
15. Shaw, P.X., Horkko, S., Chang, M.K., Curtiss, L.K., Palinski, W., Silverman, G.J., and Witztum, J.L. (2000) Natural Antibodies with the T15 Idiotype May Act in Atherosclerosis, Apoptotic Clearance and Protective Immunity. *J. Clin. Investig. 105*, 1731–1740.
16. Cheng, H.M., and Sundram, K. (1999) Oxidized LDL, Diet, and Natural Antibodies. *Am. J. Clin. Nutr. 70*, 1.
17. Aupeix, K., Weltin, D., Mejia, J.E., Christ, M., Marchal, J., Freyssinet, J.M., and Bischoff, P. (1995) Oxysterol-Induced Apoptosis in Human Monocytic Cell Lines. *Immunobiology 194*, 415–428.
18. Vine, D.F., Mamo, C.L., Beilin, L.J., Mori, T.A., and Croft, K.D. (1998) Dietary Oxysterols Are Incorporated in Plasma Triglyceride-Rich Lipoproteins, Increase Their Susceptibility to Oxidation and Increase Aortic Cholesterol Concentration of Rabbits. *J. Lipid Res. 39*, 1995–2004.
19. Staprans, I., Pan, X.M., Rapp, J.H., Grunfeld, C., and Feingold, K.R. (2000) Oxidized Cholesterol in the Diet Accelerates The Development of Atherosclerosis in LDL Receptor- and Apolipoprotein E-Deficient Mice. *Arterioscler. Thromb. Vasc. Biol. 20*, 708–713.
20. Alving, C.R., and Wassef, N.M. (1999) Naturally Occurring Antibodies to Cholesterol: A New Theory of LDL Cholesterol Metabolism. *Immunology Today 20*, 362–366.

Chapter 32

Tocopherol and Tocotrienol Effects on Normal Mammary Epithelial Cell Growth and Apoptosis

Paul W. Sylvester

College of Pharmacy, University of Louisiana at Monroe, Monroe, LA 71209–0470

Introduction

Vitamin E compounds are recognized as important antioxidants, which regulate peroxidation reactions and control free-radical production within the body (1). Uncontrolled production of free-radical products is associated with damage to cell structures and functions, and implicated as the cause of various diseases including arteriosclerosis and some types of cancer (1–3). Vitamin E is a generic term that refers to an entire class of compounds, which is further divided into two subgroups called tocopherols and tocotrienols. Tocopherols are commonly found in high concentrations in a wide variety of foods, whereas tocotrienols are relatively rare and found in appreciable levels only in a few specific vegetable fats, such as palm oil (4,5). Previous studies demonstrated that high dietary intake of crude palm oil, in contrast to other high-fat diets, suppressed carcinogen-induced mammary tumorigenesis in experimental animals (5–7). Similarly, dietary supplementation with the tocotrienol-rich fraction (TRF) of palm oil has also been shown to inhibit mammary tumorigenesis (8). However, when tocotrienols were removed from palm oil, the protective effects of high palm oil diets against mammary tumorigenesis were no longer observed (8). In contrast, studies investigating the anticancer activity of tocopherols have shown negative results for the most part.

The exact reason why tocotrienols display greater anticancer activity than tocopherols is still under investigation. Tocopherols and tocotrienols have the same basic chemical structure characterized by a long phytyl chain attached at the 1-position of a chromane ring structure (Fig. 32.1). However, tocopherols have a saturated phytyl chain, whereas that of tocotrienols is unsaturated. Each subgroup of vitamin E contains several isoforms, and individual tocopherol and tocotrienol isoforms differ from each other on the basis of the number of methyl groups bound to their chromane ring. Specifically, α-tocopherol and α-tocotrienol contain methyl groups at the 5-, 7-, and 8-positions, whereas their γ-isoforms lack the methyl group at the 5-position, and their δ-isomers lack methyl groups at the 5- and 7-positions on the chromane ring. Therefore, it is possible that the level of phytyl chain saturation and/or chromane ring methylation may be critical in determining the antiproliferative and cytotoxic activity of individual tocopherol and tocotrienol isoforms.

Although a great deal of information has been published regarding the effects of tocopherols and tocotrienol on various types of cancer cell lines, very little is known

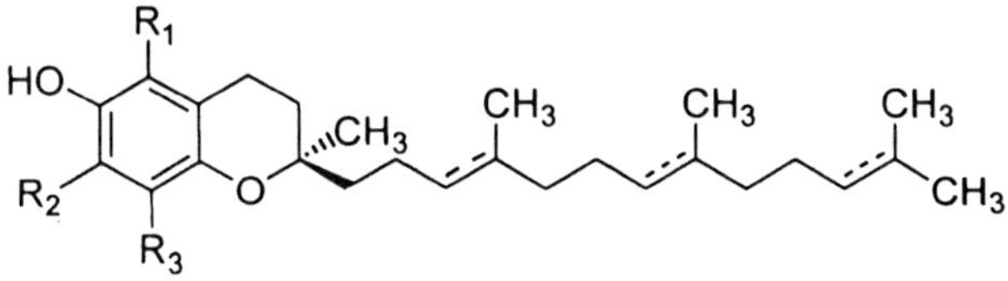

Compound	R_1	R_2	R_3	Phytyl chain
α-Tocopherol	CH_3	CH_3	CH_3	Saturated
γ-Tocopherol	H	CH_3	CH_3	Saturated
δ-Tocopherol	CH_3	H	H	Saturated
α-Tocotrienol	CH_3	CH_3	CH_3	Unsaturated
γ-Tocotrienol	H	CH_3	CH_3	Unsaturated
δ-Tocotrienol	H	H	CH_3	Unsaturated

Fig. 32.1. Generalized structure of vitamin E compounds.

about the effects of these vitamin E compounds on the growth and viability of normal cells. Therefore, the following studies were conducted to characterize the antiproliferative and apoptotic effects of specific tocopherol and tocotrienol isoforms on normal mouse mammary epithelial cells grown in primary culture and maintained in serum-free media containing 10 ng/mL epidermal growth factor (EGF).

EGF is a potent mitogen for both normal and neoplastic mammary epithelial cells (9,10). The mitogenic actions of EGF are mediated through specific membrane-bound tyrosine kinase receptors (11–14). EGF-dependent mitogenesis in normal mammary epithelial cells grown in primary culture is associated with the activation of phospholipid-dependent protein kinase C (PKC). Treatments that enhance PKC activation stimulate EGF-induced mammary epithelial cell proliferation, whereas treatments that inhibit PKC activation have an inhibitory effect (9,10,15,16). Because tocotrienols inhibit EGF-dependent mitogenesis, studies were also conducted to determine the effects of tocopherols and tocotrienols on EGF receptor (EGF-R) levels, EGF-dependent EGF-R tyrosine kinase activity, and PKC activation. Additional studies investigated the relationship between biopotency and the magnitude of cellular accumulation for the various tocopherol and tocotrienol isoforms.

Experimental Model and Methodology

Mammary epithelial cells were isolated and prepared for culture as previously described (10). Briefly, mammary glands from BALB/c mice in midpregnancy were removed, minced, and subjected to collagenase followed by pronase E digestion. Mammary epithelial cell organoids were isolated by a series of filtrations through sterile filters, and then plated within rat-tail collagen gels, and maintained in serum-free media. Serum-free control or treatment media consisted of Dulbecco's modified Eagle's media (DMEM)/F12 containing 5 mg/mL bovine serum albumin (BSA), 10 μg/mL transferrin, 100 U/mL soybean trypsin inhibitor, 100 U/mL penicillin, 0.1 mg/mL streptomycin, 10 ng/mL EGF, and 10 μg/mL insulin. Vitamin E compounds were conjugated to BSA as previously described (17), and appropriate amounts were added to the treatment media. Mammary epithelial cell number was determined by the (3[4,5-dimethylthiazol-2-yl]-2,5-diphenyltetrazolium bromide (MTT) colorimetric assay as described previously (10); it was determined that various doses (0–250 μmol/L) of specific tocopherols or tocotrienols did not affect the specific activity of the MTT colorimetric assay. EGF-R levels, intracellular protein tyrosine phosphorylation, and total, cytosolic, and membrane PKCα levels were determined by discontinuous gel electrophoresis and Western-blot analysis (10,12–14,17,18). Apoptosis was determined by DNA fragmentation (19) and nuclear condensation (20) assays. Cellular accumulation of tocopherols and tocotrienols was determined within each treatment group by reverse-phase high-performance liquid chromatography (HPLC) electrochemical detection using a modification of the methods previously described (21). The tocotrienol-rich fraction of palm oil (TRF) was assayed by HPLC before use in experimentation and determined to be composed of 20.2% α-tocopherol, 16.8% α-tocotrienol, 44.9% γ-tocotrienol, 14.8% δ-tocotrienol, and 3.2% of a non-vitamin E lipid-soluble contaminant. Treatment doses of TRF were then calculated on the bases of the percentage composition and molecular weights of individual vitamin isoforms within TRF. Linear regression analysis of treatment effects on viable cell number in growth and cytotoxcity studies was used to determine the 50% growth inhibitory concentration (IC_{50}) and median lethal dose (LD_{50}) for individual treatments.

Effects of Tocopherols and Tocotrienols on Normal Mammary Epithelial Cell Growth and Viability

Cells grown in serum-free control media displayed more than a twofold increase in viable cell number over the 5-d culture period, whereas supplementation of culture media with 12.5–50 μmol/L TRF significantly inhibited EGF-induced cell proliferation in a dose-responsive manner. Because TRF contains a number of vitamin E isoforms, it was not possible to determine whether one or all of these isoforms were responsible for mediating the growth inhibitory effects of TRF. Additional studies were conducted to determine the antiproliferative effects of specific tocopherol and tocotrienol isoforms on EGF-induced mammary epithelial cell proliferation in primary culture (Fig. 32.2). After 5 d of culture, treatment with 0–120 μmol/L α- or γ-tocopherol had no effect (Fig. 32.2A, B), whereas treatment with 100-120 μmol/L δ-tocopherol significantly inhibited mammary epithelial cell growth compared with controls (Fig. 32.2C). Treatment with 50–60 μmol/L α-tocotrienol (Fig. 32.2D), 8–14 mμol/L γ-tocotrienol (Fig. 32.2E) or δ-tocotrienol (Fig. 32.2F) was also found to significantly inhibit mammary epithelial cell growth compared with controls.

The effects of a 24-h treatment exposure to various concentrations of tocopherols, tocotrienols, or TRF on viable cell number are shown in Figure 32.3. Acute treatment with 0–250 μmol/L of α-, γ-, or δ-tocopherol had no significant affect on mammary epithelial cell viability (Fig. 32.3). In contrast, 24 h of exposure to 100–250 μmol/L TRF, 140–250 μmol/L α-tocotrienol, 25–100 μmol/L γ- or δ-tocotrienol caused a significant

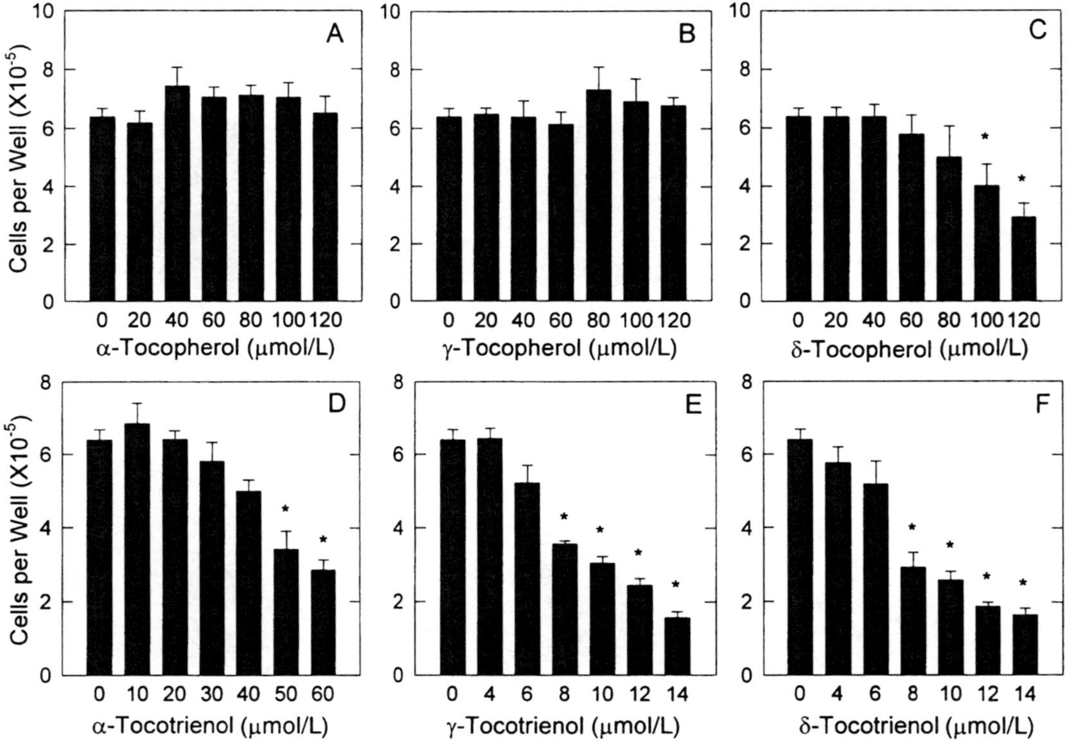

Fig. 32.2. Effects of various doses of individual tocopherol and tocotrienol isoforms on normal mammary epithelial cell proliferation in primary culture. Vertical bars represent mean cell count/well ± SEM, $n = 6$ replicates/treatment group after 5 d in culture. $*P < 0.05$ vs. controls. (*Source*: Ref. 17.)

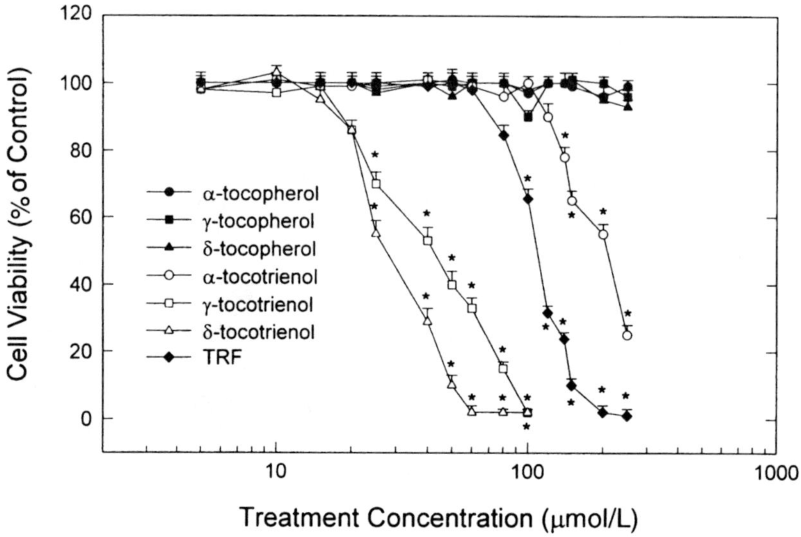

Fig. 32.3. Mammary epithelial cell viability after a 24-h exposure period to various doses of the tocotrienol-rich fraction (TRF) of palm oil, or individual tocopherol and tocotrienol isoforms. Cells in each treatment group were grown in primary culture and maintained in control media for 5 d before exposure to their respective treatments. Data points indicate the percentage of viable cells/well ± SEM, $n = 6$ replicates/treatment group. $^*P < 0.05$ vs. controls. (*Source*: Ref. 17.)

dose-responsive decrease in viable cell numbers, with 100 μmol/L γ-tocotrienol and 60–100 μmol/L δ-tocotrienol reducing viable cell numbers to undetectable levels (Fig. 32.3). Table 32.1 summarizes the relative potencies of TRF and specific tocopherol and tocotrienol isoforms on normal mammary epithelial cell growth and viability.

These results demonstrate that individual tocopherols and tocotrienols display differential potencies in their antiproliferative and cytotoxic activity in normal mammary epithelial cells grown in primary culture. Direct comparisons between the two vitamin E subclasses show that tocotrienols are significantly more potent than tocopherols. Furthermore, the biopotency of specific isoforms displayed a consistent relationship corresponding to δ-tocotrienol ≥ γ-tocotrienol > α-tocotrienol > δ-tocopherol ≥ γ- and α-tocopherol.

Effects of Tocopherols and Tocotrienols on EGF-Dependent Mitogenic Signaling

Various signaling pathways have also been suggested for mediating the antiproliferative and cytotoxic effects of vitamin E (22–29). Although dose-response studies showed that IC_{50} doses of individual tocotrienol isoforms were 5–6 times lower than the corresponding LD_{50} doses, it remains unclear whether the antiproliferative and cytotoxic effects of vitamin E are mediated through similar or independent signaling mechanisms.

TABLE 32.1 Effects of Various Vitamin E Compounds on Mammary Epithelial Cell Growth (IC_{50}) and Viability (LD_{50})[a]

	IC_{50}	LD_{50}
Vitamin E	(μmol/L)	
TRF	25	110
α-Tocopherol	>120	>250
γ-Tocopherol	>120	>250
δ-Tocopherol	94	>250
α-Tocotrienol	45	238
γ-Tocotrienol	8	46
δ-Tocotrienol	7	36

[a]Abbreviations: IC_{50}, 50% inhibitory concentration; LD_{50}, median lethal dose.

It is well known that the EGF-receptor is a receptor tyrosine kinase, and the initial response to receptor activation is autophosphorylation, which is required for receptor interaction and tyrosine phosphorylation of intracellular substrates (11). Therefore, studies were conducted to determine whether the antiproliferative effects of specific tocopherols and tocotrienols in mammary epithelial cells results from a reduction in EGF-R levels and/or EGF-induced EGF-R tyrosine kinase activity. Normal mammary epithelial cells were grown in primary culture for 5 d in serum-free control or treatment media containing either the maximum dose tested or specific IC_{50} doses for individual tocopherols or tocotrienols. Cells were then isolated from collagen gels and whole-cell lysates were prepared for subsequent assay of EGF-R levels in each treatment group by Western-blot analysis. Results showed that treatment with growth inhibitory doses of tocopherols and tocotrienols had no effect on EGF-R levels in these cells.

Additional studies were conducted to determine the effects of IC_{50} doses of specific tocopherols and tocotrienols on EGF-induced EGF-R tyrosine kinase activity. Normal mammary epithelial cells were grown in primary culture for 5 d in serum-free control or treatment media containing either the maximum dose tested or specific IC_{50} doses for individual tocopherols or tocotrienols. Cells were then washed and fed their respective treatment media minus EGF for 3 h, to allow intracellular protein tyrosine phosphorylation to return to basal levels. Cells were then placed on ice and exposed to 0 or 100 ng EGF for 5 min; then, whole-cell lysates were prepared for subsequent assay of EGF-dependent intracellular protein phosphotyrosine intensity as determined by Western-blot analysis. Results showed that before EGF exposure, there was a similar basal level of intracellular protein tyrosine phosphorylation in all treatment groups. After exposure to EGF, a similar increase in intracellular tyrosine phosphorylation in controls and treatment groups was observed. These results demonstrate that tocotrienol inhibition of EGF-dependent mammary epithelial cell proliferation does not result from a reduction in EGF-R levels or a decrease in EGF-R tyrosine kinase activity. These findings suggest that the antiproliferative effects of tocotrienols occur downstream from the EGF-receptor.

EGF-dependent mitogenesis in normal mammary epithelial cells grown in primary culture is associated with the activation of phospholipid-dependent PKC (9,10,15,16), and tocopherols and tocotrienols have also been shown to inhibit PKC activity in other cell types (22–25). Therefore, it is possible that the antiproliferative effects of tocotrienols in normal mammary epithelial cells may result from an inhibition of PKCα activity. Normal mammary epithelial cells were grown in primary culture for 5 d in serum-free control or treatment media containing either the maximum dose tested or specific IC_{50} doses for individual tocopherols or tocotrienols. Cells were then isolated from collagen gels, and whole-cell lysates were prepared for subsequent assay of PKCα levels in each treatment group by Western-blot analysis. Results showed that treatment with growth inhibitory doses of tocopherols and tocotrienols had no effect on total intracellular levels of PKCα.

Additional studies were conducted to determine the effects of growth inhibitory doses of tocopherols and tocotrienols on EGF-induced PKCα activation, as indicated by a translocation from the cytosolic to the membrane fraction in normal mammary epithelial cells. Cells were grown in primary culture for 5 d in serum-free control or treatment media containing either the maximum dose tested or specific IC_{50} doses for individual tocopherols or tocotrienols. Cells were washed and then fed their respective treatment medium minus EGF for 3 h, to allow intracellular cytosolic and membrane PKCα levels to return to basal levels. Cells in each treatment group were then exposed to 100 ng EGF, and aliquots of cells from each treatment group were collected at 0, 15, 30, 45, and 60 min after EGF exposure. Cytosolic and membrane fractions were then prepared for subsequent assay of PKCα by Western-blot analysis. Results showed that after exposure to EGF, PKCα show a time-dependent translocation from the cytosolic to the membrane fraction in controls. Treatment with 120 μmol/L α- or γ-tocopherol had no effect, whereas treatment with IC_{50} doses of δ-tocopherol or α-, γ-, and δ-tocotrienol attenuated EGF- induced PKCα translocation in these cells. These results indicate that tocotrienol inhibition of EGF-dependent mammary epithelial cell proliferation may result, at least in part, from the inhibition of PKCα activation.

Comparative Apoptotic Effects of Tocopherols and Tocotrienols in Normal Mammary Epithelial Cells

Vitamin E compounds have also been shown to play an important role in modulating several intracellular signaling pathways involved with apoptosis (26–30). Studies were conducted to determine the dose-response and time-course effects of growth inhibitory (IC_{50}) and cytotoxic (LD_{50}) doses of TRF on the initiation of apoptosis, as indicated by DNA fragmentation, in normal mammary epithelial cells grown in primary culture. Before exposure to TRF, cells grown in control serum-free media for

5 d did not show appreciable levels of DNA fragmentation (Fig. 32.4). However, after exposure to 25 µmol/L TRF (IC_{50}), mammary epithelial cells displayed detectable levels of DNA fragmentation 48 h after the start of treatment (Fig. 32.4). In contrast, exposure to 110 µmol/L TRF (LD_{50}) resulted in a rapid and intense DNA laddering response within 12 h and continuing for 48 h after the start of treatment (Fig. 32.4). These results demonstrate that although treatment with the LD_{50} dose of TRF induced a more rapid and intense response, treatment with the IC_{50} dose of TRF also induced an appreciable amount of apoptosis in normal mammary epithelial cells.

The effects of a 24-h exposure to IC_{50} or maximum doses previously tested for individual tocopherols and tocotrienols on DNA fragmentation in mammary epithelial cells are shown in Figure 32.5. DNA isolated from untreated controls showed little fragmentation or laddering (Fig. 32.5, lane C). Similarly, treatment for 24 h with 120 µmol/L α- or γ-tocopherol had little effect on DNA fragmentation in these cells (Fig. 32.5, lanes αT and γT, respectively). Similar treatments with IC_{50} doses of δ-tocopherol (94 µmol/L), α-tocotrienol (45 µmol/L), γ-tocotrienol (8 µmol/L), or δ-tocotrienol (7 µmol/L) induced intense DNA fragmentation in mammary epithelial

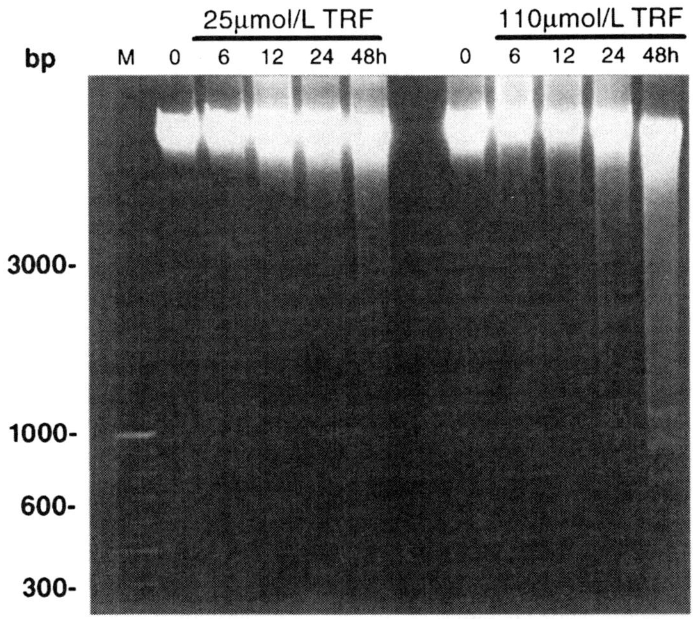

Fig. 32.4. Mammary epithelial cell internucleosomal DNA fragmentation during a 48-h period after exposure to either 25 µmol/L (IC_{50}) or 110 µmol/L (LD_{50}) of the tocotrienol-rich fraction (TRF) of palm oil. Cells were cultured in control media for 5 d and then exposed to their respective treatments. Lane M contains DNA laddering markers. (*Source*: Ref. 17.)

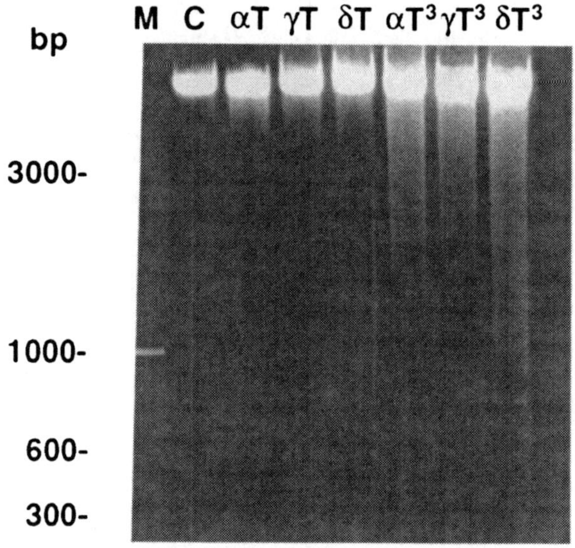

Fig. 32.5. Mammary epithelial cell internucleosomal DNA fragmentation after a 24-h exposure period to control media (lane C), 120 µmol/L α-tocopherol (lane αT), 120 µmol/L γ-tocopherol (lane γT), 94 µmol/L δ-tocopherol (lane δT), 45 µmol/L α-tocotrienol (lane αT^3), 8 µmol/L γ-tocotrienol (lane γT^3), or 7 µmol/L δ-tocotrienol (lane δT^3). Lane M contains DNA laddering markers. (*Source*: Ref. 17.)

cells (Figure 32.5, lanes δT, αT^3, γT^3, and δT^3, respectively). These findings again demonstrate that treatment with growth inhibitory doses of tocopherols and tocotrienols induced apoptosis in normal mammary epithelial cells.

Additional studies were conducted to determine the effects of 24 h of treatment with 0 (controls), 25 (IC_{50}), or 110 mol/L (LD_{50}) TRF on *in situ* nuclear condensation, as determined by ethidium bromide epifluorescence staining in mammary epithelial cells. Brightfield photomicrographs of untreated control mammary epithelial cell organoids were characterized by duct-like branching that extended throughout the collagen gel. Epifluorescence photomicrographs of the same field showed a small amount of epifluorescence staining. Cells grown in primary culture have a finite life span, and it is expected that some portions of these cells are undergoing apoptosis. Treatment for 24 h with 25 µmol/L TRF (IC_{50}) resulted in a noticeable change in mammary epithelial cell organoid morphology that was characterized by a slight fragmentation in ductal branching in brightfield photomicrographs, and an increase in epifluorescence intensity. Brightfield photomicrographs of mammary epithelial cell organoids treated for 24 h with 110 µmol/L TRF (LD_{50}) were characterized by severe fragmentation in ductal morphology, and a corresponding large increase in epifluorescence intensity.

Taken together, these findings raise the possibility that the growth inhibitory effects of vitamin E isoforms result from an increase in the total number of cells undergoing programmed cell death and not from an inhibition of EGF-dependent mitogenesis. Additional studies are required to clarify whether the antiproliferative and apoptotic effects of specific vitamin E compounds are mediated through similar or independent mechanisms.

Normal Mammary Epithelial Cell Uptake of Specific Tocopherols and Tocotrienols

Another important factor determining tocopherol and tocotrienol isoform biopotency is the ease or preference with which these compounds are taken up by mammary epithelial cells. Therefore, studies were conducted to determine cellular accumulation of specific tocopherol and tocotrienol isoforms in mammary epithelial cells treated for 24 h with 25 μmol/L (IC_{50}) or 110 μmol/L (LD_{50}) TRF. Cellular levels of α-tocopherol and α-, γ-, and δ-tocotrienol were undetectable 15 min after exposure to 25 or 110 μmol/L TRF. However, a time-dependent and dose-responsive increase in cellular levels of these compounds was observed. The relative magnitude of cellular accumulation of tocotrienol isoforms was greater than that of α-tocopherol, even though the concentration of α-tocopherol present in the TRF treatment media was higher than the concentrations of α- and δ-tocotrienol.

Similar studies examined the cellular accumulation of specific tocopherol and tocotrienol isoforms throughout the 24-h treatment period. Treatment with 250 μmol/L α-, γ-, or δ-tocopherol resulted in a time-dependent increase in cellular levels during the 24-h exposure period (Fig. 32.6, upper panel). However, cellular accumulation of individual tocopherol isoforms was not equal and was characterized as $\delta > \gamma > \alpha$ (Fig. 6, upper panel). Similarly, exposure to 45 μmol/L α-, γ-, and δ-tocotrienol also showed a time-dependent increase in cellular accumulation and a greater cellular accumulation of individual tocotrienol isoforms characterized as $\delta > \gamma > \alpha$ (Fig. 32.6, lower panel). These findings demonstrate that different isoforms within each tocopherol and tocotrienol subgroup displayed individual differences in cellular accumulation, which is directly related to its biopotency. Specifically, α-isoforms of tocopherols and tocotrienols are more highly methylated than their corresponding γ- or δ-isoforms, and cellular accumulation and biopotency of α-tocopherol and α-tocotrienol were not as great as those of their respective γ- and δ-isoforms.

It is possible that specific structural characteristics are responsible for a less restricted passage of tocotrienols through the mammary epithelial cell membrane. Tocotrienols differ from tocopherols in that they contain an unsaturated phytyl chain. The presence of double bonds in the tocotrienol phytyl chain would create a less planar molecular conformation that could allow for enhanced interaction and uptake at the surface of the cell membrane. Furthermore, data suggest that cellular uptake of tocopherols and tocotrienols is most likely determined by nonspecific factors such as molecular conformation and lipid solubility, rather than selective uptake mechanisms involving specific transporter or carrier proteins. Because mammary epithelial cells preferentially take up tocotrienols over tocopherols, higher levels of these compounds are present at their intracellular sites of action and are thereby able to induce

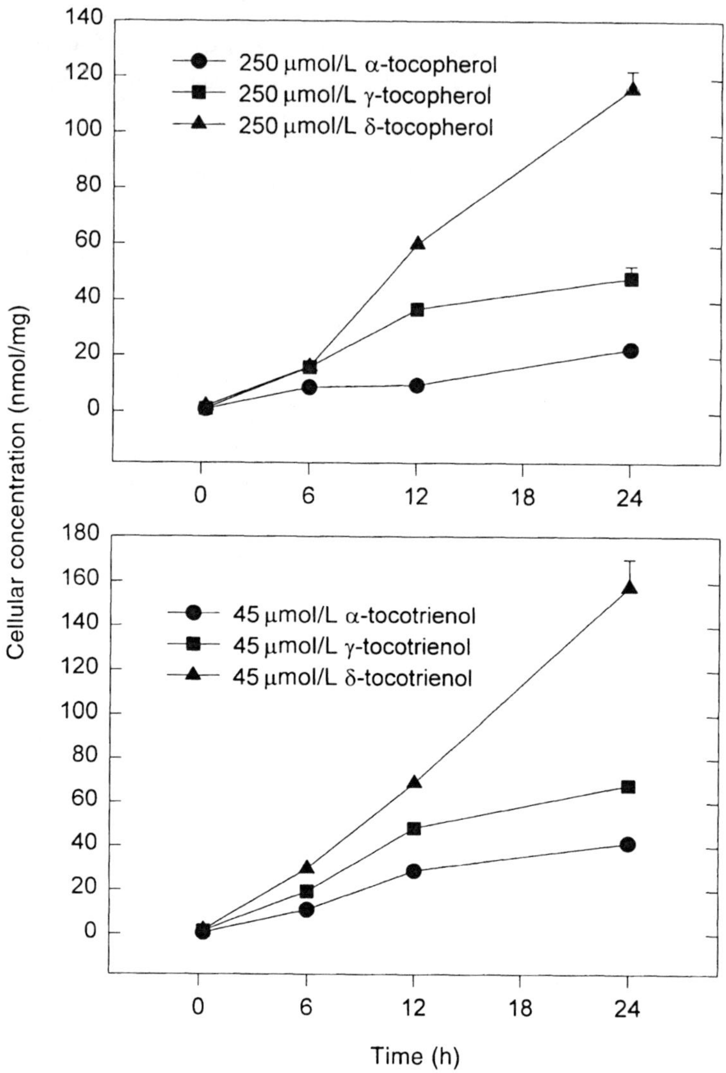

Fig. 32.6. Cellular accumulation of individual tocopherol and tocotrienol isoforms in normal mammary epithelial cells grown in primary culture during a 24-h exposure to either 250 μmol/L α-, γ-, or δ-tocopherol, or 45 μmol/L α-, γ-, or δ-tocotrienol. Data points indicate mean cellular concentration ± SEM, *n* = 4 replicates/group containing 1×10^7 cells per time point. (*Source*: Ref. 17.)

a greater biological response.

Experimental evidence also indicates that tocotrienols are inherently more potent than tocopherols in their antiproliferative and apoptotic activity. Results showed that similar cellular levels of corresponding tocopherol and tocotrienol isoforms could be obtained in mammary epithelial cells with 250 μmol/L α-, γ-, and δ-tocopherol and 45 μmol/L of α-, γ-, and δ-tocotrienol. However, treatment doses that produced similar intracellular levels of tocopherols and tocotrienols did not cause the same antiproliferative and apoptotic response in these cells. These findings indicate that tocotrienol isoforms are more potent than their corresponding tocopherol isoforms in activating the intracellular mechanisms responsible for inhibiting growth and inducing apoptosis in normal mammary epithelial cells.

Discussion

These results demonstrate that individual tocopherols and tocotrienols display differential antiproliferative and apoptotic potencies in normal mammary epithelial cells grown in primary culture. Direct comparisons between the two vitamin E subclasses show that tocotrienols are significantly more potent than tocopherols. Furthermore, the biopotency of specific isoforms displayed a consistent relationship corresponding to δ-tocotrienol ≥ γ-tocotrienol > α-tocotrienol > δ-tocopherol ≥ γ- and α-tocopherol. As stated above, treatments that inhibit PKC activation attenuate EGF-dependent mitogenesis in normal mammary epithelial cells grown in primary culture. Studies have also shown that the inhibition of PKC activity results in an increase in intracellular levels of proapoptotic vs. antiapoptotic proteins, which can result in the initiation of apoptosis (31–33). Therefore, it is possible that the antiproliferative and apoptotic effects of tocopherols and tocotrienols may result from the inhibition of PKCα activation.

It was also shown that the biopotency of individual tocotrienol and tocopherol isoforms is directly related to the ease and/or preference with which these compounds accumulate within mammary epithelial cells. Tocotrienols display greater biopotency than tocopherols at least in part because of their greater cellular uptake and enhanced ability to activate the antiproliferative and/or apoptotic signaling pathways. Nevertheless, it is well established that absorption of individual tocopherol and tocotrienol isoforms is limited by the specificity and saturability of specific transfer proteins and transport mechanisms within the body that display significant preference for α-tocopherol (34). Although it remains to be determined whether the high biopotency displayed by individual tocotrienol isoforms *in vitro* is also evident in the intact mammary gland, the present findings provide evidence to suggest that the highly biopotent γ- and δ-tocotrienol isoforms may play a physiologic role in modulating normal mammary gland growth, function, and/or remodeling.

References

1. Packer, L. (1991) Protective Role of Vitamin E in Biological Systems. *Am. J. Clin. Nutr. 53*, 1050S–1055S.
2. Elson, C.E. (1992) Tropical Oils: Nutritional and Scientific Issues. *Crit. Rev. Food Sci. Nutr. 31*, 79–102.
3. Kimmick, G.G., Bell, R.A., and Bostick, R.M. (1997) Vitamin E and Breast Cancer: A Review. *Nutr. Cancer 27*, 109–117.

4. Cottrell, R.C. (1991) Introduction: Nutritional Aspects of Palm oil. *Am. J. Clin.. Nutr. 53*, 989S–1009S.
5. Sundram, K., Khor, H.T., Ong, A.S., and Pathmanathan, R. (1989) Effect of Dietary Palm Oils on Mammary Carcinogenesis in Female Rats Induced by 7,12-Dimethylbenz(a)anthracene. *Cancer Res. 49*, 1447–1451
6. Sylvester, P.W., Russell, M., Ip, M.M., and Ip, C. (1986) Comparative Effects of Different Animal and Vegetable Fats Fed Before and During Carcinogen Administration on Mammary Tumorigenesis, Sexual Maturation, and Endocrine Function in Rats. *Cancer Res. 46*, 757–762.
7. Gould, M.N., Haag, J.D., Kennan, W.S., Tanner, M.A., and Elson, C.E. (1991) A Comparison of Tocopherol and Tocotrienol for the Chemoprevention of Chemically Induced Rat Mammary Tumors. *Am. J. Clin. Nutr. 53*, 1068S–1070S.
8. Nesaretnam, K., Khor, H.T., Ganeson, J., Chong, Y.H., Sundram, K., and Gapor, A. (1992) The Effects of Vitamin E Tocotrienols from Palm Oil on Chemically Induced Mammary Carcinogenesis in Female Rats. *Nutr. Res.12*, 879–892.
9. Imagawa, W., Bandyopadhyay, G.K., and Nandi, S. (1990) Regulation of Mammary Epithelial Cell Growth in Mice and Rats. *Endocr. Rev. 11,* 494–523.
10. Sylvester, P.W., Birkenfeld, H.P., Hosick, H.L., and Briski, K.P. (1994) Fatty Acid Modulation of Epidermal Growth Factor-Induced Mouse Mammary Epithelial Cell Proliferation In Vitro. *Exp. Cell Res. 214*, 145–153.
11. Ullrich, A., and Schlessinger, J. (1990) Signal Transduction by Receptors with Tyrosinekinase Activity. *Cell 61*, 203–212.
12. McIntyre, B.S., Birkenfeld, H.P., and Sylvester, P.W. (1995) Relationship Between Epidermal Growth Factor Receptor Levels, Autophosphorylation and Mitogenic Responsiveness in Normal Mouse Mammary Epithelial Cells In Vitro. *Cell Prolif. 28*, 45–56.
13. McIntyre, B.S., and Sylvester, P.W. (1998) Genistein and Erbstatin Inhibition of Normal Mammary Epithelial Cell Proliferation Is Associated with EGF-Receptor Downregulation. *Cell Prolif. 31*, 35–46.
14. McIntyre, B.S., Briski, K.P., Hosick, H.L., and Sylvester, P.W. (1998) Effects of Protein Tyrosine Phosphatase Inhibitors on EGF- and Insulin-Dependent Mammary Epithelial Cell Growth. *Proc. Soc. Exp. Biol. Med. 217*, 180–187.
15. Birkenfeld, H.P., McIntyre, B.S., Briski, K.P., and Sylvester, P.W. (1996) Protein Kinase C Isoenzyme Expression in Normal Mouse Mammary Epithelial Cells Grown in Primary Culture. *Proc. Soc. Exp. Biol. Med. 213*, 65–70.
16. Birkenfeld, H.P., McIntyre, B.S., Briski, K.P., and Sylvester, P.W. (1996) Role of Protein Kinase C in Modulating Epidermal Growth Factor- and Phorbol Ester-Induced Mammary Epithelial Cell Growth in Vitro. *Exp. Cell Res. 223*, 183–191.
17. McIntyre, B.S., Briski, K.P., Tirmenstein, M.A., Fariss, M.W., Gapor, A., and Sylvester, P.W. (2000) Antiproliferative and Apoptotic Effects of Tocopherols and Tocotrienols on Normal Mouse Mammary Epithelial Cells. *Lipids 35*, 171–180.
18. McIntyre, B.S., Briski, K.P., Gapor, A., and Sylvester, P.W. (2000) Antiproliferative and Apoptotic Effects of Tocopherols and Tocotrienols on Preneoplastic and Neoplastic Mouse Mammary Epithelial Cells. *Proc. Soc. Exp. Biol. Med. 224*, 292–301.
19. Tepper, C.G., and Studzinski, G.P. (1992) Teniposide Induces Nuclear but Not Mitochondrial DNA Degradation. *Cancer Res. 52*, 3384–3390.

20. Tsangaris, G.T., Moschovi, M., Mikraki, V., Vrachnou, E., and Tzortzatou-Stathopoulou, F. (1996) Study of Apoptosis in Peripheral Blood of Patients with Acute Lymphoblastic Leukemia During Induction Therapy. *Anticancer Res. 16*, 3133–3140.
21. Tirmenstein, M.A., Watson, B.W., Haar, N.C., and Fariss, M.W. (1998) Sensitive Method for Measuring Tissue α-Tocopherol and α-Tocopheryl Oxybutyric Acid by High-Performance Liquid Chromatography with Fluorometric Detection. *J. Chromatogr. B Biomed. Sci. Appl. 707*, 308–311.
22. Chatelain, E., Boscoboinik, D.O., Bartoli, G.M., Kagan, V.E., Gey, F.K., Packer, L., and Azzi, A. (1993) Inhibition of Smooth Muscle Cell Proliferation and Protein Kinase C Activity by Tocopherols and Tocotrienols. *Biochim. Biophys. Acta 1176*, 83–89.
23. Stauble, B., Boscoboinik, D., Tasinato, A., and Azzi, A. (1994) Modulation of Activator Protein-1 (AP-1) Transcription Factor and Protein Kinase C by Hydrogen Peroxide and D-α-Tocopherol in Vascular Smooth Muscle Cells. *Eur. J. Biochem. 226*, 393–402.
24. Turley, J.M., Ruscetti, F.W., Kim, S.J., Fu, T., Gou, F.V., and Birchenall-Roberts, M.C. (1997) Vitamin E Succinate Inhibits Proliferation of BT-20 Human Breast Cancer Cells: Increased Binding of Cyclin A Negatively Regulates E217 Transactivation Activity. *Cancer Res. 57*, 2668–2675.
25. Fazzio, A., Marilley, D., and Azzi, A. (1997) The Effect of α-Tocopherol and β-Tocopherol on Proliferation, Protein Kinase C Activity and Gene Expression in Different Cell Lines. *Biochem. Mol. Biol. Int. 41*, 93–101.
26. Turley, J.M., Fu, T., Ruscetti, F.W., Mikovits, J.A., Bertolette, D.C., III, and Birchenall-Roberts, M.C. (1997) Vitamin E Succinate Induces Fas-Mediated Apoptosis in Estrogen Receptor- Negative Human Breast Cancer Cells. *Cancer Res. 57*, 881–890.
27. Zhao, B., Yu, W., Qian, M., Simmons-Menchaca, M., Brown, P., Birrer, M.J., Sanders, B.G., and Kline, K. (1997) Involvement of Activator Protein-1 (AP-1) in Induction of Apoptosis by Vitamin E Succinate in Human Breast Cancer Cells. *Mol. Carcinog. 19*, 180–190.
28. Yu, W., Sanders, B.G., and Kline, K. (1997) *RRR*-α-Tocopheryl Succinate Inhibits EL4 Thymic Lymphoma Cell Growth by Inducing Apoptosis and DNA Synthesis Arrest. *Nutr. Cancer 27*, 92–101.
29. Yu, W., Heim, K., Qian, M., Simmons-Menchaca, M., Sanders, B.G., and Kline, K. (1997) Evidence for Role of Transforming Growth Factor-β in *RRR*-α-Tocopheryl Succinate- Induced Apoptosis of Human MDA-ME-435 Breast Cancer Cells. *Nutr. Cancer 27*, 267–278.
30. Sigounas, G., Anagnostou, A., and Steiner, M. (1997) *dl*-α-Tocopherol Induces Apoptosis in Erythroleukemia, Prostate, and Breast Cancer Cells. *Nutr. Cancer 28*, 30–35.
31. Carroll, M.P., and May, W.S. (1994) Protein Kinase C-Mediated Serine Phosphorylation Directly Activates Raf-I in Murine Hematopoietic Cells. *J. Biol. Chem. 269*, 1249–1256.
32. Chen, C.Y., and Faller, D.V. (1999) Selective Inhibition of Protein Kinase C Isozymes by Fas Ligation. *J. Biol. Chem. 274*, 15320–15328.
33. Ruvolo, P.P., Deng, X., Carr, B.K., and May, W.S. (1998) A Functional Role for Mitochondrial Protein Kinase Cα in Bcl2 Phosphorylation and Suppression of Apoptosis. *J. Biol. Chem. 273*, 25436–25442.
34. Hosomi, A., Arita, M., Sato, Y., Kiyose, C., Ueda, T., Igarashi, O., Arai, H., and Inoue, K. (1997) Affinity for α-Tocopherol Transfer Protein as a Determinant of the Biological Activities of Vitamin E Analogs. *FEBS Lett. 409*, 105–108.

Chapter 33

γ- vs. α-Tocopherol–Rich Edible Oils and Their Relevance for Low Density Lipoprotein Oxidation in Humans

I. Elmadfa, R. Tomasch, and K.-H. Wagner

Institute of Nutritional Sciences, University of Vienna, 1090 Vienna, Austria

Introduction

Reactive oxygen species are known to be the basis for toxic effects of oxygen in human metabolism and development of chronic diseases. The oxygen radical–induced modification of low density lipoproteins (LDL) and their subsequent unregulated uptake by macrophages in the subendothelial space of the arteries by using scavenger receptor–mediated pathways promote lipid deposition in the arterial wall and induce foam cell formation, thereby playing an important role in the progress of atherosclerosis (1,2). The increased intake of nutritive antioxidants, mainly as supplements, has been shown to be correlated with protection against various diseases, including cancers and cardiovascular diseases (3,4). Even though it is not known precisely which dietary constituents are responsible for this association, it is often assumed that antioxidants contribute to the protection (5–7). However, the effect of increased consumption of foods rich in antioxidants on overall antioxidant status is not known, and the results of intervention trials have not been conclusive regarding protection with particular antioxidants. Rather, the beneficial effects of high antioxidant intake may result from a concerted action of a combination of different antioxidants present in the normal diet. LDL is the carrier of several lipophilic antioxidative substances that are able to protect atherogenic lipoproteins against oxidative damage and modification. Quantitatively the most important antioxidants present in LDL are α-tocopherol, γ-tocopherol, β-carotene, and lycopene (8). Studies investigating the oxidative susceptibility of human LDL show that the physical and chemical characteristics, the particle size, and the particle antioxidant concentration of LDL, in particular, are inversely correlated with oxidative susceptibility. Convincing evidence for the atherogenicity of oxidized LDL and preventive effects of antioxidants was established on the basis of data from animal studies, which found vitamin E to be the most important and active antioxidant (1,9). The protective effect of vitamin E in preventing chronic diseases has been attributed to its ability to function highly efficiently as a lipid-soluble antioxidant and free radical scavenger to prevent lipid oxidation especially of unsaturated fatty acids in cell membranes (10). Of all compounds with vitamin E activity, α-tocopherol and γ-tocopherol are the principal vitamers found in human and animal diets and comprise most of the vitamin E content of tissues;

however, α-tocopherol is the most effective lipid-soluble antioxidant *in vivo*. The antioxidative activity ratio of α- to γ-tocopherol examined in vivo is calculated to be 4:1 (11) or lower (12). However, γ-tocopherol is a better antioxidant than α-tocopherol when assessed *in vitro*.

Several studies found an increased resistance against oxidative modifications in LDL after antioxidant supplementation (13,14). Only a few studies, however, have been able to describe the relationship between antioxidants from a mixed diet and the oxidative LDL modification and the total antioxidative capacity (TAC). This study was designed to determine human plasma and LDL antioxidant capacity of diets containing either γ-tocopherol–rich corn oil (CO) or an α-tocopherol–rich mixture of olive/sunflower oil (MO), providing similar α-tocopherol contents but different α-tocopherol equivalents (α-TE)/diene equivalents (DE) ratios due to their varying fatty acid patterns. The edible oils were incorporated into isoenergetic mixed diets of healthy volunteers as their main fat source.

Material and Methods

Study Subjects. Male subjects ($n = 28$), aged between 19 and 31 y, mean age 23.7 y, living in the area of Vienna, Austria, participated in this randomized study. All participants were in good health as determined by a medical history questionnaire and results of clinical laboratory tests. They were nonsmokers, free of acute or chronic illness, in the normal range of body mass index (BMI; 20.3 ± 2.3 kg/m^2), and not taking any medications, mineral or vitamin supplements for 4 wk before the start or during the study. They were informed about the purpose, nature, and potential risks

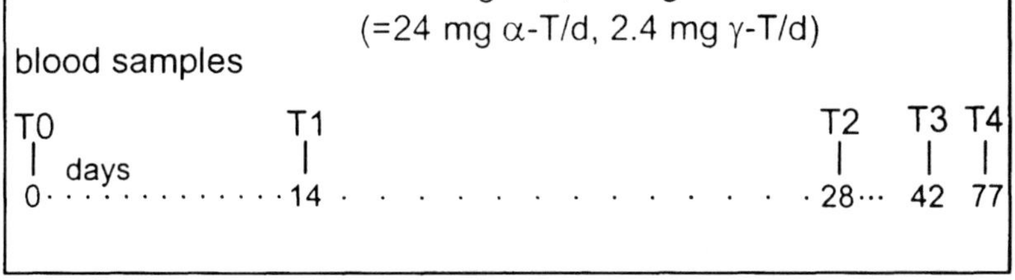

Fig. 33.1. Study design. Abbreviations: α- and γ-T, α- and γ-tocopherol; OO, olive oil; SFO, sunflower oil.

of the study and gave consent in writing. The study protocol was approved by the Ethic Committee of the Medical Faculty, University of Vienna.

Investigation Trail and Diets. The crossover design of the study consisted of an adjustment period and two diet periods of 2 wk each (Fig. 33.1). During the 2-wk adjustment period (T1), all participants consumed the same diets including the same fat source (olive/sunflower mixture, Ø energy value 11.6 MJ, Ø fat intake ~105g/d, 12 mg α-TE/d). For the intervention trial (T2), the volunteers were randomized evenly into two groups (CO and MO), $n = 14$. Both groups received the same diets except for the fat sources, i.e., the CO group received a diet with 80 g corn oil/d [saturated (S)/monounsaturated (M)/polyunsaturated (P) = 28:33:39, 20 mg α-tocopherol/d + 100 mg γ-tocopherol/d] and the MO group a mixture of 68 g olive and 12 g sunflower oil/d (S/M/P = 28:49:23, 24 mg α-tocopherol/d and 2.4 mg γ-tocopherol/d) as the main fat source (for fat specifications, see Table 33.1). At wk 5, a crossover was carried out and the trial ended after wk 6 (T3). Five weeks after the end of the intervention, the last blood samples were taken (T4) to observe the development of plasma variables after the intervention.

The daily meals during the respective study periods were prepared in accordance with dietary guidelines of the new DACH reference values of Germany, Austria, and Switzerland, with total energy consisting of 50–55% carbohydrate, 15% protein, and 30–35% fat (15).

Including the food fat, the total daily fat intake during the test period was 110 g/d (31 en%). The plant oils were used as the main fat source (80 g of 110 g/d) of normal mixed diets commonly used in Austria. The exact nutrient intake was calculated by weighed dietary records during the entire study. Plasma and LDL concentrations of α-tocopherol, γ-tocopherol, carotenoids, ascorbic acid, malondialdehyde (MDA), cholesterol, and plasma- and LDL TAC were assessed in all volunteers every 2 wk at T0–T3 and finally at T4. Additionally, the LDL tocopherol content was determined to observe the incorporation of tocopherols into the lipoproteins. Excretion of α- and γ-tocopherol in 24-h stools was analyzed by high-performance liquid chromatography (HPLC) after reduction to consider the oxidized tocopherol compounds as well.

TABLE 33.1 Content of Tocopherols and Fatty Acid Pattern in Plant Oils Used During the Study Period

	Tocopherols (T) (mg/100 g)		Fatty acids (% of total fatty acids)						
	α-T	α-T	$C_{16:0}$	$C_{16:1}$	$C_{18:0}$	$C_{18:1}$	$C_{18:2}$	$C_{18:3}$	$C_{20:0}$
Corn oil	24.6	126.2	10.0	0.5	2.4	31.1	50.0	0.9	0.5
Sunflower oil	85.3	8.8	6.2	0.5	4.8	21.9	60.2	0.5	0.5
Olive oil	20	1.7	10.8	1.5	2.4	71.7	8.0	0.9	0.5
Butter	2.1	—	21.0	1.8	9.7	20.1	1.8	1.2	0.1

Blood Preparation. Blood samples were obtained by venipuncture into heparin-containing vacuum tubes (Vacuette; Greiner, Vienna, Austria) from volunteers who had fasted overnight. Platelet-poor plasma for tocopherol, carotene, and MDA determinations was separated by centrifugation at 1111 g for 10 min and frozen in aliquots at −80°C until used. An appropriate portion of platelet-rich plasma was collected for the estimation of ascorbic acid. Lipoprotein fractionation was done from frozen plasma within 1 wk after blood was drawn. Plasma and lipoprotein concentrations of α-, γ-tocopherol, α-, and β-carotene were determined by reversed-phase HPLC according to the method of Jakob and Elmadfa (16). Ascorbic acid was detected photometrically by the method of Denson and Bowers (17). MDA was determined by HPLC, using the method of Wong *et al.* (18). Total cholesterol in plasma was measured colorimetrically by the method of Siedel *et al.* (19), using a test kit from Boehringer-Mannheim GmbH. LDL and plasma TAC were measured by a modification of the photometric method according to Rice-Evans and Miller (20).

Isolation of Lipoproteins. Lipoproteins were separated according to procedures described by Nelson (21) and Foremann *et al.* (22). The density gradients were examined by NaCl solutions [d = 1.0063 to separate very low density lipoprotein (VLDL) and d = 1.1816 to separate LDL]. The sample was spun with a Sorvall UZ ULTRA 80 ultracentrifuge with a fixed angle T865 rotor for VLDL isolation and a TV865 vertical rotor for LDL separation. To separate LDL particles by size and shape, nondenaturing polyacrylamide gradient gel electrophoresis was used to identify the major LDL peak particle (Lipidophor all in 12, Fa. IMMUNO AG, Vienna, Austria).

Fatty Acid Composition of LDL. LDL fatty acids were converted into methyl esters and analyzed with gas chromatography by using an Auto-System Gas Chromatograph (Perkin Elmer, Vienna, Austria) equipped with a split/splitless capillary injector. Fatty acid methyl esters were separated by a 30 m × 0.25 mm i.d. fused silica column (RTx-2330) and detected with a flame ionization detector (FID); the FID temperature was set to 250°C. The fatty acid pattern was analyzed in duplicate as described previously (23).

Statistical Analysis. The statistical significance of differences between the two groups was determined by analysis of variance (ANOVA) of repeated samples and double-tailed Student's *t*- test for dependent samples. The Mann-Whitney U test was used for comparison between the two diet groups. The area under the curve (AUC) of TAC in plasma and LDL was used to determine significant differences between the groups. Pearson correlation coefficients and multiple regression analysis were conducted using SPSS 8.0 for Windows (Chicago, IL). Values were expressed as means ± SEM; differences were considered to be significant at a value of $P < 0.05$.

Results

Neither side effects due to ingestion of the diets nor changes in body weight were reported throughout the study. The mean daily energy intake and the composition of the different diets, as determined by food records, were in good agreement with the calculated diet composition. After the 2-wk adjustment period (T1), no significant differences between the two test groups in BMI, antioxidant content of tocopherols, carotenes, MDA, and TAC in plasma and lipoproteins were determined (Table 33.2). The plasma tocopherol content of all subjects was found to be within normal range (α-tocopherol, 20.4 – 2.4 μmol/L; γ-tocopherol, 1.3 ± 0.4 μmol/L); lipoprotein α-tocopherol was 2.51 ± 0.78 μmol/mmol cholesterol and lipoprotein γ-tocopherol was 0.14 ± 0.06 μmol/mmol cholesterol.

After 2 wk of consumption of the test diet with CO, enhanced by the high intake of γ-tocopherol, significant differences between plasma α-, and γ-tocopherol contents, compared with the MO, were found (α-tocopherol: CO, 18.9 ± 3.7 μmol/L vs. MO, 23.2 ± 4.3 μmol/L, $P < 0.005$). As expected, the plasma γ-tocopherol content of the CO group (0.51 ± 0.11 μmol/L) increased significantly ($P < 0.001$), in contrast to the MO group (1.1 ± 0.4 μmol/L) (Table 33.2). The daily intake of γ-tocopherol from corn oil was nearly 50-fold higher than the intake with the mixed olive/sunflower oil regimen. The main carriers for tocopherol transport in blood were LDL (41–49% for γ-tocopherol; 51–59% for α-tocopherol). A significant increase in LDL α-tocopherol content was measured within the test period with the MO, but not with the CO diet. The CO diet increased LDL transported γ-tocopherol relatively (41% T1 vs. 49% T2) and absolutely ($P < 0.001$) up to fourfold (0.54 ± 0.11 μmol/mmol cholesterol) compared with the depletion phase (T1) (Table 33.2). A significant correlation ($r^2 = 0.73$; $P < 0.001$) was found between plasma and LDL γ-tocopherol concentrations in the corn oil group; however, there was no correlation between plasma and LDL α-tocopherol concentration (Fig. 33.2).

Dietary compliance was also controlled by monitoring the fatty acid pattern of the lipoprotein fractions LDL and high density lipoprotein (HDL), which ranged from $C_{14:0}$ to $C_{24:1}$. The fatty acids detected were calculated as a percentage of total fatty acids and structured into saturated (SFA), monounsaturated (MUFA) and polyunsaturated fatty acids (PUFA). The average ratio of oleic acid (18:1n-9) to linoleic acid (18:2n-6) in LDL was 0.46 ± 0.08 in the adjustment diet. The CO diet had a significantly ($P < 0.001$) lower ratio (0.3 ± 0.02) than the MO diet (0.51 ± 0.06). The LDL-MUFA content of the MO diet increased by 34% ($P < 0.001$) over the baseline diet (T1), whereas SFA and PUFA concentration were reduced compared with T1. In contrast, the CO diet increased the PUFA content by 26% compared with the depletion phase ($P < 0.001$), based on the high content of linoleic acid in the corn oil (Table 33.2). In the HDL fraction, PUFA increased significantly ($P < 0.05$) in the CO group, whereas no change in fatty acid pattern was found in the MO group. A significant correlation between LDL cholesterol and an increased level of LDL PUFA was determined in the CO group ($r = 0.69$, $P < 0.01$).

TABLE 33.2 Plasma (Pl) and Low Density Lipoprotein (LDL) Levels of Tested Tocopherols, Carotenoids, Malondialdehyde (MDA), Total Antioxidative Capacity (TAC), and Cholesterol at Baseline (T0), After Adjustment Diet (T1), Corn Oil (CO) Diet, Mixed Oil (MO) Diet (T2), and 5 wk After the Intervention (T4)

			T2			
	T0 $n = 28$	T1 Adjustment $n = 28$	Group A (CO) $n = 14$	Group B (MO) $n = 14$	T4 $n = 28$	P[a]
Pl α-tocopherol (μmol/L)	21.1 ± 3.8	20.4 ± 2.4	18.9 ± 3.7	23.2 ± 4.3	21.2 ± 3.8	$P < 0.005$
Pl γ-tocopherol (μmol/L)	1.48 ± 0.51	1.28 ± 0.35	4.01 ± 0.92	1.09 ± 0.42	1.55 ± 0.43	$P < 0.001$
Pl retinol (μmol/L)	1.48 ± 0.09	1.18 ± 0.07	1.29 ± 0.11	1.25 ± 0.07	1.34 ± 0.07	NS[b]
Pl β-carotene (μmol/L)	0.57 ± 0.17	0.51 ± 0.15	0.38 ± 0.15	0.43 ± 0.19	0.55 ± 0.23	NS
Pl lycopene (μmol/l)	0.71 ± 0.21	0.43 ± 0.20	0.37 ± 0.09	0.37 ± 0.07	0.57 ± 0.14	NS
Pl cholesterol (mmol/l)	4.3 ± 0.9	4.9 ± 0.9	4.3 ± 0.7	4.5 ± 0.7	4.4 ± 0.9	NS
LDL α-tocopherol (μmol/ mmol cholesterol)	3.46 ± 0.53	2.51 ± 0.78	2.56 ± 0.74	3.32 ± 0.81	3.41 ± 0.55	$P < 0.001$
LDL γ-tocopherol (μmol/ mmol cholesterol)	0.21 ± 0.07	0.14 ± 0.06	0.51 ± 0.11	0.13 ± 0.04	0.19 ± 0.07	$P < 0.001$
Pl MDA (μmol/L)	1.04 ± 0.39	0.86 ± 0.29	0.77 ± 0.27	0.75 ± 0.21	1.12 ± 0.42	NS
Pl TAC (mM) 0.63 ± 0.13	0.51 ± 0.08	0.55 ± 0.09	0.68 ± 0.13	0.62 ± 0.11	NS	
LDL TAC [(nmol/L)·mg protein^{-1}]	32.4 ± 7.76	34.5 ± 6.51	37.2 ± 5.87	38.6 ± 7.01	33.5 ± 6.78	NS

[a]For differences between groups at T2.
[b]NS, not significant.

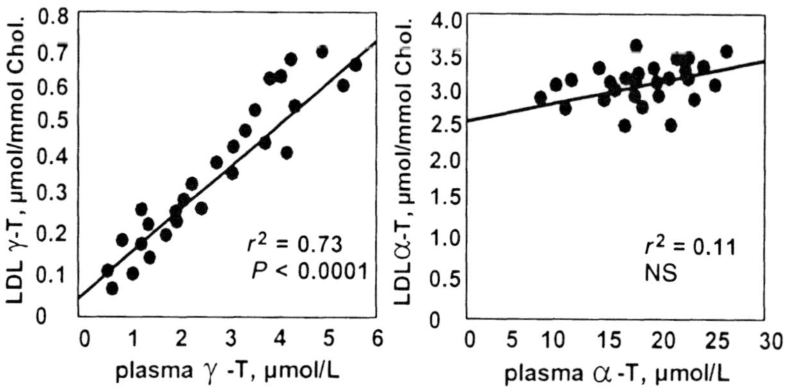

Fig. 33.2. Correlation between plasma and low density lipoprotein (LDL) tocopherol (-T) levels of corn oil diet group after 2 wk of intervention at T2.

Plasma MDA concentration, as one marker for susceptibility against lipid peroxidation, tended to decrease throughout the study period. After the adjustment period (T1), plasma MDA values were within normal range at 0.9 ± 0.3 µmol/L. During the test diet period, independently of the oil source, MDA decreased to a mean value of 0.8 ± 0.3 µmol/L. Differences between the CO diet and the MO diet could not be found. However, MDA values of the first (T0) and the last (T4) blood examination showed a significant increase ($P < 0.05$) over those at T2. A similar trend was observed during the study for TAC, which can be improved by tocopherol-rich plant oil diets. Despite the different α-/γ-tocopherol ratios (CO, 100 mg γ-tocopherol; α-/γ-tocopherol = 1:5; MO, 24 mg α-tocopherol; α-/γ-tocopherol = 10:1; see Table 33.3) in the oils, no significant difference in TAC could be confirmed between the two groups. The determinations concerning the antioxidative capacity in LDL clearly confirm the results of the plasma investigations. A slight improvement in the antioxidative situation of LDL, as well as the nonsignificant difference in TAC between the two oil groups, was discernible after the intervention diet (T2). The corn oil group reached a LDL-TAC of 96% in relation to the mixed oil group (described as AUC) (Fig. 33.3). Plasma cholesterol levels of all subjects were within normal range during the study period. The increase in plasma cholesterol during the adjustment phase can be explained by the use of butter in the diet to keep the intake of tocopherol low. However, butter was not used in the test diets. Differences between the two oil groups in circulating plasma cholesterol levels after the 2-wk investigation trial were not significant at T2, but became significant after the crossover at T3 (CO, 3.9 ± 0.8 mmol/L; MO, 4.6 ± 0.7 mmol/L; $P < 0.05$). At T4, 5 wk after the intervention, plasma cholesterol contents of the corn oil group had returned to their initial values (Table 33.2).

TABLE 33.3 Circulating Tocopherols Between the Oil Groups in Relation to Fatty Acid Composition[a]

	Corn oil	Mixed oil
Daily consumption (g/d)	80	80
SFA/MUFA/PUFA	13:33:54	14:69:17
P/S ratio	4.2	1.2
α-Tocopherol intake (mg/d)	20	24
γ-Tocopherol intake (mg/d)	100	2.4
α-/γ-Tocopherol ratio	1:5	1:0.1
α-Tocopherol equivalents (mg α-TE/d)[b]	45	24.6
α-TE excretion (mg α-TE/d)	20.8	7.6
α-TE retention (mg $\alpha\text{-TE}_{ret}$/d)	24.2	17
Diene acid equivalents (g DE/d)*c*	44	15
$\alpha\text{-TE}_{ret}$/DE ratio (mg/g)	0.55	1.13

[a]Abbreviations: SFA, saturated fatty acids; MUFA, monounsaturated fatty acids; PUFA; polyunsaturated fatty acids; P/S ratio, polyunsaturated/monounsaturated fatty acid ratio.
[b]TE = α-tocopherol equivalents = mg α-tocopherol + 0.25 × mg γ-tocopherol.
[c]DE = diene acid equivalents = 0.025 × monoene acids + 1 × diene acids + 2 × triene acids + 4 × tetraene acids.

Discussion

This study was conducted among healthy, nonsmoking young men to compare the effects of γ-tocopherol–rich corn oil and α-tocopherol–rich olive/sunflower oil, as main dietary fats in normal diets, on antioxidative capacity. The two test diets were

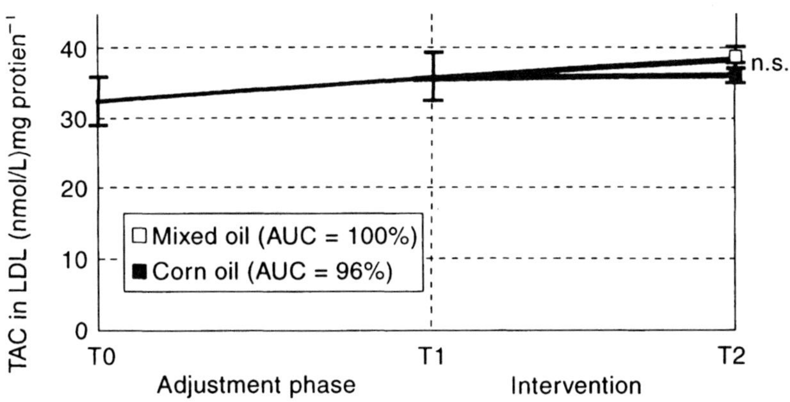

Fig. 33.3. Total antioxidative capacity (TAC) of low density lipoprotein [LDL; (nmol/L)·mg protein^{-1}] after adjustment period (T1) and 2 wk of consumption of the corn oil vs. mixed oil diet (T2). Abbreviation: AUC, area under the curve.

selected for their natural sources of tocopherols and differed in γ-tocopherol level, the percentage of MUFA and PUFA, and also in their calculated α-TE/DE ratio. At an equal daily intake of 80 g corn oil or a mixture of olive/sunflower oil, and almost equal intake of γ-tocopherol (20 mg/d with the CO diet; 24 mg/d with the MO diet), the CO diet group had significantly lower α-tocopherol in plasma and LDL than the mixed oil group after 2 wk of consuming the test diet (T2). This result may be due to the high PUFA content of the corn oil (P/S ratio = 4.2). An increased uptake of PUFA may also affect vitamin E status, either by impairing the absorption of the antioxidants (24) or by causing increased vitamin E oxidation in plasma and tissues due to enhanced lipid peroxidation (25,26). Nevertheless, due to the additional intake of γ-tocopherol (100 mg/d) in the corn oil group, γ-tocopherol plasma and LDL values increased significantly. Considering the efficiency of γ-tocopherol as reported in the literature (≤25% of α-tocopherol), the subjects of the CO group reached a daily intake of 45 mg α-TE, and those of the MO group, 24.6 mg α-TE. Results of feces investigations revealed an excretion rate for α- and γ-tocopherol between 23 and 35% and 61 and 68%, respectively. The calculated bioeffective share of α-TE between concentration and consumption to prevent lipid oxidation can be used as an indicator of the truly available amount of tocopherols. Due to the high P/S ratio of corn oil (4.2), the calculated diene equivalents of the corn oil group were 44 g, and those of the olive/sunflower oil group 15 g. Considering the absorption of vitamin E (20.8 mg excretion of α-T), the daily available amount of α-TE (retention = $\alpha\text{-TE}_{ret}$) of the CO group was 24.2 mg, whereas the MO group reached a bioeffective amount of 17.0 mg $\alpha\text{-TE}_{ret}$ (7.6 mg excretion of α-T). The calculated $\alpha\text{-TE}_{ret}$/DE ratio of the CO group was 0.55; that of the MO group was 1.13 (Table 3). The latter ratio gives information about susceptibility to lipid oxidation. The higher the ratio, the better is the protection by vitamin E of PUFA in the diet. This means that the protection by vitamin E in the mixed oil diet was theoretically twice as high as that in the corn oil diet. In determinations of TAC, variables that are strongly related to the antioxidative efficiency of the two plant oil diets were investigated. The determination of TAC permits a differentiation between several antioxidative substances and potencies. MDA, which is present as a MDA-thiobarbituric acid complex, is another parameter with which to measure the extent of peroxidation in biological systems. To increase the selectivity of MDA determination, HPLC was used to separate compounds with a reversed-phase column.

Due to the results showing a high stability in antioxidative substances through use of diets that were similar except for the plant oils, we focused on the tocopherols, which were the most significantly variable during the study period, with the main free radical scavengers as the next most significant variable. Considering LDL as the main transport fraction of tocopherols, their antioxidative capacity is more sensitive than the plasma antioxidative activity due to the high number of water-soluble reducing substances in plasma, such as ascorbic acid, uric acid, albumin, or bilirubin. It is obvious that the diet groups were not comparable in their fatty acid composition. In addition, there were unsaponifiable compounds in the corn oil that are not contained in the olive/sunflower oil mixture, especially flavonids, ubiquinones, or other phenolic compounds. Nevertheless, concerning these fats specifications, and in spite of the lower ratio of biologically active α-TE_{ret}/DE of the CO group (0.55 vs. 1.13 mg/g for MO), no significant difference was found between the groups concerning TAC and MDA values in plasma and LDL. Both diets, the γ-tocopherol–dominated PUFA-rich CO diet (P/S ratio = 4.2) and the α-tocopherol–dominated MO diet (P/S ratio = 1.2), had the same antioxidative potency. No accelerated oxidation was measurable in the high-PUFA CO diet. Consequently, given the equality of the diets except for the fat consumed, one protective factor against oxidation processes was the high antioxidative potency of γ-tocopherol. These results strongly suggest that the γ-tocopherol in the CO diet was responsible for the results and therefore has a higher antioxidative capacity than has been considered in the published literature. Many studies show a higher or at least an equal antioxidative capacity of γ-tocopherol to α-tocopherol when assessed *in vitro*. Recently, several investigations have shown that γ-tocopherol is superior to α-tocopherol in reducing reactive nitrogen species (27,28) and in prolonging oil shelf life (29). On the basis of the results obtained in this study, a synergistic effect between α- and γ-tocopherol must be considered because of the approximately equal content of α-tocopherol in the two diets but the much higher P/S ratio of the CO diet.

The plant oil–defined diets did not affect plasma concentrations of ascorbic acid, α-, and β-carotene, or other carotenoids (data not shown), which all influence the susceptibility of LDL to oxidation in vivo.

The daily intake of cholesterol with the two diets was rather constant (cholesterol intake, 191–335 mg/d). The only difference between the two diets was the oil source. LDL cholesterol levels decreased significantly during the CO diet compared with the MO diet. HDL cholesterol levels did not change significantly during the entire study period. VLDL cholesterol decreased significantly during the corn oil diet, but not with the mixed oil diet. These results agree with results of Dreon *et al.* (30) and Insull *et al.* (31) who investigated the effects of plant oils on cholesterol metabolism. These observations are discussed in connection with the different plant oil fatty acid composition and furthermore with the high amount of unsaponifiables in the corn oil.

In conclusion, the results of this study suggest that considering the retention of tocopherol, a combination of γ-tocopherol with α-tocopherol in a CO diet is more effective as a free radical scavenger *in vivo* than the high MUFA MO diet. Despite the low retention of γ-tocopherol and the high P/S ratio with the high n-6 PUFA corn oil diet, which therefore requires a higher level of protection, no significant difference was determined for plasma and LDL oxidation. This study further shows that LDL cholesterol is lowered significantly by the highly unsaturated corn oil diet, without influencing HDL cholesterol. Further analysis is warranted to give clear insight into the *in vivo* activity of γ-tocopherol and the synergistic interaction between γ-tocopherol and α-tocopherol.

References

1. Esterbauer, H., Gebicki, J., Puhl, H., and Jürgens, G. (1992) The Role of Lipid Peroxidation and Antioxidants in Oxidative Modification of LDL. *Free Radic. Biol. Med. 13*, 341–390.
2. Steinberg, D., Parthasaranthy, S., Carew, T.E., Khoo, J.C., and Witztum, J.L. (1989) Beyond Cholesterol. Modifications of LDL That Increase Its Atherogenicity. *N. Engl. J. Med. 320,* 915–924.
3. Steinmetz, K.A., and Potter, J.D. (1996) Vegetables, Fruit and Cancer Prevention: A Review. *J. Am. Diet. Assoc. 96,* 1027–1039.
4. Rimm, E.B., Ascherio, A., Giovannucci, E., Spiegelman, D., Stampfer, M.J., and Wilett, W.C. (1996) Vegetable, Fruit and Cereal Fiber Intake and Risk of Coronary Heart Disease Among Men. *J. Am. Med. Assoc. 275,* 447–451.
5. Gey, K.F. (1990) The Antioxidant Hypothesis of Cardiovascular Diseases: Epidemiology and Mechanisms. *Biochem. Soc. Trans. 18,* 1041–1045.
6. Gey, K.F., Puska, P., Jordan, P., and Moser, U.K. (1991) Inverse Correlation Between Plasma Vitamin E and Mortality from Ischemic Heart Disease in Cross-Cultural Epidemiology. *Am. J. Clin. Nutr. 53,* 326S–334S.
7. Buring, J.E., and Hennekens, C.H. (1997) Antioxidant Vitamins and Cardiovascular Disease. *Nutr. Rev. 55,* 53S–60S.
8. Esterbauer, H., Dieber-Rotheneder, M., Waeg, G., Striegl, G., and Jürgens, G. (1990) Biochemical, Structural and Functional Properties of Oxidized Low Density Lipoprotein. *Chem. Res. Toxicol. 3,* 77–92.
9. Bendich, A., and Machlin, L.J. (1988) Safety of Oral Intake of Vitamin E. *Am. J. Clin. Nutr. 48,* 612–619.
10. Van Poppel, G., and Van Den Berg, H. (1997) Vitamins and Cancer. *Cancer Lett. 114,* 195–202.
11. Schäfer, H., and Elmadfa, I. (1984) Bioactivity of Alpha- and Gamma-Tocopherol Calculated from Respiration Parameters in Rat Liver Mitochondria. *Ann. Nutr. Metab. 28,* 297–304
12. Brubacher, G., Stahelin, H.B., and Vuilleumier, J.P. (1974) Relation Between Beta-Lipoprotein Content in Serum and Plasma Vitamin E Content. A Contribution to the Question of the Estimation of the Vitamin E Status in Man. *Int. J. Vitam. Nutr. Res. 44,* 521–526.
13. Reaven, P.D., Khouw, A., Belz, W.F., Parthasaranthy, S., and Witztum J.L. (1993) Effect of Dietary Antioxidant Combination in Humans. *Arterioscler. Thromb. Vasc. Biol. 13,* 590–600.
14. Princen, H.M.G., van Duyvenvoorde, W., Buytenhek, R., van der Laarse, A., van Poppel, G., Gevers Leuven, J.A., and van Hinsbergh, V.W. (1995) Supplementation with Low Doses of Vitamin E Protects LDL from Lipid Peroxidation in Men and Women. *Artherioscler. Thromb. Vasc. Biol. 15,* 325–333.
15. D-A-CH-Referenzwerte für die Nährstoffzufuhr (Deutsche Gesellschaft für Ernährung, Österreichische Gesellschaft für Ernährung, Schweizerische Gesellschaft für Ernährungsforschung, Schweizerische Vereinigung für Ernährung), 1. Auflage, Umschau Braus Verlag, Frankfurt am Main, 2000.
16. Jakob, E., and Elmadfa, I. (1995) Rapid HPLC-Assay for Assessment of Vitamin K1, A, E and Beta-Carotene Status in Children (7–19 Years). *Int. J. Vitam. Nutr. Res. 65,* 31–35.

17. Denson, Y.W., and Bowers, E.F. (1961) The Determination of Vitamin C in White Blood Cells. *Clin. Sci. 21,* 157–160.
18. Wong, S.H.Y., Knight, J.A., Hopfer, S.M., Zaharia, O., Leach, C.N., and Sunderman, F.W. (1987) Lipoperoxides in Plasma as Measured by Liquid-Chromatographic Separation of Malondialdehyde-Thiobarbituric Adduct. *Clin. Chem. 33,* 214–220.
19. Siedel, J., Hägele, E.O., Ziegenhorn, J., and Wahlefeld, A.W. (1983) Reagent for the Enzymatic Determination of Serum Total Cholesterol with Improved Lipolytic Efficiency. *Clin. Chem. 29,* 1075–1078.
20. Rice-Evans, K., and Miller, N.J. (1994) Total Antioxidative Status in Plasma and Body Fluids. *Methods Enzymol. 234,* 279–293.
21. Nelson, R.A. (1993) Rapid, Single-Spin Fractionation of Serum Lipoproteins by Density Gradient Ultracentrifugation in Sorvall Vertical Rotors. *Sorvall Application Brief B-001.*
22. Foremann, J.R., Karlin, J.B., and Edelstein, C. (1982) Fractionation of Human Serum Lipoproteins by Single-Spin Gradient Ultracentrifugation. *J. Lipid Res. 18,* 759–767.
23. Wagner, K-H., Auer, E., and Elmadfa, I. (2000) Content of *Trans* Fatty Acids in Margarines, Plant Oils, Fried Products and Chocolate Spreads in Austria. *Eur. Food Res. Technol. 210,* 237–241.
24. Meydani, S.N., Shapiro, A.C., Meydani, M., Macauley. J.B., and Blumberg J.B. (1987) Effect of Age and Dietary Fat (Fish, Corn, and Coconut Oils) on Tocopherol Status of C57BL/6Nia Mice. *Lipids 22,* 345–350.
25. Van den Berg, J.J.M., de Fouw, N.J., Kuypers, F.A., Roelofsen, B., Houtsmuller, U.M.T., and Op den Kamp, J.A.F. (1991) Increased n-3 Polyunsaturated Fatty Acid Content of Red Blood Cells from Fish Oil-Fed Rabbits Increases *In Vitro* Lipid Peroxidation, but Decreases Hemolysis. *Free Radic. Biol. Med. 11,* 393–399.
26. Elmadfa, I., and Bosse, W. (1985) *Vitamin E.* Wissenschaftliche Verlagsgesellschaft mbH, Stuttgart.
27. Cooney, R.V., Franke, A.A., Harwood, P.J., Hatch-Pigott, V., Custer, L.J., and Morgan, L.J. (1993) γ-Tocopherol Detoxification of Nitrogen Dioxide: Superiority to α-Tocopherol. *Proc. Natl. Acad. Sci. USA 90,* 1771–1775.
28. Christen, S., Woodall, A.A., Shingenaga, M.K., Southwell-Keely, P.T., Duncan, M.W., and Ames, B.N. (1997) γ-Tocopherol Traps Mutagenic Electrophiles Such as No_x and Complements α-Tocopherol: Physiological Implications. *Proc. Natl. Acad. Sci. USA 94,* 3217–3222.
29. Wagner, K-H., and Elmadfa, I. (2000) Effects of Tocopherols and Their Mixtures on the Oxidative Stability of Olive Oil and Linseed Oil Under Heating. *Eur. J. Lipid Sci. Technol.,* in press.
30. Dreon, D.M., Fernstrom, H.A., Campos, H., Blanche, B., Wiliams, P.T., and Krauss, M. (1998) Change in Dietary Saturated Fat Intake Is Correlated with Change in Mass of Large Low Density Lipoprotein Particles in Men. *Am. J. Clin. Nutr. 67,* 282–836.
31. Insull, W., Silvers, A., Hicks, L., and Probstfield, J.L. (1994) Plasma Lipid Effects of Three Common Vegetable Oils In Reduced Fat Diets of Free Living Adults. *Am. J. Clin. Nutr. 60,* 195–202.

Chapter 34

Effect of Tocotrienols on Estrogen Metabolism in MCF-7 and MDA-MB-231 Human Breast Cancer Cell Lines

Kalanithi Nesaretnam and Kanga Rani Selvaduray

Malaysian Palm Oil Board, Kuala Lumpur 50720, Malaysia.

Introduction

Breast cancer is the most common cancer in women worldwide. Estrogens have been shown to play an important role in promoting the development of breast cancer (1). Estrone sulfate (E_1S) is present in high concentrations in breast tissue, ~15–25 times higher than in plasma (2). High levels of E_1S in breast tumors serve as a huge reservoir of active estrogens (1). The stimulatory effect of E_1S in breast tumor progression is due to the conversion of E_1S to estrone (E_1) by the enzyme, estrone sulfatase (3). In breast cancer tissues, estrone sulfatase activity is 10–100 times higher than aromatase activity, suggesting that most of the estradiol (E_2) present in breast cancer tissue originates from the enzymatic hydrolysis of E_1S (2).

Estradiol-17β-hydroxysteroid dehydrogenase (E_2DH) catalyzes the interconversion between the less active estrogen, E_1, and the more potent estrogen, E_2. E_2DH activity is higher in cancerous tissues compared with normal breast tissue (4). Increased reductive activity of E_2DH in breast cancer cells leads to increased estradiol levels in breast cancer cells.

Vitamin E compounds (tocopherols and tocotrienols) are well recognized for their effective inhibition of lipid oxidation in foods and biological systems (5). Because vitamin E is synthesized only by plants, it is a very important dietary nutrient for humans and animals. Although tocopherols are generally present in nuts (almonds) and the common vegetable oils, tocotrienols are found in high concentrations in cereal grains (oat, barley, and rye) and certain vegetable oils (palm oil and rice bran oil) (6).

Tocotrienols have been the focus of active research in the last 5–10 y, not as secondary forms of vitamin E but as unique nutritional compounds (7). Nesaretnam *et al.* (8–10) showed previously that tocotrienols can inhibit the growth of several human breast cancer cell lines, including MDA-MB-435, MCF-7, and ZR-75-1. The tocotrienol-rich fraction (TRF) of palm oil was clearly able to inhibit growth of the MCF-7 cells in the presence of estrogen. In the absence of estrogen, TRF could also serve to antagonize the action of residual estrogen in the cell or restore estrogen memory effects. However, TRF appeared to be unable to alter the expression of the estrogen-regulated pS2 gene in MCF-7 cells, which is a well-established marker of estrogen receptor–mediated action (11). Furthermore, if TRF were acting on cell growth in the absence of estrogen to inhibit residual estrogen effects, it would be expected that

TRF would act in a dose-dependent manner such that even lower levels of TRF would be required to inhibit cancer growth in the absence of estrogen. However, this was clearly not the case because inhibition of MCF-7 cell growth was found to require a similar concentration of TRF whether estrogen was present or not. The overall evidence would seem to suggest that tocotrienols do not act by an estrogen receptor–mediated mechanism.

The aim of this study was to assess the effect of TRF on estrogen metabolism, namely, estrone sulfatase and E_2DH activities, in the MCF-7 estrogen receptor (ER)-positive and MDA-MB-231 ER-negative human breast cancer cell lines. Increasing the understanding of the effects of TRF in the different breast cancer cell lines will help toward developing more effective treatment strategies for breast cancer.

Material and Methods

Materials. The TRF was obtained from the Malaysian Palm Oil Board (MPOB). [6,7-^{3}H(N)]-E_1S, ammonium salt (specific activity 1.96 TBq/mmol), [6,7-^{3}H(N)]-E_1, ammonium salt (1.48 TBq/mmol), [6,7-^{3}H(N)]-E_2, ammonium salt (48 Ci/mmol), 4-^{14}C-E_1 (2.1 GBq/mmol) and 4-^{14}C-E_2 (1.96 GBq/mmol) were purchased from New England Nuclear (Boston, MA). The unlabeled steroids E_1 and E_2 were obtained from Sigma Chemical (St. Louis, MO). Dulbecco's modified Eagle medium (DMEM) and fetal bovine serum were purchased from GIBCO BRL (Grand Island, NY). Coulter Counter Z1, Zap-oglobin II and Isoton III were purchased from Coulter. (Miami, FL). Thin-layer chromatography (TLC) sheets/silica gel 60 F_{254} were purchased from Merck (Darmstadt, Germany).

Culture of Stock Cells. The hormone-dependent MCF-7 McGrath human breast cancer cells were kindly provided by Dr. K. Osborne (12). Stock cells were grown as monolayer cultures in DMEM supplemented with 5% fetal calf serum (FCS), 10^{-8} mol/L estradiol in a humidified atmosphere of 10% carbon dioxide in air at 37°C. 17-β-Estradiol was dissolved in ethanol and diluted 1:10,000 in culture medium. MDA-MB-231 human breast cancer cells were obtained from the American Tissue Culture Collection (Manassas, VA). Stock cells were grown similarly to MCF-7 cells with the omission of estradiol.

Estrone Sulfatase Assay. Cells were plated in 12-well plastic tissue culture plates with seeding densities of ~0.2×10^6 cells and 1.2×10^6 cells for the MCF-7 cell line and between 0.2×10^6 and 0.8×10^6 cells for the MDA-MB-231 cell line. Cell numbers at these concentrations had a strong linear relationship with enzyme activity. The cells were grown for 3 d at 37°C and 10% CO_2. The medium was then removed and new medium, containing 5% dextran/charcoal-stripped FCS and 2 mmol/L glutamine, was added to each well. TRF was added to each well to obtain final concentrations of 10, 20, and 30 μg/mL. All treatments were done in triplicate. Estrone sulfatase was measured as previously described (13,14) with minor modifications.

The cell monolayers were washed with PBS and incubated with serum-free medium and 10 μL $^3H-E_1S$ (200,000 dpm) for 4 h at 37°C and 10% CO_2. Medium (1 mL) from each well was pipetted into glass tubes containing 4 mL toluene and vortex-mixed for 30 s. Toluene (2 mL) was then transferred into glass vials and the tritiated product formed was counted using a liquid scintillation counter. Results were expressed as fmol product/(4 h·10^6 cells).

E_2DH Assay. The cell monolayers were washed with PBS and incubated with serum-free medium containing 200,000 dpm $^3H-E_1$ (reductive) or $^3H-E_2$ (oxidative) for 4 h at 37°C and 5% CO_2. Medium (1 mL) from each 12-well dish was pipetted into glass-stoppered tubes individually; these contained unlabeled E_2 (2 g/L) and 50 μL $^{14}C-E_2$ (5000 dpm) (reductive assay) or $^{14}C-E_1$ (oxidative assay). Diethyl ether (5 mL) was added and the tubes were vortexed-mixed for 2 min. Diethyl ether (3 mL) was transferred to a new tube and evaporated to dryness. The extracted E_1 and E_2 were resuspended in 2 × 0.1 mL ether and spotted onto TLC plates/silica gel 60 F_{254} using Pasteur pipettes. TLC was then carried out using toluene/ethanol (90:10, vol/vol) as the solvent system. The position of the unlabeled estrogen was localized under ultraviolet light. The area containing E_2 (for reductive assay) or E_1 (for oxidative assay) was cut out and eluted with methanol. The radioactivity was determined using a liquid scintillation counter. Results were expressed as fmol product/(4 h·10^6 cells).

Cell Counting. After the cell monolayers had been incubated with the tritiated estrogen sulfate for 4 h and a portion of medium removed for the estrone sulfatase assay, the cell monolayer was washed rigorously *in situ* with phosphate buffered-saline, and then lysed in 0.5 mL of 0.01 mol/L HEPES buffer/1.5 mmol/L $MgCl_2$ plus 2 drops of zapo-globin solution for 5 min. The nuclei released were counted in Isoton III on a Coulter counter. All cell counts were carried out in triplicate and results calculated as the mean ± SD.

Statistics. Differences between cells treated with different tocotrienol concentrations and the control cells were analyzed using the unpaired Student's t test. Results were considered to be significant when $P < 0.05$.

Discussion

Estrogen receptor (ER)-negative breast cancers are normally hormone independent. They tend to be more poorly differentiated and behave more aggressively than ER-positive breast cancers. Studies have shown that these cell types differ from each other in their secretion and response to different stimulatory and inhibitory growth factors, as well as in their enzyme activities involved in estrogen synthesis. Most (~95%) breast cancer cells in the initial stages are ER-positive and depend on estrogens for their growth (15). However, with the progression of the disease, one third to one half of these cells lose their estrogen receptors and become independent

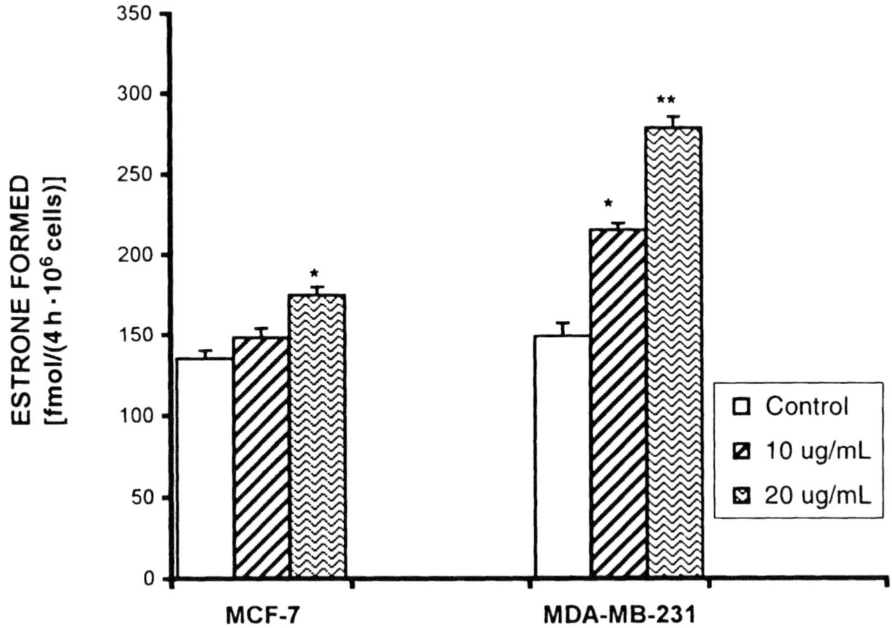

Fig. 34.1. Effect of the tocotrienol-rich fraction (TRF) of palm oil on estrone sulfatase activity in the MCF-7 and MDA-MB-231 cell lines. Estrone sulfatase activities are expressed as means of triplicate determinations + 1 SD. $*P < 0.05$, $**P < 0.01$ vs. control.

of estrogen and less responsive to hormonal treatment. The mechanism involved in the transformation of breast cancers from hormone dependence to independence is not yet well understood. Interest has been focused on the differences in estrogen metabolism in these types of cells, particularly those that involve estrone sulfatase and E_2DH.

The importance of E_1S in breast tumor progression is due to its conversion to E_1 by the enzyme, estrone sulfatase (3). TRF stimulated estrone sulfatase activity in the MCF-7 (Fig. 34.1) and, to a greater extent, in the MDA-MB-231 (Fig. 34.1) cell lines. The stimulation of estrone sulfatase activity results in the production of more E_1, which can then be converted to the potent estrogen, E_2. This would increase the risk of breast cancer.

It is interesting to note that TRF at 10 µg/mL can inhibit reductive E_2DH (Fig. 34.2) activity in the MCF-7 cells. The mechanism may be through an antioxidation effect of tocotrienols on cofactors that are necessary for E_2DH activity. The inhibition of E_2DH activity in the MCF-7 cell line was accompanied by growth inhibition (Fig. 34.3). It has been shown that the addition of oxidized cofactor NAD+ increased the activity of E_2DH, and reduced availability of this cofactor decreased E_2DH activity in estrogen-dependent MCF-7 (16) and T47-D (17) breast cancer cell lines. Reed *et al.* (16) noted that the availability of the cofactors was not found to be limiting but governed the direction (reductive or oxidative) in which E_2DH acts.

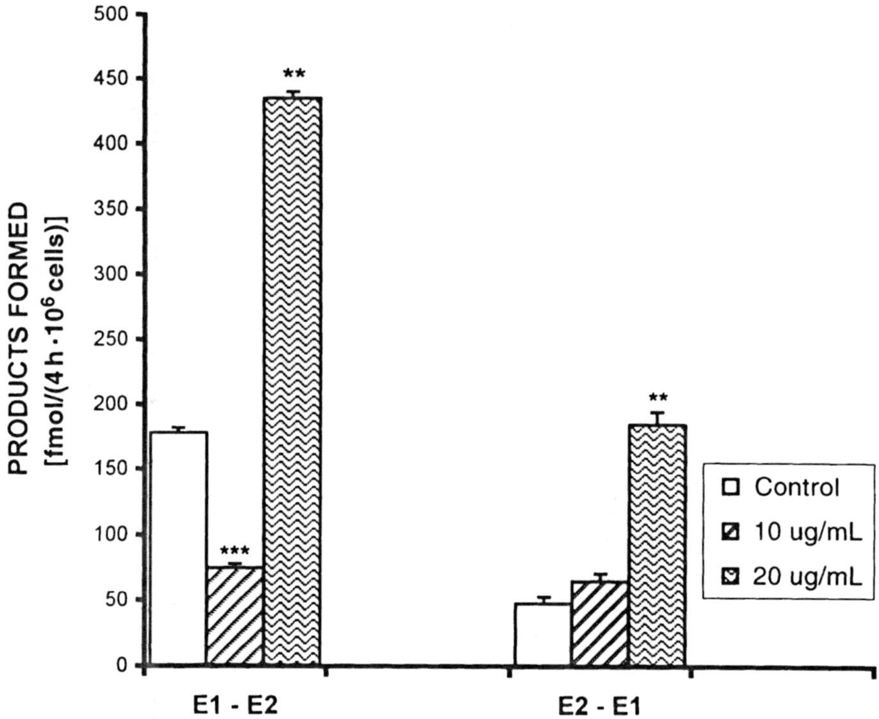

Fig. 34.2. Effect of the tocotrienol-rich fraction (TRF) of palm oil on reductive [estrone (E_1) to estradiol (E_2)] and oxidative (E_2 to E_1) E_2DH activity in the MCF-7 cell line. Results are expressed as means of triplicate determinations + 1 SD. $**P < 0.01$, $***P < 0.001$ vs. control.

At a higher TRF concentration of 20 µg/mL, the reductive E_2DH activity in the MCF-7 cell line was stimulated (Fig. 34.2). The stimulation of reductive E_2DH activity was also accompanied by growth inhibition (Fig. 34.3). TRF at 20 µg/mL also stimulated oxidative E_2DH activity in the MCF-7 cell line. Stimulation of reductive E_2DH activity was accompanied by an increase in the oxidative E_2DH activity. The net result was that there was no increase in the local production of the potent estrogen, estradiol, which increases the proliferation of the MCF-7 cell line. In the MDA-MB-231 cells, there was a slight but significant increase in the reductive oxidative E_2DH activity (Fig. 34.4). It was again accompanied at 20 µg/mL by an increase in the oxidative E_2DH activity, thereby converting the potent estrogen to the weak estrone.

In conclusion, the study has shown that tocotrienols inhibit growth of the ER-positive MCF-7 and ER-negative MDA-MB-231 human breast cancer cell lines (Fig. 34.3), which confirms our previous findings (8–10). Increased E_2 formation as a result of increased estrone sulfatase and reductive E_2DH activities, which may potentially increase the risk of breast cancer, was accompanied by a simultaneous conversion to the weak estrone in both cell lines. The net result was growth inhibition

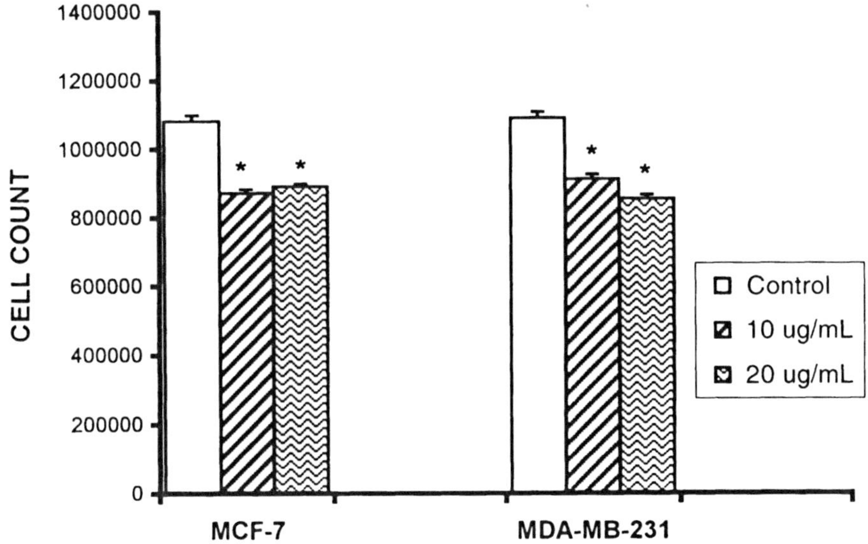

Fig. 34.3. Effect of the tocotrienol-rich fraction (TRF) of palm oil on cell growth of MCF-7 and MDA-MB-231 cells. Cell counts are expressed as means of triplicate determinations + 1 SD. *$P < 0.05$ vs. control.

in both cell lines by the TRF. Because the MDA-MB-231 cell line is estrogen independent and unresponsive to estrogens, the alterations in estrogen concentrations are unlikely to contribute to the changes of cell growth in this cell line. On the other hand, control of the production of the potent estrogen estradiol by TRF in the MCF-7 cells could open new possibilities in the treatment of hormone-dependent breast cancer.

References

1. Pasqualini, J.R., Gelly, C., Nguyen, B.L., and Vella, C. (1989) Importance of Estrogen Sulfates in Breast Cancer. *J. Steroid Biochem. 34*, 155–163.
2. Pasqualini, J.R., Chetrite, G., Nguyen, B.L., Maloche, C., Delalonde, L., Talbi, M., Feinstein, M.C., Blacker, C., Botella, J., and Pains, J. (1995) Estrone Sulfate-Sulfatase and 17 Beta-Hydroxy Steroid Dehydrogenase Activities: A Hypothesis for Their Role in the Evolution of Human Breast Cancer from Hormone-Dependence to Hormone Independence. *J. Steroid Biochem. Mol. Biol. 53*, 407–412.
3. Santner, S.J., Ohlsson-Wilhelm, B., and Santner, R.J. (1993) Estrone Sulfate Promotes Human Breast Cancer Cell Replication and Nuclear Uptake of Estradiol in MCF-7 Cell Cultures. *Int. J. Cancer 54*, 119–124.
4. Labrie, C., Martel, C., Dufour, J. M., Levesque, C., Merand, Y., and Labrie, F. (1992) Novel Compounds Inhibit Estrogen Formation and Action. *Cancer Res. 52*, 610–615.
5. Kamal-Eldin, A., and Appelqvist, L.A. (1996) The Chemistry and Antioxidant Properties of Tocopherols and Tocotrienols. *Lipids 31*, 671–701.

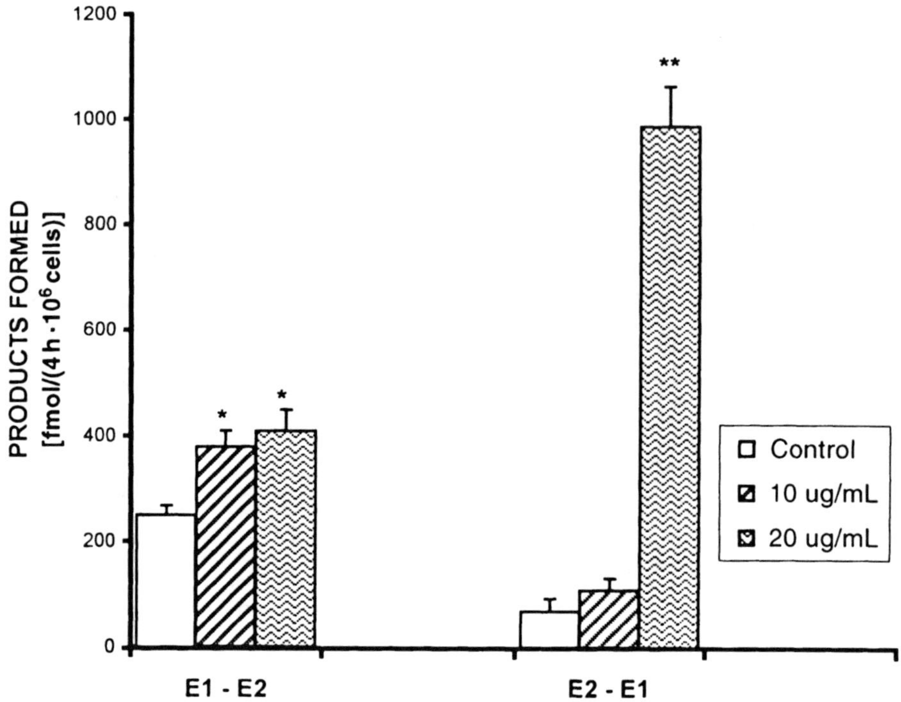

Fig. 34.4. Effect of the tocotrienol-rich fraction (TRF) of palm oil on reductive [estrone (E_1) to estradiol (E_2)] and oxidative (E_2 to E_1) E_2DH activity in the MDA-MB-231 cell line. Results are expressed as means of triplicate determinations + 1 SD. *$P <$ 0.05, **$P < 0.01$ vs. control.

6. Combs, G.F. (1992) *The Vitamins: Fundamental Aspects in Nutrition and Health*, Academic Press, San Diego.
7. Theriault, A., Chao, J.T., Wang, Q., Gapor, A., and Adeli, K. (1999) Tocotrienol: A Review of Its Therapeutic Potential. *Clin. Biochem. 32*, 309–319.
8. Nesaretnam, K., Guthrie, N., Chambers, A.F., and Carroll, K.K. (1995) Effect of Tocotrienols on the Growth of Human Breast Cancer Cell Line in Culture. *Lipids 30*, 1139–1143.
9. Nesaretnam, K., Stephen, R., Dils, R., and Darbre, P. (1998) Tocotrienols Inhibit the Growth of Human Breast Cancer Cells Irrespective of Estrogen Receptor Status, *Lipids 33*, 461–469.
10. Nesaretnam, K., Selvarajan, D., and Darbre, P. (2000) Tocotrienols Inhibit the Growth of ZR-75-1 Human Breast Cancer Cells. *Int. J. Food Sci. Nutr., 51,* S95–S103.
11. Masiakowski, P., Breathnach, R., Bloch, J., Gannon, F., Krust, A., and Chambon, P. (1982) Cloning of cDNA Sequences of Hormone-Regulated Genes from the MCF-7 Human Breast Cancer Cell Line. *Nucleic Acids Res. 10*, 7895–7903.
12. Osborne, C.K., Hobbs, K., and Trent, J.M. (1987) Biological Differences Among MCF-7 Human Breast Cancer Cell Lines from Different Laboratories. *Breast Cancer Res. Treat. 9*, 111–121.

13. Purohit, A., and Reed, M.J. (1992) Oestrone Sulphatase Activity in Hormone Dependent and Hormone Independent Breast Cancer Cells: Modulation by Steroidal and Non-Steroidal Therapeutic Agents. *Int. J. Cancer. 50*, 901–905.
14. Adams, E.F., Coldham, N.G., and James, V.H.T. (1988) Steroidal Regulation of Estradiol-17β-Hydroxysteroid Dehydrogenase Activity of Human Breast Cancer Cell Line MCF-7. *J. Endocrinol. 188*, 149–154.
15. Henderson, B.E., Ross, R., and Bernstein, L. (1988) Estrogens as a Cause of Human Cancer: The Richard Hinadau Rosenthal Foundation Award Lecture. *Cancer Res. 48*, 246–253.
16. Reed, M.J., Duncan, L.J., and Parker, M.G. (1994) Regulation of Estradiol 17β-Hydroxysteroid Dehydrogenase Expresion and Activity by Retinoic Acid in T47D Breast Cancer Cells. *Endocrinol. 135,* 4–9.

Chapter 35

Antioxidants Modulate the Course of Carotid Atherosclerosis: A Four-Year Report

Dawn K. Kooyenga,[a] Tom R. Watkins,[a] Martin Geller,[b] and Marvin L. Bierenbaum[a]

[a]Kenneth L. Jordan Research Group, Montclair, NJ 07042
[b]Department of Neurology, Elmhurst Medical Center, Queens, NY

Introduction

In recent studies, an association between oxygen-derived free radicals and the activation and promotion of atherosclerosis has been demonstrated. The function of oxidatively modified low density lipoprotein (LDL) in the propagation of carotid atherosclerosis has been shown in various studies (1–4). For >40 y, antioxidants, especially those from the vitamin E family, have received much attention as potential protectors from the process of atherogenesis. A number of recent reports have demonstrated the ability of antioxidants to protect LDL, preventing both *ex vivo* and *in vitro* LDL oxidation, which in turn, would potentially stop the development of atherosclerotic lesions (5–8). Epidemiologic studies have linked the dietary intake of vitamin E and other antioxidants with a reduced risk of coronary heart disease (9,10), ischemic heart disease (11), ischemic stroke (12), coronary mortality (13), and coronary artery disease (14), and with a decrease in carotid artery wall thickness (15,16). Because tocopherols and tocotrienols both have antioxidant effects, an investigation of their use as a treatment modality for carotid atherosclerotic regression in poststroke patients was warranted.

Materials and Methods

The methodology was described previously (17) and was continued throughout this entire period of observation. For the first 3 y of the study, the supplement used was extracted from palm oil; because of a change in research support, for y 4, the source was rice bran oil (RBO). The rice bran oil had additional sterols with an antioxidant content very similar to that of palm oil. Each capsule (Rangsit Biotech, Bangkok) provided 52 mg of tocotrienol, 60 mg of α-tocopherol, and 76 mg of other nonsaponifiables. The placebo capsules contained 300 mg oil. The vehicle was composed of 17.5% palmitic and stearic acids, 42.5% oleic acid, and 40% linoleic acid (by weight), a total of 112 mg. No one in either group reported side effects such as headache, intestinal upset, muscle weakness, or persistent liver function abnormalities.

Results

Patients being supplemented with tocopherol and tocotrienols for 48 mo approximately doubled their serum α-tocopherol levels compared with baseline (22.1 ± 2.3 to 41.8 ± 3.9 μmol/L; $P < 0.01$). The levels in the placebo group did not change significantly (19.0 ± 1.6 to 26.7 ± 3.7 μmol/L).

After 48 mo, both antioxidant supplement (16.9 ± 2.4 Ω to 24.4 ± 3.1 Ω; $P < 0.05$) and placebo (17.7 ± 2.5 Ω to 27.2 ± 2.5 Ω; $P < 0.01$) groups showed an increase of collagen-induced platelet aggregation compared with baseline (Table 35.1). The platelet ATP response to thrombin did not change in either the placebo group (1.02 ± 0.08 to 0.97 ± 0.13 μmol/L) or the tocol group (0.99 ± 0.09 to 1.09 ± 0.16 μmol/L). At acceptance into the study, all subjects were started on a daily regimen of aspirin [a majority were already doing so (see Table 35.2)]. It appears that the increase seen in platelet aggregation resulted from resumption of smoking by some subjects ($n = 3$ in placebo group; $n = 4$ in treatment group) (18).

Data on the effect of the mixed tocopherol and tocotrienols vs. placebo in lowering serum lipid oxidation products is shown in Table 35.3. Serum thiobaribituric acid–reactive substance (TBARS) values after 48 mo for patients receiving antioxidants decreased from (mean ± SEM) 1.08 ± 0.14 to 0.59 ± 0.12 μmol/L ($P < 0.01$), whereas placebo subjects' values showed no significant change (0.99 ± 0.16 to 0.78 ± 0.10 μmol/L). At baseline, a difference was seen in hydroperoxide levels (Table 35.3). The fatty acid hydroperoxides (LOPS) increased nonsignificantly, rising from 4.59 ± 2.22 to 4.99 ± 1.38 μmol/L after 48 mo in the test group. In the placebo group, the LOPS rose from 2.27 ± 0.23 to 5.30 ± 1.40 μmol/L ($P < 0.05$).

As reported earlier, treatment with the same daily dosage of refined palm oil tocopherols and tocotrienols had no significant effect on serum lipids for the first 36

TABLE 35.1 Whole Blood Platelet Responses for 48 mo[a]

	Treatment, $n = 25$					
	Baseline	6	12	24	36	48
	(mo)					
Collagen (Ω)	16.9 ± 2.4	9.52 ± 1.7	12.0 ± 1.8	25.5 ± 3.0[b]	25.9 ± 3.7[c]	24.4 ± 3.12[c]
ATP (μmol/L)	0.99 ± 0.09	0.92 ± 0.09	1.24 ± 0.15	1.24 ± 0.09	0.87 ± 0.09	1.09 ± 0.16
	Placebo, $n = 25$					
Collagen, Ω	17.7 ± 2.5	14.9 ± 2.0	12.0 ± 1.6	28.8 ± 3.0[d]	26.7 ± 3.3[c]	27.2 ± 2.5[d]
ATP (μmol/L)	1.02 ± 0.08	0.99 ± 0.14	1.04 ± 0.15	0.91 ± 0.08	1.05 ± 0.14	0.97 ± 0.13

[a]Data are means ± SEM, Student's *t* test.
[b]$P < 0.03$ vs. respective baseline value.
[c]$P < 0.05$ vs. respective baseline value.
[d]$P < 0.01$ vs. respective baseline value.

TABLE 35.2 Comparison of Patient Characteristics at Study Entry by Treatment Group[a]

Patient characteristic	Treatment $n = 25$	Placebo $n = 25$	P
Age (y)	66.4	66.7	NS
Gender (F/M)	13/12	14/11	NS
Antiplatelet (aspirin) use (n)[b]	15	11	NS
Anticoagulant use (n)[b]	21	24	NS
Hypertensive (n)	9	14	NS
Diabetic (n)	5	2	NS
Abnormal EKG (n)[c]	16	15	NS
Abnormal chest X-ray (n)[c]	7	12	NS
Smoker (n)	5	4	NS
Height, in (m)	64.8 ± 4.2 (1.65 ± 0.1)	64.4 ± 3.5 (1.63 ± 0.1)	NS
Weight, lb (kg)	152.8 ± 39.5 (69.4 ± 17.9)	150.8 ± 26.9 (68.6 ± 12.2)	NS
BMI[d] (kg/m^2)	25.2 ± 5.4	26.3 ± 4.0	NS
Systolic blood pressure (mm Hg)	138.6 ± 14.4	147.8 ± 20.0	NS
Diastolic blood pressure (mm Hg)	82.4 ± 9.7	81.2 ± 9.6	NS
>49% carotid stenosis (n)	15	11	NS

[a]Data are means ± SD; NS, not significant.
[b]Therapy regimen was maintained for each patient according to current medical practice throughout the study, as indicated.
[c]Abnormal for cardiovascular pathology.
[d]BMI, body mass index.

TABLE 35.3 Serum TBARS and LOPS Values of Subjects Given Tocols or Placebo for 48 mo[a,b]

	Treatment, $n = 25$					
	Baseline	6	12	24	36	48
	(mo)					
TBARS (μmol/L)	1.08 ± 0.14	0.68 ± 0.11	0.80 ± 0.11	0.80 ± 0.14[c]	0.44 ± 0.09[d]	0.59 ± 0.12[e]
LOPS (μmol/L)	4.59 ± 2.22	4.52 ± 1.3	3.50 ± 1.5	2.85 ± 0.55	3.33 ± 1.22	4.99 ± 1.38
	Placebo, $n = 25$					
TBARS (μmol/L)	0.99 ± 0.16	1.01 ± 0.14	1.26 ± 0.11	1.06 ± 0.07	0.83 ± 0.21	0.78 ± 0.10
LOPS (μmol/L)	2.27 ± 0.23	2.10 ± 0.32	3.60 ± 1.90	3.02 ± 0.62	3.06 ± 0.62	5.30 ± 1.40[c]

[a]Data are means ± SEM, Student's t test.
[b]Abbreviations: TBARS, thiobarbituric acid–reactive substances, an indicator of peroxidation. See text. LOPS, fatty acid hydroperoxides, an indicator of oxygen-damaged fat. See text.
[c]$P < 0.05$ vs. respective baseline value.
[d]$P < 0.001$ vs. respective baseline value.
[e]$P < 0.01$ vs. respective baseline value.

mo (17,19). However, we did observe a change from 36 to 48 mo while the subjects were consuming rice bran oil containing sterols, tocopherols, and tocotrienols (Table 35.4). Treatment group cholesterol values decreased 14.1% from 6.18 ± 0.33 to 5.31 ± 0.20 mmol/L ($P < 0.05$). LDL cholesterol (LDL-C) values also decreased 20.6% from 4.28 ± 0.37 to 3.40 ± 0.18 mmol/L ($P < 0.05$). In the same interval, total and LDL-C levels in the placebo group remained stable at 5.70 ± 0.21 and 6.06 ± 0.32 mmol/L and 3.95 ± 0.18 and 4.05 ± 0.31 mmol/L (Table 35.4). Serum high density lipoprotein (HDL) cholesterol (HDL-C) values rose with the RBO with nonsaponifiables (RBN) treatment, improving the ratio of HDL-C/cholesterol from 0.17 ± 0.02 to 0.24 ± 0.02 mmol/L ($P < 0.025$). RBN feeding produced a decrease in triglyceride values. The triglyceride/HDL-C ratio decreased from 2.16 ± 0.35 to 1.21 ± 0.21 mmol/L ($P < 0.05$) in the RBN group. Placebo group values were stable, going from 1.54 ± 0.31 to 1.55 ± 0.20 mmol/L.

The percentage change of carotid stenosis in patients by category differed in the treatment and placebo groups after 48 mo of observation. The data indicated (Table 35.5) that eight (32%) of the subjects supplemented with antioxidants for 48 mo moved one category to a lesser apparent degree of stenosis; two (8%) improved

TABLE 35.4 Lipid Responses of Subjects to Supplementation for 48 mo[a,b]

	Treatment, n = 25					
	Baseline	6	12	24	36	48
	(mo)					
Cholesterol (mmol/L)	6.05 ± 0.25	6.15 ± 0.31	6.17 ± 0.33	5.95 ± 0.26	6.18 ± 0.33	5.31 ± 0.20[c]
LDL-C (mmol/L)	4.27 ± 0.21	4.39 ± 0.30	4.39 ± 0.29	4.11 ± 0.21	4.28 ± 0.37	3.40 ± 0.18[c]
HDL-C (mmol/L)	0.98 ± 0.06	0.92 ± 0.04	1.00 ± 0.07	1.07 ± 0.10	1.03 ± 0.10	1.24 ± 0.12
Triglyceride[d] (mmol/L)	2.19 ± 0.30	2.73 ± 0.46	2.11 ± 0.25	2.02 ± 0.27	2.30 ± 0.35	1.77 ± 0.27
	Placebo, n = 25					
Cholesterol (mmol/L)	5.90 ± 0.33	5.68 ± 0.28	5.67 ± 0.26	5.77 ± 0.23	5.70 ± 0.21	6.06 ± 0.32
LDL-C (mmol/L)	4.19 ± 0.28	4.00 ± 0.27	4.01 ± 0.27	4.03 ± 0.22	3.95 ± 0.18	4.05 ± 0.31
HDL-C (mmol/L)	1.10 ± 0.05	1.10 ± 0.05	1.15 ± 0.06	1.15 ± 0.09	1.18 ± 0.09	1.30 ± 0.09
Triglyceride[d] (mmol/L)	1.82 ± 0.32	1.90 ± 0.35	1.50 ± 0.14	1.52 ± 0.20	1.51 ± 0.18	1.90 ± 0.25

[a]Data are means ± SEM; Student's t test.
[b]LDL-C, low density lipoprotein cholesterol; HDL-C, high density lipoprotein cholesterol.
[c]$P < 0.05$ vs. 36-mo values.
[d]Average molecular weight, 914 Da.

TABLE 35.5 Comparison of Change in Carotid Stenosis in Groups Receiving Tocols (T) or Placebo (P) at 6, 36, and 48 mo[a,b]

	T	P	T	P	T	P
	6 mo		36 mo[c]		48 mo[d]	
MR	1	0	1	0	2	0
R	5	0	7	0	8	2
NC	18	20	15	13	12	8
P	1	2	2	8	3	11
MP	0	3	0	4	0	4
Total number	25	25	25	25	25	25

[a]Data are expressed as the number of subjects per category.
[b]Abbreviations: MR, marked regression; R, regression; NC, no change; P, progression; MP, marked progression.
[c]$P < 0.001$; Mann-Whitney test.
[d]$P < 0.001$; Mann-Whitney test.

by two categories, suggesting marked regression. Because there had been no earlier changes in lipids, we attributed this to the accumulated effect of the antioxidant intake. Only three (12%) subjects from this group exhibited progression of carotid atherosclerosis. The remaining 48% manifested no change in disease state. In contrast, eleven (44%) of the placebo group showed progression, and four (16%) showed marked progression of carotid stenosis. Only two (8%) subjects in this group showed regression of carotid stenosis. The remaining 32% showed no change in degree of stenosis. Previous stenosis data were presented in earlier publications (17,19). During the 4 y of the study, three patients from each group were referred to surgery according to original admission criteria. Due to the surgical intercession, they were maintained in the "no change category" as in fact was the case.

Discussion

The objective of this clinical study was to test the effect of mixed tocotrienols and tocopherols in patients with carotid atherosclerosis. After following the antioxidant supplementation study for 48 mo with analysis of the results of 50 subjects, we found no measurable improvement in blood lipids during the first 36 mo, although we did observe an apparent improvement in blood flow in the carotid arteries of 10 of 25 patients. This suggests that although blood lipids might affect arterial wall status, they may not change blood flow. In contrast, Qureshi *et al.* (20,21) reported a reduction in both serum total cholesterol and LDL-C in human hyperlipidemics supplemented with tocotrienols. Wahlqvist *et al.* (22), however, observed hemostatic serum responses to both tocopherol and, to a lesser extent, tocotrienol supplementation in humans, without any change in serum lipids. In preliminary trials with a rat model, we observed a hypolipidemic effect with γ-tocotrienol (23); however, our results in rats were not confirmed by the outcome in patients consuming uncontrolled diets who were taking a variety of medications. From the previous data, a decrease in serum cholesterol was not a prerequisite in the 10 patients suggested to have reduced carotid atherosclerosis. This result is in contrast to coronary atherosclerosis, as we reported earlier (24). On balance, serum cholesterol is a poor predictor of carotid, compared with coronary, plaque thickness. Miettinen *et al.* (25) reported that although no significant decrease in coronary risk was measured when clofibrate was given with probucol, no stroke cases were observed in the 1200-subject study. Mao *et al.* (7) demonstrated that a concomitant reduction in serum cholesterol levels was not present with the attenuation of atherosclerotic lesions in Watanabe rabbits by a probucol analog. Similarly, Bocan *et al.* (26), using Japanese hypercholesterolemic quail, demonstrated that probucol use decreased the incidence of atherosclerotic lesions without altering the plasma total or lipoprotein cholesterol levels. These investigators attributed this effect to the antioxidant properties of probucol. In view of the recent finding that the use of probucol for hypercholesterolemia results in lowered HDL_{2b} levels (27), probucol use in atherosclerosis must be viewed with caution. In two recent meta-analyses of randomized, controlled trials using middle-aged male subjects (28,29), the authors found that lowering serum cholesterol through modified diets or medications did not decrease stroke mortality or morbidity. These results were further substantiated by an even more recent Swedish report (30), which showed no difference in carotid-intima-media thickness or plaque status in a group with comprehensive risk reduction (including a 9% LDL-C decrease) after 3.5 y of observation. Similar results were found and reported in the EVA study (31), once again showing the close relationship of antioxidant status and early atherosclerosis without associated serum lipid changes. Not to be overlooked, however, Bucher *et al.* (32) concluded that β-hydroxyl-β-methyl glutarate (HMG)CoA reductase inhibitors reduce the risk for fatal and nonfatal stroke, accompanied by serum lipid reduction.

Although we observed no change in serum lipids in the first 36 mo, we did see a change from mo 36 to 48. In this period, significant decreases were noted in serum cholesterol, LDL-C, and triglyceride levels with a concomitant increase in HDL-C. Thus, the decrements noted in serum cholesterol with a small daily intake of RBN (without other dietary change) occurred against a background of unchanging cholesterol values over a 3-y period when subjects were consuming refined palm oil tocotrienols and tocopherols (17,19,22,33). Ingestion of palm tocotrienols and tocopherols led to improved carotid artery stenosis (17,19). Therefore, although the tocotrienols and tocopherols were largely responsible for the improvement of the carotid arteries, we have inferred that the sterols in the RBO, which are lacking in palm oil, were responsible for the hypocholesterolemic effect that we observed after y 3.

The hypocholesterolemic potency of RBO when fed as ≥10% of dietary energy has been documented in rats (34), monkeys (35), and humans (36). Our subjects received <0.5% of energy as RBN; therefore, we suspected activity in fractions other than the oil. Oryzanols, cycloarterenols, 24-methyl-cycloartenol, β-sitosterol, and other ferulates have been studied (37–39). The data presented do not allow assignment of the hypocholesterolemic effect seen here to a particular fraction(s).

Consumption of RBN also resulted in significantly lower LDL-C levels. This major atherosclerotic risk factor determines, in part, the antioxidant need (5). The LDL-C values decreased significantly, suggesting an improved antioxidant economy. Patterson (40) noted that the typical U.S. diet provides only modest antioxidant supplies. A supplementation of RBN allowed a realistic solution to restore antioxidant levels in the tissues.

The encapsulated RBN also led to increased HDL/cholesterol values. Though RBO use led to improved HDL in monkeys (35) and humans (36), these data showed that the benefit of the active principles may be taken without the oil.

Over a 1-y period, an inverse correlation was observed between plasma antioxidant levels (vitamin E, β-carotene, selenium) and the increase in carotid intima-media thickness in a population of hypercholesterolemic Eastern Finnish men (41). Similarly, Kritchevsky *et al.* (15) found an inverse relationship between dietary antioxidant intake (α-tocopherol, ascorbic acid, β-carotene) and carotid artery wall thickness in both men and women. The precise mechanism(s) responsible for plaque regression appears to be ambiguous and has yet to be explained fully. Earlier work from this laboratory documented the effective inhibition of platelet aggregation by antioxidants in hyperlipemic patients (42). After taking into account that one measure of the thrombogenicity of the blood was altered equally in the two groups, and that the serum lipid profiles remained stable for the first 3 y, it appears that the level of serum TBARS may provide a clue concerning the mode of action of these antioxidants. The decrease we observed in serum peroxidation as measured by TBARS in the tocotrienol group appears to be the pathway of improvement of blood flow in the study group because changes occurred within y 1. Elegant studies aptly support the theory that antioxidants curtail the levels of blood lipid peroxides, and blunt the formation of the atherosclerotic lesion. Esterbauer *et al.* (5) demonstrated that vitamin E was very effective in preventing *in vitro* oxidation of LDL, and Carew *et al.* (6) showed that the antioxidant probucol inhibited the progression of atherosclerotic lesions in LDL receptor–deficient rabbits. We have inferred from the data presented from this cohort that the dynamics of both serum lipids and the endothelium are modulated by daily tocotrienols and tocopherols in the latter and nonsaponifiables in the former. These represent a promising adjunct therapy in cardiovascular patients, especially the poststroke patient.

Summary

In summary, our results highlight the potential of antioxidants such as mixed tocopherols and tocotrienols in preventing and possibly reversing the progressive course of carotid atherosclerosis, probably independently of serum lipid levels. Other moieties in RBN, which are absent in palm oil, may be responsible for the hypolipidemic effect in the subjects. Finding a hypolipidemic effect of a vitamin E–rich fraction of rice bran oil with sterols intact is a significant bonus and may provide additional protection against coronary heart disease.

Acknowledgment

The KL Jordan Research Group gratefully acknowledges the support in these studies of Rangsit Biotech, Thailand.

References

1. Salonen, J.T., Yla-Hertuala, S., Yamamoto, R., Butler, S., Korpella, H., Salonen, R., Nyyssonen, K., Palinski, W., and Witztum, J.L. (1992) Autoantibody Against Oxidized LDL and Progression of Carotid Atherosclerosis. *Lancet 339*, 883–887.
2. Witztum, J.L. (1994) The Oxidative Hypothesis of Atherosclerosis. *Lancet 344*, 793–795.
3. Steinberg, D., and Workshop Participants (1992) Antioxidants in the Prevention of Atherosclerosis. *Circulation 85*, 2338–2344.
4. Salonen, J.T., Nyyssonen, K., Salonen, R., Porkkala-Saratano, E., Tuomainen, T.P., Diczfalusy, U., and Bjorkhem, I. (1997) Lipoprotein Oxidation and Progression of Carotid Atherosclerosis. *Circulation 95*, 840–845.
5. Esterbauer, H., Dieber-Rotheneder, M., Striegel, G., and Waeg, G. (1991) Role of Vitamin E in Preventing the Oxidation of Low-Density Lipoprotein. *Am. J. Clin. Nutr. 53*, 314S–321S.
6. Carew, T.E., Schwenke, D.C., and Steinberg, D. (1987) Antiatherogenic Effect of Probucol Unrelated to Its Hypocholesterolemic Effect: Evidence That Antioxidants *In Vivo* Can Selectively Inhibit Low Density Lipoprotein Degradation in Macrophage-Rich Fatty Streaks and Slow the Progression of Atherosclerosis in the WHHL Rabbit. *Proc. Natl. Acad. Sci. USA 84*, 7725–7729.
7. Mao, S.J.T., Yates, M.T., Parker, R.A., Chi, E.M., and Jackson, R.L. (1991) Attenuation of Atherosclerosis in a Modified Strain of Hypercholesterolemic Watanabe Rabbit with Use of a Probucol Analogue (MD29, 311) That Does Not Lower Serum Cholesterol. *Arterioscl. Thromb. 11*, 1266–1275.
8. Princen, H.M.G., van Duyvenvoorde, W., Buytenhek, R., van der Laarse, A., van Poppel, G., Gevers Leuven, J.H., and van Hinsbergh, V.W. (1995) Supplementation with Low Doses of Vitamin E Protects LDL from Lipid Peroxidation in Men and Women. *Arterioscl. Thromb. Vasc. Biol. 15*, 325–333.
9. Rimm, E.B., Stampfer, M.J., Ascherio, A., Giovanucci, E., Colditz, G.A., and Willett, W.C. (1993) Vitamin E Consumption and the Risk of Coronary Heart Disease in Men. *N. Engl. J. Med. 328*, 1450–1456.
10. Stampfer, M.J., Hennekens, C.H., Manson, J.E., Colditz, G.A., Rosner, B., and Willett, W.C. (1993) Vitamin E and Risk of Coronary Disease in Women. *N. Engl. J. Med. 328*, 1444–1449.
11. Gey, K.D. (1995) Ten-Year Retrospective on the Antioxidant Hypothesis of Arteriosclerosis. *J. Nutr. Biochem. 6*, 206–236.
12. Bonner, L.L., Kanter, D.S., and Manson, J.E. (1995) Primary Prevention of Stroke. *N. Engl. J. Med. 333*, 1392–1400.
13. Stephens, N.G., Parsons, A., Schufield, P.M., Kelly, F., Cheeseman, K., Mitchinson, N.J., and Brown, M.J. (1996) Randomized Controlled Trial of Vitamin E in Patients with Coronary Disease: Cambridge Heart Antioxidant Study (CHAOS). *Lancet 347*, 781–786.

14. Hodis, H.N., Mack, W.J., LaBree, L., Gashin-Hemphill, L., Sevanian, A., Johnson, R., and Azen, S. (1995) Serial Coronary Angiographic Evidence That Antioxidant Vitamin Intake Reduces Progression of Coronary Artery Atherosclerosis. *J. Am. Med. Assoc. 173*, 1849–1854.
15. Kritchevsky, S.B., Shimakawa, T., Dennis, B., Eckfeldt, J., Carpenter, M., and Heiss, G. (1995) Dietary Antioxidants and Carotid Artery Wall Thickness: ARIC Study. *Circulation 92*, 2142–2150.
16. Azen, S.P., Qian, D., Mack, W.J., Sevanian, A., Selzer, R.H., Liu, C.R., Liu, C.H., and Hodin, H.N. (1996) Effect of Supplementary Antioxidant Vitamin Intake on Carotid Arterial Wall Intima-Media Thickness in a Controlled Clinical Trial of Cholesterol Lowering. *Circulation 94*, 2369–2372.
17. Tomeo, A.C., Geller, M., Watkins, T.R., Gapor, A., and Bierenbaum, M.L. (1995) Antioxidant Effects of Tocotrienols in Patients with Hyperlipidemia and Carotid Stenosis. *Lipids 30*, 1179–1183.
18. Bierenbaum, M.L., Fleischman, A.I., Steir, A., Somol, H., and Watson, P.B. (1978) Effect of Cigarette Smoking upon *In Vivo* Platelet Function in Man. *Thromb. Res. 12*, 1051–1057.
19. Kooyenga, D.K., Geller, M., Watkins, T., and Bierenbaum, M.L. (1995) Palm Oil Antioxidants: Effects in Patients with Hyperlipidemia and Carotid Stenosis. *Asia Pac. J. Clin. Nutr. 6*, 72–75.
20. Qureshi, A.A., Bradlow, B.A,. Brace, L., Manganello, J., Peterson, D.M., Pearce, B.C., Wright, J.J.K., Gapor, A., and Elson, C.E. (1995) Response of Hypercholestrerolemic Subjects to Administration of Tocotrienols. *Lipids 30*, 1171–1177.
21. Qureshi, A.A., Bradlow, B.A., Salser, W.A., and Brace, L.D. (1997) Novel Tocotrienols of Rice Bran Modulate Cardiovascular Disease Risk Parameters of Hypercholesterolemic Humans. *J. Nutr. Biochem. 8*, 290–298.
22. Wahlqvist, M.L., Krivokuca-Bogtic, V., Lo, C.S., Hage, B., Smith, R., and Lukito, W. (1992) Differential Serum Responses of Tocopherols and Tocotrienols During Vitamin Supplementation in Hypercholesterolemic Individuals Without Change in Coronary Risk Factors. *Nutr. Res. 12*, S181–S201.
23. Watkins, T.R., Lenz, P., Gapor, A., Struck, M., Tomeo, A., and Bierenbaum, M.L. (1993) γ-Tocotrienol as a Hypocholesterolemic and Antioxidant Agent in Rats Fed Atherogenic Diets. *Lipids 28*, 1113–1118.
24. Bierenbaum, M.L., Fleischman, A.I., Raichelson, R.I., Hayton, T., and Watson, P.B. (1973) Ten-Year Experience of Modified-Fat Diets on Younger Men with Coronary Heart Disease. *Lancet 2*, 1404–1407.
25. Miettinen, T.A., Huttunen, J.K., Naukkaunien, V., Strandberg, T., and Watson, B.P. (1986) Long-Term Use of Probucol in the Multifactorial Primary Prevention of Vascular Disease. *Am. J. Cardiol. 57*, 49H–54H.
26. Bocan, T.M.A., Mazur, M.J., Mueller, S.B., Charlton, G., Keift, K.A., and Krause, B.R. (1994) Atherosclerotic Lesion Development in Hypercholesterolemic Japanese Quail Following Probucol Treatment: A Biochemical and Morphological Evaluation. *Pharmacol. Res. 29*, 65–76.
27. Johansson, J., Olsson, A., Bergstrand, L., Elinder, L.S., Nilsson, S., Erikson, U., Molgaard, J., Holme, I., and Waldius, G. (1995) Lowering of HDL_{2b} by Probucol Partly Explains the Failure of the Drugs to Affect Femoral Atherosclerosis in Subjects with Hypercholesterolemia. *Arterioscl. Vasc. Biol. 15*, 1049–1056.

28. Atkins, D., Psaty, B.M., Koepsell, T.D., Longstreth, W.T., and Larson, E.B. (1993) Cholesterol Reduction and the Risk of Stroke in Men. A Meta-Analysis of Randomized, Controlled Trials. *Ann. Intern. Med. 119*, 136–145.
29. Herbert, P.R., Gaziano, J.M., and Hennekens, C.H. (1995) An Overview of Trials of Cholesterol Lowering and Risk of Stroke. *Arch. Intern. Med. 155*, 50–55.
30. Suurküla, M., Agewall, S., Fagerberg, B., Wedehag, I., and Wikstrand, J. on Behalf of the Risk Intervention Study (RIS) Group (1996) Multiple Risk Intervention in High-Risk Hypertensive Patients. *Arterioscl. Thromb. Vasc. Biol. 16*, 462–470.
31. Bonithon-Kopp, C., Coudray, C., Berr, C., Touboul, P., Fève, J.M., Favier, A., and Ducimetière, P. (1997) Combined Effects of Lipid Peroxidation and Antioxidant Status on Carotid Atherosclerosis in a Population Aged 59-71 y: The EVA Study. *Am. J. Clin. Nutr. 65*, 121–127.
32. Bucher, H.C., Griffith, L.E., and Guyatt, G.H. (1998) Effect of HMGCoA Reductase Inhibitors on Stroke. A Meta-Analysis of Randomized, Controlled Trials. *Ann. Intern. Med. 128*, 89–95.
33. Antila, A., Atroshi, F., Sankari, S., Treuthardt, J., Hakomaa, S., Gapor, A., and Westermarck, T. (1991) Palm Oil-Vitamin E Therapy in Hypercholesterolemia. *Proc. of Trends in Biomed.: Free Radic., Diet Trace Elem., Vitamins* 2, 36.
34. Sharma, R.D., and Rukmini, C. (1985) Rice Bran Oil and Hypocholesterolemia in Rats. *Lipids 21*, 715–717.
35. Nicolosi, R.J., Ausman, L., and Hegsted, D.M. (1991) Rice Bran Oil Lowers Serum Total and Low Density Lipoprotein Cholesterol and Apo-B Levels in Non-Human Primates. *Atherosclerosis 88*, 133–142.
36. Lichtenstein, A.H., Ausman, L.M., Carrasco, W., Gualtieri, L.J., Jenner, J.L., Ordovas, J.M., Nicolosi, R.J., Goldin, B.R., and Schaefer, E.J. (1994) Rice Bran Oil Consumption and Plasma Lipid Levels in Moderately Hypercholesterolemic Humans. *Atheroscler. Thromb. 14*, 549–658.
37. Seetaramaiah, G.S., and Chandrasehara, N. (1988) Hypocholesterolemic Activity of Oryzanol in Rats. *Nutr. Rep. Int. 38*, 927–935.
38. Rong, N., Ausman, L.M., and Nicolosi, R.J. (1997) Oryzanol Decreases Cholesterol Absorbtion and Aortic Fatty Streaks in Hamsters. *Lipids 32*, 303–309.
39. Ikeda, I., Nakashima-Yoshida, K., and Sugano, M. (1985) Effect of Cycloartenol on Absorption and Serum Levels of Cholesterol in Rats *J. Nutr. Sci. Vitaminol. 31*, 375–384.
40. Patterson, B.H., and Block, G.A. (1991) Fruit and Vegetable Consumption: National Survey Data, in *Micronutrients in Health and in Disease Prevention* (Butterworth, C.E., and Bendich, A., eds.), pp. 409–436, M. Dekker, New York.
41. Salonen, J.T., Nyssonen, K., Parviainen, M., Kantola, M., Korpela, H., and Salonen, R. (1993) Low Plasma β-Carotene, Vitamin E and Selenium Levels Associated with Accelerated Carotid Atherogenesis in Hypercholesterolemic Finnish Men. *Circulation. 87*, 2 (abstr.).
42. Bierenbaum, M.L., Reichstein, R.P., Bhagavan, H.N., and Watkins, T.R. (1992) Relationship Between Serum Lipid Peroxidation Products in Hypercholesterolemic Subjects and Vitamin E Status. *Biochem. Int.* 28, 57–66.

Chapter 36

Human Vitamin E Requirements: Is α-Tocopherol the Only Form That Is Required?

Maret G. Traber

Linus Pauling Institute, Oregon State University, Corvallis, OR and Department of Internal Medicine, University of California, Davis, CA

Introduction

The Food and Nutrition Board (FNB), Institute of Medicine of the National Academy of Science has published recommended nutrient intakes approximately every 10 y since the 1940s. Recently, the FNB has developed a new approach to these recommendations (1). The goal is to provide dietary advice for normal, healthy people consuming North American diets to obtain optimal health. These recommendations are based principally upon published, peer-reviewed studies carried out in humans. There are four different dietary reference intakes (DRI) for each nutrient studied. These include the following: EAR, estimated average requirement; RDA, recommended dietary allowance; AI, average intake; and UL, upper limit. Ideally, the EAR is amount of nutrient that prevents an adverse health effect in 50% of the population; then, the RDA is based on the EAR plus an estimated amount that should ensure an adequate intake for almost all of the population. If insufficient data are available, sometimes it is necessary to use an AI as the recommended amount—this category is frequently used to make recommendations for the nutrient intake of infants consuming human milk. Finally, the UL is set to indicate the maximum amount of a nutrient that can be consumed without adverse effect. The UL is not a goal, but rather a limitation that should not be exceeded.

Vitamin E Recommendation

The vitamin E DRI were published by the FNB in April 2000 (2). The RDA for adults is 15 mg α-tocopherol. This new recommendation has two important aspects, i.e., form and amount. With respect to form, the new recommendation differentiates between the various forms of vitamin E that have similar antioxidant activities. Although there are eight different naturally occurring forms, including α-, β-, γ-, and δ- tocopherols and α-, β-, γ-, and δ-tocotrienols, only one form, α-tocopherol, was recognized by the FNB to meet the human vitamin E requirement. The FNB recommended α-tocopherol because it is maintained in the plasma as a result of the function of the α-tocopherol transfer protein. Humans with a defect in the gene for this protein become vitamin E deficient (3); supplementation with α-tocopherol reverses or halts their deficiency symptoms (4). The α-tocopherol transfer protein selects α-tocopherol in preference to the other forms of vitamin E and facilitates its secretion into plasma (5). The absence of this protein causes vitamin E deficiency (6). Thus, it is clear that humans require α-tocopherol.

Other dietary forms of vitamin E were not included in the new RDA (2). The FNB decided that there was insufficient evidence in humans that other forms of vitamin E are equivalent to α-tocopherol. Furthermore, there was insufficient evidence for health benefits of these other forms to make any specific dietary recommendations. The new RDA differ from the 1989 RDA, which were in units of α-tocopherol equivalents (7). These units included, for example, 10% of the amount of γ-tocopherol in the diet. However, subsequent to that recommendation, studies in humans demonstrated that although γ-tocopherol was absorbed, it disappeared rapidly from the plasma (8). These data suggested that the α-tocopherol transfer protein did not maintain plasma γ-tocopherol and that, unlike α-tocopherol, there was no specific evidence demonstrating that γ-tocopherol was required.

The FNB specified not only that α-tocopherol meets the human vitamin E requirement, it further specified that only the 2*R*-forms of α-tocopherol met the requirement. The "2*R*-" indicates that the orientation of the phytyl tail where it meets the chromanol ring must be in the *R* conformation, as occurs in nature. Natural and synthetic α-tocopherols are not chemically identical. Synthetic (*all-rac,* or as it is commercially labeled, *dl*) α-tocopherol contains eight different stereoisomers of α-tocopherol that vary at the three chiral centers in the molecule. The naturally occurring stereoisomer of α-tocopherol is *RRR*, whereas *all-rac* contains eight stereoisomers (*RRR, RSR, RRS, RSS, SRR, SRS, SSR, SSS*). The human body retains the *RRR*-, RSR-, RRS-, RSS-α-tocopherols, but not *SRR*, *SRS*, *SSR*, *SSS* (9). Therefore, the synthetic has only half the activity of an equal amount of *RRR*-α-tocopherol (2).

With respect to amounts, the DRI are based on prevention of erythrocyte hemolysis (2). Is 15 mg α-tocopherol enough? With respect to obvious vitamin E deficiency, the amount of vitamin E consumed by most Americans is sufficient to prevent vitamin E deficiency symptoms, e.g., peripheral neuropathy. But, the actual quantities of α-tocopherol consumed by most Americans has been estimated to be closer to 8 mg, as assessed from survey studies (2). These low intakes may be real or they may result from underreporting of fat intakes. However, if intakes are about half the requirement, it may be that many people do not consume sufficient α-tocopherol. Moreover, it is not clear whether chronic diseases are a hallmark of long-term suboptimal α-tocopherol intakes.

It is especially noteworthy that studies examining vitamin E function at the molecular level demonstrate that α-tocopherol modulates pathways important in heart disease (10). Additionally studies in animal models demonstrate that α-tocopherol can decrease atherosclerotic lesion formation (6,11). However, the studies in humans given vitamin E supplements to observe α-tocopherol effects on heart attack risk have resulted in conflicting outcomes, i.e., beneficial effects (12,13), limited effects (14), and no benefit (15). It has been suggested that in the clinical trials in which vitamin E has had the greatest benefit, the subjects consuming the placebo had a higher occurrence of cardiovascular incident; perhaps subjects with greater oxidative stress are more likely to benefit from vitamin E (13).

It is likely that the benefit arising from vitamin E supplementation results from its ability to interfere with clot formation. This is an important function in the prevention of thrombosis, which can lead to heart attacks or stroke. However, this effect also points out the potential risks. Supplemental vitamin E may increase bleeding tendencies. Additionally, vitamin E may potentiate the effects of aspirin with respect to blood clotting (16). Certainly, the UL set by the FNB of 1000 mg α-tocopherol should not be exceeded by supplement users.

Tocotrienol Supplementation Study—An Investigation of Health Benefits

In an effort to assess the health benefits of vitamin E other than α-tocopherol, O'Byrne *et al.* (17) carried out a double-blind, placebo-controlled investigation in hypercholesterolemic humans of the effects of supplements containing α-, γ-, or δ-tocotrienyl acetates. *In vitro* tocotrienols (T3), like tocopherols, have potent antioxidant activity; in addition, T3 can inhibit cholesterol synthesis by suppressing 3-hydroxy-3-methylglutaryl-CoA (HMG-CoA) reductase (18–21). Because hypercholesterolemia is a major risk factor for coronary artery disease, and oxidative modification of low density lipoprotein (LDL) may be involved in atherogenesis, these authors investigated whether daily supplements (250 mg) of α-, γ-, or δ-tocotrienyl acetates would alter serum cholesterol or LDL oxidative resistance.

Hypercholesterolemic subjects were randomly assigned to the study groups as follows: placebo (n = 13), α- (n = 13), γ- (n = 12), or δ- (n = 13) tocotrienyl acetates. The placebo group was given gel-capsules identical in appearance to treatment capsules that contained tocotrienol- free, medium-chain triglyceride oil. All subjects followed a low-fat diet for 4 wk, then took the capsules with dinner for the following 8 wk while continuing the low-fat diet.

As expected, the supplements had no effect on plasma α- or γ-tocopherol concentrations (Fig. 36.1). Plasma T3 were undetectable initially in all groups and always undetectable in the placebo group. After supplementation, there were detectable plasma concentrations of the respective tocotrienols as follows: α-T3, 0.98 ± 0.80; γ-T3, 0.54 ± 0.45' and δ-T3, 0.09 ± 0.07 μmol/L (Fig. 36.2).

Lipid and Lipoprotein Profiles

Presupplementation lipid and lipoprotein profiles of subjects were not significantly different between groups (not shown). After 4 wk of adherence to the American Heart Association (AHA) Step 1 diet, serum cholesterol decreased by ~4–5%. The addition of tocotrienyl acetate supplements to the diet failed to lower total or LDL cholesterol (LDL-C) compared with the placebo group (Fig. 36.3). In contrast, the δ-tocotrienyl acetate supplement resulted in a significant *increase* in total cholesterol and LDL-C levels ($P < 0.05$). No significant changes in serum HDL-C, LDL-C/HDL-C ratio, or in triglycerides were observed in any group.

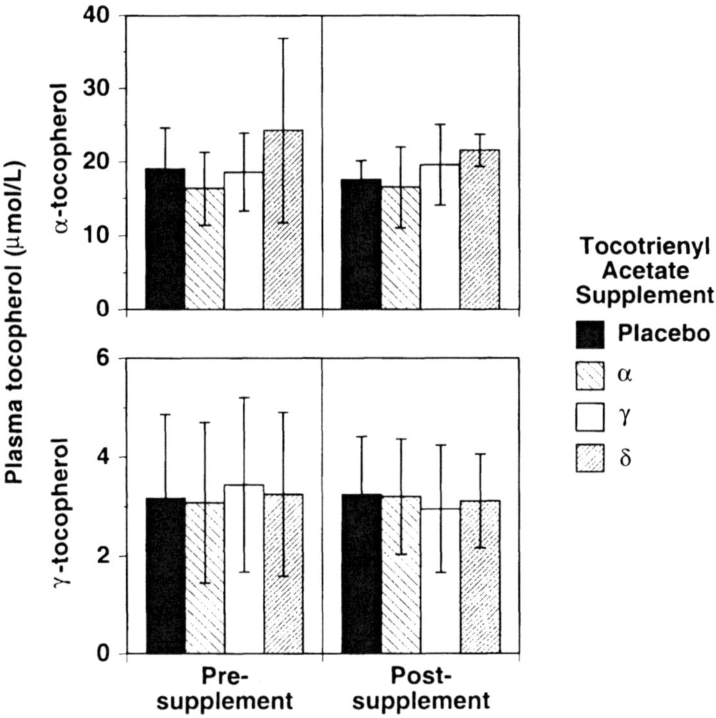

Fig. 36.1. Plasma α- and γ-tocopherol concentrations before and after tocotrienol supplementation. Fasting plasma was obtained before and after subjects consumed 250 mg/d placebo or individual tocotrienyl acetate supplements for 8 wk while adhering to the American Heart Association (AHA) Step 1 diet. Shown are the means ± SD of the plasma α- and γ-tocopherol concentrations (μmol/L) for the presupplementation and the postsupplementation phases for the following groups: placebo (n = 13); α-tocotrienyl acetate (n = 13); γ-tocotrienyl acetate (n = 12); and δ-tocotrienyl acetate (n = 13).

Apolipoprotein (apo) B concentrations were not altered by tocotrienyl acetate supplements, indicating that the number of circulating LDL particles was unchanged. Furthermore, α-, γ-, and δ-tocotrienyl acetate supplements did not modify the cholesterol content of the LDL particles, as reflected by the LDL-C/apoB ratios.

LDL Oxidative Profiles

The ability of T3 supplements to protect LDL against Cu^{2+}-induced oxidation was measured *ex vivo*, and assessed by the length of time before onset of conjugated diene formation (lag time), rate of oxidation, and the maximum concentration of conjugated dienes formed during the 5-h incubation. No significant differences were detected in the LDL oxidation profile between groups during the presupplementation phase, although it should be noted that the group receiving α-tocotrienyl acetate

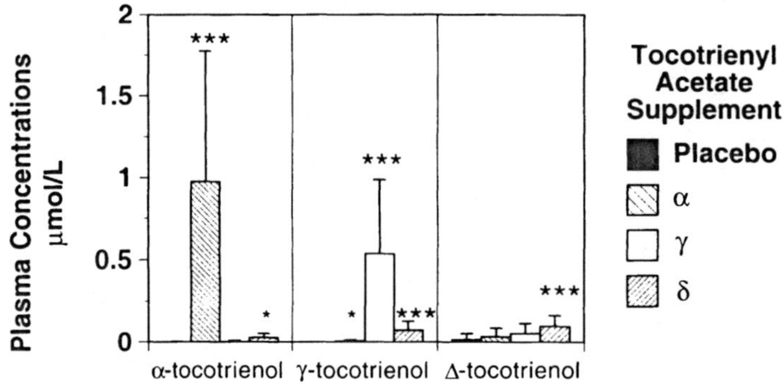

Fig. 36.2. Plasma tocotrienol concentrations after tocotrienol supplementation. Plasma tocotrienol concentrations (µmol/L, means ± SD) in the subjects shown in Figure 36.1 after supplementation. Presupplementation plasma T3 concentrations were below the limits of detection. $^*P < 0.05$, $^{***}P < 0.001$ indicates significant differences in postsupplementation plasma T3 concentrations compared with placebo.

supplements had slightly shorter lag times and greater oxidation rates than the other groups.

The change in LDL oxidation profile was calculated for each of the parameters from the difference between postsupplementation and presupplementation values. Supplementation with placebo, α-, γ- and δ-tocotrienyl acetates resulted in 4.7, 22, 8.8, and 11.6% increases in lag time, respectively; however, only α-tocotrienyl acetate

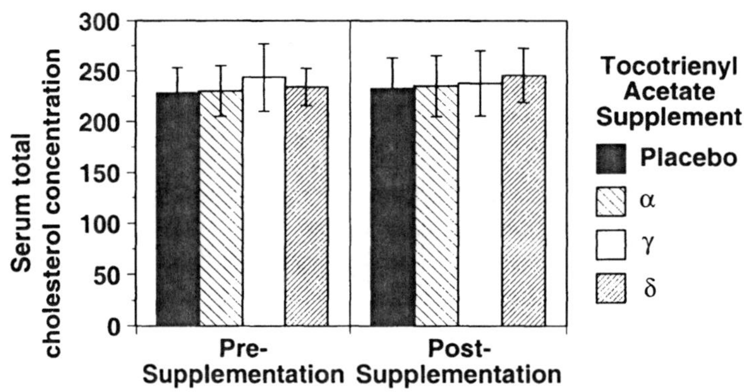

Fig. 36.3. Serum total cholesterol concentrations before and after tocotrienol supplementation. Serum total cholesterol concentrations (mg/dL, means ± SD) in the subjects shown in Figure 36.1 before and after tocotrienol supplementation. Tocotrienyl acetate supplements compared with placebo did not lower total cholesterol. However, the δ-tocotrienyl acetate supplement resulted in a significant increase in total cholesterol levels ($^*P < 0.05$).

supplements resulted in significantly greater increases in lag time compared with changes observed in the placebo group ($P < 0.001$). α-Tocotrienyl acetate supplements also significantly reduced the rate of LDL oxidation ($P < 0.01$). The effect of γ-tocotrienyl acetate on the oxidative indices of LDL supplements did not significantly differ from that of placebo. δ-Tocotrienyl acetate supplements resulted in significantly greater reductions in the rate of LDL oxidation and the amount of conjugated dienes formed, compared with the placebo group ($P < 0.05$). Serum cholesterol, LDL-C, and apoB were not significantly decreased by tocotrienyl acetate supplements.

Summary

In summary, tocotrienyl acetate supplements are hydrolyzed, absorbed, and detectable in human plasma, albeit at minimal concentrations (<1 μmol/L). Despite evidence to the contrary in tissue culture systems and in experimental animal models, tocotrienyl acetate supplements do not lower cholesterol in hypercholesterolemic subjects consuming low-fat diets, although α-T3 was somewhat effective in decreasing LDL oxidizability. However, with respect to human vitamin E requirements, no clear health benefit of tocotrienyl acetate supplements could be documented. Thus far, only α-tocopherol has been demonstrated to reverse human vitamin E deficiency symptoms; it remains the only form of vitamin E that the FNB has recommended to meet human vitamin E requirements.

References

1. Yates, A.A., Schlicker, S.A., and Suitor, C.W. (1998) Dietary Reference Intakes: The New Basis for Recommendations for Calcium and Related Nutrients, B Vitamins, and Choline. *J. Am. Diet* Assoc., *98,* 699–706.
2. Food and Nutrition Board, Institute of Medicine (2000) *Dietary Reference Intakes for Vitamin C, Vitamin E, Selenium, and Carotenoids*, p. 506, National Academy Press, Washington, DC.
3. Cavalier, L., Ouahchi, K., Kayden, H.J., Di Donato, S., Reutenauer, L., Mandel, J.L., and Koenig, M. (1998) Ataxia with Isolated Vitamin E Deficiency: Heterogeneity of Mutations and Phenotypic Variability in a Large Number of Families. *Am. J. Hum. Genet. 62,* 301–310.
4. Sokol, R.J. (1993) in, *Vitamin E in Health and Disease,* (Packer, L., and Fuchs, J., eds.) pp. 815–849, Marcel Dekker, New York.
5. Hosomi, A., Arita, M., Sato, Y., Kiyose, C., Ueda, T., Igarashi, C., Arai, H., and Inoue, K (1997) Affinity for Alpha-Tocopherol Transfer Protein as a Determinant of the Biological Activities of Vitamin E Analogs. *FEBS Lett. 409,* 105–108.
6. Terasawa, Y., Ladha, Z., Leonard, S., Morrow, J., Newland, D., Sanan, D., Packer, L., Traber, M.G., and Farese, R.V., Jr. (2000) Increased Atherosclerosis in Hyperlipidemic Mice Deficient in α–Tocopherol Transfer Protein and Vitamin E. *Proc. Natl. Acad. Sci. USA*, *97,* 13830–13834.
7. Food and Nutrition Board, National Research Council (1989) *Recommended Dietary Allowances,* 10th edn., National Academy of Sciences Press, Washington, DC.

8. Taber, M.G., Burton, G.W., Hughes, L., Ingold, K.U., Hidaka, H., Malloy, M., Kane, J., Hyams, J., and Kayden, H.J. (1992) Discrimination Between Forms of Vitamin E by Humans with and Without Genetic Abnormalities of Lipoprotein Metabolism. *J. Lipid Res. 33*, 1171–1182.
9. Kiyose, C., Muramatsu, R., Kameyama, Y., Ueda, T., and Igarashi, O. (1997) Biodiscrimination of Alpha-Tocopherol Stereoisomers in Humans After Oral Administration. *Am. J. Clin. Nutr. 65,* 785–789.
10. Devaraj, S., and Jialal, I. (1998) The Effects of Alpha Tocopherol on Crucial Cells in Atherogenesis. *Curr. Opin. Lipidol. 9,* 11–15.
11. Pratico, D., Tangirala, R.K., Rader, D.J., Rokach, J., and FitzGerald, G.A. (1998) Vitamin E Suppresses Isoprostane Generation In Vivo and Reduces Atherosclerosis in ApoE-Deficient Mice. *Nat. Med. 4,* 1189–1192.
12. Stephens, N.G., Parsons, A., Schofield, P.M., Kelly, F., Cheeseman, K., and Mitchinson, M.J. (1996) Randomised Controlled Trial of Vitamin E in Patients with Coronary Disease: Cambridge Heart Antioxidant Study (CHAOS). *Lancet 347,* 781–786.
13. Boaz, M., Smetana, S., Weinstein, T., Matas, Z., Gafter, U., Iaina, A., Knecht, A., Weissgarten, Y., Brunner, D., Fainaru, M., and Green, M.S. (2000) Secondary Prevention with Antioxidants of Cardiovascular Disease in Endstage Renal Disease (SPACE): Randomised Placebo-Controlled Trial, *Lancet 356,* 1213–1218.
14. GISSI-Prevenzione Investigators (1999) Dietary Supplementation with n-3 Polyunsaturated Fatty Acids and Vitamin E After Myocardial Infarction: Results of the GISSI-Prevenzione Trial. *Lancet 354*, 447–455.
15. Yusaf, S., Dagenais, G., Pogue, J., Bosch, J., and Sleight, P. (2000) Vitamin E Supplementation and Cardiovascular Events in High-Risk Patients. The Heart Outcomes Prevention Evaluation Study Investigators. *N. Engl. J. Med. 342,* 154–160.
16. Steiner, M., Glantz, M., and Lekos, A. (1995) Vitamin E Plus Aspirin Compared with Aspirin Alone in Patients with Transient Ischemic Attacks. *Am. J. Clin. Nutr. 62,* 1381S–1384S.
17. O'Byrne, D., Grundy, S., Packer, L., Devaraj, S., Baldenius, K., Hoppe, P., Kramer, K., Jialal, I., and Traber, M.G. (2000) Studies of LDL Oxidation Following Alpha-, Gamma- or Delta-Tocotrienyl Acetate Supplementation in Hypercholesterolermic Humans, *Free Radic. Biol. Med., 29,* 834–845.
18. Pearce, B.C., Parker, R.A., Deason, M.E., Qureshi, A.A., and Wright, J.J. (1992) Hypocholesterolemic Activity of Synthetic and Natural Tocotrienols. *J. Med. Chem. 35,* 3595–3606.
19. Parker, R.A., Pearce, B.C., Clark, R.W., Gordon, D.A., and Wright, J.J. (1993) Tocotrienols Regulate Cholesterol Production in Mammalian Cells by Post-Transcriptional Suppression of 3-Hydroxy-3-methylglutaryl-Coenzyrne A Reductase. *J. Biol. Chem 268,* 11230–11238.
20- Pearce, B.C., Parker, R.A., Deason, M.E., Dischino, D.D., Gillespie, E., Qureshi, A.A., Volk, K., and Wright, J.J. (1994) Inhibitors of Cholesterol Biosynthesis. 2. Hypocholesterolemic and Antioxidant Activities of Benzopyran and Tetrahydronaphthalene Analogues of the Tocotrienols. *J. Med. Chem. 37,* 526–541.
21. Theriault, A., Wang, Q., Gapor, A., and Adeli, K. (1999) Effects of γ-Tocotrienol on ApoB Synthesis, Degradation, and Secretion in HepG2 Cells. *Arterioscler. Thromb. Vasc. Biol. 19*, 704–712.

Chapter 37

Oxidative Damage Induced by Peroxynitrite/Singlet Oxygen in Rat Liver Mitochondria and Its Inhibition by Tocotrienols from Palm Oil

J.P. Kamat,[a] K.K. Boloor,[a] T.P.A. Devasagayam,[a] K.Nesaretnam,[b] and Y.Basiron[b]

[a]Cell Biology Division, Bhabha Atomic Research Centre, Mumbai-400 085, India
[b]Palm Oil Research Institute of Malaysia, 43650 Bandar Baru Bangi, Selangor Darul Ehsan, Malaysia

Introduction

The pivotal role of oxygen/nitrogen–derived reactive species in several human degenerative diseases is well documented (1–3). In view of their relevance in human health, studying the effect of such reactive oxygen/nitrogen species (ROS/RNS) in relation to their biological and biomedical ramifications has become an active area of interest in recent years. Incomplete reduction of oxygen produces ROS such as superoxide ($O_2^{-\bullet}$), hydrogen peroxide (H_2O_2), and the hydroxyl radical ($^\bullet OH$), whereas its energy absorption process generates singlet oxygen ($^1O_2$) (4).The reaction of nitric oxide ($NO^\bullet$) with $O_2^{-\bullet}$ favors the formation of peroxynitrite ($ONOO^-$) (5,6). Peroxynitrite is a potent oxidant of biological interest; it is produced by endothelial cells, Kupffer cells, neutrophils, and macrophages during phagocytosis (7). The peroxynitrite mediates oxidation of large numbers of crucial cellular molecules. This includes oxidation of nonprotein/protein (8), lipids (9), DNA (10), as well as nitration of aromatic amino acids (5). Cellular membranes, due to the high degree of unsaturated fatty acids in lipids and hydrophobic regions of proteins, are potential sinks for these species, resulting in highly deleterious reactions such as lipid peroxidation and protein oxidation (11,12). The structural and functional alterations occurring due to damage to lipid, protein, and DNA can account for the changes associated with oxidative stress (12). Oxidative reactions in the body are generally neutralized by biologically established antioxidants, vitamins C, E, glutathione (GSH), and enzymatic defenses (11,13). However, their availability is limited especially under conditions in which overexpression of ROS is occurring due to endogenous or exogenous agents (5,11). Therefore, the study of naturally occurring dietary antioxidants in relation to oxidative stress has attracted immense interest in recent years.

In our studies we have focused our attention on palm oil, an edible vegetable oil rich in vitamin E (having both tocotrienol and tocopherol) because of its popularity in human diets in all parts of the world. Additionally, palm oil exhibits multifunctional properties against several human diseases (14,15). The tocotrienol-rich fraction (TRF) from palm oil is considered to be an economical substitute for α-tocopherol, and as palm vit E capsule, it has been used as a nutritional supplement with potential therapeutic applications (15–17). Hypocholesterolemic action, together with inhibition of hydroxymethylglutaryl (HMG) coenzyme A (CoA) reductase, was indicated as a possible reason for protection by TRF against atherosclerosis. On the other hand, its anticancer action is linked to its role in limiting the availability of cholesterol in membrane formation in proliferating tissues and possible interference in signal transduction (17). The mechanism of TRF action against diseases in relation to its antioxidant ability is not yet clearly understood. In addition to studies concerning RNS-mediated nitration reactions, the essential antioxidant role of TRF, particularly during peroxynitrite-induced oxidative damage in mitochondrial membranes, remains to be explored.

These studies concern the effect of TRF on oxidative damage induced by peroxynitrite as well as singlet oxygen in rat liver mitochondria. The studies demonstrated that TRF is an effective antioxidant against such damage in lipids and proteins and it was more efficient than α-tocopherol.

Materials and Methods

Materials. 2-Thiobarbituric acid, methylene blue, α-tocopherol, 2-4-dinitrophenylhydrazine, guanidine hydrochloride, sodium azide, GSH, glutathione reductase, dithiobisnitrobenzoic acid, epinephrine, and superoxide dismutase (SOD) were purchased from Sigma Chemical, St. Louis, MO. TRF from palm oil was obtained from the Palm Oil Research Institute of Malaysia.

Isolation of Mitochondria. Liver mitochondria were prepared from 3-month-old female Wistar rats (250 ± 20 g) (18). Lipid peroxidation and protein oxidation were induced by exposure of mitochondria to peroxynitrite/singlet oxygen. Products of peroxidation were measured as thiobarbituric acid reactive substances (TBARS), conjugated dienes (CD), and lipid hydroperoxides (LOOH) (18–21). The protein oxidation (12), activity of SOD and GSH were also measured (22). Generation of singlet oxygen was carried out as described earlier (20). Peroxynitrite was synthesized according to the method of Pryor *et al.* (9). Briefly, a gas stream from an ozonator (5% ozone in oxygen, 100 mL/min) was bubbled through a glass-frit into 100 mL of 0.1 mol/L sodium azide in water (pH 12) and chilled to 0–4°C for 2 h. The concentration of peroxynitrite was determined spectrophotometrically by measuring the absorbance at 302 nm using an extinction coefficient of 1670 $M^{-1}cm^{-1}$.

Results

Figure 37.1A demonstrates the results on lipid peroxidation induced by peroxynitrite as a function of its concentration. The effect of peroxynitrite in a concentration range up to 1000 μmol/L was examined in terms of TBARS formation, one of the stable products of lipid peroxidation. Peroxynitrite effectively enhanced the formation of TBARS at a concentration of 100 μmol/L. The damage was maximum at 300 μmol/L,

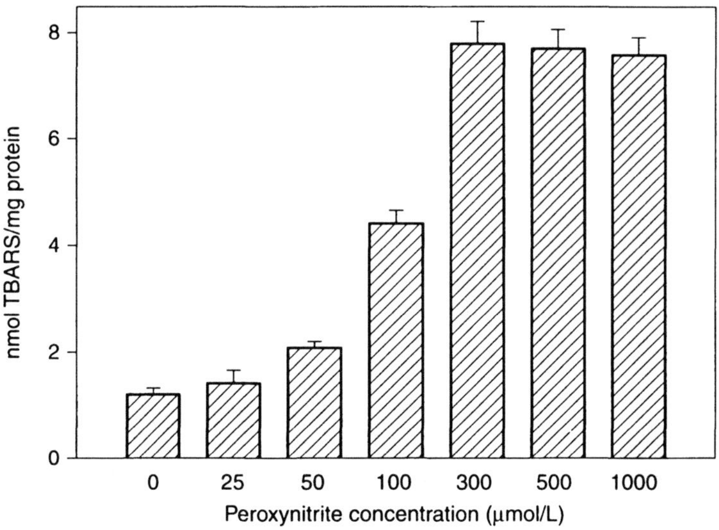

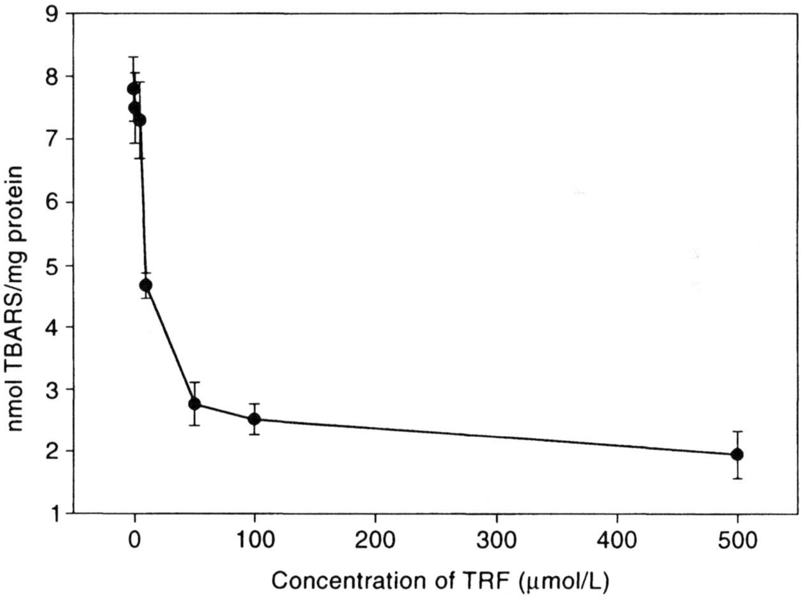

Fig. 37.1. (a) Lipid peroxidation induced by peroxynitrite as a function of concentration and (b) the effect of tocotrienol-rich fraction (TRF) on peroxynitrite-induced formation of thiobarbituric acid reactive substances (TBARS). Lipid peroxidation was induced in rat liver mitochondria (2 mg protein/mL) by exposure to peroxynitrite at various concentration up to1000 μmol/L. The effect of TRF at 1–500 μmol/L was examined in the presence of 300 μmol/L peroxynitrite, and the formation of TBARS was measured. Values are means ± SEM, n = 5 experiments.

TABLE 37.1 Peroxynitrite (PXN)-Induced Lipid Peroxidation and Protein Oxidation and Its Prevention by Tocotrienol-Rich Fraction (TRF)[a,b]

Treatment	Lipid peroxidation CD[a] (nmol product/mg protein)	Lipid peroxidation LOOH[b] (nmol product/mg protein)	Protein oxidation
None	8.82 ± 0.38	36.10 ± 0.10	1.38 ± 0.21
25 μmol/L PXN	16.20 ± 0.42	47.97 ± 4.80	1.33 ± 0.31
300 μmol/L PXN	67.20 ± 0.60	67.95 ± 5.80	4.33 ± 0.39
1000 μmol/L PXN	67.30 ± 7.85	52.91 ± 3.10	4.50 ± 0.21
300 μmol/L PXN + 10 μmol/L TRF	50.10[c] ± 2.50	29.50[c] ± 1.50	1.90 ± 0.21

[a]Values are means ± SEM, $n = 5$ experiments.
[b]Abbreviations: CD, conjugated dienes; LOOH, lipid hydroperoxides.
Significant difference up to $P < 0.001$ level.

beyond which no further enhancement was observed. The inhibitory effect of TRF on peroxynitrite-induced formation of TBARS is presented in Figure 37.1B. As little as 10 μmol/L TRF was sufficient to significantly inhibit TBARS. The inhibition was μmol/L ~40% at 10 mol/L, whereas that obtained at 50 μmol/L was 65%. Above 50 μmol/L, TRF did not further enhance protection.

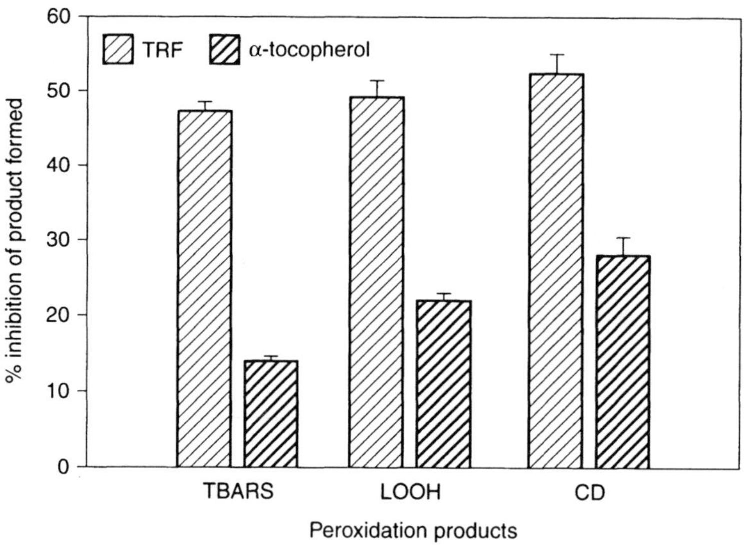

Fig 37.2. Inhibitory effect of tocotrienol-rich fraction (TRF) on photosensitization-induced lipid peroxidation in comparison with α-tocopherol. Lipid peroxidation was induced in rat liver mitochondria (0.5 mg protein/mL) by photosensitization, and the effect of TRF/α-tocopherol was examined in terms of thiobarbituric acid reactive substances (TBARS). Values are means ± SEM, $n = 5$ experiments. Abbreviations: LOOH, lipid hydroperoxides; CD, conjugated dienes.

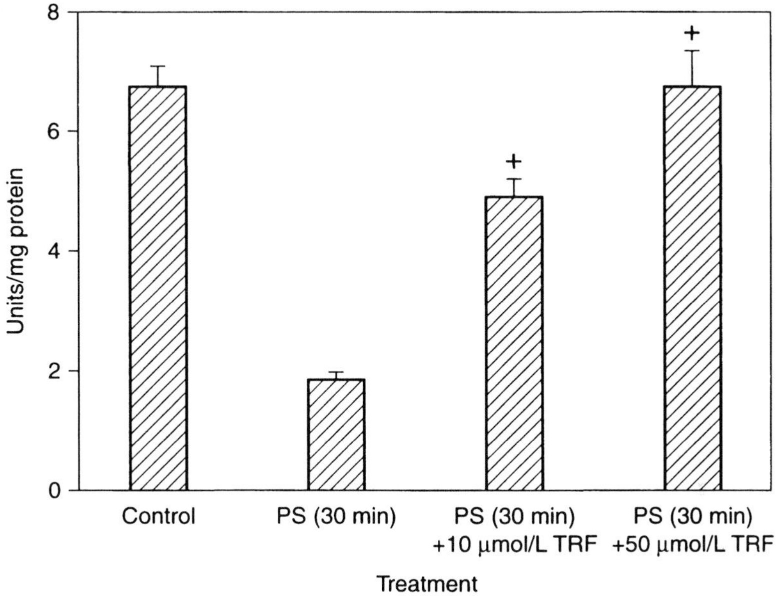

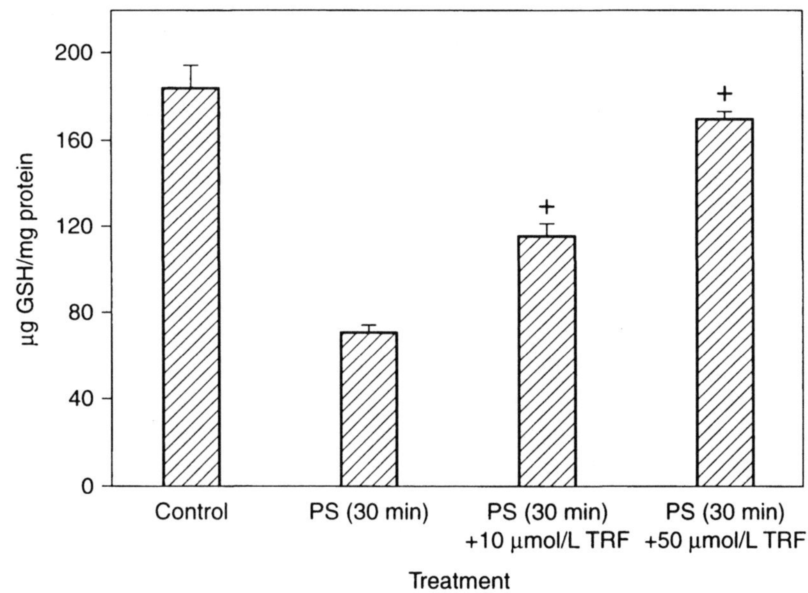

Fig 37.3. Measurement of (a) superoxide dismutase (SOD) and (b) glutathione (GSH) in methylene blue + visible light–induced photosensitization (PS) in rat liver mitochondria. Rat liver mitochondria were isolated, exposed to photosensitization (0.5 mg protein/mL) for 30 min. and levels of SOD/GSH were examined. Values are means ± SEM, $n = 5$ experiments. $^{+}P < 0.01$ compared with PS-treated sample.

The peroxynitrite-induced dose-dependent increase in the other two products of lipid peroxidation, i.e., CD and LOOH, as well as protein oxidation is shown in Table 37.1. It is clear from the table that CD, the initial lipid peroxidation product formed by the abstraction of a hydrogen atom in the lipid chain by free radical attack, is increased effectively up to 300 μmol/L. Similar enhancement was also demonstrated in the formation of LOOH, the product formed by the addition of oxygen to the lipid radical, which was induced by exposure to peroxynitrite ranging from 25 to 300 μmol/L. The increase obtained in the formation of CD at 1000 μmol/L was the same as that obtained at 300 μmol/L. Peroxynitrite-induced damage observed in the case of LOOH was comparatively higher than that of CD at 25 μmol/L peroxynitrite. Its formation was further reduced at 1000 μmol/L. It is evident from the table that, similar to lipid peroxidation, peroxynitrite is also able to enhance the formation of protein oxidation in a dose-dependent manner. We observed an increase in protein oxidation up to 300 μmol/L (more than threefold), beyond which saturation occurred. TRF at a concentration of 10 μmol/L could prevent this damage effectively, bringing the elevated activity of protein oxidation to near control levels. The protection afforded by TRF for CD, LOOH, and protein oxidation was 25, 56, and 56%, respectively. Thus equal protection by TRF was observed with LOOH and protein oxidation.

The inhibitory effect of TRF on photosensitization-induced lipid peroxidation in comparison with α-tocopherol is given in Figure 37.2. TRF effectively reduced the formation of all three products of lipid peroxidation, i.e., TBARS, LOOH, and CD. The protection observed was ~50% for all three products. The inhibitory effect of TRF was observed to be about twice that of α-tocopherol. Thus efficacy of TRF against oxidative damage is better than that of α-tocopherol. The protective effect was relatively less with CD.

Our results dealing with photosensitization experiments demonstrate that methylene blue + light-induced photosensitization reactions are also equally damaging (5,6). We studied two antioxidant defenses, namely, enzymatic SOD (Fig. 37.3A) and nonenzymatic GSH (Fig. 37.3B) by exposure to photosensitization with methylene blue as a sensitizer in the presence of visible light. The results showed that the activity of SOD was decreased significantly by photosensitization. The depleted level of this enzyme was 70% and that of GSH was 60%. TRF at 10 μmol/L was effective in restoring the impaired activity of SOD as well as that of GSH. However, the effect was more pronounced at higher concentrations of TRF (50 μmol/L), showing almost complete restoration in both cases.

Discussion

The discovery that nitric oxide (NO•) reacts with superoxide (5,6) to form peroxynitrite and the proof that this reaction occurs *in vivo* hold enormous implications for the understanding of RNS in biological systems. Similarly, the profound damaging effects of ROS with respect to human health are well known (1,2). Several reports have provided evidence of the reactivity of peroxynitrite toward cellular biomolecules as well as its pathophysiologic role in shock, inflammation, ischemia-reperfusion, and other diseases (2,3,5,6). Therefore, detailed understanding of the oxidative and nitration reactions in the membrane system will provide new insight into the development of therapeutic strategies to minimize such damage. Our studies demonstrate the damaging effect of peroxynitrite on the mitochondrial membrane components, lipid and protein. The damaging effect acts in a concentration-dependent way. Such observations were also supported by other evidence on the reaction of peroxynitrite with lipid, leading to its peroxidation (malondialdehyde and conjugated diene formation) (23) and the formation of nitrito-nitrosoperoxo and or/nitrated lipid oxidation adduct (3). In addition, peroxynitrite has been shown to cause direct damage to pulmonary surfactant protein (24), nitration of aromatic amino acids (5), and inactivation of mitochondrial enzymes, which increases the amount of hydrogen peroxide generated by the mitochondria responsible for cellular injury (25). Peroxynitrite-induced lipid peroxidation may be occurring due to the abstraction of a hydrogen atom in the lipid chain, whereas that observed in the case of protein oxidation may be by oxidative modification of proteins as well as its side chains of amino acids. The inhibitory effect of TRF on oxidative damage induced by peroxynitrite against lipid peroxidation/protein oxidation could be the result of radical recycling ability (26). TRF inhibits peroxynitrite-induced formation of LOOH and protein oxidation in comparison with CD, indicating that its action is at the levels of secondary (LOOH) and end-product formation (protein oxidation) but not at the primary level (CD). However, in the case of photosensitization, the effect was the same for the three products of peroxidation. Thus, the action of TRF may be at both the primary and secondary levels. The extent of oxidation as well as its protection by TRF seemed to differ in peroxynitrite- and $^1O_2$-induced reactions. This may be due to the difference in the potency of the two species, $ONOO^-$ and $^1O_2$, and their scavenging action with TRF.

We showed that $^1O_2$ generated during photosensitization involving methylene blue plus light is a damaging agent in cellular systems (18–21). Restoration of depleted levels of SOD and GSH during photosensitization further supports the scavenging action of TRF toward $^1O_2$. The protection of GSH as well as that of SOD is less at the lower concentration of TRF used. This indicates that there may be a greater number of oxidized SH groups and that their restoration to reduced forms requires a greater concentration of TRF. Our earlier studies showed that the reactivity of $^1O_2$ toward other antioxidants in the form of nicotinamide (22) and chlorophyllin (27) clearly established the quenching action of these compounds as shown by the histidine destruction assay. It may be that TRF also has similar reactivity with this molecule. Studies on quenching of $^1O_2$ and that of $ONOO^-$ by TRF may provide additional information in connection with the mechanistic aspects of protection by TRF against oxidative damage.

The activity of vitamin E is associated with its well-defined antioxidant property, especially against lipid peroxidation in biological membranes (15). Our present results demonstrate higher antioxidant ability of TRF compared with α-tocopherol. This can be explained by the fact that the molecular mobility of polyenoic lipids in the membrane bilayer is much higher than that of saturated lipids. Hence, tocotrienols could be more mobile than tocopherol in their interaction with lipid radicals in membranes (21,26). TRF has multifunctional roles. It has been shown to possess novel hypocholesterolemic effects, together with an ability to reduce the atherogenic apolipoprotein (apo) B and lipoprotein (a) plasma levels. Among its isomers, γ-tocotrienol stimulates apoB degradation more, possibly due to decreased apoB translocation into the endoplasmic reticulum lumen (28). Naturally occurring tocotrienols are also effective apoptotic inducers for human cancer cells (29). In addition, tocotrienol has been suggested to have antithrombotic and antitumor effects, indicating that tocotrienol may serve as an effective agent in the prevention and/or treatment of cardiovascular diseases and tumor promotion/chemical carcinogenesis (14,16,29–31). Our earlier *in vivo* and *in vitro* (32,33) studies on TRF as an antioxidant in rat subcellular fractions against other reactive species further support the present finding concerning oxidative damage induced by peroxynitrite. These observations suggest additional therapeutic properties of TRF.

Summary

Our studies showed that TRF from palm oil effectively protects rat liver mitochondria against oxidative damage induced by peroxynitrite and $^1O_2$. TRF may have potential applications as a dietary supplement in preventing humans against the effects of ROS/RNS.

Acknowledgments

The authors acknowledge the encouragement and helpful suggestions by Dr. (Mrs.) A.M. Samuel, Director Bio-Medical Group and Dr. K.B. Sainis, Head, Cell Biology Division of the Bhabha Atomic Research Centre. I also would like to acknowledge the financial support from organizers of the meeting on Micronutrients and Health: Molecular Biological Mechanisms and Bhabha Atomic Research Centre.

References

1. Ames, B.N. (1983) Dietary Carcinogens and Anticarcinogens, Oxygen Radicals and Degenerative Diseases. *Science 221*, 1256–1264.
2. Szabo, C. (1996) The Pathophysiological Role of Peroxynitrite in Shock, Inflammation, and Ischemia-Refusion Injury. *Shock 6,* 79–88.
3. Muijsers, R.B.R., Folkerts, G., Henricks, P.A.J., Sadeghi-Hashjin, G., and Niikamp, F.P. (1997) Peroxynitrite: A Two-Faced Metabolite of Nitric Oxide. *Life Sci. 60,* 1833–1845.
4. Paillous, N., and Ferry-Forgues, S. (1994) Interest of Photochemical Methods for Induction of Lipid Peroxidation. *Biochemie 76*, 355–368.
5. Halliwell, B., Zhao, K., and Whiteman, M. (1999) Nitric Oxide and Peroxynitrite, the Ugly, the Uglier and the Not So Good. *Free Radic. Res. 31*, 651–669.
6. Beckman, J.S., Beckman, T.W., Chen, J., Marshall, P.A., and Freeman, B.A. (1990) Apparent Hydroxyl Radical Production by Peroxynitrite: Implication for Endothelial Injury from Nitric Oxide and Superoxide. *Proc. Natl. Acad. Sci. USA 87,* 1620–1624.

7. Briviba, K., Roussyn, I., Sharov, V.S., and Sies, H. (1996) Attenuation of Oxidation and Nitration Reactions of Peroxynitrite by Selenomethionine, Selenocystine and Ebselen. *Biochem. J. 319*, 13–15.
8. Radi, R., Beckman, J.S., Bush, K.M., and Freeman, B.A. (1991) Peroxynitrite Oxidation of Sulfhydryls: The Cytotoxic Potential of Superoxide and Nitric Oxide. *J. Biol. Chem. 266*, 4244–4250.
9. Kanski, J., Koppal, T., and Butterfield, A. (1999) Investigation of Peroxynitrite Induced Oxidative Stress in Red Blood Cells Monitored by Luminal Dependent Chemiluminescence. *Anal. Lett. 32*, 1183–1192.
10. Salgo, M.G., Stone, K., Squadrito, G.L., Battista, J.R., and Pryor, W.A. (1995) Peroxynitrite Causes DNA Nicks in Plasmid pBR322. *Biochem. Biophys. Res. Commun. 210*, 1025–1030.
11. Sies, H. (1991) *Oxidative Stress: Oxidants and Antioxidants*, Academic Press, New York.
12. Palamanda, J.R., and Kehrer, J.P. (1992) Inhibition of Protein Carbonyls and Lipid Peroxidation in Rat Liver Microsomes. *Arch. Biochim. Biophys. 293*, 103–109.
13. Sies, H. (1996) *Antioxidants in Diseases, Mechanisms and Therapy*, Academic Press, New York.
14. Ong, A.S.H., and Packer, L., eds. (1997) *Lipid Soluble Antioxidants: Biochemistry and Clinical Applications*, Birkhauser Verlag, Basel.
15. Gurr, M.I. (1997) Oil Palm Lipids, Edible Oils with Interesting Nutritional Attributes. *Lipid Technol.*, April–June, 62–69.
16. Goh, S.H., Hew, N.F., Norhanonm, A.W., and Yadav, M. (1994) Inhibition of Tumour Promotion by Various Palm Oil Tocotrienols. *Int. J. Cancer 57*, 529–531.
17. Ong, A.S.H., Niki, E., and Packer, L. (1995) *Nutrition, Lipids, Health and Disease*, AOCS Press, Champaign, IL.
18. Kamat, J.P., Ghosh, A., and Devasagayam, T.P.A. (2000) Vanillin as an Antioxidant in Rat Liver Mitochondria: Inhibition of Protein Oxidation and Lipid Peroxidation Induced by Photosensitization. *Mol. Cell. Biochem. 209*, 47–53.
19. Kamat, J.P., and Devasagayam, T.P.A. (1995) Tocotrienols from Palm Oil as Potent Inhibitors of Lipid Peroxidation and Protein Oxidation in Rat Brain Mitochondria. *Neurosci. Lett. 195*, 179–182.
20. Kamat, J.P., and Devasagayam, T.P.A. (1996) Methylene Blue Plus Light-Induced Lipid Peroxidation in Rat Liver Microsomes: Inhibition by Nicotonamide (Vitamin B_3). *Chem.-Biol. Interact. 99*, 1–16.
21. Kamat, J.P., Sarma, H.D., Devasagayam, T.P.A., Nesaretnam, K., and Basiron, Y. (1997) Tocotrienols from Palm Oil as Effective Inhibitors of Protein Oxidation and Lipid Peroxidation in Rat Liver Microsomes. *Mol. Cell. Biochem. 170*, 131–138.
22. Kamat, J.P., Boloor, K.K., Devasagayam, T.P.A., Jayashree, B., and Kesavan, P.C. (2000) Differential Modification by Caffeine of Oxygen-Dependent and Independent Effects of γ-Irradiation on Rat Liver Mitochondria. *Int. J. Radiat. Biol.*, in press.
23. Radi, R., Beckman, J.S., Bush, K.M., and Freeman, B.A. (1997) Peroxynitrite-Induced Membrane Lipid Peroxidation: The Cytotoxic Potential of Superoxide and Nitric Oxide. *Arch. Biochem. Biophys. 288*, 481–487.
24. Haddad, I.Y., Crow, J.P., Hu, P., Ye, Y., Beckman, J., and Matalon, S. (1994) Concurrent Generation of Nitric Oxide and Superoxide Damage Surfactant Protein. *Am. J. Physiol. 267*, L242–L249.

25. Radi, R., Rodriguez, M., Castro, L., and Telleri, R. (1994) Inhibition of Mitochondrial Electron Transport by Peroxynitrite. *Arch. Biochem. Biophys. 308*, 89–95.
26. Serbinova, E., Kagan, V., Han, D., and Packer, L. (1991) Free Radical Recycling and Intramembrane Mobility in the Antioxidant Properties of Alpha-Tocopherol and Alpha Tocotrienols. *Free Radic. Biol. Med. 10,* 263–275.
27. Kamat, J.P., Boloor, K.K., and Devasagayam, T.P.A. (2000) Chlorophyllin as an Effective Antioxidant Against Membrane Damage *in vitro* and *ex vivo. Biochim. Biophys. Acta,* in press.
28. Theriault, A., Wang, Q., Gapor, A., and Adeli, K. (1999) Effect of Gamma-Tocotrienol on ApoB Synthesis, Degradation and Secretion in HepG2 Cells. *Arterioscler. Thromb. Vasc. Biol. 19,* 704–712.
29. Yu, W., Simmons-Menchaca, M., Gapor, A., Sanders, B.G., and Kline, K. (1999) Induction of Apoptosis in Human Breast Cancer Cells by Tocopherols and Tocotrienols. *Nutr. Cancer 33*, 26–32.
30. Nasaretnam, K., Stephen, R., Dils, R., and Darbre, R. (1998) Tocotrienols Inhibit the Growth of Human Breast Cancer Cells Irrespective of Estrogen Receptor Status. *Lipids 33,* 461–469.
31. Theriault, A., Chao, J.T., Wang, Q., and Adeli, K. (1999) Tocotrienol: A Review of Its Therapeutic Potential. *Clin. Biochem. 32*, 309–319.
32. Kamat, J.P., and Devasagayam, T.P.A. (1995) Tocotrienol from Palm Oil as Potent Inhibitors of Lipid Peroxidation and Protein Oxidation in Rat Brain Mitochondria. *Neurosci. 195,* 179–182.
33. Nesaretnam, K., Devasagayam, T.P.A., Singh, B.B., and Basiron, Y. (1993) Influence of Palm Oil or Its Tocotrienol-Rich Fraction on the Lipid Peroxidation Potential of Rat Liver Mitochondria and Microsomes. *Biochem. Mol. Biol. Int. 30,* 159–167.

Index

CPSIA information can be obtained at www.ICGtesting.com
Printed in the USA
LVOW092252120412

277428LV00002B/4/P